PERFORATOR FLAPS
Anatomy, Technique,
& Clinical Applications

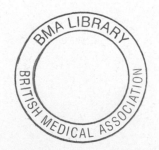

PERFORATOR FLAPS

Anatomy, Technique, & Clinical Applications

SECOND EDITION

EDITED BY

Phillip N. Blondeel, MD, PhD, FCCP
Professor in Plastic Surgery, Department of Plastic and Reconstructive Surgery,
University Hospital Gent, Gent, Belgium

Steven F. Morris, MD, MSc, FRCSC
Professor of Surgery, Professor of Anatomy and Neurobiology, Department of Surgery,
Anatomy and Neurobiology, Dalhousie University, Halifax, Nova Scotia, Canada

Geoffrey G. Hallock, MD, FACS
Consultant in Plastic and Reconstructive Surgery, Sacred Heart Hospital
and The Lehigh Valley Hospital, Allentown, Pennsylvania;
St. Luke's Hospital, Bethlehem, Pennsylvania

Peter C. Neligan, MB, FRCS(I), FRCSC, FACS
Professor, Department of Surgery, University of Washington, Seattle, Washington

WITH ILLUSTRATIONS BY
Jennifer C. Darcy, MS, CMI

Quality Medical Publishing, Inc.

ST. LOUIS, MISSOURI
2013

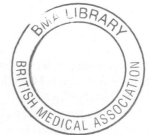

This book presents current scientific information and opinion pertinent to medical professionals. It does not provide advice concerning specific diagnosis and treatment of individual cases and is not intended for use by the layperson. The author and publisher have made every attempt to check dosages and medical content for accuracy. Because the science of pharmacology is continually advancing, our knowledge base continues to expand. Therefore we recommend that the reader always check product information for changes in dosage or administration before administering any medication. This is particularly important with new or rarely used drugs. If you have any questions about the information contained in the book, contact the manufacturer of specific drugs for clarification before making a final decision. The authors and publisher will not be responsible for any errors or liable for actions taken as a result of information or opinions expressed in this book.

PUBLISHER Karen Berger
EDITORIAL DIRECTOR Michelle Berger
SENIOR ASSOCIATE EDITOR Amy Debrecht
DIRECTOR OF EDITING Suzanne Wakefield
MANUSCRIPT EDITOR Rebecca Sweeney
VICE-PRESIDENT OF PRODUCTION AND MANUFACTURING Carolyn Reich
DIRECTOR OF GRAPHICS Brett C. Stone
GRAPHICS PRODUCTION Ngoc-Thuy Khuu
DIRECTOR OF MEDICAL ILLUSTRATION Amanda Yarberry Behr
ADDITIONAL ILLUSTRATORS Briar Lee Mitchell, Jennifer Gentry, Helen A. Macfarlane, Joan M.K. Tycko, Vicki Friedman, William Scavone, Jennifer Parsons Brumbaugh, Amanda Yarberry Behr
LAYOUT ARTISTS Elaine Kitsis, Susan Trail, Carol Hollett

Quality Medical Publishing, Inc.
2248 Welsch Industrial Court
St. Louis, Missouri 63146
Telephone: 800-348-7808; 314-878-7808
Website: *http://www.qmp.com*

LIBRARY OF CONGRESS CATALOGING-IN-PUBLICATION DATA

Perforator flaps : anatomy, technique & clinical applications / editors, Phillip N. Blondeel ... [et al.]. -- 2nd ed.
    p. ; cm.
  Includes bibliographical references and index.
  ISBN 978-1-57626-317-4 (hardcover)
  I. Blondeel, Phillip N.
  [DNLM: 1. Surgical Flaps. 2. Arteries--anatomy & histology. 3.
Reconstructive Surgical Procedures--methods. 4. Surgical Flaps--blood supply. WO 610]

  617.9'5--dc23
                        2012030389
QM/L/L

5 4 3 2 1

To my mother, Hilde Spruyt; my wife, Karlien;
and my children, Laurence, Jonathan, and Victoria.

Phillip N. Blondeel

To my mother, Lorraine, who has always been enthusiastically supportive;
my wife, Kay, who has been a stable, loving force in my life;
and my wonderful children, Alexander and Leah, who continually amaze me.

Steven F. Morris

Without the impetus and constant persuasion of Karen Berger, this book would not exist. Yet she has been gentle when compared to my father, Houghton Ross Hallock, the West Point engineer, who made me understand the discipline necessary to build things. Even this project would have made him proud.

Most important has been my wife, Patty, my high school sweetheart, who continues to tolerate my transgressions, correct my misspellings, and lets me know when I have been particularly stupid. She also feeds my Dachshunds when I am not there—too often—a joy of life we share together.

Geoffrey G. Hallock

To my wife, Gabrielle, and my children, Kate and David,
who are unflagging in their love and support.

Peter C. Neligan

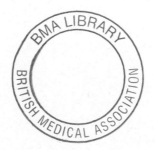

CONTRIBUTORS

Reza Ahmadzadeh, MD
Department of Surgery, Division of Plastic Surgery,
Dalhousie University, Halifax, Nova Scotia, Canada

Ammar S. Al Dhamin, MBChB, MRCSI
Fellow Staff, Department of Surgery,
Division of Plastic Surgery, Dalhousie University,
Queen Elizabeth II Health Sciences Centre,
Halifax, Nova Scotia, Canada

Faisal M. Al-Mufarrej, MB, BCh
Assistant Professor of Surgery, College of Medicine,
Mayo Clinic; Fellow, Division of Plastic Surgery,
Department of Surgery, Mayo Clinic, Rochester,
Minnesota

Mohammad M. Al-Qattan
Professor of Plastic Surgery, Department of Surgery,
King Saud University, Riyadh, Saudi Arabia

Robert J. Allen, Sr., MD
Clinical Professor, Institute of Reconstructive Plastic
Surgery, New York University Langone Medical
Center, New York, New York

Robert Johnson Allen, Jr., MD
Resident, Institute of Reconstructive Plastic Surgery,
New York University Langone Medical Center, New
York, New York

Patricio Andrades, MD, FACS
Associate Professor, Division of Plastic Surgery,
Department of Surgery, University of Chile Clinical
Hospital; Staff Member, Department of Maxillofacial
Surgery, Hospital del Trabajador de Santiago,
Santiago, Chile

Claudio Angrigiani, MD
Chief, Department of Plastic Surgery, Hospital
Santojanni, Buenos Aires, Argentina

Mark W. Ashton, MBBS, MD, FRACS
Senior Research Fellow, The Taylor Lab,
Reconstructive Plastic Surgery Research Unit,
Department of Anatomy and Neurosciences,
University of Melbourne, Parkville, Victoria,
Australia

Phillip N. Blondeel, MD, PhD, FCCP
Professor in Plastic Surgery, Department of Plastic
and Reconstructive Surgery, University Hospital
Gent, Gent, Belgium

Willy Boeckx, MD, PhD
Professor, Department of Plastic and Reconstructive
Surgery, Brugmann Hospital, U.L.B. Free University
of Brussels, Brussels, Belgium

Constance M. Chen, MD, MPH
Attending Surgeon, Division of Plastic and
Reconstructive Surgery, Lenox Hill Hospital;
Attending Surgeon, Department of Plastic and
Reconstructive Surgery, New York Eye and Ear
Infirmary, New York, New York

Hung-Chi Chen, MD, MHA, FACS
Professor, Department of Plastic Surgery, China
Medical University Hospital, Taichung, Taiwan

Ming-Huei Cheng, MD, MBA, FACS
Vice President and Professor, Department of Plastic
and Reconstructive Surgery, Chang Gung Memorial
Hospital, Taoyuan, Taiwan

Carmen Navarro Coll, MD
Plastic Surgeon, Department of Plastic Surgery,
Hospital de la Santa Creu i Sant Pau (Universitat
Autonoma de Barcelona), Barcelona, Spain

Ashish Davalbhakta, MBBS, MS Mch(Plast), FRCS
Chief Consultant, Chairman, and Managing
Director, Department of Aesthetic Plastic Surgery,
Aesthetics Medispa; Assistant Professor, Department
of Plastic Surgery, Bharati Vidyapeeth Deemed
University; Honorary Consultant, Aesthetic Plastic
Surgeon, Ruby Hall Clinic, Oyster and Pearl
Hospital, Noble Hospital, Pune, Maharastra, India

Frederick J. Duffy, Jr., MD
Assistant Clinical Professor, Department of Plastic
Surgery, University of Texas–Southwestern, Dallas,
Texas

Karen Kim Evans, MD
Assistant Professor, Department of Plastic Surgery,
Georgetown University Medical Center,
Washington, DC

Misako Fujitsu, MD
Chief, Department of Plastic Surgery, Kanmon
Medical Center, Shimonoseki, Yamagichi, Japan

Christopher R. Geddes, MD, MSc
Chief Resident, Division of Orthopaedic Surgery,
University of Toronto, Toronto, Ontario, Canada

Patrick J. Gullane, CM, MB, FRCSC, FACS,
Hon FRACS, Hon FRCS, Hon FRCSI
Professor and Chair, Department of Otolaryngology–
Head and Neck Surgery, University of Toronto;
Otolaryngologist-in-Chief, Wharton Chair,
Department of Otolaryngology–Head and Neck
Surgery, University Health Network,
Toronto, Ontario, Canada

Amit Gupta, MD, FRCS
Clinical Associate Professor, Department of
Orthopedic Surgery, University of Louisville;
Director, Louisville Arm and Hand,
Louisville, Kentucky

Geoffrey G. Hallock, MD, FACS
Consultant in Plastic and Reconstructive Surgery,
Sacred Heart Hospital and The Lehigh Valley
Hospital, Allentown, Pennsylvania; St. Luke's
Hospital, Bethlehem, Pennsylvania

John B. Hijjawi, MD, FACS
Associate Professor, Department of Plastic and
Reconstructive Surgery, Medical College of
Wisconsin, Milwaukee, Wisconsin

Stefan O.P. Hofer, MD, PhD, FRCSC
Associate Professor, Department of Surgery,
Division of Plastic Surgery, University Health
Network; Associate Professor, Department of
Surgical Oncology, University Health Network,
Toronto, Ontario, Canada

Charlotte Holm, MD, PhD
Clinical Professor of Plastic Surgery, Department of
Plastic and Aesthetic Surgery, ATOS Clinic Munich,
Munich, Germany

Joon Pio Hong, MD, PhD, MMM
Professor and Department Chair, Department of
Plastic Surgery, Asan Medical Center, University
of Ulsan, Seoul, Korea

Philippe Houtmeyers, MD
Medical Doctor, Department of Plastic Surgery,
University Hospital, Ghent University,
Ghent, Belgium

Jung-Ju Huang, MD
Assistant Professor, Department of Plastic and
Reconstructive Surgery, Chang Gung Memorial
Hospital, Taoyuan, Taiwan

Hiko Hyakusoku, MD, PhD
Professor, Department of Plastic, Reconstructive,
and Aesthetic Surgery, Nippon Medical School,
Tokyo, Japan

Seng-Feng Jeng, MD, FACS
Professor Surgery, Department of Plastic Surgery,
E-Da Hospital, I-Shou University,
Kaohsiung City, Taiwan

Shuji Kayano, MD, PhD
Plastic Surgeon, Division of Plastic and
Reconstructive Surgery, National Cancer Center
Hospital, Tokyo, Japan

Jeong Tae Kim, MD, PhD
Professor, Chief of Department, Department of
Plastic and Reconstructive Surgery, Hanyang
University Medical Center, Seoul, Korea

Yoshihiro Kimata, MD, PhD
Professor and Chairman, Department of Plastic
and Reconstructive Surgery, Okayama University,
Graduate School of Medicine, Dentistry and
Pharmaceutical Sciences, Okayama City,
Okayama, Japan

Naohiro Kimura, MD
Director, Tsukiji Dermatology, Plastic, and Hand
Surgery Clinic, Tokyo, Japan

Isao Koshima, MD
Professor and Chief, Department of Plastic
and Reconstructive Surgery, The University of
Tokyo, Tokyo, Japan

Joshua L. Levine, MD
Surgeon Director, Department of Surgery, New York
Eye and Ear Infirmary, New York, New York

Anita A. Liem, MD, MRCS(Glasg), FRCSGlasg(Plast)
Canniesburn Plastic Surgery Unit, Glasgow
Royal Infirmary, Glasgow, United Kingdom;
Previous Microsurgical Fellow, Department of
Plastic Surgery, China Medical University Hospital,
Taichung, Taiwan

Chih-Hung Lin, MD
Professor and Chairman, Department of Plastic
Surgery, Chang Gung Memorial Hospital,
Taoyuan, Taiwan

Joan E. Lipa, MD, MSc, FRCSC, FACS
Associate Professor, Department of Surgery,
University of Toronto; Associate Professor, Division
of Plastic and Reconstructive Surgery, Sunnybrook
Health Sciences Centre, Toronto, Ontario, Canada

Maria M. LoTempio, MD
Assistant Professor, Department of Surgery, Medical
University of South Carolina, Charleston, South
Carolina; Assistant Adjunct Professor, Department
of Plastic Surgery, New York Eye and Ear Infirmary,
New York, New York

Debra A. Lutz, RN
Division of Plastic Surgery, Sacred Heart Hospital,
Allentown, Pennsylvania

Alejandro Maciel-Miranda, MD
Plastic Surgeon, Department of Surgery, Anatomy,
and Neurobiology, Dalhousie University; Plastic
Surgeon, Division of Plastic Surgery, Queen
Elizabeth II Health Sciences Centre, Halifax, Nova
Scotia, Canada

Samir Mardini, MD
Professor of Surgery, Program Director, Division of
Plastic Surgery, Department of Surgery, Mayo Clinic,
Rochester, Minnesota

Jaume Masia, MD, PhD
Professor and Chairman, Department of Plastic
Surgery, Hospital de la Santa Creu i Sant Pau
(Universitat Autonoma de Barcelona),
Barcelona, Spain

Musa Mateev, MD, PhD
Professor, National Hospital in Kyrgyzstan,
Department of Plastic and Reconstructive
Microsurgery and Hand Surgery, Kyrgyz State
Medical Academy, Bishkek, Kyrgyzstan

David W. Mathes, MD, FACS
Associate Professor, Department of Surgery,
University of Washington, Seattle, Washington

James L. Mayo, MD
Resident, Division of Plastic and Reconstructive
Surgery, Department of Surgery, Louisiana
State University Health Sciences Center,
New Orleans, Louisiana

Makoto Mihara, MD
Assistant Professor, Department of Plastic and
Reconstructive Surgery, The University of Tokyo,
Tokyo, Japan

Michael J. Miller, MD
Chair, Department of Plastic Surgery, Ohio State
University, Columbus, Ohio

Stan J. Monstrey, MD, PhD, FCCP
Professor and Chairman, Department of Plastic
Surgery, Ghent University Hospital, Ghent, Belgium

Steven F. Morris, MD, MSc, FRCSC
Professor of Surgery, Professor of Anatomy and
Neurobiology, Department of Surgery, Anatomy and
Neurobiology, Dalhousie University, Halifax,
Nova Scotia, Canada

Colin M. Morrison, MSc, FRCSI(Plast)
Consultant, Department of Plastic and
Reconstructive Surgery, St. Vincent's University
Hospital, Dublin, Ireland

Masahiro Nakagawa, MD, PhD
Chief, Division of Plastic and Reconstructive
Surgery, Shizuoka Cancer Center Hospital,
Nagaizumi, Shizuoka, Japan

Mitsunaga Narushima, MD
Lecturer, Department of Plastic and Reconstructive
Surgery, The University of Tokyo, Tokyo, Japan

Peter C. Neligan, MB, FRCS(I), FRCSC, FACS
Professor, Department of Surgery, University
of Washington, Seattle, Washington

Dung H. Nguyen, MD
Clinical Assistant Professor, Department of Surgery,
Division of Plastic and Reconstructive Surgery,
USC Keck School of Medicine; Faculty, Plastic and
Reconstructive Surgeon, Department of Surgery,
Division of Plastic and Reconstructive Surgery,
Cedars Sinai Medical Center, Los Angeles, California

Milomir Ninkovic, MD, PhD
Professor, Head, Department of Plastic,
Reconstructive, Hand and Burn Surgery, Academic
Hospital Munich Bogenhausen, Technical University
Munich, Munich, Germany

Niri Niranjan, MS, FRCS(Plast)
Consultant Plastic Surgeon, St. Andrews Centre
for Plastic and Burn Surgery, Broomfield Hospital,
Chelmsford, Essex, United Kingdom

Christine B. Novak, PT, PhD
Associate Professor, Department of Surgery, Division
of Plastic and Reconstructive Surgery, University
of Toronto; Research Associate, Toronto Western
Hospital Hand Program and Wharton Head and
Neck Centre, University Health Network, Toronto,
Ontario, Canada

Rei Ogawa, MD, PhD, FACS
Associate Professor, Department of Plastic,
Reconstructive, and Aesthetic Surgery, Nippon
Medical School, Tokyo, Japan

Vani Prasad, MBBS, MRCSEd
Research Fellow, Department of Surgery, Dalhousie
University, Halifax, Nova Scotia, Canada;
Department of Plastic and Reconstructive Surgery,
School of Medicine, University of Tasmania, Hobart,
Tasmania, Australia

Julian J. Pribaz, MD
Professor, Department of Surgery, Harvard Medical
School, Boston, Massachusetts

David C. Rice, BS
Physician Extender, Division of Plastic Surgery,
Sacred Heart Hospital, Allentown, Pennsylvania

**Warren M. Rozen, MBBS, BMedSc,
PGDipSurgAnat, PhD**
Senior Research Fellow, The Taylor Lab,
Reconstructive Plastic Surgery Research Unit,
Department of Anatomy and Neurosciences,
University of Melbourne, Parkville, Victoria,
Australia

S. Raja Sabapathy, MS(Gen), MCh(Plast), DNB(Plast), FRCS(Ed), MAMS
Chairman, Division of Plastic Surgery, Hand and Microsurgery and Burns, Ganga Hospital, Coimbatore, Tamil Nadu, India

Michel Saint-Cyr, MD, FRCSC
Associate Professor, Division of Plastic Surgery, Mayo Clinic, Rochester, Minnesota

Kazufumi Sano, MD, PhD
Associate Professor, Department of Orthopaedic Surgery, Dokkyo Medical University Koshigaya Hospital, Saitama, Japan

Luis R. Scheker, MD
Associate Clinical Professor of Plastic and Reconstructive Surgery, Department of Surgery, Division of Plastic and Reconstructive Surgery, University of Louisville School of Medicine, Louisville, Kentucky; Associate Consulting Professor of Surgery, Division of Plastic, Reconstructive, and Maxillofacial Surgery, Duke University Medical Center, Durham, North Carolina

Rossella Sgarzani, MD
Plastic Surgeon, Plastic Surgery Unit, Policlinico S. Orsola Malpighi, Bologna, Italy

Minoru Shibata, MD, PhD
Professor, Department of Plastic and Reconstructive Surgery, Graduate School of Medical and Dental Sciences, Niigata University, Niigata-shi, Niigata, Japan

Filip B. Stillaert, MD, FCCP
Plastic Surgeon, Department of Plastic and Reconstructive Surgery, University Hospital Gent, Gent, Belgium

Narushi Sugiyama, MD
Lecturer, Department of Plastic Surgery, Okayama University, Okayama City, Okayama, Japan

Maolin Tang
Department of Anatomy, Wenzhou Medical College, Wenzhou University-Town, Wenzhou-Zhejiang, China

G. Ian Taylor, AO, MD, FRACS, FRCS, FACS
Professor, Department of Plastic Surgery, Royal Melbourne Hospital, Melbourne, Australia

Tiew Chong Teo, MB, ChB, MD(Hons), FRCS(Ed), FRCS(Plast)
Consultant Plastic and Reconstructive Surgeon, Department of Plastic Surgery, The Queen Victoria Hospital, East Grinstead, West Sussex, United Kingdom

Binu Prathap Thomas, MBBS, D.ORTH, M.S.ORTH, PDFHS
Professor and Head, Dr. Paul Brand Centre for Hand Surgery, Christian Medical College and Hospital, Vellore, Tamil Nadu, India

Juan A. Clavero Torrent, MD
Radiologist, Department of Radiology, Clinica Creu-Blanca, Barcelona, Spain

Tetsuji Ucmura, MD
Professor, Department of Plastic and Reconstructive Surgery, Saga University, Saga City, Saga Prefecture, Japan

Shigeko Ushio, MD
Lecturer, Department of Plastic Surgery, Tohoku University, Sendai, Japan

Koenraad Van Landuyt, MD, PhD
Professor, Department of Plastic and Reconstructive Surgery, University Hospital Gent, Gent, Belgium

Stephen M. Warren, MD, FACS
Associate Professor of Plastic Surgery, Department of Plastic Surgery, New York University Langone Medical Center, New York, New York

Fu-Chan Wei, MD, FACS
Professor, Department of Plastic Surgery, Chang
Gung Memorial Hospital, Taoyuan, Taiwan

Klaus-Dietrich Wolff, MD, DMD, PhD
Professor, Department of Maxillofacial Surgery,
Klinikum rechts der Isar, Technical University
of Munich, Munich, Germany

Takumi Yamamoto, MD
Resident, Department of Plastic and Reconstructive
Surgery, The University of Tokyo, Tokyo, Japan

Daping Yang, MD
Division of Plastic Surgery, The Second Hospital of
Harbin Medical University, Harbin, China

Jenny Fei Yang, BSc
Medical Student, Yale University School of Medicine,
New Haven, Connecticut

FOREWORD

TO THE FIRST EDITION

Sir Harold Gillies, the father of plastic surgery, often lamented that "tissue transfer is a constant battle between blood supply and beauty" when, with artistic flair, he repaired the horrific defects of those poor unfortunates who were mutilated during the two Great Wars. This dilemma was because Gillies designed his skin flaps on a trial-and-error basis without knowledge of the underlying blood supply of the region, assigning rigid length-to-breadth ratios to his flap procedures.

The pioneering work of Ian McGregor and Ian Jackson answered his plea. They focused our attention on skin flaps supplied by named axial vessels that perforated the outer layer of the deep fascia and coursed parallel to the skin for long distances. This culminated in their publication of a description of the "groin flap" for local or pedicled transfer. After initial failed attempts by Buncke and Antia in 1971, we successfully transplanted this flap in one stage in 1973 using microsurgery and coined the phrase "the free flap" for the procedure.

This microsurgical technique demanded a reappraisal of the basic vascular and neurovascular anatomy of the body for future transplants. Consequently, this led to the design of various free flaps based on either direct cutaneous perforators that passed from their source arteries and veins between the deep structures to pierce the outer layer of the deep fascia as *fasciocutaneous* flaps, or indirect cutaneous perforators that were derived from vessels supplying the deep structures, usually as musculocutaneous flaps.

These musculocutaneous free flaps were bulky because of the obligatory muscle and often imposed a greater morbidity on the donor site when compared with their fasciocutaneous counterparts. This problem stimulated Bob Allen and Phillip Blondeel to dissect these indirect musculocutaneous perforators, tracing them to their underlying source vessels to provide a sleeker flap and at the same time to preserve muscle function. They first targeted the perforators of the deep inferior epigastric artery. As other musculocutaneous flaps were reexamined, the concept of "perforator flaps" evolved and was expanded to include the direct fasciocutaneous vessels.

The editors of these two volumes of text have made a valuable contribution to reconstructive surgery. Not only have they combined their own particular clinical and research expertise as leaders in the field, but they have also captured an "arm full of bullfrogs" of flamboyant contributors, all skilled in the art of free tissue transfer.

With any multiauthored book it is difficult to avoid overlap and to provide continuity and a logical sequence to the text. The editors have achieved this by coauthoring 27 of the 64 chapters, standardizing the illustrations, and introducing each region with superb cadaver studies of the cutaneous perforators and underlying source vessels. Steven Morris, who I am proud to say spent 2 years with me in the 1990s examining with

Mark Gianoutsos the neurovascular territories of the skin and muscles, has reexamined our angiosome territories of the cutaneous perforators with his team in Halifax. He has confirmed our results and gone a step farther in several regions, subdividing some perforator territories. Phillip Blondeel and Peter Neligan have combined their pioneering technical skills, their tips and pitfalls, and Geoff Hallock has not only simplified terminology with a clear analytical mind, but has also compiled an exhaustive list of references in the Appendix on perforator flaps that are state of the art today.

Although designed specifically for microsurgeons performing free tissue transfers, *Perforator Flaps: Anatomy, Technique, & Clinical Applications* provides valuable anatomic data for any reconstructive surgeon who breaches the vascular network of the skin with an incision or who designs a flap in the area for local repair.

It is noteworthy that some of the contributors believe that "big is beautiful" as they trace the cutaneous perforators to their sizeable source vessels for transplantation, whereas others exhibit their microsurgical skills using "supermicrosurgery" to reconnect tiny cutaneous perforators. It will be interesting to see which techniques will survive and which will be relegated to the bookshelves. Having been involved for more than 30 years with free tissue transfers, I have come to the conclusion that for the average surgeon, long pedicles with large vessels have the highest success rate. This is why the radial forearm skin flap is so popular in Western countries, whereas in Taiwan, for example, where the forearm is always exposed because of the hot climate, lateral thigh flaps based on the large descending branch of the later femoral circumflex vessels are favored because the donor site is more easily concealed.

The abbreviated nomenclature for these perforator flaps may pose a problem for the future. When John Palmer and I published our angiosome concept, we identified an average of 374 direct or indirect cutaneous perforators of greater than 0.5 mm diameter. Even though most were represented bilaterally, there are still at least 187 possible perforators to which an individual abbreviation may be attributed. It will be interesting to see which of these will remain in common use.

In the preface of this book, the authors describe how they intend it to be used in clinical practice. The clinical problem is presented to the reader, and then the clinical application chapter is consulted for various options. The reader can learn how to perform the flap in the relevant sections in Part II.

The DVDs that accompany the books show the harvesting of the most popular flaps. This is a nice addition and might be very valuable for the surgeon attempting a flap for the first time. The clinical case reports and photographs are impressive and tie in well with the text.

I believe these volumes will become an important reference that no doubt will be revised from time to time as new techniques evolve. It has been a monumental task done in a time of flux. Above all, the editors have made us focus on the most important factor that determines flap survival: the anatomy of the blood supply of the transplant. Both they and all of their invited contributors to the various chapters are to be congratulated on their achievement.

G. Ian Taylor, AO, MD, FRACS, FRCS, FACS
Professor, Department of Plastic Surgery,
Royal Melbourne Hospital, Melbourne, Australia

PREFACE

TO THE SECOND EDITION

In the first edition of *Perforator Flaps: Anatomy, Technique, & Clinical Applications*, we cautiously stated that perforator flaps were the latest advance in the continuing evolution of flap choices for reconstructive purposes. Seven years have passed, and now we can enthusiastically state that perforator flaps have become mainstream. Their impact on reconstructive surgery is pervasive. The table of contents of every plastic surgery or microsurgery journal and every plastic surgery meeting today invariably includes at least one article or presentation discussing a topic within the realm of perforator flaps. There has been a veritable explosion of information about this topic, which has led to the most rapid development of flap options in the history of plastic surgery.

As editors of the first textbook on the subject of perforator flaps, we have been invited together to all corners of this planet to help educate our colleagues worldwide about the special techniques and advantages of perforator flaps for improving not only the functional but also the aesthetic result of any reconstructive procedure. We continue those efforts to spread the word in this new edition. Injection studies and anatomic dissections presented throughout this book delineate the pertinent perforators so that a donor site can now be chosen that truly has the attributes of replacing "like with like."

Whereas the first edition emphasized the microsurgical transfer of tissues, this second edition encompasses current applications for local flap transfer. Today, more and more local perforator flaps such as propeller and peninsular flaps have been found to be equally valuable as simpler alternatives that do not depend on microvascular anastomoses; we have included detailed coverage of these local flap options. However, we also continue to emphasize the critical role of microsurgical skills in allowing atraumatic dissection of the perforators. These dissection techniques for a variety of perforator flaps have been elegantly demonstrated by the expert contributors who are featured on the four DVDs and 23 operative videos that accompany this edition.

Our contributors are the leading experts in the field of perforator flap surgery. Many of them are trailblazers and primary innovators who have graciously given their time to update their opinions by showing us how their thought processes and techniques have evolved from their continuing experience. We have also included some of the younger members of this worldwide phenomenon whose new ideas prove that they will be the bright future of reconstructive surgery. We have tried to maintain a consistent format for each chapter, appreciating full well that each author has his or her own voice and views that must be respected. The publisher has ensured an essential continuity by providing consistency in the superb color illustrations and layout.

Although much is new in this second edition, the basic organization remains the same; it consists of two volumes that are divided into four parts. Part I focuses on the fundamentals of perforator flap surgery, providing the essentials of basic anatomy and physiology, appropriate preoperative planning, an approach to the correct surgical technique, and anticipation of complications to minimize their occurrence. Lest we forget, the controversial topic of nomenclature is discussed, which explains our conventions throughout the book that we deem necessary for surgeons to properly communicate with each other.

Part II lists the currently available flaps by body region based on the source vessel to that territory. Part III takes a different approach, focusing on defect analysis in each body region with guidance for selecting the best flap solutions for particular problems. Part IV presents a collection of important, pragmatic thoughts that may be key to future explorations in the field and subsequent editions of this work. Our final chapter, "Concluding Thoughts," summarizes our personal opinions and philosophies, which continue to evolve through our collaborative visions.

In addition, we have included the first edition's Appendix with references on DVD 4 for readers who want to access these, as well as the most current references, which are included in the Appendix to this second edition.

It is not our intent to provide immutable answers to every question in this new edition; rather, we view it as a guide, taking the reader along a path he or she wants to follow. Our goal is to contribute a valuable resource that can be used in the daily practice of reconstructive surgery, no matter how subspecialized it has become. Of course, there will continue to be controversy and debate about everything said and written between these covers. This we encourage strongly, because that is how we will grow, as demonstrated by the undercurrent of interest that has prompted us to write this edition about what is today such an important topic in our field. The fundamental quest is to determine how best perforator flaps may be used to serve our patients and how their applications can serve as a stimulus for even better alternatives in the future.

Phillip N. Blondeel
Steven F. Morris
Geoffrey G. Hallock
Peter C. Neligan

PREFACE

TO THE FIRST EDITION

Perforator flaps represent the latest milestone in the evolution of reconstructive flap surgery. As our understanding of the vascular anatomy of perforators has advanced, we have come to recognize the large network of perforator vessels present throughout the body and their potential for flap dissection. We now understand that any skin flap can be harvested, as long as it incorporates a perforator vessel that can be dissected. So, instead of first searching for the perforator and then determining the skin island overlying the vessel, we can now select a donor skin island that is a match to the recipient site in skin, color, thickness, texture, and subcutaneous fat quality, and then identify a nourishing perforator in the deeper tissues. The implications of this discovery are of major import to all reconstructive surgeons. We are no longer bound by the traditional conventions of flap surgery. More attention can be paid to the aesthetic quality of the reconstruction at the recipient site. Thus, with perforator flaps, we have progressed from the era of simply closing defects to that of customizing our reconstructions to achieve the best functional and aesthetic result in the reconstructed site as well as the donor site.

Although interest in perforator flap technique is growing worldwide, there is a relative paucity of reference materials to guide the surgeon interested in learning about these flaps and their clinical applications. This book has been written to fill that void. We have long been aware of the special advantages of perforator flaps and the need to educate our colleagues about this reconstructive advance. Thus we have collaborated on this project, combining our anatomic research and clinical experience, to provide an up-to-date reference that covers the entire spectrum of perforator flap applications known worldwide. We hope this work will convey our enthusiasm for these flaps and their potential for reconstructive surgery.

Our contributors are leading experts in the field of perforator flap surgery; they have added tremendous depth to this project. Many are the pioneers who blazed the trails to bring us to this point in the development of the perforator flap technique. Although as editors we are well aware of the organizational challenges that a multiauthored, two-volume textbook presents, we have made every effort to avoid potential weaknesses and build on obvious strengths. Thus great care has been taken to develop consistent formats for the chapters in each section and to create artwork and present anatomic studies that serve as a unifying theme throughout. We have also attempted to preserve the special voice and character of each contributor. We regard their divergent views and approaches as a distinct advantage for the reader, a culmination of expertise drawn from a worldwide perspective.

This book is unique in its coverage. For the first time all current information about existing perforator flaps has been gathered in one comprehensive work. The goal is to provide the reader with an overview of all skin flaps available today and their potential applications in daily clinical practice. We have standardized the nomenclature throughout the chapters to facilitate improved and consistent communication and to guide future research. The anatomic injection studies throughout the book demonstrate the vast number of flaps that can be harvested on perforators throughout the body. If one masters the technique for freeing the perforator vessels from surrounding tissues, the only limitations to the development of new perforator flaps will be the individual surgeon's ingenuity, creativity, and surgical skill. Equipped with this anatomic knowledge, we hope that others will be inspired to create, develop, and share new methods for tissue transfer.

This book is divided into four parts. Part I focuses on the fundamentals of perforator flap surgery. It includes a historical overview as well as chapters on anatomy, nomenclature, physiology, basic technique, planning, and complications. We regard this introductory section as essential reading for the neophyte surgeon learning basic technique as well as the experienced reconstructive surgeon seeking to refine and enhance skills. Of particular note are the technical considerations described in Chapters 6 and 7, which are intended to help the reader avoid numerous potential pitfalls associated with perforator flap surgery. Part II is a region-by-region guide to the anatomy and surgical technique used for obtaining specific flaps from the head and neck, upper extremity, trunk, and lower extremity. Chapters in this section provide a thorough review of all currently described perforator flaps. Part III focuses on clinical applications for the various flaps for reconstructing defects in each body region. Part IV is an amalgam of unusual, unique, or futuristic topics. It includes innovations in flap design, free-style free or pedicled flaps, supermicrosurgery, and nonmuscle perforator flaps. In the final chapter, "Concluding Thoughts," we discuss the current state of the art and philosophize about future directions. As has been true throughout the book, it is a collaborative vision.

This book is meant to be used in daily surgical practice as an invaluable and practical tool for the surgeon planning a reconstructive procedure. Thus if the surgeon is confronted with a soft tissue defect in a certain area of the body, he or she need only turn to the clinical applications section to review the various options for reconstruction. Once a specific flap has been selected as most appropriate, a step-by-step guide on how to harvest a flap can then be found in Part II. If a reader has a preference for a particular flap, the possible applications for each flap are also described in Part II.

A DVD is included with the book to enhance the learning experience. These videos graphically depict techniques for harvesting the most popular flaps used today. They also emphasize the theoretical and anatomic information necessary to put these techniques into practice in the operating room. Although techniques may vary from surgeon to surgeon, we hope that these flap demonstrations will help the reader gain perspective on the intraoperative decision-making and basic surgical principles involved with harvesting perforator flaps.

The reader will find controversy and debate within these pages, as should be expected and encouraged in a publication that explores a new and evolving field. Ultimately, you will reach your own conclusions as to what constitutes a perforator, whether perforator flap surgery is actually a novel technique or an extension of what we already do, or even whether perforator flaps are worthwhile. We firmly believe, however, that by learning about perforator flaps you will gain access to a vast array of new reconstructive options that will benefit your practice and your patients. It is our hope that the anatomic information contained herein will serve as a stimulus for innovation in developing new, exciting flap options for the future.

Steven F. Morris
Geoffrey G. Hallock
Peter C. Neligan
Phillip N. Blondeel

ACKNOWLEDGMENTS

The success of this second edition of *Perforator Flaps: Anatomy, Technique, & Clinical Applications* is built on a great team. All team members have been equal in their contribution, and I can only express my deepest respect and gratitude to all of them. Without Geoff, Peter, and Steve, such an undertaking would have been unthinkable. Our friendship gave this book the power to excel. In addition, my gratitude to all our colleagues throughout the world who have contributed chapters based on their own expertise; they have made this the most comprehensive didactic tool on the market today.

Karen Berger, Michelle Berger, Amy Debrecht, Taira Keele, Suzanne Wakefield, Carolyn Reich, Amanda Behr, and all the other medical illustrators and coworkers at Quality Medical Publishing have been very patient with us and have once more put together a work of art.

My fellows, residents, and young students have been crucial to the writing process: constantly picking my brain, pushing me to distill and refine the thought processes and the surgical technique. Passing down our knowledge and skills is for me a great passion and should be for everybody involved in teaching. The greatest honor for a teacher is that his students surpass him. This book will help those eager, aspiring, and enthusiastic young lions to further develop the field of reconstructive surgery.

Phillip N. Blondeel

No scientific work is created without the efforts of countless previous investigators. Surgical work is similar, since our evolution depends on the pioneering efforts of our surgical forefathers and mentors. In my case, Ian Taylor stands out as the individual who shaped my thinking and approach to surgery more than any other. To this day, Ian continues to stimulate his former fellows and trainees with original and thought-provoking questions and hypotheses. Professor Taylor's contributions to plastic surgery are probably unrivalled and have truly enriched our specialty. Thus many of the principles and concepts presented herein may have the Taylor signature.

I have been very fortunate in having a series of superb trainees work with me who have produced the bulk of the anatomic work presented in this text. The tireless efforts of these individuals have improved our understanding of the vascular basis of flap design.

Gradually over the past two decades, we have seen a significant, growing acceptance of the importance of vascular supply to flaps, and in fact, to a variety of aspects of our specialty. I would like to thank these scientists and surgeons for their contributions to this work: Daping Yang, Chris Geddes, Maolin Tang, Binu Thomas, Reza Ahmadzadeh, Ammar Al Dhamin, and Alejandro Maciel-Miranda. To each, a special thank you.

Finally, the helter-skelter of the normal day at work doesn't really allow the time necessary for clinical work, committee work, teaching, research, and so on. Yet my wonderful assistant, Heather DeWolfe, cheerfully manages all with complete confidence and thoroughness.

Steven F. Morris

As I reflect on the 7 years since our first edition of this book on "just perforator flaps," I am overwhelmed at all the new memories I have collected. My fellow editors, Steve, Peter, and Phillip, don't hesitate to remind me that I am the senior member of this quaternion, and I have the gray hairs to prove it. I cherish these individuals as well as our collegiality.

Without a doubt, perforator flaps require microsurgery skills, for which I continue to be indebted to my assistant, David C. Rice, with whom I learned de novo, and we are still together some three decades later. My office nurse, Debra A. Lutz, has been with me for just as long; she has redirected my footsteps when I get lost, and kept my patients happy, which is why we do this. Similarly, I cannot forget my long-term colleagues, special nurses, and truly all my friends at the inner city sanctum of Sacred Heart Hospital, who have been a blessing and refuge in my final days as a solo private practitioner.

Rather than today sitting in a rocking chair at the rehabilitation center, my involvement in this exciting field at the end of my career has provided an unparalleled euphoria, sense of excitement, and the opportunity to travel together with my fellow editors to visit the world to spread this gospel, to lecture and to listen, to find novelty in the dissection lab, and to discover life, sometimes inadvertently. For a quiet person from a small town and smaller community hospital, to be among so many professors of title and so many curious and wonderful students we've met, this has been the adventure of a lifetime—all possible just by writing a few words on a piece of paper. Truly amazing that life can be so! May it only continue, and I look forward to the *tenth edition* if Karen Berger and the team at Quality Medical Publishing have the patience to have us, and the willingness to continue to turn our rough drafts into a silk purse.

Geoffrey G. Hallock

I have dedicated this book to my family, who have supported me throughout my career. I must also acknowledge Karen Berger, President of QMP, without whose friendship, perseverance, and encouragement this edition would not have happened. The whole team at QMP have supported us, and I am grateful for their encouragement, dedication, and professionalism throughout this project. Amy Debrecht is a master of diplomacy and manages to needle without nagging. Michelle Berger is the soul of efficiency and tact. Amanda Behr has once again shown her artistic mastery, and Suzanne Wakefield managed to put us back to work when we thought we had finished! My partners in the Division of Plastic Surgery at the University of Washington, under the leadership of Nick Vedder, generate such a positive atmosphere that work is a pleasure, and the enthusiasm of our residents and fellows keeps me on my toes. Finally, I would like to thank my fellow editors, Phil, Steve, and Geoff, for their friendship and for the bond between us that writing and editing these books has generated.

Peter C. Neligan

CONTENTS

VOLUME II

Lower Extremity

Part III   Clinical Applications

Head and Neck

VIDEO CONTENTS

PART I

Fundamentals

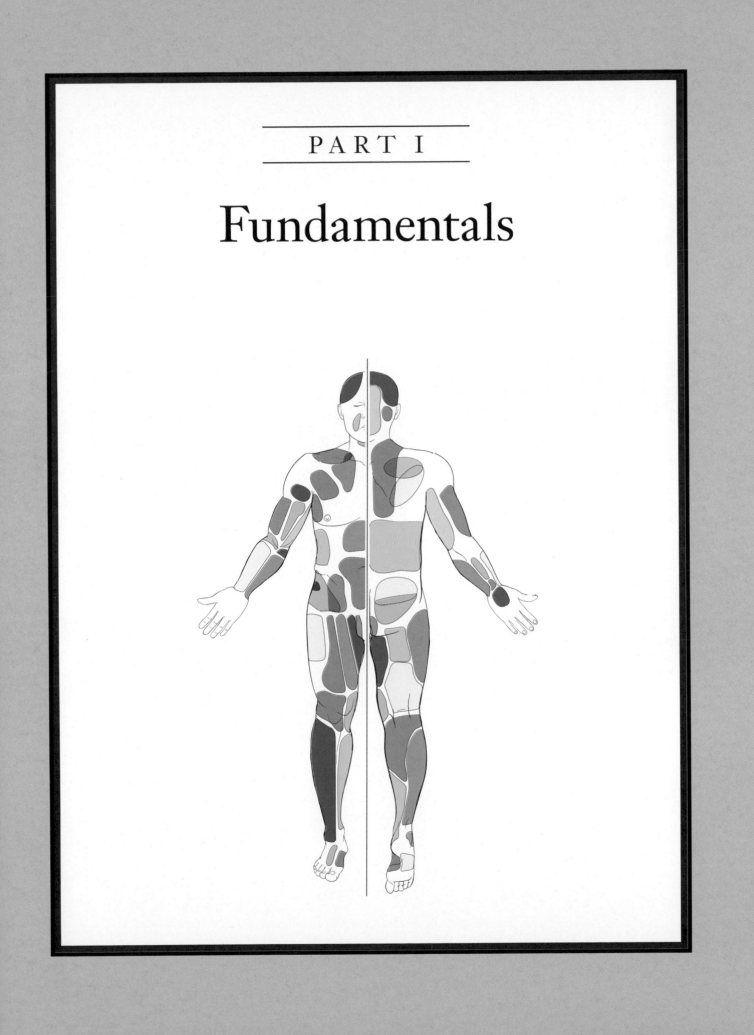

1

History of
Perforator Flap Surgery

Steven F. Morris
Alejandro Maciel-Miranda
Geoffrey G. Hallock

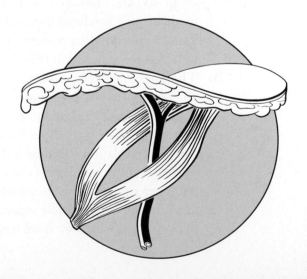

EARLY HISTORY

The history of flap surgery mirrors that of the specialty of plastic and reconstructive surgery. From the earliest times, surgeons have treated patients with complex wounds and sought to solve these challenges with wound closure or tissue transfers. The early attempts were woefully inadequate and often resulted in poor results. Nevertheless, the advantages of obtaining early wound coverage became increasingly appreciated. However, significant gaps in basic knowledge, especially regarding the vascular supply of tissue transfers, hindered progress. Our understanding of the anatomic territories of individual perforators to the skin and their crucial role in flap design and survival developed excruciatingly slowly until the last two decades, when our understanding of this concept grew exponentially (see Appendix). Based on this knowledge, some flaps used throughout the last century could be considered as perforator flaps. The concept of flaps and their transfer will continue to evolve as more sophisticated techniques develop. In this chapter, we review the origin of perforator flaps and highlight the importance of understanding the vascular anatomy as an integral component in their evolution.

600 BC The writings of Sushruta[1] appear to contain the first account of skin flaps performed in India. Sushruta described using a cheek flap to reconstruct amputated noses. Estimates vary considerably on the exact dates of Sushruta's work, but Nehru[2] noted that although Sushruta lived several hundred years before Christ, his work became widely known and applied about 400 AD. The flap described by Sushruta was later modified by Indian medicine as a forehead flap and was the first account of a local axial flap. This so-called Indian rhinoplasty is still used clinically as a workhorse flap for nasal reconstruction (Fig. 1-1).

30 AD   The ancient Greek philosopher Aulus Cornelius Celsus[3] (25 BC to 50 AD) reported on techniques for lip reconstruction using advancement flaps for a quadrangular defect. He also proposed a surgical procedure to reshape the defect to allow closure with an advancement flap. The first English translation (original in Latin), by Spencer,[4] states, "The method of treatment is as follows: the mutilation is enclosed in a square; from the inner angles of this incisions are made across, so that the part on the quadrilateral is completely separated from that on the opposite side. Then the two flaps, which we have freed, are brought together."

400 AD Oribasius of Alexandria[5,6] (320 to 400 AD), a Greek medical writer and the personal physician of the Roman emperor Julian the Apostate, described skin flaps for reconstructing defects in the ears, nose, lips, and forehead. In his books, he recorded the "plastic" operations of Galen and Antyllus, among others (Fig. 1-2).

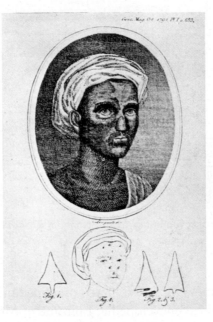

Fig. 1-1 Sushruta's technique of nose reconstruction. (From *Gentleman's Magazine of Calcutta*, October 1794.)

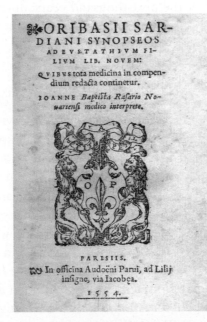

Fig. 1-2 Oribasius' *Chirurgia ex Greco in Latinum Conversa*. (Courtesy Historical Collections and Services, Claude Moore Health Sciences Library, University of Virginia. Available at http://historical. hsl.virginia.edu/treasures/images/R126_O7_S93_1554_title_big.jpg.)

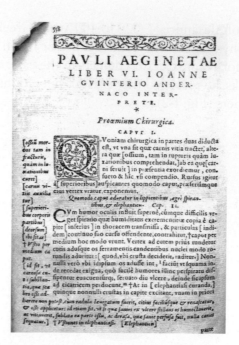

Fig. 1-3   Cover for the sixth of seven books from *Epitome of Medicine,* attributed to Paulus of Aegineta and published in 1528.

650 AD   Paulus Aegineta (625 to 690 AD) practiced medicine in Alexandria and wrote a medical encyclopedia, Epitome of Medicine, in seven books. It included discussions on reconstructing "maimed parts," such as mutilated ears and lips, and described dissection below flaps for better advancement (Fig. 1-3).[7,8] Over the next thousand years, during the "dark" or Middle Ages, there were essentially no further flap innovations until the Renaissance period.

RENAISSANCE PERIOD

In 1597, Tagliacozzi[9] described a random-pattern upper arm, distally based skin flap for nasal reconstruction. Through his efforts, this flap became widely applied. During the Renaissance period, the study of human anatomy became widespread throughout Europe, and several key anatomists contributed extensively to its understanding. Leonardo da Vinci and Andreas Vesalius, in particular, produced significant works that increased our understanding of this anatomy. Leonardo da Vinci's beautiful anatomic illustrations (Fig. 1-4) and other artwork redefined anatomy. His principles of research and methodologies warranted his title as the "father of modern science."[10] A new willingness to question previously held truths and search for new answers resulted in a period of major scientific advancements. Andreas Vesalius published the book *De Humani Corporis Fabrica*[11] (On the Workings of the Human Body) in 1543, which, when first printed, significantly elevated the roles of dissection, observation, and the mechanistic view of anatomy, giving surgeons more confidence[12] (Fig. 1-5). Perhaps the most significant development of the era was not a specific new observation, but rather a process for discovery and the recognition of the scientific method.[12]

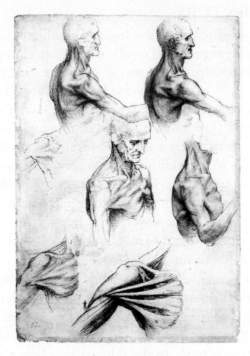

Fig. 1-4 From the unpublished works of Leonardo da Vinci.

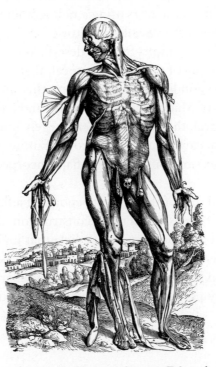

Fig. 1-5 From an original woodcut in *De Humani Corporis Fabrica* by Andreas Vesalius, published in 1543.

NINETEENTH CENTURY

Carpue[13] (1764 to 1846) rediscovered the Indian rhinoplasty technique flap during a trip to India in 1816. He reported good results using the technique in two patients and published a monograph entitled *An Account of Two Successful Operations for Restoring a Lost Nose Including Description of the Indian and Italian Methods.* This generated renewed interest in flap surgery in Europe and the United States. With the increasing awareness of anatomy in the sixteenth through eighteenth centuries, transferring tissues to reconstruct traumatic wounds, particularly war injuries, gradually evolved into the nineteenth century, when 280 articles were published on flap reconstruction.[14]

Despite rapid growth in our understanding of the anatomy of the human body, implementation of this new information by surgeons was painfully slow. Carl Manchot[15] (1889) performed extensive anatomic dissections of the vascular supply to the skin and theorized quite appropriately about the vascular territories of the human body, without the benefit of any radiologic technique. In 1893, Spalteholz[16] published an important paper on the origin, course, and distribution of cutaneous perforators. He injected several cadavers with a solution of the "finest French gelatin," to which he added pigments. He concluded that there are two major types of vessels to the skin: (1) arteries that supply another structure, usually muscle, and then only indirectly provide branches to the skin, and (2) arteries that course directly to the skin, passing between the tissues. The two types of vessels to the skin then anastomose and branch within the deepest layers of the skin to form a "cutaneous plexus." Michel Salmon[17] published extensive anatomic works in the 1930s comprising four books on the vascular anatomy of the skin and soft tissues of the body. He studied fifteen cadavers using a radiographic technique with lead oxide injection and further defined the vascular territories of the skin, summarizing important anatomic concepts. For example, Salmon described the law of equilibrium, which notes that the vascular supply of tissue is reciprocal; that is, if one vessel supplying an area is large, then a corresponding vessel supplying the same area is smaller, and vice versa. Though the works of Manchot,[15] Spalteholz,[16] and Salmon[17] were extensive and very relevant to flap survival, their findings went largely unrecognized by the surgical community. However, this awareness of the role of individual vessels supplying the skin provided the basis for surgeons to design flaps incorporating these vessels, today known as *perforators*.

Sabattini[18] published one of the earliest reports of a flap based on a specific vascularized pedicle in 1838. He described the reconstruction of an upper lip defect using a flap from the lower lip based on a narrow pedicle that included the labial vessels. In 1898, Abbé[19] published his work on the transposition of a pedicle flap from the lower lip to the upper lip—a flap that now bears his name. Vascularized flaps based on known vessels were subsequently performed to reconstruct wounds in different parts of the body, thereby achieving greater rates of success. Gersuny[20] of Vienna performed a submandibular cutaneous flap to repair a cheek defect in 1887. In 1898, Monks[21] presented the island temporal skin flap based on a subcutaneous pedicle that is tunneled superficial or deep to the zygomatic arch for reconstruction of the oral cavity. Remarkably in 1906, Tansini[22] reported on a latissimus dorsi flap supplied by the thoracodorsal artery. This was an important landmark paper in the evolution of flaps, because it led to the further description of many flaps from the thoracic region.

TWENTIETH CENTURY

Wars have caused a multitude of wounds that require reconstruction, and by necessity, have served as an important stimulus for flap innovation. Distant flaps are a good example. These include the cross-leg flap, described by Hamilton[23] in 1854 for covering a chronic ulcer; the tube flap described by Filatov[24] from Odessa, Russia in 1917, taken from the neck for lower eyelid reconstruction (Fig. 1-6); and others used by Esser[25] in the Austrian war. Daniel and Kerrigan[26] credited Esser[27] with the concept of axial-pattern flaps. These were described by Esser as early as 1918 as "biological" flaps, having a narrow pedicle that included the requisite vessels, to demonstrate that a flap could survive as long as it had an arterial pedicle.

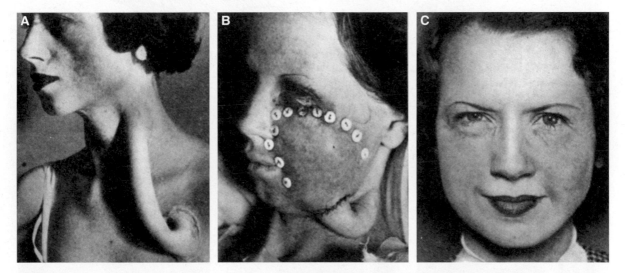

Fig. 1-6   A-C, A compound flap from the neck to the face. (From Smith AE. Reconstructive plastic and oral surgery. Cal West Med 42:432, 1935.)

In 1917, Harold Gillies[28] used tube flaps to reconstruct several facial burns, and later published his book, *Plastic Surgery of the Face,*[29] based on his experiences treating patients in London during the First World War. Gillies, whom some consider the "father of modern plastic surgery,"[30] also insisted that all operations be carefully documented with drawings and illustrations. This improved planning, assisted in the development of new methods, and was a useful teaching tool (Fig. 1-7).[31]

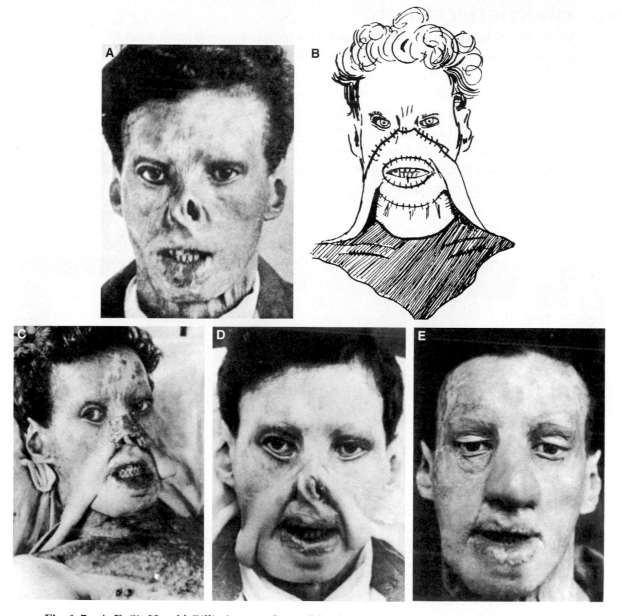

Fig. 1-7   A-E, Sir Harold Gillies' case at Queen Mary's Hospital Sidcup. (From Gillies H, Millard DR Jr, eds. *The Principles and Art of Plastic Surgery.* Boston: Little Brown, 1957. Current copyright held by Lippincott Williams & Wilkins.)

Over the period of flap development from the 1920s through the 1960s, several new flaps were introduced, but surgeons relied on maneuvers such as delay and tube flaps to ensure better flap survival. In 1921, Blair[32] described a forehead flap based on the superficial temporal vessels, and in 1929 Esser published the landmark book, *Artery Flaps*.[33] Shaw and Payne[34] (1946) performed island tube flaps based on the superficial epigastric vessels to cover the back of a patient's hand. McGregor and Jackson[35] later used these flaps in the groin area (Fig. 1-8).

In 1955, Owens[36] documented the successful transfer of skin and muscle together as a flap to reconstruct major facial defects. It comprised the sternocleidomastoid muscle, overlying platysma, subcutaneous tissue, and skin. In 1968, Hueston and McConchie[37] performed a musculocutaneous pectoralis major flap to repair a sternal defect. The flap was better described by Ariyan[38] in 1979 as a musculocutaneous flap based on the thoracoacromial artery. In 1964, Converse[39] presented his classification schema of dermatocutaneous flaps, in which he listed the type of anatomic vascular basis as the most accurate point of differentiation. He divided flaps into cutaneous, arterial, and island flaps.

In 1965, Bakanjiam[40] described the deltopectoral flap based on intercostal perforators from the internal mammary artery for immediate coverage of defects after laryngopharyngectomy surgeries. A second stage was required to divide the base of the flap

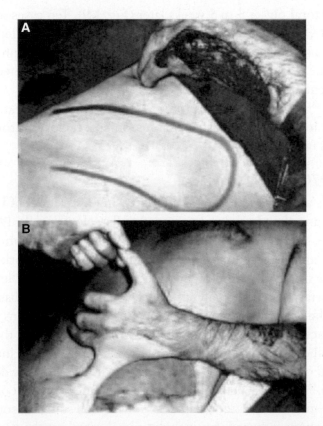

Fig. 1-8 A and **B,** Original photographs of the McGregor flap. (From Smith PJ, Foley B, McGregor IA, Jackson IT. The anatomical basis of the groin flap. Plast Reconstr Surg 49:42, 1972. Courtesy of Plastic and Reconstructive Surgery.)

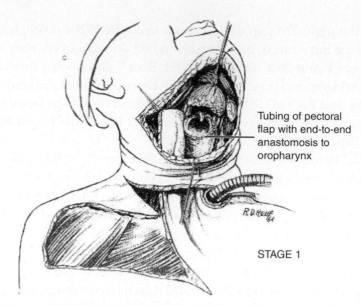

Tubing of pectoral
flap with end-to-end
anastomosis to
oropharynx

STAGE 1

Fig. 1-9 A drawing from Bakamjiam's original article. (From Bakamjian VY. A two-stage method for pharyngoesophageal reconstruction with a primary pectoral skin flap. Plast Reconstr Surg 36:176, 1965. Courtesy of Plastic and Reconstructive Surgery.)

and close the pectoral outlet 3 to 5 weeks later (Fig. 1-9). Ten cases were published in his original article, where the word "perforator" is specifically spelled out! The delto-pectoral flap was used for reconstructing pharynx and cervical esophagus defects, and rapidly became the workhorse for reconstructing head and neck defects before the era of local musculocutaneous or free flap options.

In 1971, Ger[41] used muscle flaps to treat traumatic and ulcerative lesions of the lower extremity, including the gastrocnemius, soleus, flexor digitorum longus, and abductor hallucis muscles.

1960s AND 1970s

During the 1960s and 1970s, there was an increasing awareness of both the vascular anatomy of flaps and the physiologic response to flap elevation. In 1970, Milton[42] disproved the notion of a relationship between the width and the anticipated surviving length of a skin flap. He based his landmark work on previous work of Manchot and studied the blood supply of skin flaps in pigs, concluding that the "length to breadth" ratio is not important when a cutaneous artery is included in the base of the flap.[34,43] He also studied the delay phenomenon.[44,45] In a series of publications in 1972 and 1973, McGregor and Jackson[35] and Smith and colleagues[46,47] established the concept of flap axiality and described the groin flap. The earliest axial-pattern flaps included the hypogastric flap (based on the superficial inferior epigastric artery),[48] the deltopectoral flap, and the groin flap.[35,46] The island flap arose from further development of the axial pattern flap. The axial element of the island flap was reduced to a subcutaneous pedicle. These pioneering surgeons recognized that including axial vessels at the flap base provided a superior blood supply. These vessels generally arose from the source arteries, traversed the intermuscular septa, and then ran horizontally in the subcutaneous tissues for long distances. As surgeons began to realize the benefit of including a known axial vessel

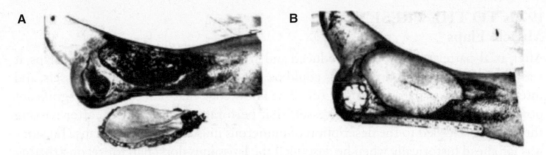

Fig. 1-10   A and **B,** The first successful free flap, described by Taylor and Daniel. (From Taylor GI, Daniel RK. The free flap: composite tissue transfer by vascular anastomosis. Aust N Z J Surg 43:1, 1973. With permission from John Wiley & Sons.)

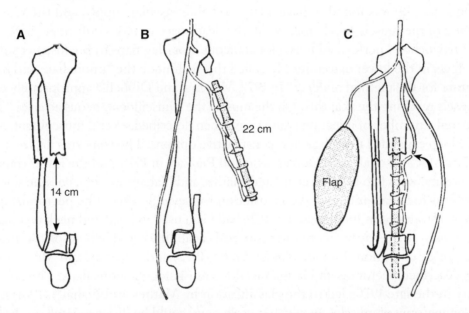

Fig. 1-11   A-C, The free vascularized bone graft introduced by Taylor and colleagues. (From Taylor GI, Miller GD, Ham FJ. The free vascularized bone graft. A clinical extension of microvascular techniques. Plast Reconstr Surg 55:538, 1975. Courtesy of Plastic and Reconstructive Surgery.)

in their flaps, the importance of knowing the precise vascular anatomy of the skin for better flap design became increasingly apparent. The resulting flaps were more reliable, and surviving lengths were more consistent.

The era of reconstructive microsurgery was born in the 1970s. There were already successful reports of tissue transplantation (kidney and liver), but the vessels anastomosed were much larger than the small cutaneous vessels required for skin transfer. There were experimental animal studies of free tissue transfer and some unsuccessful clinical attempts. However, the first successful clinical case of a free microvascular composite tissue transfer is attributed to Taylor and Daniel,[49] who performed a groin "free flap" to reconstruct an ankle soft tissue defect in 1973 (Fig. 1-10).

Since that era, dozens of free microvascular transfers of skin, muscle, bone, nerve, tendon, and various other combinations have been described and perfected. Taylor and colleagues[50,51] introduced the vascularized iliac crest and later the fibula as alternatives for an osseous flap (Fig. 1-11).

1970s TO THE PRESENT
Muscle Flaps

After axial-pattern flaps were introduced and around the time of the first free flaps, it was generally understood that flaps could be raised completely on known vessels, and interest in further anatomic study grew. The knowledge that skin receives a significant portion of its blood supply from vessels that perforate the deep fascia after passing through muscles led to the description of numerous musculocutaneous flaps. Tansini[22] was far ahead historically when he described the latissimus dorsi flap for reconstructing radical mastectomy deformities in 1906. Muscle and musculocutaneous flaps became popular through the work of McCraw,[52] McCraw and Arnold,[53] Mathes and Nahai,[54-56] and many others in the 1970s and 1980s. Muscle flaps were initially popular, because muscle generally was found to have a large reliable vascular supply, and the vascularized bulk of the muscle flap helped to fill the dead space of large, soft tissue defects. In 1972, Orticochea[57] performed musculocutaneous cross-leg flaps to reconstruct soft tissue defects in the lower extremity. He called this technique the "immediate and heroic substitute for the method of delay." In 1977, McCraw and Dibbell[58] appropriately called the vessels reaching the skin through the muscle the "musculocutaneous arteries." They conducted a number of injection studies, and then described several musculocutaneous flaps, which expanded the range of reconstructive options. The trapezius flap first published by McCraw et al[59] and Demergasso and Piazza[60] in 1979, and the lower trapezius musculocutaneous flap by Baek et al[61] and Mathes and Nahai[62] in 1980, became standard procedures for head and neck reconstruction for several years. The pectoralis major flap was introduced in 1968[37] and, by 1979, had been used in head and neck reconstruction extensively by Ariyan[38] until microsurgical capabilities gradually displaced this flap as the preferred option. Publications by Ger[63] (1972) and Hueston and McConchie[37] (1968) described pectoralis and latissimus dorsi musculocutaneous flaps. This flurry of activity in the late 1970s led to the classification by Mathes and Nahai[54] (1981) of the vascular anatomy of muscles, in which muscle types could be differentiated on the basis of their circulation patterns, leading to a more direct, safer surgical approach. Mathes and Nahai[55,56] also published two textbooks on muscle and musculocutaneous flaps, which made the field accessible for surgeons around the world.

Fasciocutaneous Flaps

Despite the popularity of muscle flaps, some disadvantages were immediately apparent, including excessive bulk, unpredictable atrophy, and functional impairment caused by sacrificing the muscle. Pontén[64] in (1981) reintroduced another option for securing a large cutaneous flap that totally omitted muscle. Basically, he maintained the deep fascia with the overlying skin and subcutaneous tissues, postulating that this resulted in greater reliability of these "super flaps" in the lower leg. Today these flaps are known as *fasciocutaneous flaps*. Pontén never delineated the intrinsic blood supply to the "fascial plexus" found between the epidermis and deep fascia, and some today might refer to these as variations of neurocutaneous flaps.[65] Tolhurst et al[66] expanded this idea to show that fasciocutaneous flaps could be used for reconstruction in the upper limbs and trunk, proving that a deep fascia existed not only in the lower leg.

Although the deep fascia is relatively avascular, a subfascial and suprafascial plexus exist. This plexus alone can sustain the "fascial feeder" flaps introduced by Niranjan.[67] These can be distally based fasciocutaneous flaps, fascia-only flaps, adipofascial flaps, and adiposal flaps (numerous variations of fasciocutaneous flaps in which the fascia itself does not need to be included). Nakajima et al[68] theorized that six perforators of the deep fascia supply this fascial plexus, including musculocutaneous, septocutaneous, and axial cutaneous perforators. Further anatomic studies by Cormack and Lamberty[69] provided the basis for their classification of fasciocutaneous flaps. The same authors published a landmark book, *The Arterial Anatomy of Skin Flaps*,[70] that contains a concise appraisal of the history, anatomy, and clinical aspects of skin flap surgery, including fasciocutaneous flaps. Hallock[71] emphasized the importance of this concept in his book, *Fasciocutaneous Flaps*.

Perforator Flaps

Through the long history of flap development, perforator flaps are the most sophisticated application of flap vascular anatomy. As our knowledge of vascular anatomy improved, surgeons gradually began to understand that a certain amount of tissue was not required to successfully transfer a flap; an isolated source artery and vein were all that was needed. This led to greater precision in flap design, improved results by diminishing bulk, and less donor site morbidity. Perforator flaps arose because surgeons wanted to maintain the excellent vascularity of the large vessels supplying muscle flaps and avoid the bulk of musculocutaneous flaps and the functional loss caused by harvesting muscle.

In 1987, Taylor and Palmer[72] created the concept of "angiosomes" or vascular territories, and choke vessels. This opened the door for creating myriad flaps based on a perforator artery. Taylor and colleagues[73-75] argued that the direct vessels are the primary cutaneous supply, and it is irrelevant if they have first traversed intermuscular or intramuscular septa, because their main destination is always the skin.

The definition of a *perforator flap* has been extensively discussed. Strictly defined, it is a vascularized tissue transfer nourished by a musculocutaneous perforator; clinically, it is a vascularized tissue transfer nourished by an adequate cutaneous perforator (musculocutaneous, septocutaneous, or direct axial vessel).[76]

The earliest pioneers of perforator flap surgery reported cases in which they dissected through the muscle fascia to harvest vessels supplying the overlying skin. The impact of perforator flaps has been immense. Approximately 400 cutaneous perforators have been described in the human body.[77] A perforator flap could conceivably be based on any suitable perforator where the donor site is acceptable. Therefore the technique has increased to include flap options for reconstruction. New reports and modifications are being reported at an exponential rate. However, the perforator flaps that have made very significant impact include the deep inferior epigastric artery perforator (DIEAP) flap,[78,79] the thoracodorsal artery perforator (TDAP) flap,[80] anterolateral thigh flap or lateral circumflex femoral artery perforator–vastus lateralis (LCFAP-*vl*),[81] submental artery perforator (SMAP) flap,[82] the superior gluteal artery (SGAP) perforator flap,[83] and inferior gluteal artery perforator (IGAP) flaps,[84] and the superficial circumflex iliac artery perforator (SCIAP) flap.[85] The DIEAP flap is perhaps the most widely used perforator flap in the world.

In 1989, Koshima and Soeda[78] reported on a skin flap based only on a perforating vessel of the deep fascia, from the deep inferior epigastric artery, demonstrating that it is possible to harvest the flap without sacrificing the rectus abdominis muscle. Allen and Treece[79] described its use in breast reconstruction in 1994 (Fig. 1-12), and Blondeel and colleagues[86-88] made extensive refinements.

Taylor et al[89] described the posterior tibial artery perforator (PTAP) flap (Fig. 1-13), and Kroll and Rosenfield[90] described the paraspinal perforators used for reconstruct-

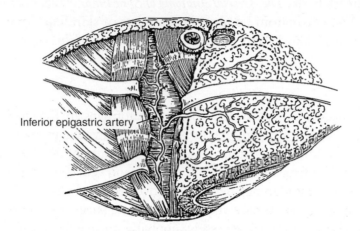

Fig. 1-12   The DIEAP flap for breast reconstruction, described by Allen and Treece. (From Allen RJ, Treece P. Deep inferior epigastric perforator flap for breast reconstruction. Annals of Plastic Surgery 32:32-38, 1994.)

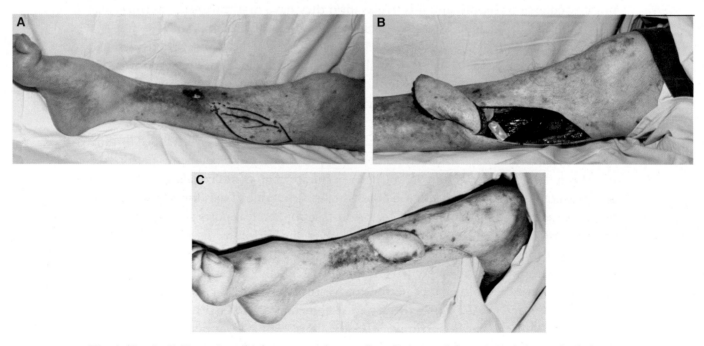

Fig. 1-13   A-C, Posterior tibial artery perforator flap. (Reprinted from British Journal of Plastic Surgery, Volume 43, Taylor GI, Doyle M, McCarten G, The Doppler probe for planning flaps: anatomical study and clinical applications, pages 1-16, copyright 1990, with permission from Elsevier.)

ing low posterior midline defects (Fig. 1-14). All of these surgeons contributed seminal works in which they isolated individual perforators and harvested free or pedicle tissue transfers based on these vessels. In 1998, Koshima et al[91] introduced the paraumbilical perforator (PUP) flap, which they initially used for breast reconstruction (Fig. 1-15).

The TDAP flap was first described by Angrigiani et al.[80] They proposed the possibility of raising the cutaneous island of the latissimus dorsi musculocutaneous flap without muscle, based only on one cutaneous perforator. This has become a popular pedicle flap option for regional reconstruction of the axilla and breast, and is also widely used as a free flap.

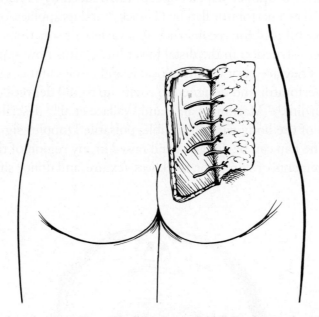

Fig. 1-14   Paraspinal perforators. (From Kroll SS, Rosenfield L. Perforator-based flaps for low posterior midline defects. Plast Reconstr Surg 81:561, 1988. Courtesy of Plastic and Reconstructive Surgery.)

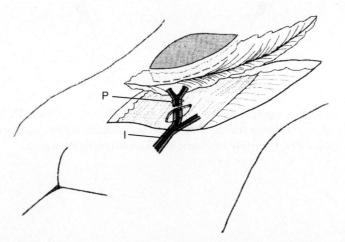

Fig. 1-15   The paraumbilical perforator flap described by Koshima and colleagues. *P* is the muscle perforator, and *I* is the deep inferior epigastric vessel. (From Koshima I, Inagawa K, Urushibara K, Moriguchi T. Paraumbilical perforator flap without deep inferior epigastric vessels. Plast Reconstr Surg 102:1055, 1998. Courtesy of Plastic and Reconstructive Surgery.)

The anterolateral thigh flap, introduced by Song et al,[81] and has become very popular as a reliable large cutaneous flap for reconstruction throughout the body. Wei et al[92] described this as the "ideal flap." It can provide skin, fascia, muscle, or any of these in combination.

The SMAP flap, first reported by Martin et al,[82] is a reliable regional or free flap for facial defects. It matches the color, texture, and thickness of facial skin, with a good aesthetic result at the donor site. The flap can be used inferiorly based on the submental and facial arteries or as a superiorly based reverse-pattern submental flap based on the distal facial vessels[93,94] (Fig. 1-16).

The perforator propeller flap, a concept introduced by Hyakusoku et al,[95] was originally described as a perforator flap by Hallock,[96] and its applications were expanded by Teo.[97] It is a useful tool for reconstructing a variety of soft tissue defects. Initially performed for reconstruction in the distal lower limb,[98] it is now applied in every part of the body.[99-101] They are very versatile local island fasciocutaneous flaps based on a single dissected perforator and designed to rotate up to 180 degrees (Fig. 1-17).

Wei and Mardini,[102] Mardini et al,[103] and Wallace et al[104] described free-style free flaps. Any region of the body with an audible, pulsatile Doppler signal can be chosen as a donor site. The flap can be designed and raised in any region of the body that suits the unique requirements of skin color, thickness, texture, and donor site morbidity.[104-106]

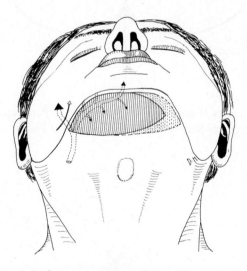

Fig. 1-16 Submental flap, original representation. (From Martin D, Pascal JF, Baudet J, et al. The submental island flap: a new donor site. Anatomy and clinical applications as a free pedicled flap. Plast Reconstr Surg 92:868, 1993. Courtesy of Plastic and Reconstructive Surgery.)

The uses for perforator flaps are continuously expanding. Masia and colleagues[107,108] have been developing an imaging technique for planning perforator flaps, particularly for breast reconstruction (Fig. 1-18), and more recently through the use of noncontrast MRI.[109] Novadaq SPY imaging (Novadaq Technologies, Inc., Bonita Springs, Florida) is a fluorescent angiography system that provides simple and efficient intraoperative real-time surface angiographic imaging, has augmented our understanding of the physiology of these flaps. This technology is helpful for evaluating vascular anastomosis and flap perfusion intraoperatively and facilitates surgical decision making.[110]

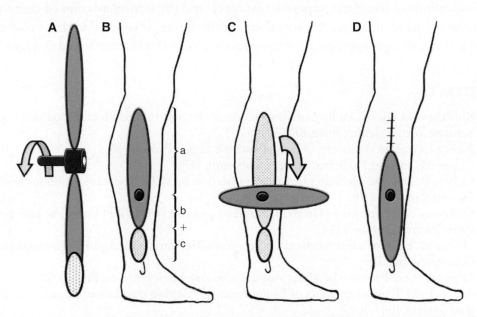

Fig. 1-17 **A-D,** Propeller flap concept. (Reprinted from Clinics in Plastic Surgery, Volume 37, Teo TC, The Propeller Flap Concept, pages 615-626, Copyright 2010, with permission from Elsevier.)

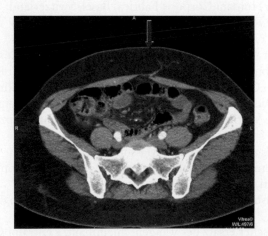

Fig. 1-18 CT is commonly used for planning perforator flaps. (Reprinted from J Plast Reconstr Aesthet Surg, Volume 59, Masia J, Clavero JA, Larrañaga JR, Alomar X, Pons G, Serret P, Multidetector-row computed tomography in the planning of abdominal perforator flaps, pages 594-599, copyright 2006, with permission from Elsevier.)

CONCLUSION

What can we expect in the future? We anticipate more precisely defined limits of vasculature, including branching patterns, to achieve more predictable results. As more of our experiences are reported, recommendations for specific flaps for specific problems should become evidence based. Methods of augmenting flow through perforator vessels are needed. These advancements will allow us to customize methods for solving more-complex clinical problems with improved imaging and an enhanced understanding of all vascular territories and their respective vessels.

Perforator flap surgery had undergone tremendous growth in recent years with the innovations of free flaps, supramicrosurgery, and the transplantation of composite tissues of the hand and face, among others. In the future, it is possible that every conceivable tissue with an appropriate arteriovenous system can be transferred as a free flap.

References

1. Bhishagratna KJ, ed. An English Translation of the Sushruta Samhita, Based on Original Sanskrit Text. Calcutta: Bose, 1907-1916.
2. Nehru J, ed. The Discovery of India. Calcutta: Signet Press, 1946.
3. Celsus AC, ed. De Medicina. Firenze: Laurentii, 1478.
4. Celsus AC, ed. De Medicina [English translation by W.G. Spencer]. London: William Heinemann Ltd, 1938.
5. Oribasius, ed. Chirurgia ex Greco in Latinum Conversa [Vido Vidi Florentino, Interprete]. Paris: Pierre Gaultier, 1544.
6. Oribasius, ed. Oribasius Sardiani Collectorum Medicinalium. Apud B Turrisanum sub Official Aldina. Paris, 1555.
7. Aegineta P, ed. Epitome of Medicine (seven books). Venice: Aldine Press, 1528.
8. Adams F, ed. The Seven Books of Paulus Aegineta [English translation]. London: Syndenham Society, 1844-1847.
9. Tagliacozzi G, ed. De Curtorum Chirurgica per Insitionem. Venetiis: G Bindonus, 1597.
10. Capra F, ed. The Science of Leonardo: Inside the Mind of the Great Genius of the Renaissance. New York: Doubleday, 2007.
11. Vesalius A, ed. De Humani Corporis Fabrica. Basel, Switzerland: Joannis Oporini, 1543.
12. Brotton J, ed. The Renaissance: A Very Short Introduction. New York: Oxford University Press, 2006.
13. Carpue JC, ed. An Account of Two Successful Operations for Restoring a Lost Nose Including Description of the Indian and Italian methods. London: Longman, 1816.
14. Mazzola FR, Lupo G. Evolving concepts in lip reconstruction. Clin Plast Surg 2:583, 1984.
15. Manchot C, ed. Die Hautarterien de Menschlichen Korpers. Leipzig: FCW Vogel, 1889.
16. Spalteholz W. Die Vertheilung der Blutgefässe in der Haut. Leipzig: Arch Anat Entwicklungsgesch, 1893.
17. Salmon M. Artères de la Peau. Paris: Masson, 1936.
18. Sabattini P, ed. Cenno Storico dell'Origine e Progressi della Rinoplastica e Cheiloplastica. Bologna: Belle Arti, 1838.
19. Abbé R. A new plastic operation for the relief of deformity due to double harelip. Med Rec 53:447, 1898.
20. Gersuny R. Plastischer ersatz der wangenschleimhaut. Zentralbl Chir 14:706, 1887.
21. Monks GH. Correction by operation of some nasal deformities and disfigurements. Boston Med Surg J 139:262, 1898.
22. Tansini I. Sopra il mio nuovo processo di amputazione della. Gazz Med Ital 57:141, 1906.

23. Hamilton FH, ed. Elkoplasty or Anaplasty Applied to the Treatment of Old Ulcers. New York: Holman Gray, 1854.

24. Filatov VP. Plastic procedure using a round pedicle. Vestnik Oftalmol 34:149, 1917.

25. Esser JF. General rules used in simple plastic work on Austrian war-wounded soldiers. Surg Gynecol Obstet 34:737, 1917.

26. Daniel RK, Kerrigan CL. Principles and physiology of skin flap surgery. In McCarthy JG, ed. Plastic Surgery. Philadelphia: WB Saunders, 1990.

27. Esser JF. Schwerer verschluss einer brustwand perforation. Berl Klin Wochenschr 55:1197, 1918.

28. Gillies HD. The tubed pedicle in plastic surgery. NY Med J 111:1, 1920.

29. Gillies HD, ed. Plastic Surgery of the Face: Based on Selected Cases of War Injuries of the Face Including Burns. London: Henry Frowde, Oxford University Press, and Hodder and Stoughton, 1920.

30. Hallock GG. The plastic surgeon of the 20th century. Plast Reconstr Surg 107:1014, 2001.

31. Gillies H, Millard DR Jr, eds. The Principles and Art of Plastic Surgery. Boston: Little Brown, 1957.

32. Blair VP. The delayed transfer of long pedicle flaps in plastic surgery (face). Surg Gynecol Obstet 33:261, 1921.

33. Esser JF, ed. Artery Flaps. Antwerp: De Vos–van Kleef, 1929.

34. Shaw D, Payne RL Jr. One stage tubed abdominal flaps; single pedicle tubes. Surg Gynecol Obstet 83:205, 1946.

35. McGregor IA, Jackson IT. The groin flap. Br J Plast Surg 25:3, 1972.

36. Owens N. Compound neck pedicle designed for the repair of massive facial defects: formation, development and application. Plast Reconstr Surg 15:369, 1955.

37. Hueston JT, McConchie IH. A compound pectoral flap. Aust N Z J Surg 38:61, 1968.

38. Ariyan S. The pectoralis major myocutaneous flap. A versatile flap for reconstruction in the head and neck. Plast Reconstr Surg 63:73, 1979.

39. Converse JM, ed. Skin Flaps. Reconstructive Plastic Surgery. Philadelphia: WB Saunders, 1964.

40. Bakanjiam VY. A two-stage method for pharyngoesophageal reconstruction with a primary pectoral skin flap. Plast Reconstr Surg 36:173-184, 1965.

41. Ger R. The technique of muscle transposition in the operative treatment of traumatic and ulcerative lesions of the leg. J Trauma 11:502, 1971.

42. Milton SH. Pedicled skin-flaps: the fallacy of the length: width ratio. Br J Surg 57:502, 1970.

43. Milton SH. Experimental study on island flaps. I. Surviving length. Plast Reconstr Surg 48:574, 1971.

44. Milton SH. The effects of "delay" on the survival of experimental pedicled skin flaps. Br J Plast Surg 22:244, 1969.

45. Milton SH. Experimental study on island flaps. II. Ischaemia and delay. Plast Reconstr Surg 49:444, 1973.

46. Smith PJ, Foley B, McGregor IA, et al. The anatomical basis of the groin flap. Plast Reconstr Surg 49:41-47, 1972.

47. Smith PJ. Vascular basis of axial pattern flaps. Br J Plast Surg 26:150, 1973.

48. D'Hooghe P, Hendrickx EE. Protection of femoral vessels with a de-epithelialized hypogastric flap. Case report. Plast Reconstr Surg 55:87, 1975.

49. Taylor GI, Daniel RK. The free flap: composite tissue transfer by vascular anastomosis. Aust N Z J Surg 43:1, 1973.

50. Taylor GI, Townsend P, Corlett R. Superiority of the deep circumflex iliac vessels as the supply for free groin flap. II. Clinical work. Plast Reconstr Surg 64:745, 1979.

51. Taylor GI, Miller GD, Ham FJ. The free vascularized bone graft: a clinical extension of microvascular techniques. Plast Reconstr Surg 55:533-544, 1975.

52. McCraw JB. The recent history of myocutaneous flaps. Clin Plast Surg 7:3, 1980.

53. McCraw JB, Arnold PG, eds. McCraw and Arnold's Atlas of Muscle and Musculocutaneous Flaps. Norfolk, VA: Hampton Press, 1986.

54. Mathes SJ, Nahai F. Classification of the vascular anatomy of muscles: experimental and clinical correlation. Plast Reconstr Surg 67:1177, 1981.

55. Mathes SJ, Nahai F, eds. Clinical Atlas of Muscle and Musculocutaneous Flaps. St Louis: CV Mosby, 1979.

56. Mathes SJ, Nahai F, eds. Clinical Applications for Muscle and Musculocutaneous Flaps. St Louis: CV Mosby, 1982.

57. Orticochea M. The musculocutaneous flap method: an immediate and heroic substitute for the method of delay. Br J Plast Surg 25:106, 1972.

58. McCraw JB, Dibbell DG. Experimental definition of independent myocutaneous vascular territories. Plast Reconstr Surg 60:212, 1977.

59. McCraw JB, Magee WP, Kalwaic H. Uses of the trapezius and sternomastoid myocutaneous flaps in head and neck reconstruction. Plast Reconstr Surg 63:49, 1979.

60. Demergasso F, Piazza MV. Trapezius myocutaneous flap in reconstructive surgery for head and neck cancer: an original technique. Am J Surg 138:533, 1979.

61. Baek SM, Biller HP, Krespi YP, et al. The lower trapezius island myocutaneous flap. Ann Plast Surg 5:108, 1980.

62. Mathes SJ, Nahai F. Muscle flap transposition with functional preservation: technical and clinical considerations. Plast Reconstr Surg 66:242, 1980.

63. Ger R. Surgical management of ulcerative lesions in the leg. Curr Probl Surg Mar:1-52, 1972.

64. Pontén B. The fasciocutaneous flap: its use in soft tissue defects of the lower leg. Br J Plast Surg 34:215-220, 1981.

65. Hallock GG. Direct and indirect perforator flaps: the history and the controversy. Plast Reconstr Surg 111:855, 2003.

66. Tolhurst DE, Haeseker B, Zeeman RJ. The development of the fasciocutaneous flap and its clinical applications. Plast Reconstr Surg 71:597, 1983.

67. Niranjan NS, Price RD, Govilkar P. Fascial feeder and perforator-based V-Y advancement flaps in the reconstruction of lower limb defects. Br J Plast Surg 53:679, 2000.

68. Nakajima H, Fujino T, Adachi S. A new concept of vascular supply to the skin and classification of skin flaps according to their vascularization. Ann Plast Surg 16:1, 1986.

69. Cormack GC, Lamberty BG. A classification of fascia-cutaneous flaps according to their patterns of vascularization. Br J Plast Surg 37:80, 1984.

70. Cormack GC, Lamberty BG, eds. The Arterial Anatomy of Skin Flaps. Edinburgh: Churchill Livingstone, 1986.

71. Hallock GG. Fasciocutaneous Flaps. Boston: Blackwell Scientific Publications, 1992.

72. Taylor GI, Palmer JM. The vascular territories (angiosomes) of the body: experimental study and clinical observation. Br J Plast Surg 40:113, 1987.

73. Taylor GI, Palmer JH, McManamny D, eds. The vascular territories of the body (angiosomes) and their clinical applications. In McCarthy JG, ed. Plastic Surgery, vol 1. Philadelphia: WB Saunders, 1990.

74. Taylor GI. Foreword. In Manchot C, ed. The Cutaneous Arteries of the Human Body. New York: Springer-Verlag, 1983.

75. Taylor GI. The blood supply of the skin. In Aston SJ, Beasley RW, Thorne CH, eds. Grabb and Smith's Plastic Surgery. Philadelphia: Lippincott-Raven, 1997.

76. Geddes CR, Morris SF, Neligan PC. Perforator flaps: evolution, classification, and applications. Ann Plast Surg 50:90, 2003.

77. Morris SF, Tang M, Almutairi K, et al. The anatomic basis of perforator flaps. Ann Plast Surg 37:553-570, 2010.

78. Koshima I, Soeda S. Inferior epigastric artery skin flap without rectus abdominis muscle. Br J Plast Surg 42:645, 1989.

79. Allen RJ, Treece P. Deep inferior epigastric perforator flap for breast reconstruction. Ann Plast Surg 32:32, 1994.

80. Angrigiani C, Grilli D, Siebert J. Latissimus dorsi musculocutaneous flap without muscle. Plast Reconstr Surg 96:1608, 1995.

81. Song YG, Chen GZ, Song YL. The free thigh flap: a new free flap concept based on the septocutaneous artery. Br J Plast Surg 37:149, 1984.

82. Martin D, Pascal JF, Baudet J, et al. The submental island flap: a new donor site. Anatomy and clinical applications as a free of pedicled flap. Plast Reconstr Surg 92:867, 1993.

83. Fujino T, Harashina T, Aoyagi F. Reconstruction for aplasia of the breast and pectoral region by microvascular transfer of a free flap from the buttock. Plast Reconstr Surg 56:178, 1975.

84. Paletta CE, Bostwick J III, Nahai F. The inferior gluteal free flap in breast reconstruction. Plast Reconstr Surg 84:875, 1989.

85. Koshima I, Nanba Y, Tsutsui T, et al. Superficial circumflex iliac artery perforator flap for reconstruction of limb defects. Plast Reconstr Surg 113:233, 2004.

86. Blondeel PN, Boeckx WD. Refinements in free flap breast reconstruction: the free bilateral deep inferior epigastric perforator flap anastomosed to the internal mammary artery. Br J Plast Surg 47:495, 1994.

87. Blondeel PN. One hundred free DIEP flap breast reconstructions: a personal experience. Br J Plast Surg 52:104, 1999.

88. Blondeel PN, Hijjawi J, Depypere H, et al. Shaping the breast in aesthetic and reconstructive breast surgery: an easy three-step principle. II. Breast reconstruction after total mastectomy. Plast Reconstr Surg 123:794, 2009.

89. Taylor GI, Doyle M, McCarten G. The Doppler probe for planning flaps: anatomical study and clinical applications. Br J Plast Surg 43:1, 1990.

90. Kroll SS, Rosenfield L. Perforator-based flaps for low posterior midline defects. Plast Reconstr Surg 81:561, 1988.

91. Koshima I, Inagawa K, Urushibara K, et al. Paraumbilical perforator flap without deep inferior epigastric vessels. Plast Reconstr Surg 102:1052, 1998.

92. Wei FC, Jain V, Celik N, et al. Have we found an ideal soft-tissue flap? An experience with 672 anterolateral thigh flaps. Plast Reconstr Surg 109:2219, 2002.

93. Kim JT, Kim SK, Koshima I, et al. An anatomical study and clinical applications of the reversed submental perforator-based island flap. Plast Reconstr Surg 109:2204, 2002.

94. Tang M, Ding M, Almutairi K, Morris, SF. Three-dimensional angiography of the submental artery perforator flap. J Plast Reconstr Aesthet Surg 64:608, 2011.

95. Hyakusoku H, Yamamoto T, Fumiiri M. The propeller flap method. Br J Plast Surg 44:53, 1991.

96. Hallock GG. The propeller flap version of the adductor muscle perforator flap for coverage of ischial or trochanteric pressure sores. Ann Plast Surg 56:540, 2006.

97. Teo TC. The propeller flap concept. Clin Plast Surg 37:615, 2010.

98. Teo TC. Perforator local flaps in lower limb reconstruction. Cir Plas Iberolatinoam 32:287, 2006.

99. Smeets L, Hendrickx B, Teo TC. The propeller flap concept used in vaginal wall reconstruction. J Plast Reconstr Aesthet Surg, 2011 Nov 29. [Epub ahead of print]

100. Oh TS, Hallock G, Hong JP. Freestyle propeller flaps to reconstruct defects of the posterior trunk: a simple approach to a difficult problem. Ann Plast Surg 68:79, 2012.

101. Pignatti M, Ogawa R, Hallock GG, et al. The "Tokyo" consensus on propeller flaps. Plast Reconstr Surg 127:716, 2011.

102. Wei FC, Mardini S. Free-style free flaps. Plast Reconstr Surg 114:910, 2004.

103. Mardini S, Tsai FC, Wei FC. The thigh as a model for free style free flaps. Clin Plast Surg 30:473, 2003.

104. Wallace CG, Kao HK, Jeng SF, et al. Free-style flaps: a further step forward for perforator flap surgery. Plast Reconstr Surg 124:e419, 2009.

105. Eom JS, Sun SH, Hong JP. Use of the upper medial thigh perforator flap (gracilis perforator flap) for lower extremity reconstruction. Plast Reconstr Surg 127:731, 2011.

106. Eom JS, Hong JP. Lower back defect coverage using a free-style gluteal perforator flap. Ann Plast Surg 67:516, 2011.

107. Masia J, Clavero JA, Larrañaga JR, et al. Multidetector-row computed tomography in the planning of abdominal perforator flaps. J Plast Reconstr Aesthet Surg 59:594, 2006.

108. Masia J, Kosutic D, Clavero JA, et al. Preoperative computed tomographic angiogram for deep inferior epigastric artery perforator flap breast reconstruction. J Reconstr Microsurg 26:21, 2010.

109. Masia J, Kosutic D, Cervelli D, et al. In search of the ideal method in perforator mapping: noncontrast magnetic resonance imaging. J Reconstr Microsurg 26:29, 2010.

110. Pestana IA, Coan B, Erdmann D, et al. Early experience with fluorescent angiography in free-tissue transfer reconstruction. Plast Reconstr Surg 123:1239, 2009.

2

Vascular Territories of the Integument

Steven F. Morris

G. Ian Taylor

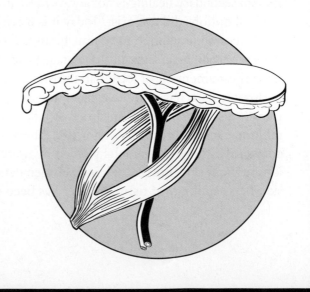

Our knowledge of the vascular supply to the skin has evolved over the past century.[1] This process has been driven by the culmination of two main forces: the work of researchers who have sought to further our understanding of human anatomy and the innovation of surgeons who have either applied or expanded this knowledge as they provided surgical solutions to wound-closure problems. This evolution has not been a process of steady, cumulative learning; the development has been sporadic, sometimes stimulated by the need for surgical solutions to difficult problems. However, at other times researchers have worked to define the vascular anatomy of the integument without a clear plan to use this information in the surgical setting. Our accumulation of knowledge of the vascular supply to the skin has been characterized by both discovery and rediscovery, which is often the case when significant contributors work independently and publish in various languages. As Cormack and Lamberty[1] noted, often what is new in reconstructive surgery can be traced back to earlier work that was either overlooked or ignored until the clinical need arose. Clearly, there is an ongoing need for detailed vascular anatomic information to assist surgeons in devising improved methods of tissue transfer.

It is likely that surgeons have always faced the dilemma of closing a wound where tissue is missing and where local tissue laxity does not permit primary closure. In the absence of exposed vital structures, most wounds will eventually heal secondarily. Although secondary healing is not always ideal, it would have sufficed at a time when better surgical options did not exist. Today it is often preferable from a functional, economic, and/or cosmetic standpoint to transfer tissues of suitable thickness and contour into the defect to facilitate closure in a one-stage procedure. Advances in the design of skin flaps, from the refinement of local flap transfer to the use of regional, distant, free, and now perforator flaps have successively equipped surgeons with an ever-increasing ability to transfer tissue of desirable qualities, to tailor that tissue to the defect in question, and to minimize morbidity at the donor site. This process has been a surgical evolution, with constantly improving results yielded by increasingly more sophisticated procedures. Throughout this process, the link between detailed anatomic knowledge and successful skin flap planning for tissue transfer has been clear.

The survival of any skin flap is related to factors such as the patient's age and co-morbidities, skin flap physiology, flap design, and probably most important, the anatomy of the underlying vasculature. The physiologic effects of the surgical elevation and transfer of skin flaps have been clarified by Milton,[2-4] Pang et al,[5-7] Sasaki and Pang,[8] and Kerrigan and Daniel,[9-11] among others.

In this chapter we will review the vascular anatomy of the integument and place the historical development of this important field into perspective. The history of the study of the anatomy of the integument and the history of skin flaps are intimately but not directly associated.

STUDY OF THE VASCULAR ANATOMY OF THE INTEGUMENT

In 1628 William Harvey provided the earliest accurate description of the vascular supply to the skin in his landmark publication, *An Anatomical Disputation Concerning the Movement of the Heart and Blood in Living Creatures.*[12] Wladimir Tomsa[13] of Kiev (1873) and Werner Spalteholz[14] of Leipzig (1893) added important early works on the anatomy and physiology of the cutaneous vasculature. Tomsa completed injection studies to describe the subdermal and dermal plexuses of vessels in the skin. Spalteholz used gelatin and pigment (ultramarine, lampblack) injection studies to define direct and indirect perforators to the skin. Spalteholz divided the arteries to the skin into two types. The first type of artery is the *pure* or *direct* artery, which branches directly to the skin. These vessels typically travel through the intermuscular septa and primarily supply blood to the skin. Some of these vessels travel for long distances in the subcutaneous tissues, sending multiple branches to the surrounding skin. These were among the first vessels noticed by surgeons for their ability to supply large axial pattern skin flaps (for example, the forehead flap). The second type of artery to the skin is the *impure* or *indirect* artery. These vessels are perforators that primarily supply the deeper tissues, particularly muscle, and then emerge to supply the skin. This distinction implies that the most direct perforators are septocutaneous in nature, and that the most indirect perforators are musculocutaneous. It is now known that many anatomic variations of this theme exist, which has spawned a wide variety of classifications of the blood supply to the skin.[15-22]

In the 1880s, Carl Manchot[23,24] sought to clarify the vascular anatomy of the skin in a systematic and comprehensive fashion. As a medical student and while at the Kaiser-Wilhelm University Medical School in Strassburg, Manchot completed a monumental review of the cutaneous vasculature before the discovery of x-rays by Roentgen in 1895. Manchot is credited with the first detailed description of the human cutaneous blood supply. He identified distinct skin territories, each receiving its blood supply from a source vessel. This work was published in diagrammatic form in his book, *Die Hautarterien des Menschlichen Korpers (The Skin Arteries of the Body)*, in 1889[23] (Fig. 2-1). The detail of his work is remarkable, considering that he did not have the benefit of radiographic contrast studies. His anatomic descriptions of the skin's vascular territories, although not completely accurate, are impressive. His work became known to some, influencing flap design for a few surgeons, and was subsequently published in English.[24]

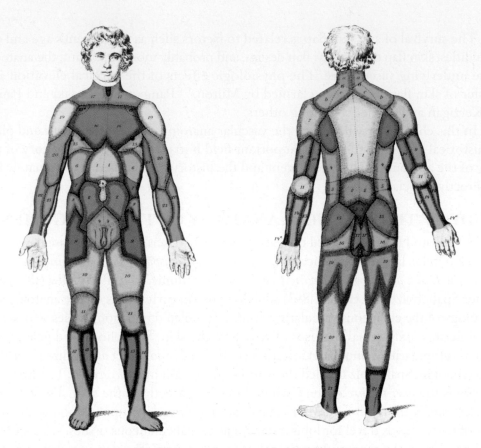

Fig. 2-1   The cutaneous arteries of the human body. This figure is based on Carl Manchot's dissections in the 1880s clarifying the vascular anatomy of skin of the body. This work was published initially in German and subsequently translated to English. (Modified from Manchot C, ed. Die Hautarterien des Menschlichen Korpers. Leipzig: FCW Vogel, 1889; Manchot C, ed. The Cutaneous Arteries of the Human Body. New York: Springer-Verlag, 1982.)

Manchot's work was later reappraised by Michel Salmon[25,26] in the 1930s in a series of anatomic studies. Salmon developed an intravascular injection technique using lead oxide, gelatin, phenol, and water, which he used on fresh human cadavers to identify and describe the vascular anatomy of skin and muscles of the body. His studies produced impressive images, allowing a more detailed description than Manchot was able to achieve. In his 1936 book, *Artères de la Peau*, Salmon[25,27] described approximately twice the number of vascular territories as originally proposed by Manchot (Fig. 2-2). Salmon published three additional books: *The Arteries of the Muscles of the Limbs and the Trunk*,[26] *Arteries of the Muscles of the Head and Neck*, and *The Arterial Anastomotic Networks of the Limbs*.

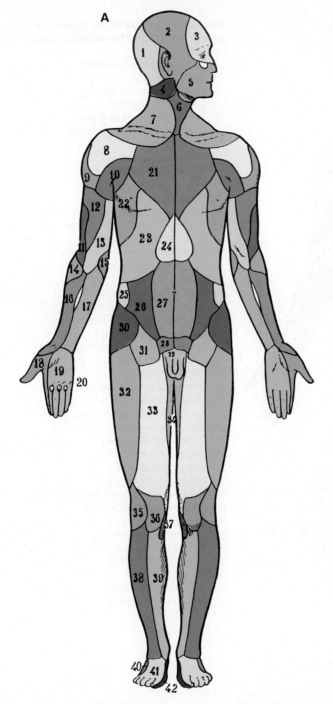

Schematic summary of the cutaneous arterial territory of the ventral surface of the body.
1. Occipital artery
2. Superficial temporal artery
3. Ophthalmic artery
4. Sternocleidomastoid artery
5. Facial artery
6. Thyroid arteries
7. Transverse cervical and suprascapular arteries
8. Deltoid branch of the acromiothoracic trunk
9. Circumflex humeral arteries
10. Small thoracic branches of the acromiothoracic trunk
11. Profunda brachii artery
12. Brachial artery (muscular branches)
13. Brachial artery (direct branches)
14. Epicondylar arteries
15. Epitrochlear arteries
16. Radial artery
17. Ulnar artery
18. Deep palmar arch
19. Superficial palmar arch
20. Anterior interosseous artery
21. Internal mammary artery
22. External mammary (lateral thoracic) and subscapular arteries
23. Intercostal arteries
24. Superficial superior epigastic artery
25. Lumbar arteries
26. Inferior superficial epigastric artery
27. Deep epigastric artery
28. External superior pudendal artery
29. External inferior pudendal artery
30. Superficial circumflex iliac artery
31. Femoral artery
32. Artery to the vastus lateralis muscle
33. Superficial femoral artery
34. Artery to the adductor muscles
35. Lateral articular branches
36. Medial articular branches
37. Genus descendens artery
38. Anterior tibial artery
39. Posterior tibial artery
40. Peroneal artery
41. Dorsalis pedis artery
42. Medial plantar artery

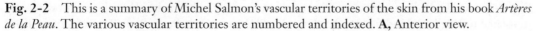

Fig. 2-2   This is a summary of Michel Salmon's vascular territories of the skin from his book *Artères de la Peau.* The various vascular territories are numbered and indexed. **A,** Anterior view.

Continued

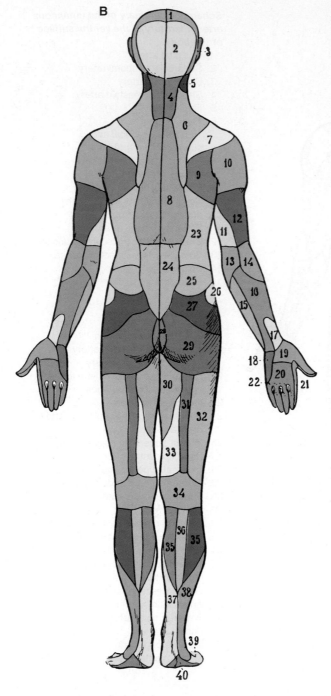

Schematic summary of the cutaneous arterial territories of the dorsal surface of the body.

1. Superficial temporal artery
2. Occipital artery
3. Posterior auricular artery
4. Deep cervical artery
5. Sternocleidomastoid artery
6. Deep branch of the transverse cervical artery
7. Suprascapular artery
8. Dorsospinal branch of the intercostal artery
9. Subscapular artery
10. Posterior circumflex humeral artery
11. Brachial artery (medial collateral branches)
12. Profunda brachii artery
13. Posterior recurrent ulnar artery
14. Radial recurrent artery
15. Ulnar artery
16. Posterior interosseous artery
17. Anterior interosseous artery
18. Dorsal branch of the ulnar artery
19. Dorsal carpal artery
20. Posterior interosseous arteries
21. Deep palmar arch
22. Digital arteries
23. Intercostal arteries (perforating branches)
24. Lumbar arteries (dorsospinal branches)
25. Lumbar arteries (perforating branches)
26. Superficial circumflex iliac artery
27. Superior gluteal artery
28. Internal pudendal artery
29. Inferior gluteal artery
30. Artery to the adductors
31. Artery accompanying the sciatic nerve
32 and 33. Perforating arteries
34. Popliteal artery
35. Gastrocnemius arteries
36. Small saphenous artery
37. Posterior tibial artery
38. Peroneal artery
39. Dorsalis pedis artery
40. Medial plantar artery

Fig. 2-2, cont'd   B, Posterior view. This work was initially published in French and subsequently translated to English. (Modified from Salmon M, ed. Artères de la Peau. Paris: Masson et Cie, 1936; Salmon M, Taylor GI, Tempest MN, eds. Arteries of the Skin. London: Churchill Livingstone, 1988.)

Much of Salmon's work remains accurate and applicable to modern flap design, and his techniques have served as a template for subsequent anatomic studies. Some of Salmon's anatomic insights regarding the placement of surgical incisions and skin flap orientation are remarkable. He stated in 1936 that in reconstructive surgery, the base of any flaps that are raised must include the arterial pedicle. In the preface to *Artères de la Peau*, Raymond Grégoire notes: "This new work by Michel Salmon is a painstaking study that no surgeon from now on can ignore and few anatomists would have had the courage to undertake."

MICROCIRCULATION OF THE INTEGUMENT

The histologic aspects of the microcirculation of the integument have been extensively studied.[28-32] The main architecture of the skin's microvascular supply includes arterioles, terminal arterioles, precapillary sphincters, capillaries, postcapillary venules, collecting venules, and muscular venules.[1] The arterioles arise from direct or indirect arterial branches to the skin. The skin's microcirculation delivers oxygen and nutrients, removes waste products, and provides thermoregulation.

The vasculature of the skin and subcutaneous tissue is arranged in five vascular plexuses: the subepidermal plexus, dermal plexus, subdermal plexus, subcutaneous plexus, and fascial plexus (prefascial and subfascial) (Fig. 2-3). Each plexus consists of a fine meshwork of interconnecting vessels that runs in a horizontal sheet at the anatomic level corresponding to the name of the plexus. The result of this arrangement is an enormous cumulative vascular length, facilitating the skin's significant capacity for distribution of

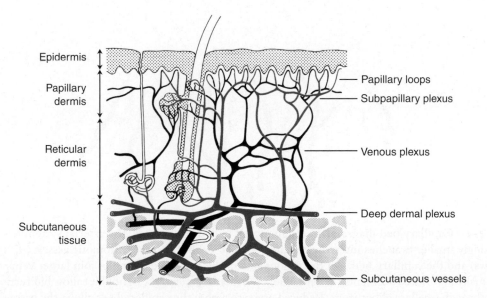

Fig. 2-3 The vascular plexuses of the integument. This figure shows the different vascular plexuses of the skin, according to Cormack and Lamberty. (From Cormack GC, Lamberty BG. The Arterial Anatomy of Skin Flaps. Edinburgh: Churchill Livingstone, 1986.)

blood flow and thermoregulation across the capillary bed (Fig. 2-4). Thermoregulation is achieved primarily by the relatively muscular arteriolar vessels of the dermal plexus, and nutrient exchange occurs through the thin-walled capillaries of the subepidermal plexus. Throughout the body there is a vast array of interconnected arcades of vessels connected through reduced-caliber choke anastomotic vessels, arteriovenous shunts, across capillaries, and through oscillating bidirectional venous segments (see Fig. 2-4). This system effectively distributes blood flow evenly and responds to physiologic mechanisms controlling blood flow.

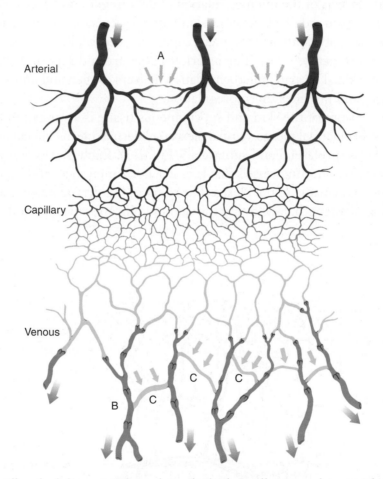

Fig. 2-4 Capillary bed diagram. Throughout the body in all tissues, the arterial system has increasingly smaller branches interconnected by reduced-caliber choke anastomotic vessels (*A*, small arrows) and the capillary bed. On the venous side of the capillaries, venules join larger veins and eventually join valved segments (*B*, dark blue). Avalvular segments (*C*, light blue) allow bidirectional flow through smaller caliber veins. Reduced pressure within the capillary beds allows the passage of nutrients and oxygen.

Numerous perforating arteries supply the plexus arrangement of vessels above the fascia. These perforators arise from the source arteries below the fascia and approach the skin by passing through muscle and then perforating the overlying fascia (musculocutaneous perforators), or by passing around the muscles through the intermuscular septa as septocutaneous perforators (Fig. 2-5). Many authors differentiate between direct cutaneous (axial) vessels and septocutaneous perforators. However, both types of perforator supply the skin, and the differentiation is probably semantic. Spalteholz,[14] Salmon,[26,27] and Taylor and colleagues[33,34] defined cutaneous vessels as either direct or indirect. Musculocutaneous perforators compose the largest group of indirect vessels. Overall, the distribution of these two types of vessels in the body is approximately 60% indirect musculocutaneous and 40% septocutaneous or direct cutaneous (axial). Salmon stated that vessels supply vascular branches to each structure they pass, which helps us to understand the vascular architecture of the soft tissues.

The relative contribution of each type of vessel depends on the anatomic region. In the torso, musculocutaneous perforators dominate, with many of these vessels penetrating the large, flat muscles of the chest and abdomen. In the head and neck, direct cutaneous vessels are more common. In the extremities, where numerous long thin muscles predominate, septocutaneous perforators are common, winding their way toward the skin by passing around the muscles and through the many intermuscular septa.

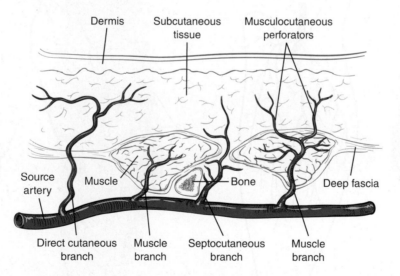

Fig. 2-5 Direct cutaneous, septocutaneous, and musculocutaneous perforators to the integument. Approximately 40% of the skin's perforators are direct cutaneous or septocutaneous, whereas approximately 60% are indirect musculocutaneous.

Musculocutaneous Flaps

Musculocutaneous flaps became widely used in the 1970s and 1980s because of their reliable vascularity and bulk, which facilitates wound closure.[35,36] The large vessels supplying muscles were identified to reliably perfuse the overlying skin portion of musculocutaneous flaps. The Mathes and Nahai classification of vascular anatomy of muscles differentiates muscles into five groups according to the pattern of vascular supply[37-39] (Fig. 2-6). Type I muscles are supplied by one main vascular pedicle (for example, tensor fascia lata and gastrocnemius muscles). Type II muscles have a dominant pedicle and minor pedicle (for example, gracilis, biceps femoris, trapezius, and soleus muscles). Type III muscles have two main vascular pedicles, each arising from a separate regional vessel (for example, gluteus maximus, rectus abdominis, and serratus anterior muscles). Type IV muscles have multiple segmental vascular pedicles (for example, sartorius, external oblique, and tibialis anterior muscles). Type V muscles derive their vascular supply from one main vascular pedicle and multiple secondary pedicles (for example, latissimus dorsi and pectoralis major muscles). We have identified the perforators emerging from each muscle; therefore it is possible to determine the likely source vessel for musculocutaneous perforators, depending on the muscle and region of muscle.[40]

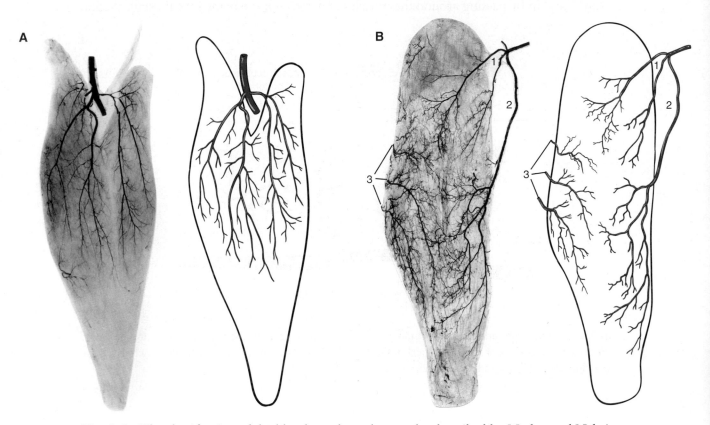

Fig. 2-6   The classification of the blood supply to the muscles described by Mathes and Nahai consists of five vascular patterns. **A**, Type I muscle. The medial and lateral gastrocnemius muscles are each supplied by a single vascular pedicle from the popliteal artery. **B**, Type II muscle. The vastus lateralis muscle is mainly supplied by the lateral circumflex femoral artery (*1*, Transverse branch and *2*, descending branch) and by perforating arteries from the profunda femoral artery as minor pedicles *(3)*.

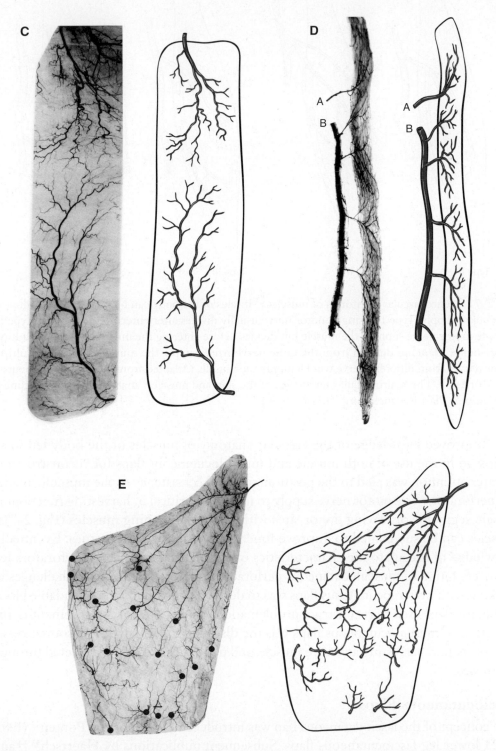

Fig. 2-6, cont'd C, Type III muscle. The rectus abdominis muscle receives its blood supply from two main sources: the superior and inferior epigastric arteries. **D,** Type IV muscle. The sartorius muscle has a segmental vascular supply from the lateral circumflex femoral artery *(A)* and the superficial femoral artery *(B)*. **E,** Type V muscle. The latissimus dorsi muscle has a dominant pedicle from the thoracodorsal artery, and several secondary segmental pedicles from the posterior intercostal arteries *(dots)*.

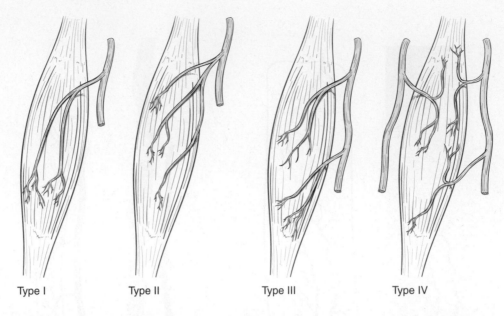

Type I   Type II   Type III   Type IV

Fig. 2-7   Neurovascular territories of muscles. Muscles of the body can be classified according to their nerve supply. Type I: A single motor nerve usually divides after entering the muscle; Type II: A single motor nerve supplies the muscle but divides before entering the muscle; Type III, Multiple motor nerve branches derived from the same nerve trunk supply the muscle; Type IV: Multiple motor nerves from different nerve trunks supply the muscle. (Adapted from Taylor GI, Gianoutsos MP, Morris SF. The neurovascular territories of the skin and muscles: anatomic study and clinical implications. Plast Reconstr Surg 94:1-36, 1994.)

Improved knowledge of the vascular anatomy of muscles of the body led to an explosion in the use of both muscle and musculocutaneous flaps for reconstruction. Greater attention was paid to the position, size, and consistency of the musculocutaneous perforators. The motor nerve supply to muscles is critical in harvesting functioning muscle segments or leaving donor sites with intact functioning muscles (Fig. 2-7).[41] Muscles can be subdivided to improve functional or aesthetic outcomes. Eventually, knowledge of the anatomic characteristics of the musculocutaneous perforators led to the evolution of musculocutaneous perforator flaps. One of the main challenges of working with musculocutaneous flaps was to derive a consistent and dependable blood supply for flaps used to reconstruct problematic wounds. A major advancement in the evolution of musculocutaneous flaps was the discovery that including a source vessel did not require harvesting an entire muscle, and perforators could be dissected through the muscle.

Fasciocutaneous Flaps

The concept of the fasciocutaneous flap was introduced in a report by Ponten[42] (1981) on 23 lower leg fasciocutaneous flaps. Subsequent publications by Haertsch[43,44] and Barclay et al[45] enhanced the understanding of the vascular basis of the fasciocutaneous flap. The major advantage of fasciocutaneous flaps over their predecessor, the random skin flap, is the inclusion of fascia, which contains a source vessel and its cutaneous branches. Cormack and Lamberty[20] described in detail fascial structures throughout the body. They classified fasciocutaneous flaps into four main types (Fig. 2-8). Type A flaps have multiple fasciocutaneous vessels entering at the base of the flap. These are oriented

GENERAL SCHEME OF VASCULARIZATION

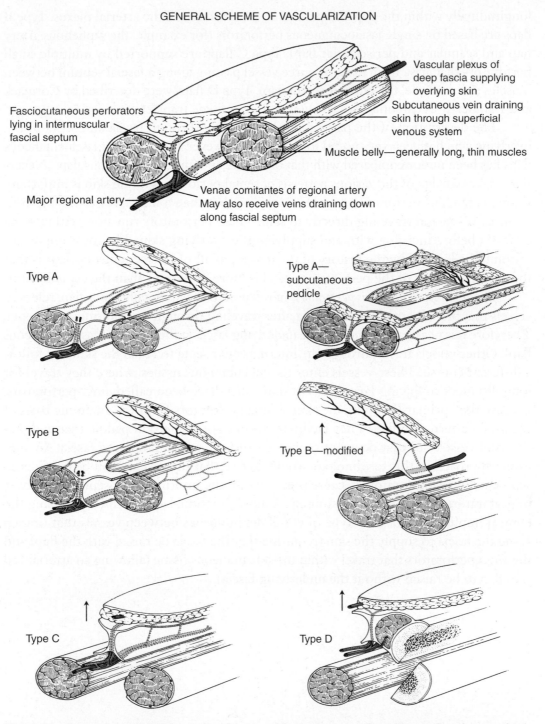

Fig. 2-8 Cormack and Lamberty's classification of fasciocutaneous flaps. Type A flaps have multiple fasciocutaneous vessels entering at the base of the flap, which are oriented longitudinally within the flap and parallel to the direction of the arterial plexus. Type B flaps are based on a single fasciocutaneous perforator. Type C flaps are supported by multiple small perforators, which arise from a main source vessel passing along a fascial septum between muscles. Type D flaps are osteomyofacial cutaneous free tissue transfers. (Modified from Cormack GC, Lamberty BG, eds. The Arterial Anatomy of Skin Flaps. Edinburgh: Churchill Livingstone, 1986.)

longitudinally within the flap and parallel to the direction of the arterial plexus. Type B flaps are based on single fasciocutaneous perforators (for example, the saphenous artery flap and scapular and periscapular flap). Type C flaps are supported by multiple small perforators that arise from a main source vessel passing along a fascial septum between muscles (for example, the radial forearm flap). Type D flaps were described by Cormack and Lamberty[1] as osteomyofascial cutaneous free tissue transfer.

The description of the pattern of blood supply through fascia and septa to the overlying skin has been very useful for surgeons; however, the impact of fasciocutaneous flaps has been minor compared with that of muscle and musculocutaneous flaps. Nevertheless, knowledge of the various patterns of septal perforators to the skin is important. Direct cutaneous perforators may be anything other than a direct vessel arising from a source vessel and traveling directly to skin. These perforators run along either septa or fascia before merging with and supplying the overlying skin. The most important lesson to be learned by the history of the development of fasciocutaneous flaps is that the actual anatomy of the perforating vessel is more important than the classification.

The term *septocutaneous perforators*, in relation to the fasciocutaneous flap, refers to vessels that branch out along the fascia after traveling through the intermuscular septa. Therefore it is necessary to include the underlying fascia in the skin flap (fasciocutaneous flap). Other vessels travel through the intermuscular septa to reach the skin and follow a different course. These vessels enter the subcutaneous tissues, where they travel for long distances supplying large areas of skin. They have been called *direct* perforators, because they primarily supply the skin. These perforators form the anatomic basis of the axial pattern skin flap. They facilitate the elevation of a skin paddle that includes the axial vessel, but that does not require inclusion of the underlying fascia. An anatomic approach to this terminology would dictate that these vessels all be considered septocutaneous perforators because they traverse the intermuscular septa, in contrast to perforators that pass through muscle. A more functional approach emphasizing the clinical implications of each type of vessel distinguishes between vessels that branch along the fascia to supply the skin (requiring that the fascia be raised with the flap) and the *direct* perforators that travel within the subcutaneous tissue (allowing an arterialized skin flap to be raised without the underlying fascia).

ANGIOSOME CONCEPT

The angiosome concept is largely the work of Ian Taylor of Melbourne, Australia, who for more than 30 years has comprehensively documented the vascular anatomy of the human body and has described the results in a long series of landmark papers and presentations. Among these accomplishments are the first reports of a free tissue transfer,[46] free fibular transfer,[47] free iliac crest transfer,[48] vascularized nerve grafts,[49] Doppler imaging in planning flaps,[50] and—probably most significant—the angiosome concept.[33,34,51,52]

As the result of multiple studies including cadaver dissection, ink injection, and contrast injection, Taylor and colleagues developed a comprehensive three-dimensional concept of the vascular anatomy of the body, particularly the skin. This work followed reports on the *angiotome* by Behan and Wilson,[53] who defined this as "the area of skin that can be cut as a flap which is supplied by an axial vessel but may be extended by its communication with branches of an adjacent vessel." Cormack and Lamberty[54] expanded the concept of angiotomes. They used the terms *anatomical*, *dynamic*, and *potential* to describe the various types of vascular territories that could be included in a skin flap based on a single vessel. Cormack and Lamberty[1] also described and documented the cutaneous anatomic basis of skin flaps. Taylor and Palmer[33] then combined the descriptions of vascular territories presented by Manchot[23,24] and Salmon,[25-27] the two-dimensional concept of angiotomes introduced by Behan and Wilson,[53] and the anatomic, dynamic, and potential territories described by Cormack and Lamberty[54] to conceive the three-dimensional *angiosome* concept, which was published in a landmark paper in 1987 (Fig. 2-9). Taylor and Palmer described the angiosome as a three-dimensional composite unit of tissue supplied by a given source artery. The composite building block of tissue contains muscle, nerve, connective tissue, bone, and overlying skin. Taylor divided the body into 40 angiosomes based on named source arteries, although some of these can be broken down into smaller territories. The concept of the angiosome is well accepted, but the subdivision of the angiosome is sometimes debated. The named source arteries are useful divisions of the vascular anatomy of the body, because they tend to be quite consistent from individual to individual in terms of course, size, and branches. However, individual cutaneous perforators are highly variable. For example, the deep inferior epigastric artery (DIEA) and superior epigastric artery (SEA) anastomose within the rectus abdominis muscle and give off highly variable perforators to the overlying skin[55,56] (Fig. 2-10).

TAYLOR AND PALMER'S ANGIOSOMES OF THE BODY

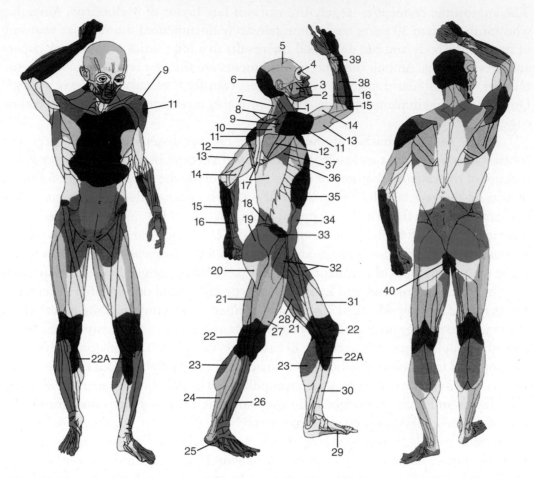

Fig. 2-9 Vascular territories of the integument of the skin are delineated according to the source vessel of the perforator. *1,* Thyroid; *2,* facial; *3,* buccal internal maxillary; *4,* ophthalmic; *5,* superficial temporal; *6,* occipital; *7,* deep cervical; *8,* transverse cervical; *9,* acromiothoracic; *10,* suprascapular; *11,* posterior circumflex humeral; *12,* circumflex scapular; *13,* profunda brachii; *14,* brachial; *15,* ulnar; *16,* radial; *17,* posterior intercostals; *18,* lumbar; *19,* superior gluteal; *20,* inferior gluteal; *21,* profunda femoris; *22,* popliteal; *22a,* descending geniculate saphenous; *23,* sural; *24,* peroneal; *25,* lateral plantar; *26,* anterior tibial; *27,* lateral femoral circumflex; *28,* adductor profunda; *29,* medial plantar; *30,* posterior tibial; *31,* superficial femoral; *32,* common femoral; *33,* deep circumflex iliac; *34,* deep inferior epigastric; *35,* internal thoracic; *36,* lateral thoracic; *37,* thoracodorsal; *38,* posterior interosseous; *39,* anterior interosseous; *40,* internal pudendal. (Reprinted from Br J Plast Surg, Volume 40, Taylor GI, Palmer JH. The vascular territories (angiosomes) of the body: experimental study and clinical applications pages 113-141, Copyright 1987, with permission from Elsevier.)

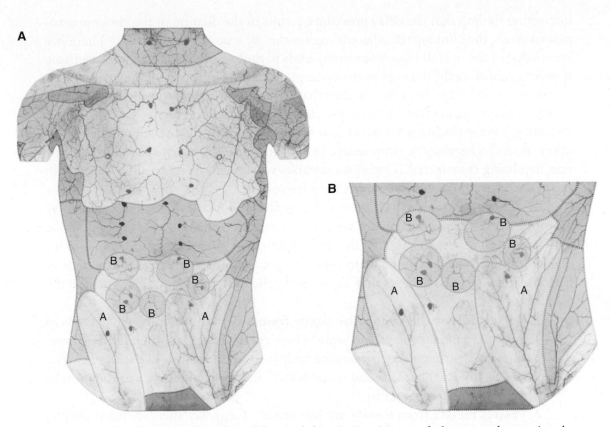

Fig. 2-10 Vascular territories of the abdominal skin. **A,** Arteriogram of a human cadaver using the lead oxide injection technique. The territory of the superficial inferior epigastric arteries is indicated by *A*. The territory of the individual perforators of the deep inferior epigastric arteries is indicated by the five circles labeled *B*. **B,** Close-up view. Note the asymmetry in the vascular supply to the abdominal skin.

The DIEA and SEA perforators are variable in size, course (musculocutaneous or septocutaneous), length, and number and are usually asymmetric within an individual and quite different from individual to individual. The vascular territory therefore is divisible depending on the level of branching of the main source artery considered. For reconstructive surgery, the reliable area of tissue harvested on a specific vessel depends on the vascular architecture of the region.

Angiosomes throughout the body are usually linked by reduced-caliber choke anastomotic vessels, but sometimes by true anastomoses without reduction in caliber. The angiosome concept and the idea that adjacent angiosomes are linked provide the basis for tissue transfers, particularly microsurgical tissue transfers.[53] The angiosome concept suggests that the watershed areas between vascular territories are important predictors of ultimate flap survival. Studies on the delay phenomenon have yielded the interesting finding that the delay procedure results in the dilation of the choke anastomotic vessels, thus linking the adjacent angiosomes by true anastomoses.[57-59] Therefore knowledge of the overall vascular anatomy leads to more defined planning of free tissue transfers. Additionally, the angiosome concept dispels the mystique of the various classifications of skin flaps, because it is clear that the main source vessel provides branches to most adjacent structures. For example, the goal of the reconstructive surgeon who is dissecting a musculocutaneous perforator flap is to carefully ligate the branches to the other tissues to harvest the main source vessel and provide adequate vascularity to the skin flap being transferred. The adjacent choke vessels will dilate to allow blood into the tissue where the source vessel has been harvested.

Taylor et al[34] also described a number of anatomic concepts based on his extensive anatomic work. These concepts are pertinent to perforator flaps, because they describe patterns of vascularity throughout the body. All anatomy varies from individual to individual, and knowledge of the main concepts is important to guide the dissection of perforator flaps. The concepts that Taylor and colleagues have described include the following:

1. **Vessels follow the connective tissue framework of the body**   The fascia of muscular compartments and septa, which connect the skin to underlying bony and fascial structures, separates the body into a honeycomb-like structure. The vessels follow the fascial and septal planes and supply branches to the muscle, nerve, bone, fascia, and fat.

2. **Vessels radiate from fixed to mobile areas**   Generally, there are many smaller vascular branches to the overlying skin in areas where the skin is fixed to underlying structures. Where the skin is mobile, long cutaneous vessels are seen.

3. **Vessels hitchhike with nerves**   There is often a chain-link system of vessels that accompanies cutaneous nerves. This combination of vessels and nerves has been used by surgeons for harvesting pedicle and free innervated neurocutaneous flaps.

4. **Vessels interconnect to form a three-dimensional network of vascular arcades**   Taylor and colleagues conceptualized the body as an array of vascular territories interconnected by choke anastomotic vessels. The outer limits of each vascular territory are defined by the position of these vessels relative to adjacent vascular territories. Taylor attributed this concept to Hunter, who described vascular arcades in the hands and feet in 1794. The angiosome concept provides a conceptual framework to consider when performing free tissue transfers such as the harvest of musculocutaneous perforator flaps.

VENOUS DRAINAGE

The venous drainage of the skin has received much less attention than it deserves, given that flap failure caused by venous compromise is probably more common than arterial problems. Venous drainage of the skin and subcutaneous tissue consists of two systems interconnected by veins without valves (oscillating or bidirectional) (Fig. 2-11).[60] The first system is the longitudinal subdermal plexus of veins. These are large vessels, such as the cephalic, basilic, saphenous, and superficial inferior epigastric veins, and they are involved with thermoregulation. They travel for long distances parallel to the skin surface and are interconnected, often by avalvular channels. These veins pierce the deep fascia near joints, including the elbow, shoulder, knee, and the groin. They are sometimes connected to deep veins by venae communicantes, which may or may not be accompanied by cutaneous arteries. Veins in this system often accompany the cutaneous nerves. The second system of veins is the longitudinal venae comitantes, which accompany the cutaneous arteries.

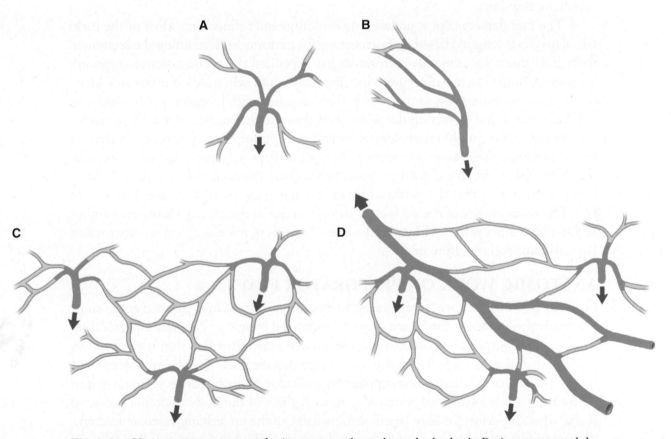

Fig. 2-11 Various arrangements of vein anatomy throughout the body. **A,** Basic venous module, which is repeated in various forms. **B,** Modified basic venous module. **C,** Network of veins that has been reorganized to form longitudinal channels. **D,** Large horizontal channel based within reticular framework. (From Taylor GI, Caddy CM, Watterson PA, et al. The venous territories (venosomes) of the human body: experimental study and clinical implications. Plast Reconstr Surg 86:185-213, 1990.)

MICROVASCULAR TISSUE TRANSFER

Perhaps the most significant advancement in reconstructive surgery has been the development and refinement of microvascular techniques in the late 1960s and early 1970s, allowing free flap reconstruction of the most challenging defects. Tissues based on vessels of suitable caliber can now be harvested from a donor site and reanastomosed to a recipient artery and vein to cover a distant defect. Advances in the necessary techniques for such transfers were pioneered by Buncke and colleagues,[61,62] whose work led to the first successful free tissue transfers by Taylor and Daniel[46] in 1973. The free flap has revolutionized modern reconstructive surgery, providing reliable options for defects in areas where there are no suitable local alternatives, either in terms of tissue quantity (for example, distal lower extremity defects) or tissue characteristics (for example, proximal esophageal defects). Presently it is common to transfer composite blocks of tissue for complex reconstructions (for example, the fibula osteocutaneous flap for mandible and floor of mouth reconstruction). These most recent advances in flap surgery have occurred because of continued interest in further delineating the anatomy of all vessels supplying the skin.

The free flap concept is undergoing evolution and refinement. Most of the early free flaps were designed based on fasciocutaneous perforators. Extending the technique to include musculocutaneous perforators has expanded the reconstructive surgeon's armamentarium. These flaps require incising the desired skin paddle for transfer, identifying the perforating vessels that supply the skin (often with Doppler or CTA imaging preoperatively), and dissecting the perforators down to the source artery. These perforators may pass through muscle (musculocutaneous perforators) or directly to skin via fascial or septal planes (septocutaneous). Perforator flaps have provided surgeons with the continued ability to tailor flaps to specific defects and minimize donor site morbidity, because the tissues that the perforators pass through (for example, muscle) remain in situ. The main impact of the perforator flap technique is the greatly increased number of flap donor site options. However, the overall results of microsurgical reconstruction have also undergone refinement.

ANATOMIC WORK ON PERFORATOR FLAPS

Over the past 30 years, we have injected a large series of fresh human cadavers to comprehensively document the location, size, origin, and course of cutaneous perforating arteries. The purpose has been to reassess known perforator flap donor sites and to study potential perforator flap donor sites. More specific goals have been to document the proportion of cutaneous skin supplied by musculocutaneous versus septocutaneous perforators. Additionally, we reviewed various regions of the body to define potential donor sites for perforator flaps based on knowledge of the underlying vascular anatomy. The anatomic techniques used for this study are described in Chapter 4. Basically, we used the lead oxide and gelatin arterial injection technique of Salmon and colleagues[25-27] as modified by Rees and Taylor,[63] and developed a new lead oxide injection technique.[57] This injection technique is the gold standard for vascular anatomic studies, because it allows simple dissection of the tissues using a bright orange color to mark the vessels and also provides excellent angiography. Using this technique, we have precisely identified the vascular territories of each perforator throughout the body. These results are shown in Chapters 10, 15, 21, and 35.

The surface area of a series of 10 fresh cadaver dissections was recorded. We defined the number of perforators 0.5 mm in diameter or larger supplying the skin. The areas in each region of the body and the area of skin supplied by each perforator were then calculated (Table 2-1). We have defined 61 vascular territories based on the dissection of these perforators. These territories are listed in Table 2-2 and illustrated in Fig. 2-12.

Table 2-1 summarizes the number of vascular territories in each region, the length and diameter of the perforators, and the ratio of musculocutaneous to septocutaneous perforators.

Table 2-1   Summary of Ten Cadaver Dissections Performed to Identify Cutaneous Perforators

Region	Number of Vascular Territories	Average Number of Perforators	Superficial Length (cm)	Diameter (mm)	MC/SC Ratio
Whole Body	61	442	3.3	0.7	3:2
Head and Neck	10	40	3.7	0.9	1:3
Scalp	4	14	4.9	1.1	1:4
Face	4	10	3.8	0.9	1:4
Neck	2	16	2.9	0.7	3:2
Upper Extremity	15	96	3.3	0.7	2:3
Shoulder and arm	7	44	3.8	0.8	2:3
Elbow and forearm	5	48	2.5	0.5	1:1
Wrist and hand	3	6*	4.4	1.3	1:4
Trunk	15	122	3.2	0.7	4:1
Chest	4	20	3.5	1.0	4:1
Abdomen	7	40	3.0	0.7	4:1
Upper back	5	48	3.1	0.8	4:1
Lumbar region	1	12	2.7	0.7	1:2
Lower Extremity	21	184	3.3	0.7	1:1
Gluteal region	3	42	2.4	0.6	9:1
Hip and thigh	5	68	3.5	0.7	3:2
Knee and leg	8	60	3.6	0.7	1:1
Ankle and foot	5	12*	2.9	0.8	1:4

*These values were calculated under the assumption that the integument of the hands and feet is supplied by only a few large direct cutaneous perforators from their respective arterial arches.
(*MC*, Musculocutaneous; *SC*, septocutaneous.)

Table 2-2 Vascular Territories

Artery	Artery Abbreviation	Artery	Artery Abbreviation
Anterior interosseous artery	AIOA	Occipital artery	OCA
Anterior tibial artery	ATA	Ophthalmic artery	OPA
Brachial artery	BA	Peroneal artery	PNA
Circumflex scapular artery	CSA	Popliteal artery	PA
Deep circumflex iliac artery	DCIA	Lateral sural artery	LSA
Deep inferior epigastric artery	DIEA	Medial sural artery	MSA
Deep palmar arch	DPAA	Posterior auricular artery	PAA
Descending genicular artery	DGA	Posterior circumflex humeral artery	PCHA
Dorsal branch of posterior intercostal artery	DPIA	Posterior interosseous artery	PIOA
Dorsal carpal arch	DCA	Posterior radial collateral artery	PRCA
Dorsal pedis artery	DPA	Posterior tibial artery	PTA
External pudendal artery	EPA	Profunda brachial artery	PBA
Facial artery	FA	Profunda femoris artery	PFA
Mental artery	MA	Radial artery	RA
Submental artery	SMA	Radial recurrent artery	RRA
Inferior gluteal artery	IGA	Superficial circumflex iliac artery	SCIA
Inferior ulnar collateral artery	IUCA	Superficial femoral artery	SFA
Infraorbital artery	IOA	Superficial inferior epigastric artery	SIEA
Internal pudendal arteries	IPA	Superficial palmar arch	SPA
Internal thoracic (mammary) artery	ITA	Superficial temporal artery	STA
Lateral branches of posterior intercostal arteries	LPIA	Superior epigastric artery	SEA
Lateral calcaneal artery	LCA	Superior gluteal artery	SGA
Lateral circumflex femoral artery	LCFA	Superior thyroid artery	STHA
Lateral inferior genicular artery	LIGA	Superior ulnar collateral artery	SUCA
Lateral plantar artery	LPA	Thoracoacromial artery	TAA
Lateral sacral arteries	LSA	Thoracodorsal artery	TDA
Lateral superior genicular artery	LSGA	Thyrocervical trunk	TCT
Lateral thoracic (mammary) artery	LTA	Dorsal scapular artery	DSA
Lumbar arteries	LA	Suprascapular artery	SSA
Medial calcaneal artery	MCA	Transverse cervical artery	TCA
Medial circumflex femoral artery	MCFA	Transverse facial artery	TFA
Medial inferior genicular artery	MIGA	Ulnar artery	UA
Medial superior genicular artery	MSGA		

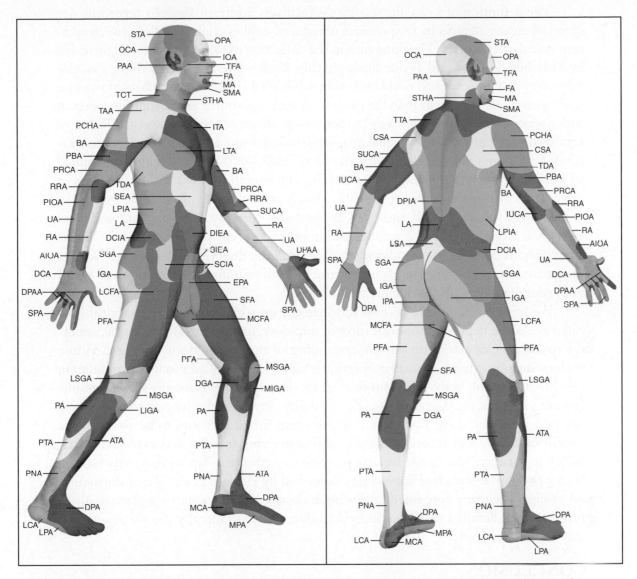

Fig. 2-12 Vascular territories of the body corresponding to source arteries that provide musculo-cutaneous or septocutaneous perforators to the skin. Vascular territories and their abbreviations are listed in Table 2-2.

The definition of a vascular territory is relatively arbitrary. Vascular territories are detected on angiograms by the presence of reduced-caliber choke vessels between adjacent vascular territories. The difference in the definition of vascular territories provided by Manchot, Salmon, and Taylor alludes to this. Taylor stated that many of the vascular territories that he described could be further subdivided. The actual numbers of vascular territories is less important than the concept that a main source artery supplies a region with a series of perforators that may be musculocutaneous or septocutaneous. The law of equilibrium suggests that the actual proportion of musculocutaneous versus septocutaneous perforators in a specific region may be variable, but the overall region is supplied by the perforator's consistent source vessels. The overall number and dimensions of perforators in a specific area are probably closely related to the physiologic "needs" of the tissues of the region and, therefore, are probably constant. However, in some cases vessel X is larger and vessel Y smaller, and in other cases the opposite is noted. This is an important concept to consider when dissecting the donor site of a perforator flap; the perforator in question may actually arise in a rather unusual orientation as a result of the degree of vascular variability in the body.

We must continuously reassess the anatomy on which we base our surgical procedures. As the degree of sophistication of microsurgery evolves (for example, supermicrosurgery), demands on our understanding of surgical anatomy increase. While performing our extensive vascular injection studies, we identified vascular variability in every region of the body. In the surgical arena, this variability is usually surmountable; however, at times, the degree of vascular variability may affect the surgery contemplated, planned, or undertaken. Therefore it is important for all surgeons to be aware of the overall vascular architecture of the skin and underlying muscles and to plan for variability in surgery. This is particularly relevant to perforator flap surgery, which often becomes the free-style free flap surgery described by Wallace et al.[64] The information on vascular anatomy contained in this book should serve as a starting place to allow further, more detailed studies of individual donor sites to identify the variations that may be encountered.

CONCLUSION

Over the past century, anatomists, surgeons, and surgeon-anatomists have made tremendous advances in defining the vascular anatomy of the skin. This progress has been directly linked to improved surgical results of tissue transfers, from axial patterned pedicle flaps to musculocutaneous flaps, fasciocutaneous flaps, free tissue transfers, and finally musculocutaneous or septocutaneous perforator flaps. The latter group is the subject of this book; however, any discussion of perforator flaps must take place in the context of the historical background and the actual anatomy available.

The anatomy described in this book helps surgeons design appropriate tissue transfers to address particular reconstructive challenges in a unique fashion. This work has not arisen overnight, nor will future challenges be solved in the next few months. The process of assessing, redefining, and expanding our knowledge of the vascular basis of tissue transfers is gradual. The tissue transfers described and discussed in this book need to be carefully assessed from both clinical and anatomic viewpoints to truly determine their role in reconstructive surgery. This continual reappraisal will strengthen this surgical field and assist in providing optimal care for our patients.

References

1. Cormack GC, Lamberty BG, eds. The Arterial Anatomy of Skin Flaps. Edinburgh: Churchill Livingstone, 1986.
   This comprehensive text presented the history of the study of the cutaneous vasculature, and described in detail its anatomy. The blood supply to the skin was presented for each region of the body, and the roles of the vascular territories in flap design were discussed.
2. Milton SH. The tubed pedicle flap. Br J Plast Surg 22:53-59, 1969.
3. Milton SH. The effects of "delay" on the survival of experimental pedicled skin flaps. Br J Plast Surg 22:244-252, 1965.
4. Milton SH. Pedicled skin flaps: the fallacy of the length:width ratio. Br J Plast Surg 57:502-508, 1970.
5. Pang CY, Forrest CR, Neligan PC, et al. Augmentation of blood flow in delayed random skin flaps in the pig: effect of length of delay period and angiogenesis. Plast Reconstr Surg 78:68-74, 1986.
6. Pang CY, Neligan PC, Nakatsuka T, et al. Pharmacologic manipulation of the microcirculation in cutaneous and myocutaneous flaps in pigs. Clin Plast Surg 12:173-184, 1985.
7. Pang CY, Morris SF, Forrest CR. Pharmacologic augmentation of skin viability in pedicled skin flaps: a working hypothesis to mimic the surgical delay phenomenon. Ann Plast Surg 22:293-304, 1989.
8. Sasaki GH, Pang CY. Hemodynamics and viability of acute neurovascular island skin flaps in rats. Plast Reconst Surg 65:152-158, 1980.
9. Kerrigan CL, Daniel RK. Pharmacologic treatment of the failing skin flap. Plast Reconstr Surg 70:541-548, 1982.
10. Kerrigan CL. Skin flap failure: pathophysiology. Plast Reconst Surg 72:766-777, 1983.
11. Kerrigan CL, Daniel RK. Critical ischemia time and the failing skin flap. Plast Reconstr Surg 69:986-989, 1982.
12. Harvey W, ed. An Anatomical Disputation Concerning the Movement of the Heart and Blood in Living Creatures. Oxford: Blackwell Scientific, 1976.
13. Tomsa W. Beitrage zur Anatomie und Physiologie der menschlichen Haut. Arch Dermatol Syphilis 5:1, 1873.
14. Spalteholz W. Die Vertheilung der Blutgefasse in der Haut. Arch Anat Entwcklngs-Gesch (Leipz) 1:54, 1893.
15. Nakajima H, Fujino T, Adachi S. A new concept of vascular supply to the skin and classification of skin flaps according to their vascularization. Ann Plast Surg 16:1-19, 1986.

16. Nakajima H, Minabe T, Imanishi N. Three-dimensional analysis and classification of arteries in the skin and subcutaneous adipofascial tissue by computer graphics imaging. Plast Reconstr Surg 102:748-760, 1998.

17. Hallock G, ed. Principles of Fascia and Fasciocutaneous Flaps. Philadelphia: Hanley & Belfus, 1999.

18. Cormack GC, Lamberty BG, eds. The fascio-cutaneous system of vessels. In The Arterial Anatomy of Skin Flaps, 2nd ed. Edinburgh: Churchill Livingstone, 1994.

19. Tolhurst DE. A comprehensive classification of flaps: the atomic system. Plast Reconstr Surg 80:608-609, 1987.

20. Cormack GC, Lamberty BG. A classification of fascio-cutaneous flaps according to their patterns of vascularisation. Br J Plast Surg 37:80-87, 1984.

21. Kim JT. New nomenclature concept of perforator flap. Br J Plast Surg 58:431-440, 2005.

22. Pignatti M, Ogawa R, Hallock GG, et al. The "Tokyo" consensus on propeller flaps. Plast Reconstr Surg 127:716-722, 2011.

23. Manchot C, ed. Die Hautarterien des menschlichen Korpers. Leipzig: FCW Vogel, 1889.

24. Manchot C, ed. The Cutaneous Arteries of the Human Body. New York: Springer-Verlag, 1982.

25. Salmon M, ed. Artères de la Peau. Paris: Masson et Cie, 1936.

26. Salmon M, ed. Artères des Muscles des Membres et du Tronc. Paris: Masson et Cie, 1936.

27. Salmon M, Taylor GI, Tempest MN, eds. Arteries of the Skin. London: Churchill Livingstone, 1988.

    This English translation of Salmon's original treatise, Artères de la Peau, contains a description of the author's injection techniques and the cutaneous arteries by region, and a discussion of the anatomic concepts related to the skin's vasculature. Multiple radiographs and drawings are included.

28. Rhodin J. The ultrastructure of mammalian arterioles and precapillary sphincters. J Ultrastr Res 18:181-223, 1967.

29. Rhodin J. Ultrastructure of mammalian venous capillaries, venules and small collecting veins. J Ultrastr Res 15:452-500, 1968.

30. Hibbs RG, Burch GE, Philips JH. The fine structure of the small blood vessels of normal human dermis and subcutis. Am Heart J 56:662-670, 1958.

31. Braverman IM, Keh-Yen A. Ultrastructure of the human dermal microcirculation. III. The vessels in the mid- and lower dermis and subcutaneous fat. J Invest Dermatol 77:297-304, 1981.

32. Braverman IM, Yen A. Ultrastructure of the human dermal microcirculation. II. The capillary loops of the dermal papillae. J Invest Dermatol 68:44-52, 1977.

33. Taylor GI, Palmer JH. The vascular territories (angiosomes) of the body: experimental study and clinical applications. Br J Plast Surg 40:113-141, 1987.

    Taylor summarized his work on the vascular anatomy of the skin, discussing his methodology, including anatomic dissection, ink injection, radiographic studies, and perforator mapping. Results were presented, culminating in several anatomic concepts and a description of the angiosome theory.

34. Taylor GI, Ives A, Dhar S. Vascular territories. In Mathes SJ, ed. Plastic Surgery, 2nd ed. Philadelphia: Saunders Elsevier, 2006.

35. McCraw JB. The recent history of myocutaneous flaps. Clin Plast Surg 7:3-7, 1980.

36. McCraw JB, Arnold PG, eds. McCraw and Arnold's Atlas of Muscle and Musculocutaneous Flaps. Norfolk, VA: Hampton Press, 1986.

37. Mathes SJ, Nahai F. Classification of the vascular anatomy of muscles: experimental and clinical correlation. Plast Reconstr Surg 67:1177-1187, 1981.

38. Mathes SJ, Nahai F, eds. Clinical Atlas of Muscle and Musculocutaneous Flaps. St Louis: Mosby, 1979.

39. Mathes SJ, Nahai F, eds. Clinical Applications for Muscle and Musculocutaneous Flaps. St Louis: Mosby, 1982.

    The authors introduced their classification of the vascular supply to the muscles of the body and illustrate the anatomic basis for numerous muscle and musculocutaneous flaps. Surgical applications and techniques were discussed.

40. Morris SF, Tang M, Almutairi K, et al. The anatomic basis of perforator flaps. Clin Plast Surg 37:553-570, 2010.

41. Taylor GI, Gianoutsos MP, Morris SF. The neurovascular territories of the skin and muscles: anatomic study and clinical implications. Plast Reconstr Surg 94:1-36, 1994.

42. Ponten B. The fasciocutaneous flap: its use in soft tissue defects of the lower leg. Br J Plast Surg 34:215-220, 1981.

43. Haertsch PA. The surgical plane in the leg. Br J Plast Surg 34:464-469, 1981.

44. Haertsch PA. The blood supply to the skin of the leg: a post-mortem investigation. Br J Plast Surg 34:470-477, 1981.

45. Barclay TL, Cardoso E, Sharpe DT, et al. Repair of lower leg injuries with fasciocutaneous flaps. Br J Plast Surg 35:127-132, 1982.

46. Taylor GI, Daniel RK. The free flap: composite tissue transfer by vascular anastomoses. Aust N Z J Surg 43:1-3, 1973.

47. Taylor GI, Miller G, Ham FJ. The free vascularized bone graft. Plast Reconstr Surg 55:533-544, 1975.

48. Taylor GI, Watson N. One stage repair of compound leg defects with revascularized flaps of groin skin and iliac bone. Plast Reconstr Surg 61:494-506, 1978.

49. Taylor GI, Ham FJ. The free vascularized nerve graft. Plast Reconstr Surg 57:413-426, 1976.

50. Taylor GI, Doyle M, McCarten F. The Doppler probe for planning flaps: anatomical study and clinical applications. Br J Plast Surg 43:1-16, 1990.

51. Taylor GI, Palmer JH, McManamay D. The vascular territories of the body (angiosomes) and their clinical applications. In McCarthy J, ed. Plastic Surgery. Philadelphia: WB Saunders, 1990.

52. Taylor GI. The angiosomes of the body and their supply to perforator flaps. Clin Plast Surg 30:331-342, 2003.

    The angiosome concept was reviewed, with particular emphasis on those angiosomes that have relevance to perforator flap design and clinical application.

53. Behan FC, Wilson JS. The principle of the angiotome—a system of linked axial pattern flaps. In Marchac D, Hueston JT, eds. Transactions of the Sixth International Congress of Plastic and Reconstructive Surgery. Paris: Masson, 1975.

54. Cormack GC, Lamberty BG. Cadaver studies of correlation between vessel size and anatomical territory of cutaneous supply. Br J Plast Surg 39:300-306, 1986.

55. Boyd JB, Taylor GI, Corlett R. The vascular territories of the superior epigastric and the deep inferior epigastric systems. Plast Reconstr Surg 73:1-16, 1984.

56. Moon HK, Taylor GI. The vascular anatomy of rectus abdominis musculocutaneous flaps based on the deep superior epigastric system. Plast Reconstr Surg 82:815-829, 1988.

57. Tang M, Geddes CR, Yang D, Morris SF. Modified lead oxide-gelatin injection technique for vascular studies. J Clin Anat 1:73-78, 2002.

58. Wallace CG, Kao HK, Jeng SF, et al. Free style free flaps: a further step forward for perforator flap surgery. Plast Reconstr Surg 124(6 Suppl):e419-e426, 2009.

59. Timmons MJ. Landmarks in the anatomical study of the blood supply of the skin. Br J Plast Surg 38:197-207, 1985.

60. Taylor GI, Caddy CM, Watterson PA, et al. The venous territories (venosomes) of the human body: experimental study and clinical implications. Plast Reconstr Surg 86:185-213, 1990.

61. Buncke HJ, Schulz WP. Total ear reimplantation in the rabbit utilising microminiature vascular anastomoses. Br J Plast Surg 19:15-22, 1966.

62. Buncke HJ Jr, Buncke CM, Schulz WP. Immediate Nicoladoni procedure in the Rhesus monkey, or hallux to hand transplantation, utilising microminiature vascular anastomoses. Br J Plast Surg 19:322-337, 1966.

63. Rees MJW, Taylor GI. A simplified lead oxide cadaver injection technique. Plast Reconstr Surg 77:141-145, 1986.

64. Wallace CG, Kao HK, Jeng SF, Wei FC. Free-style flaps: a further step forward for perforator flap surgery. Plast Reconstr Surg 124(6 Suppl):e419-e426, 2009.

3

Perforator Flaps: Overview, Classification, and Nomenclature

Peter C. Neligan
Phillip N. Blondeel
Steven F. Morris
Geoffrey G. Hallock

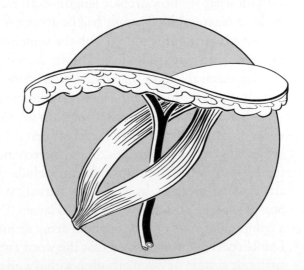

THE EVOLUTION OF CUTANEOUS FLAPS

A century ago the design of all skin flaps was essentially random. The skin was raised with no regard to a known blood supply, other than to maintain the subdermal plexus.[1,2] These flaps were distinguished from one another only in their construction, which typically related to how they were transposed (for example, an advancement or rotation flap), their shape (for example, a tubed flap), and their destination[3] (for example, a local or distant flap). Because of their limited blood supply, these flaps were restricted to rigid length:width ratios to ensure viability. A renaissance predicated on a new awareness of the anatomic basis of circulation to the skin was initiated by McGregor and Morgan[4] when they discovered that some regions of the body had discrete and relatively large subcutaneous vessels that pierced the deep fascia and then followed a predictable course. This discovery allowed the creation of comparatively huge cutaneous flaps that were safe, as long as they were oriented along the axis of that vascular pathway. These flaps were appropriately called *axial flaps*. Soon thereafter, Ger,[5] Orticochea,[6] and others reintroduced the concept of using muscle not only as a soft tissue flap, but also as a carrier of the overlying skin to create even larger musculocutaneous flaps.

As the cutaneous flap evolved over the latter part of the twentieth century, its intrinsic blood supply deservedly became recognized as the most important determinant for ensuring flap viability.[7-9] Milton[10] had correctly asserted that the vitality of any skin flap depended entirely on its means of vascularization, and had nothing whatsoever to do with what are now archaic length:width ratios. Nevertheless, another major source of the cutaneous blood supply had been completely overlooked. Ponten[11] deserves credit for reintroducing this source with the principle of *fasciocutaneous flaps*, although he was not quite sure why the inclusion of the deep fascia with his superflaps resulted in a longer flap survival length than could be predicted for random flaps of comparable width.

It is interesting in hindsight that the medical student, Manchot,[12] more than 100 years before Ponten's work was performed, was well aware that "larger cutaneous arteries . . . appear from the fissure between . . . muscles. Directly above the fascia, they divide into terminal branches . . . and interconnect." This understanding sublimely states the basis for a fascial plexus that can include the subfascial, intrafascial, and suprafascial vascular plexuses, as well as the dermal, subdermal, superficial adipofascial (above Scarpa's fascia) and deep apidofascial layers. Each plexus, or layer, in some way forms a component part of this splendid array of interconnected vessels.[13-15] Cormack and Lamberty[8] have emphasized that the word *fasciocutaneous* implies the retention of this anatomic system of vascularization within a given flap, and does not refer to any specific tissue constituents. Thus, even if the skin and/or deep fascia are excluded from a flap

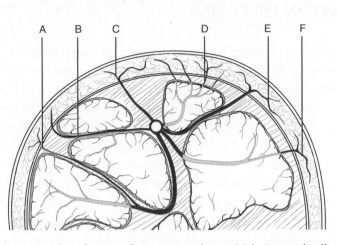

Fig. 3-1 The six distinctive deep fascia perforators according to Nakajima and colleagues are indicated. (*A*, Direct cutaneous branch of a muscular vessel; *B*, septocutaneous perforator; *C*, direct cutaneous; *D*, musculocutaneous perforator; *E*, direct septocutaneous; *F*, perforating cutaneous branch of a muscular vessel.) A separate type of fasciocutaneous flap could be named after each different perforator. (Modified from Nakajima H, Fujino T, Adachi S. A new concept of vascular supply to the skin and classification of skin flaps according to their vascularization. Ann Plast Surg 16:1-19, 1986.)

that is dependent on this fascial plexus, such a flap would still be a fasciocutaneous flap. A true fasciocutaneous flap has a defined blood supply through its fascial plexus and can be composed of any or all of the tissue layers found between the skin and deep fascia.[16]

Nakajima et al[13] methodically identified six distinctly different kinds of deep fascial perforators that, in turn, could supply this fascial plexus, and all could arise from a common source vessel (Fig. 3-1). Their direct cutaneous fascial perforators corresponded to the axial vessels of McGregor and Morgan[4] so that axial flaps could be considered just another variant of a fasciocutaneous flap. Direct septocutaneous branches followed intercompartmental septa, and more diminutive septocutaneous perforators traversed an intermuscular or intertendinous septum. Each vessel was capable, in turn, of nourishing septocutaneous flaps, although Cormack and Lamberty[17] thought that only the direct septocutaneous branches served true fasciocutaneous flaps.

The real innovative discovery by Nakajima et al[13] was of two completely new types of deep fascial perforators: (1) the direct cutaneous branch of a muscular vessel and (2) the perforating cutaneous branch of a muscular vessel. They also hypothesized that fasciocutaneous flaps could eventually be based on either branch. Using computer graphics imaging, Nakajima et al[15] later developed a three-dimensional view of the fascial plexus that demonstrated the axiality, vessel size, and suprafascial course of these vessels. They proved that the function of these two muscular vessels was to provide nutrition to the skin, and only secondarily to the involved muscle. The direct cutaneous branch of the muscular vessel is somewhat of an enigma because of its quite variable presence, although it is becoming more prevalent than anticipated.[18] However, the perforating cutaneous branch of the muscular vessel has become the backbone of the genre of muscle perforator flaps, the primary subject of this edition.

CLASSIFICATION OF FLAPS
Skin Flaps

A complete description of a skin flap must include all characteristics, as in the atomic classification system of Tolhurst.[19,20] This system incorporates the six Cs of flap design described by Cormack and Lamberty.[17] In addition to the pattern of **C**irculation, which is of paramount importance, the flap **C**onstituents (tissue composition), **C**onstruction (type of pedicle, including method of transposition), **C**onformation (geometric configuration), **C**ontiguity (location of the flap in relationship to the defect), and **C**onditioning (for example, delay maneuvers) must all be considered. For millennia, the random skin flap was the only alternative. Because all flaps then relied on the subdermal plexus for circulation, stratification of these cutaneous flaps was routinely determined by their secondary characteristics, as described above and in the introduction to this chapter.[3]

Fasciocutaneous Flaps

As the actual source of circulation feeding the subdermal plexus became better appreciated, Cormack and Lamberty[21,22] described a tripartite system of skin flaps. This consisted of the direct cutaneous (axial), musculocutaneous, and fasciocutaneous flaps and included all known skin flaps.

Cormack and Lamberty further classified fasciocutaneous flaps into three major subdivisions, according to the origin of the circulation to the fascial plexus.[22,23] Their type A flap had multiple fascial feeders, but none had to be specifically identified, and were quite reminiscent of random skin flaps. Type B flaps typically had a large, solitary perforator similar to a septocutaneous branch arising from a major source vessel. Type C flaps relied on multiple, and usually small, segmental septocutaneous branches. Elevation of type C flaps almost always necessitated inclusion of the source vessel with the flap to maintain their complete integrity.

Nakajima et al[13] contracted the overall number of cutaneous flaps, but expanded the types of fasciocutaneous flaps and described them as being based on six distinctly different perforators of the deep fascia that fed the fascial plexus of each (see Fig. 3-1). Their type I direct cutaneous flaps were identical to the axial flaps of McGregor and Morgan.[4] Their Type II direct septocutaneous flaps were the same as type B fasciocutaneous flaps, and type V septocutaneous perforator flaps were the same as type C fasciocutaneous flaps, as per the schema of Cormack and Lamberty.[21,22] Type VI musculocutaneous perforator flaps resembled traditional musculocutaneous flaps, or perhaps the capillary perforator flaps of Koshima et al.[24] The remaining two types of flaps described by Nakajima et al,[13] based on direct (type III) or perforating cutaneous branches of a muscular vessel, were excitingly different. Recognition of the latter as the type IV perforating cutaneous branch of the muscular vessel fasciocutaneous flap gave birth to a concept better known today as the *true muscle perforator flap*.[25]

Perforator Flaps

It is not by coincidence that the fasciocutaneous flap classification schemas of Cormack and Lamberty,[21,22] Nakajima et al,[13] and later, Mathes and Nahai[26] are so similar. The basis for each system is predicated on distinct differences of circulation patterns to each flap subtype. This is a pragmatic approach for the operating surgeon, because the vascular supply, if nothing else, must be correctly identified to ensure flap viability. However, even further consolidation of flap types, yet greater universality, is possible. Taylor and Palmer[27] and Taylor et al[28] credited Spalteholz with postulating as early as 1893 that all arteries to the skin could be considered as either direct or indirect branches from an underlying source vessel. Taylor and colleagues[27-29] passionately argued that the direct vessels are the primary cutaneous supply, and it is irrelevant if they first pierce intermuscular or intramuscular septa, because their main destination is always the skin. Indirect vessels are those that emerge above the deep fascia as terminal branches and have supplied deeper tissues along their course. These vessels are only a secondary means of cutaneous blood supply.[7]

If this argument is slightly modified, all the deep fascial perforators could be construed to be direct if they essentially course from the source vessel to the fascia without first passing through some other tissue intermediary; otherwise they would be indirect perforators[30,31] (Fig. 3-2). The corresponding cutaneous flaps would be direct or indirect perforator flaps. This schema, it could be argued, does the most to simplify the jargon and still encompass all presently known skin flaps.

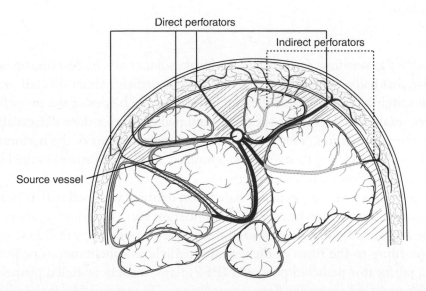

Fig. 3-2 The distinct deep fascia perforators of Nakajima and colleagues (see Fig. 3-1) can be considered more simply to be either *direct* or *indirect* perforators. All these perforators arise from the same source vessel, but only indirect perforators *(dotted lines)* first course through some other tissue intermediary (here depicted as muscle), before piercing the deep fascia. (Modified from Nakajima H, Fujino T, Adachi S. A new concept of vascular supply to the skin and classification of skin flaps according to their vascularization. Ann Plast Surg 16:1-19, 1986.)

By definition, the perforator to a muscle perforator flap must first traverse the substance of that muscle.[25] According to the preceding classification system, these flaps would all be known as indirect perforator flaps. Neurocutaneous flaps are becoming more commonly used, and are an excellent example of an indirect, nonmuscle perforator flap. Neurocutaneous flaps rely on an intrinsic and extrinsic neurocutaneous or venocutaneous vascular supply that primarily accompanies the peripheral cutaneous nerve.[31-35] Often the extrinsic vascular supply can be a true artery. Depending on the nerve, both structures can simultaneously pierce the deep fascia before proceeding within the subcutaneous tissues.[31-35] Again, the major purpose of this accompanying vascular system is to provide circulation to the nerve, and only secondarily (or indirectly) are cutaneous branches given off that will support an overlying cutaneous flap. Niranjan et al[23] have pointed out that fascial feeders and/or perforators similar to those accompanying cutaneous nerves, can also arise independently from fascioperiosteal or tenosynovial branches, which, in turn, can also supply indirect nonmuscle perforator flaps (see Chapter 73). Thus, indirect perforator flaps, more than any other cutaneous flap, deserve to be separately distinguished to ensure that the appropriate, tedious dissection through whatever is the intermediary tissue will protect the requisite vascular supply.

Another nomenclature system for describing muscle perforator flaps that adheres to the Gent consensus[36] and Canadian proposal[37] will be the focal point in the section at the end of this chapter. However, many other classification systems exist that are intended to be more complete in details that might facilitate the anatomic and surgical approach and descriptions of these flaps.[38-41] In addition, it is important to be familiar with some other commonly encountered terms used in conjunction with perforator flaps as follows here.

Propeller Flaps

The term *propeller flap* was first used in 1991 by Hyakusoku et al[42] to describe an adipocutaneous flap that had a random central subcutaneous pedicle. About this hub were two skin paddles slightly longer than wide, reminiscent of the blades of the propeller. The blades were rotated 90 degrees about the central pedicle to resurface defects after release of burn scar contractures. This idea became an important part of the perforator flap concept when Hallock[43] used a solitary skeletonized perforator instead as the hub, which now allowed rotation up to 180 degrees.

The "Tokyo" consensus on propeller flaps[44] has defined a propeller flap as any island flap, often with a propeller-like shape, that undergoes an axial rotation about its vascular pedicle as a locoregional flap to reach the proposed recipient site. These may be classified according to the form of the vascular pedicle as subcutaneous pedicled propeller flaps, perforator pedicled propeller (PPP) flaps, muscle pedicled propeller flaps, or vascular pedicled propeller flaps, according to Ogawa and Hyakusoku (see Chapter 75), the latter two being somewhat hybrid forms of perforator-based flaps. If one blade of the propeller is exceedingly long, a retained perforator at the end furthest from the hub can help augment either inflow or outflow via a microanastomosis to a recipient vessel near the defect to create a supercharged propeller flap.[44] The PPP has proved to be the most versatile variant (see Chapters 54 and 71) and is named after the source artery of the chosen perforator, or, if unknown, as in an ad hoc[45] or free-style local flap,[39] according to the muscle perforated or donor site location.[44]

Perforator-Plus Flaps

An island perforator flap remains attached to the donor site only by its perforator vascular supply. If a cutaneous attachment is retained, that locoregional flap will now have a dual source of circulation, because that of the perforator will be augmented by the neurovenocutaneous circulation through the second pedicle.[46] This base will also improve venous or lymphatic outflow.[47,48] As a hybrid fasciocutaneous flap originally introduced by Mehrotra,[49,50] this commonly has a peninsular shape, and is called a *perforator-plus flap*. These can be used as rotation, transposition, or advancement flaps where the perforator itself is dissected back to its source vessel only as necessary to permit tension-free insetting of the flap into an adjacent defect.[50] The terms *perforator-sparing*[46,51] and *perforator-assisted*[52] flap are similar in that, if during dissection of a planned fasciocutaneous flap a perforator is encountered, it is kept with the flap to obtain the same aforementioned advantages.

Septocutaneous or Direct Cutaneous Muscle Perforator Flaps

The expanding use of preoperative CTA or MRA imaging for identifying perforators has expedited and improved the reliability of perforator flaps. Particularly in breast reconstruction, a spin-off has been the identification of perforators that course around or between muscles in a direct septocutaneous course. These have been called *septocutaneous perforators*, and the flaps *septocutaneous perforator flaps*.[53-58] Typically, these are larger vessels, and, because no intramuscular dissection is required, flap elevation is easier and quicker with less donor site morbidity, including no muscle denervation because motor nerves are not at jeopardy.[54] In these imaging studies, septocutaneous perforators were present in 22% of potential deep inferior epigastric artery perforator flap candidates, 38% of either superior gluteal artery perforator or inferior gluteal artery perforator flaps, and 16% of planned transverse upper gracilis thigh flaps.[54]

However, anatomists define *intermuscular septa* as "laminae of deep fasciae which extend between and enclose muscle groups, frequently being continuous with the periosteum of the bones," which serves to separate muscle compartments.[59] These so-called septocutaneous perforators are found in the loose areolar layer between muscles,[53-56] or circumnavigate the rectus abdominis muscle.[57,58] The sheath of the rectus abdominis muscle is formed by the fusion and separation of the aponeuroses of the internal and external abdominal oblique muscles and the transversus abdominis muscle. An aponeurosis is a sheetlike tendon and not at all a septum.[61] Rather than being septocutaneous (these perforators do not really pass through a true septum), they instead are probably direct cutaneous branches of a muscular vessel, using the terminology of Nakajima et al[13] (see Fig. 3-1). These direct cutaneous branches arise from the source vessel to the given muscle, usually at its hilum, long before any muscular branches enter the muscle, and pass directly to the subdermal plexus while giving off few if any branches. True septocutaneous branches often give off multiple muscular branches to muscles on either side as they make this same journey. This distinction is often also seen in the anterolateral thigh flap, where a proximal so-called septocutaneous perforator arises deep near the takeoff of the descending branch from the lateral circumflex femoral artery proper, then passes directly to the deep fascia, perhaps passing through no or only a few wisps of vastus lateralis muscle, which is quite different from the course for more distal anterolateral thigh septocutaneous perforators.[18] These facts imply that the direct cutaneous branches of muscle vessels described by Nakajima et al[13] are much more common than expected, and certainly underreported until now. Rather than *septocutaneous perforator flaps*, this subtype of perforator flap should perhaps be better called *direct cutaneous muscle* or *paramuscular perforator flaps*.[18,62]

Combined Perforator Flaps

A compound flap has multiple, often diverse tissue components that, joined together and transferred simultaneously, allow a more efficient reconstruction. If the compound flap has multiple intrinsic sources of vascularization, usually discrete to each component, this would be a *combined flap*.[63] A combined flap can be further classified as a *chimeric* or *conjoined flap*.[64] These differ according to the physical relationship of their tissue components, yet are similar in that each part retains an independent blood supply. This pattern of circulation to either subtype can be indigenous or naturally occurring, or intentionally fabricated to advantage using microsurgical techniques.[65] Huang et al[66] first applied this nomenclature to describe strictly perforator-based chimeric flaps, but conjoined flaps based only on perforators are also possible[67] (Fig. 3-3).

Conjoined perforator flaps can be huge and consist of "multiple perforasomes, each *dependent* because of a common physical junction, but each perforasome still supplied by an *independent* perforator"[65] (Fig. 3-4). Any perforator flap raised with more than a single perforator, in essence, is a conjoined perforator flap whose perforators naturally have a common origin from the flap source vessel (Fig. 3-5). If those perforators arose from unconnected branches or even different source vessels, this would be an *independent* branch-based type of indigenous conjoined perforator flap.[67] This complicates the transfer of this subtype, because "supercharging" in some form with a microanastomosis would be required. Instead of finding a second recipient site at the defect, the mosaic flap principle of Koshima et al[67] can be used to connect one perforator to a side branch of the other to fabricate an *internal* conjoined perforator flap. If the perforators are from contiguous angiosomes, the different source vessels themselves may be similarly connected to each other to create a *congruent* conjoined perforator flap.

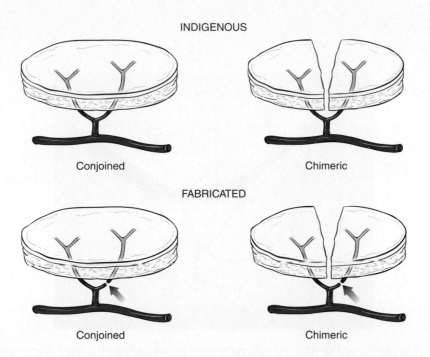

Fig. 3-3 Combined perforator flaps can be further subdivided into conjoined or chimeric perforator flaps. Either can be based on an indigenous or naturally occurring arrangement of perforators or can be fabricated by joining perforators via a microanastomosis *(arrows)*.

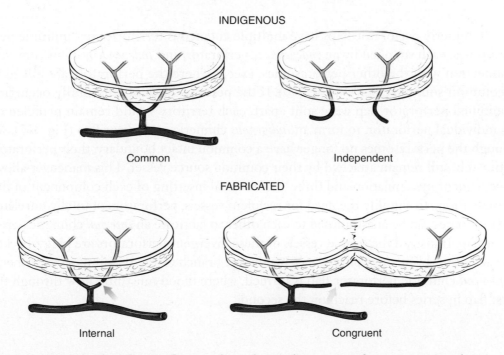

Fig. 3-4 Conjoined perforator flaps can have their indigenous perforators connected to a *common* source vessel, or they may arise from *independent* branches, or even a different source vessel. A conjoined perforator flap can be fabricated by either an *internal* microanastomosis *(blue arrow)* of perforators or microanastomosis of the source vessels to source independent source branches to form a *congruent* flap *(yellow arrow)*.

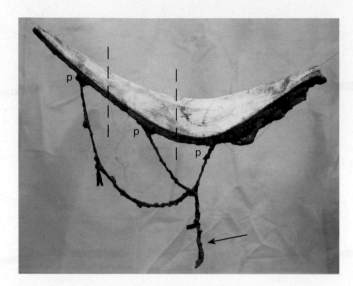

Fig. 3-5   Any perforator flap with multiple perforators *(p)* arising from the same source vessel *(arrow)* can be considered to be a *common* form of indigenous conjoined perforator flap, because the respective perforasomes of each perforator share a common boundary (here implied by the *dashed lines*).

Chimeric perforator flaps have multiple cutaneous territories or "multiple perforasomes, each supplied by an *independent* perforator, and *independent* of any physical connection with the other perforasomes, except where the perforators are linked to a common source vessel"[65] (Fig. 3-6). If the perforasomes of a naturally occurring conjoined perforator flap were split apart, each territory would remain pedicled on its individual perforator, to form an *indigenous* chimeric perforator flap (Fig. 3-7). Although the perforasomes no longer have a common intact boundary, their perforators ultimately still remain attached by their common source vessel. This maneuver allows independent manipulation and three-dimensional insetting of each component of this combination. To simplify the need for recipient vessels, perforators of totally unrelated perforasomes can be anastomosed to each other to fabricate an *internal* chimeric perforator flap. If instead the source vessels of these divergent perforators are piggy-backed to each other by an anastomosis to a major side branch or the terminus of the other, a *sequential* chimeric perforator flap is formed, where blood must first flow through the first flap in series before reaching the second.

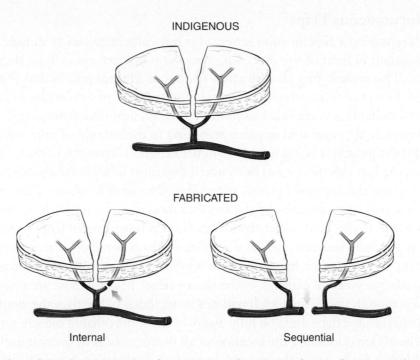

INDIGENOUS

FABRICATED

Internal   Sequential

Fig. 3-6 The independent territories of an *indigenous* chimeric perforator flap are supplied by separate perforators that are ultimately connected to a common source vessel. Anomalies may sometimes require an intraflap microanastomosis of perforators *(blue arrow)* to fabricate an *internal* chimeric flap. More commonly, to accommodate the usual paucity of potential recipient vessels, the source vessels of multiple perforator flaps can be connected to each other in a series *(yellow arrow)* to fabricate a *sequential* chimeric flap.

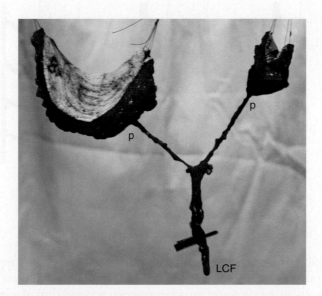

Fig. 3-7 An anterolateral thigh flap was split between two perforators *(p)* that are now connected only by the same source vessel *(LCF)*, creating an indigenous type of chimeric perforator flap. *(LCF,* Descending branch of lateral circumflex femoral.)

Musculocutaneous Flaps

Although repeating a classification schema for musculocutaneous or muscle flaps may seem redundant in light of the preceding discussion on perforator flaps, there is some relevance. The muscle flap classification system of Mathes and Nahai,[68] which has withstood the test of time, categorizes muscles on the basis of similarities in their blood supply. This schema was intended to simplify their clinical dissection (Fig. 3-8). In addition, Taylor et al[70] separated muscles according to their mode of innervation, which is critical if the muscle is being used for a dynamic muscle transfer. In these studies and during muscle flap elevation it has been noted that most musculocutaneous perforators arise near where the dominant pedicle enters the hilum of that muscle. This observation is circumstantially corroborated by the fact that most clinical applications using muscle perforator flaps to date have concentrated on the skin territories of large muscles, which have large dominant source vessels and consistently large musculocutaneous perforators near that point of entry (see Appendix). Few applications have utilized minor pedicles, or even secondary segmental pedicles, as the source vessel, because these are more difficult. Thus, even though the muscle itself will not be included in the flap, the astute student of muscle perforator flaps must be fully aware of the most reliable muscle types, which of their vessels are dominant, the location of all source vessels to every muscle, and the predictable site for locating the musculocutaneous perforators essential for inclusion in muscle perforator flaps.

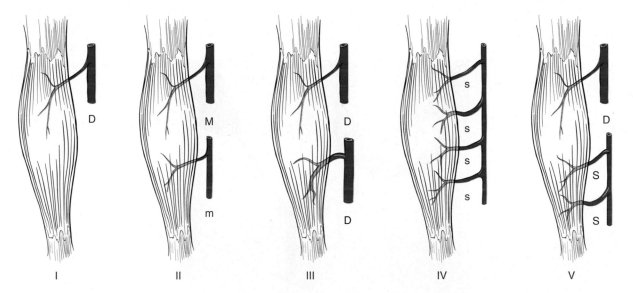

Fig. 3-8   The classical classification schema of Mathes and Nahai for the five types of muscle flaps based on the predominant vascular pattern for that muscle type. (Modified from Mathes SJ, Nahai F. Classification of the vascular anatomy of muscles: experimental and clinical correlation. Plast Reconstr Surg 67:177-187, 1981.) (*D*, Dominant pedicle; *M*, major; *m*, minor; *S*, secondary segmental; *s*, segmental.)

DEFINITION, CLASSIFICATION, AND NOMENCLATURE OF PEFORATOR FLAPS

In 1989 Koshima and Soeda were the first surgeons to name a perforator flap.[71] The superthin paraumbilical perforator (PUP) flap was based on a paraumbilical perforator of the deep inferior epigastric vessels. Very shortly thereafter, Allen and Treece[72] used a different name for a flap based on the same perforators for breast reconstruction. Within the first years of the development of perforator flaps, confusion over flap names was already present. Soon it became clear that in a totally new field of flap surgery, many surgeons were taking new initiatives to develop new flaps. In different articles, different surgeons were using different names for the same flap. For example, a perforator flap from the lower abdomen based on the deep inferior epigastric vessels was sometimes called a *paraumbilical perforator flap*, *ultrathin paraumbilical perforator-based cutaneous island flap*, or *deep inferior epigastric perforator flap*. Skin flaps derived from the thoracodorsal region were sometimes called *thoracodorsal artery perforator flaps* (with different acronyms, such as TDP flap, TAP flap, and TDAP flap), *latissimus dorsi perforator* (LDP) *flap*, *thoracodorsal perforator–based cutaneous island flap*, or *thin latissimus dorsi perforator–based free flap*. It was apparent that a simplified nomenclature was required to ease the confusion.

In 2001 during the Fifth International Course on Perforator Flaps in Gent, Belgium, the first initiative was taken to simplify the nomenclature of perforator flaps. The purpose of the meeting was to standardize flap names and facilitate communication among surgeons. During this meeting it became evident that we did not have a clear definition of perforator flaps and perforator vessels. In that meeting and in subsequent meetings in Taipei and London, the nomenclature was further discussed and simplified.

Meanwhile, different opinions had developed in various parts of the world. The European point of view formulated during the Fifth International Course in Gent involved a preliminary consensus on five different perforator vessels and five definitions of perforator vessels and perforator flaps. This consensus was later simplified to three different perforator vessels, and a clear differentiation between muscle and septal perforator flaps was made.

The Canadian proposal was summarized in an article by Geddes et al.[37] The nomenclature and abbreviations were very similar to those of the European proposal. The main difference was the use of suffixes to differentiate between muscular and septal perforator flaps. Additionally, if more than one flap could be harvested on perforators derived from the same nutrient source vessel, the abbreviation of the name of the muscle through which the perforator runs was added to the abbreviation of the source vessel.

The Asian microsurgical community had a tendency to use more complex terminology. The Korean proposal, presented at the Sixth International Course on Perforator Flaps in Taipei, Taiwan,[41] was developed to name every flap that required an intramuscular dissection after the muscle that enclosed the perforator. A more complex terminology was proposed, with the use of several adjuncts to obtain a more specific description of the surgery performed. A typical example is the *thoracodorsal perforator–based cutaneous island flap* instead of *thoracodorsal artery perforator flap*.

The complexity of the Asian terminology, the lack of published articles on this topic, and the need for a global standard nomenclature drove us to unify the Canadian, American, and European points of view and to propose a standard nomenclature.

Definition of a Perforator Flap

Defining exactly what a perforator flap is requires a clear description of a perforator vessel. Hallock[30] made a clear distinction between direct and indirect perforating vessels. Direct perforator vessels perforate only the deep fascia after they branch off the source vessel. Indirect perforators run through a specific anatomic structure before perforating the deep fascia. This anatomic structure is mostly muscle or septum but can also be nerve, bone, tendon, periosteum, perichondrium, or otherwise. Large perforators that come up from nerve, bone, tendon, periosteum, or perichondrium are relatively rare. Because mostly muscle and septal perforators are used in routine surgery, the first two definitions that follow are limited to muscle and septal perforators. However, flaps based on vessels that perforate structures other than muscle or septum are also possible.

Definition 1   A muscle or musculocutaneous perforator is a blood vessel that traverses through muscle to pierce the outer layer of the deep fascia to supply the overlying skin.

Definition 2   A septal or septocutaneous perforator is a blood vessel that traverses *only* through septum to supply the overlying skin after piercing the outer layer of the deep fascia.

The terms *musculocutaneous* and *septocutaneous* were introduced to clearly indicate the course of the perforator through the deeper structures (Fig. 3-9). This clarification is analogous to the older terms *musculocutaneous* or *musculocutaneous flaps* and *septocutaneous flaps*.

Definition 3   A perforator flap is a flap consisting of skin and/or subcutaneous fat. The vessels that supply the blood to the flap are isolated perforators. These perforators may pass from their source vessel origin, either through or between the deep tissues (mostly muscle).

With regard to the difference between direct and indirect perforators and indirect muscle and indirect septal perforators, the following definitions were given to the two most frequently used perforator flaps.

Definition 4   A skin flap vascularized by a muscle perforator is called a *muscle perforator flap* or *musculocutaneous perforator flap*.

Definition 5   A skin flap vascularized by a septal perforator is called a *septal perforator flap* or *septocutaneous perforator flap*.

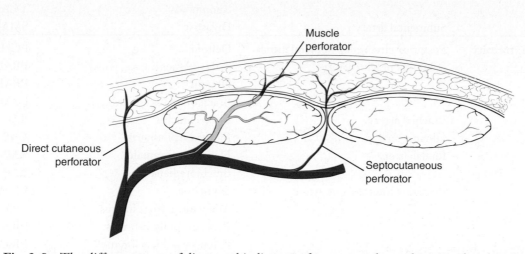

Fig. 3-9 The different types of direct and indirect perforator vessels emphasizing their surgical importance: direct perforator perforating the deep fascia only, indirect muscle perforator traveling through muscle before piercing the deep fascia, and indirect septal perforator traveling through the intermuscular septum before piercing the deep fascia.

At this time it is still not clear whether a skin flap vascularized by a direct perforator should be called a direct *perforator* flap. By doing so, all skin flaps harvested in the human body would be perforator flaps. Skin flaps vascularized by direct perforators do not require the same specific surgical technique needed to harvest indirect perforator flaps and should therefore be distinguished.

Some surgeons argue that septocutaneous perforators and direct perforators are one and the same vessel.[29,39] The protagonists argue that the dissection of a septocutaneous perforator is very similar to the dissection of a flap vascularized by a direct perforator and that it would simplify the classification. From a semantic point of view, the antagonists argue that septocutaneous perforator flaps are not the same as a flap vascularized by a direct perforator and therefore require distinction.

A few other concepts have become clear in recent years. A perforator vessel starts where it branches off its source vessel that has a common anatomic name and ends in the subdermal plexus. Generally, perforators do not have a common anatomic name. Also, the vessels of a muscle perforator flap can pierce any muscle independent of the donor morbidity created, independent of the muscle fiber direction of the muscle it perforates, and independent of the course, direction, and length of the pedicle.

Nomenclature
Table 3-1 provides a list of muscle perforator flaps with their abbreviations.

Table 3-1 Proposed Standard Nomenclature for Muscle Perforator Flaps

	Muscle Perforator Flap	Muscle Perforated	Abbreviation
Head and Neck	Transverse cervical artery	Trapezius	TCAP-*t*
		Rhomboids	TCAP-*r*
	Submental artery	Digastric	SMAP
Upper Extremity	Posterior circumflex humeral artery	Deltoid	PCHAP
	Profunda brachii artery	Triceps brachii	PBAP-*t*
		Deltoid	PBAP-*d*
		Brachioradialis	PBAP-*b*
	Brachial artery	Biceps brachii	BAP
	Ulnar artery	Flexor carpi ulnaris	UAP
	Radial artery	Flexor carpi radialis	RAP-*fcr*
		Brachioradialis	RAP-*b*
	Posterior interosseous artery	Supinator	PIOAP-*s*
		Abductor pollicis longus	PIOAP-*apl*
		Extensor pollicis brevis	PIOAP-*epb*
		Extensor pollicis longus	PIOAP-*epl*
		Extensor indicis	PIOAP-*ei*
	Anterior interosseous artery	Flexor digitorum profundus	AIOAP-*fdp*
		Supinator	AIOAP-*s*
		Pronator quadratus	AIOAP-*pq*
Thorax	Thoracoacromial artery	Pectoralis major	TAAP-*pma*
		Pectoralis minor	TAAP-*pmi*
		Deltoid	TAAP-*d*
	Suprascapular artery	Infraspinatus	SSAP-*is*
		Supraspinatus	SSAP-*ss*
	Dorsal scapular artery	Trapezius	DSAP
	Dorsal intercostal artery	Trapezius (superior)	DICAP
		Latissimus dorsi (inferior)	
	Dorsolateral intercostal artery	Latissimus dorsi	DLICAP
	Lateral intercostal artery	Serratus anterior/latissimus dorsi (superior intercostal spaces)	LICAP
		External oblique (inferior intercostal spaces)	
	Anterior intercostal artery	Pectoralis major (superior)	AICAP
		Rectus abdominis (inferior)	
	Subcostal artery	Latissimus dorsi/external oblique	SCAP
	Circumflex scapular artery	Teres major	CSAP
	Thoracodorsal artery	Latissimus dorsi	TDAP
	Internal thoracic (mammary) artery	Pectoralis major	ITAP (IMAP)
	Lateral thoracic artery	Serratus anterior	LTAP-*sa*
		Pectoralis major	LTAP-*pma*
		Pectoralis minor	LTAP-*pmi*
		Subscapularis	LTAP-*s*
	Posterior intercostal artery	Back muscles	PIAP-*n*
	Lumbar artery	Lower back muscles	LAP-*n*
	Parasacral artery	Gluteus maximus	PSAP
Abdomen	Superior epigastric artery	Rectus abdominis	SEAP
	Superficial inferior epigastric artery	Rectus abdominis	SIEAP
	Deep inferior epigastric artery	Rectus abdominis	DIEAP
Pelvis	Deep circumflex iliac artery	Transversus abdominis	DCIAP-*ta*
		Obliquus internus	DCIAP-*oi*
		Iliacus	DCIAP-*i*

	Muscle Perforator Flap	Muscle Perforated	Abbreviation
	Internal pudendal artery	Gluteus maximus	IPAP
	Superior gluteal artery	Gluteus maximus	SGAP
		Gluteus medius	
		Gluteus minimus	
		Piriformis	
	Inferior gluteal artery	Gluteus maximus	IGAP
		Gluteus medius	
		Gluteus minimus	
Lower Extremity	Common femoral artery	Sartorius	CFAP-*s*
		Vastus medialis	CFAP-*vm*
		Rectus femoris	CFAP-*rf*
		Adductor longus	CFAP-*al*
	Lateral circumflex femoral artery	Tensor fascia lata	LCFAP-*tfl*
		Vastus lateralis	LCFAP-*vl*
		Rectus femoris	LCFAP-*rf*
	Medial circumflex femoral artery	Adductor longus	MCFAP-*al*
		Gracilis	MCFAP-*g*
	Profunda femoris artery	Biceps femoris	PFAP-*bf*
		Adductor magnus	PFAP-*am*
		Adductor longus	PFAP-*al*
		Adductor brevis	PFAP-*ab*
		Gracilis	PFAP-*g*
	Superficial femoral artery	Adductor longus	SFAP-*al*
		Adductor brevis	SFAP-*ab*
		Adductor magnus	SFAP-*am*
		Gracilis	SFAP-*g*
		Vastus medialis	SFAP-*vm*
		Sartorius	SFAP-*s*
	Descending genicular artery	Vastus medialis	DGAP-*vm*
		Adductor magnus	DGAP-*am*
		Sartorius	DGAP-*s*
	Popliteal artery	Soleus	PAP
	Medial sural artery	Gastrocnemius (med.)	MSAP
	Lateral sural artery	Gastrocnemius (lat.)	LSAP
	Peroneal artery	Extensor hallucis longus	PNAP-*ehl*
		Flexor hallucis longus	PNAP-*fhl*
		Peroneus tertius	PNAP-*pt*
		Soleus	PNAP-*s*
		Tibialis posterior	PNAP-*tp*
	Anterior tibial artery	Tibialis anterior	ATAP-*ta*
		Extensor digitorum longus	ATAP-*edl*
		Extensor hallucis	ATAP-*eh*
		Peroneus tertius	ATAP-*pt*
	Posterior tibial artery	Tibialis posterior	PTAP-*tp*
		Soleus	PTAP-*s*
		Flexor digitorum longus	PTAP-*fdl*
	Medial plantar artery	Abductor hallucis	MPAP-*ah*
		Flexor digitorum brevis	MPAP-*fdb*
	Lateral plantar artery	Abductor digiti minimi	LPAP

Definition 6   To give a new perforator flap a name, certain rules should be followed. A perforator flap should be named after the main source artery supplying the flap, and not after the underlying muscle.

Following the European proposal, this sentence was originally added to the definition: "If there is a potential to harvest multiple perforator flaps from one source vessel, the name of each flap should be based upon its anatomic region or muscle." The problem with this statement is that a specific perforator can come off its source vessel and can perforate different muscles in the same region. Therefore the definition was not specific enough, and the proposal of Geddes et al[37] is more logical.

Muscle perforator flaps are named by their nutrient or source vessel (Fig. 3-10). The suffix -AP always follows the abbreviation of the source vessel (for example, DIEAP stands for deep inferior epigastric artery perforator flap). Inclusion of the A of artery makes pronunciation and semantics easier.

If this nomenclature is not specific enough, and in cases in which different flaps are based on perforators of the same source artery, the muscular origin of the perforators is abbreviated and italicized to indicate the anatomic origin of the flap. For example, LCFAP-*vl* stands for the lateral circumflex femoral artery perforator–vastus lateralis muscle, and LCFAP-*tfl* stands for the lateral circumflex femoral artery perforator–tensor fascia lata muscle (see Fig. 3-10). In the case of flaps based on source arteries that have numbered segmental origins, such as the posterior intercostal or lumbar arteries, the numbered source vessel requires notation. For example, PIAP-8 stands for the eighth posterior intercostal artery perforator.[38] Obviously, the italicized muscle or number suffix should not be added if the perforators of the source vessel can only perforate one muscle.

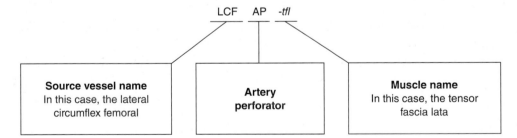

Fig. 3-10   Standardized muscle perforator flap nomenclature.

CONCLUSION

Simplification of the perforator vessels classification led to more specific definitions of musculocutaneous and septocutaneous perforator flaps, which now make up the two main groups of indirect perforator flaps. The third group comprises the direct perforator flaps. These three subgroups of flaps can be employed to classify most pedicle and free axial skin flaps used in daily practice today. Nevertheless, a small group of perforator vessels perforates structures other than muscle and septum such as bone, the parotid gland, nerve, or periosteum. For instance, in the head and neck area, many osteocutaneous perforators can be found, including the mental, infraorbital, and supraorbital vessels.

The main goal of defining a perforator flap and subclassifying three important groups is twofold. First, the term *perforator flap* indicates to the surgeon that a specific surgical technique is needed to harvest the flap. The adjuncts of *indirect musculocutaneous*, *indirect septocutaneous*, and *direct perforator flap* clearly describe which surgical approach is needed. The surgeon will have to focus on the position and the three-dimensional course of the vessel through the deeper tissues. More specifically, muscle or musculocutaneous perforator flaps will have to be raised by opening the deep fascia, splitting the donor muscle, preserving its other vascularization and motor innervation, and eventually exposing its source artery. For septal or septocutaneous perforator flaps, the perforator will be dissected within an intermuscular septum, and followed through that septum down to the source artery.

Some microsurgeons might argue that direct perforator flaps and septocutaneous perforator flaps should comprise one group. We, on the other hand, believe it is necessary to make a clear distinction between these two groups. In a direct perforator flap such as the groin flap, the perforators do not run through a specific intermuscular septum. They only pass through loose fatty tissue in the groin area and eventually perforate the deep fascia more proximally. A specific septum is not looked for, and the surgical technique is different from the technique used to harvest a septocutaneous flap. With the septocutaneous perforator, the perforator can be localized directly within the fibers of an intermuscular septum.

In the discussion of nomenclature, the definition of a source vessel is extremely important. Although everybody seems to agree with naming a perforator flap after the nutrient artery, there is some discussion around perforator flaps harvested from a source vessel that can give rise to multiple perforator flaps. Different orders of vessels are observed between the skin and the aorta with obviously different names. There is clearly still some debate over which order of branching should be used to name a perforator flap. For the time being, the closest underlying axial source vessel that has been clearly anatomically defined is used in naming the perforator flap.

References

1. Mathes S, Nahai F. The reconstructive triangle: a paradigm for surgical decision making. In Mathes S, Nahai F, eds. Reconstructive Surgery: Principles, Anatomy, & Technique. New York: Churchill Livingstone, 1997.

2. Pearl RM, Johnson D. The vascular supply to the skin: an anatomical and physiological reappraisal (Part II). Ann Plast Surg 11:196-205, 1983.

3. Daniel R, Kerrigan C, eds. Principles and Physiology of Skin Flap Surgery. Philadelphia: WB Saunders, 1990.

4. McGregor IA, Morgan G. Axial and random pattern flaps. Br J Plast Surg 26:202-213, 1973.

5. Ger R. The technique of muscle transposition in the operative treatment of traumatic and ulcerative lesions of the leg. J Trauma 11:502-510, 1971.

6. Orticochea M. The musculocutaneous flap method: an immediate and heroic substitute for the method of delay. Br J Plast Surg 25:106-110, 1972.

7. Taylor G, ed. The Blood Supply of the Skin, 5th ed. Philadelphia: Lippincott-Raven, 1997.

8. Cormack G, Lamberty B, eds. The Anatomical Basis for Fasciocutaneous Flaps. Cambridge, MA: Blackwell Scientific Publications, 1992.

9. Kunert P. Structure and construction: the system of skin flaps. Ann Plast Surg 27:509-516; discussion 27:517-518, 1991.

10. Milton SH. Pedicled skin flaps: the fallacy of the length:width ratio. Br J Surg 57:502-508, 1970.

11. Ponten B. The fasciocutaneous flap: its use in soft tissue defects of the lower leg. Br J Plast Surg 34:215-220, 1981.

12. Manchot C, Ristic J, Morain WD, et al, eds. The Cutaneous Arteries of the Human Body. New York: Springer-Verlag, 1983.

13. Nakajima H, Fujino T, Adachi S. A new concept of vascular supply to the skin and classification of skin flaps according to their vascularization. Ann Plast Surg 16:1-19, 1986.

    The authors divided the vascular systems involved in the cutaneous circulation into four categories. This allowed classification of skin flaps into five types (cutaneous, fasciocutaneous, adipofascial, septocutaneous, and musculocutaneous flaps). Fasciocutaneous flaps were further divided into six types, according to the patterns of vascular input to the fasciocutaneous plexus. This classification has been demonstrated to be related to clinical effects. Nine new free and island flaps were discussed.

14. Batchelor JS, Moss AL. The relationship between fasciocutaneous perforators and their fascial branches: an anatomical study in human cadaver lower legs. Plast Reconstr Surg 95:629-633, 1995.

15. Nakajima H, Minabe T, Imanishi N. Three-dimensional analysis and classification of arteries in the skin and subcutaneous adipofascial tissue by computer graphics imaging. Plast Reconstr Surg 102:748-760, 1998.

16. Hallock GG, ed. Principles of Fascia and Fasciocutaneous Flaps. Philadelphia: Hanley & Belfus, 1999.

17. Cormack G, Lamberty B. The fasciocutaneous system of vessels. In Cormack G, Lamberty B, eds. The Arterial Anatomy of Skin Flaps, 2nd ed. Edinburgh: Churchill Livingstone, 1994.

18. Hallock GG. The tripartite system of muscle perforators, with emphasis on the emerging importance of the direct cutaneous muscle perforator flap. J Reconstr Microsurg (submitted for publication).

19. Tolhurst DE. A comprehensive classification of flaps: the atomic system. Plast Reconstr Surg 80:608-609, 1987.

20. Tolhurst D. Fasciocutaneous flaps and their use in reconstructive surgery. Perspect Plast Surg 4:129-145, 1990.

21. Cormack GC, Lamberty BG. A classification of fasciocutaneous flaps according to their patterns of vascularisation. Br J Plast Surg 37:80-87, 1984.

22. Cormack G, Lamberty B. Alternative flap nomenclature and classification. In Cormack G, Lamberty B, eds. The Arterial Anatomy of Skin Flaps, 2nd ed. Edinburgh: Churchill Livingstone, 1994.

23. Niranjan NS, Price RD, Govilkar P. Fascial feeder and perforator-based V-Y advancement flaps in the reconstruction of lower limb defects [review]. Br J Plast Surg 53:679-689, 2000.

> *The planning and design of V-Y advancement flaps was discussed, including distinct perforator or fascial feeder vessels, which may originate from periosteum, muscle, cutaneous nerve, or large tendon sheaths. Forty cases were described in which perforator-based V-Y advancement flaps were used to cover large defects of the lower leg following excision of malignant skin lesions and in selected trauma cases that did not involve degloving injuries. The planning, operative technique, and results with case presentations were presented.*

24. Koshima I, Narushima M, Mihara M, et al. New thoracodorsal artery perforator (TAPcp) flap with capillary perforators for reconstruction of upper limb. J Plast Reconstr Aesthet Surg 64:140-145, 2010.

25. Wei FC, Jain V, Suominen S, et al. Confusion among perforator flaps: what is a true perforator flap? Plast Reconstr Surg 107:874-876, 2001.

26. Mathes S, Nahai F. Flap selection: analysis of features, modifications, and applications. In Mathes S, Nahai F, eds. Reconstructive Surgery: Principles, Anatomy, & Technique. New York: Churchill Livingstone, 1997.

27. Taylor GI, Palmer JH. The vascular territories (angiosomes) of the body: experimental study and clinical applications. Br J Plast Surg 40:113-141, 1987.

28. Taylor G, Palmer J, McManammy D. The vascular territories of the body (angiosomes) and their clinical applications. In McCarthy J, ed. Plastic Surgery. Philadelphia: WB Saunders, 1990.

29. Taylor G. Foreword. In Manchot C, ed. The Cutaneous Arteries of the Human Body. New York: Springer-Verlag, 1983.

30. Hallock GG. Direct and indirect perforator flaps: the history and the controversy. Plast Reconstr Surg 111:855-865; quiz 111:866, 2003.

> *This article emphasized the major role of the vascular supply to a cutaneous flap, explained how to predict its reliability, and outlined basic schemes for classification. The history of the evolution of cutaneous flaps was reviewed and provided insight essential for understanding a simple proposal for their classification. All fascial perforators course either directly from a source vessel or indirectly first through some other tissue to reach the suprafascial layer; therefore corresponding flaps based on any such perforators could be called either direct perforator flaps or indirect perforator flaps, respectively.*

31. Taylor GI. The "Gent" consensus on perforator flap terminology: preliminary definitions [discussion]. Plast Reconstr Surg 112:138, 2003.

32. Nakajima H, Imanishi N, Fukuzumi S, et al. Accompanying arteries of the cutaneous veins and cutaneous nerves in the extremities: anatomical study and a concept of the venoadipofascial and/or neuroadipofascial pedicled fasciocutaneous flap. Plast Reconstr Surg 102:779-791, 1998.

33. Masquelet AC, Romana MC, Wolf G. Skin island flaps supplied by the vascular axis of the sensitive superficial nerves: anatomic study and clinical experience in the leg. Plast Reconstr Surg 89:1115-1121, 1992.

34. Hallock GG. "Microleaps" in the progression of flaps and grafts. Clin Plast Surg 23:117-138, 1996.

35. Bertelli JA, Catarina S. Neurocutaneous island flaps in upper limb coverage: experience with 44 clinical cases. J Hand Surg Am 22:515-526, 1997.

36. Blondeel PN, van Landuyt KH, Monstrey SJ, et al. The "Gent" consensus on perforator flap terminology: preliminary definitions. Plast Reconstr Surg 112:1378-1383, 2003.

37. Geddes CR, Morris SF, Neligan PC. Perforator flaps: evolution, classification, and applications. Ann Plast Surg 50:90-99, 2003.

38. Hallock GG. Muscle perforator flaps: the name game. Ann Plast Surg 51:630-632, 2003.

   A consistent, simple nomenclature for muscle perforator flaps is essential to eliminate confusion in the literature and to facilitate their surgical application. A system that names flaps according to the involved muscle and its source vessel avoids confusion caused by variations in perforator origin or overlapping "mother" vessels. Such a combination readily identifies the precise anatomic location of the flap and indicates exactly which vascular pedicle must be dissected.

39. Bravo FG, Schwarze HP. Free-style local perforator flaps: concept and classification system. J Plast Reconstr Aesthet Surg 62:602-608, 2009.

   A classification schema for free-style local flaps was proposed based on the number of perforator vessels preserved with the flap and the type of flap movement. The described type I flap is similar to propeller flaps, and type III is similar to perforator plus flaps.

40. Sinna R, Boloorchi A, Mahajan AL, et al. What should define a "perforator flap"? Plast Reconstr Surg 126:2258-2263, 2010.

   Terms that better clarify the anatomy and surgical approach to any given flap would include, in this order, the vessel of origin, type or extent of vascular dissection, the muscle penetrated, and the type of perforator vessel; that is, musculocutaneous or septocutaneous. The name for the flap would list these characteristics in this order.

41. Kim JT. New nomenclature concept of perforator flap. Br J Plast Surg 58:431-440, 2005.

42. Hyakusoku H, Yamamoto T, Fumiiri M. The propeller flap method. Br J Plast Surg 44:53-54, 1991.

   This was the original article that first used the term "propeller flap." The central hub of the propeller was based on a subcutaneous pedicle with no specifically defined vascular source. Rotation about the hub could not exceed 90 degrees.

43. Hallock GG. The propeller flap version of the adductor muscle perforator flap for coverage of ischial or trochanteric pressure sores. Ann Plast Surg 56:540-542, 2006.

   The propeller flap concept introduced by Hyakusoku was modified by using a solitary perforator as the specifically identified source of perfusion to the flap. This allowed far greater rotation of the flap about the perforator, which became the hub. While the larger blade of the propeller closed the defect, the minor blade could be designed to facilitate direct closure of the former. This brought together two important concepts to increase the versatility of perforator propeller flaps as local free-style perforator flaps.

44. Pignatti M, Ogawa R, Hallock GG, et al. The "Tokyo" consensus on propeller flaps. Plast Reconstr Surg 127:716-722, 2011.

   At the first Tokyo meeting on perforator and propeller flaps, a consensus was reached on defining, classifying, and describing the versatility of primarily perforator propeller flaps as local flaps for solving cutaneous deficiencies throughout the body.

45. Waterston SW, Quaba O, Quaba AA. The ad hoc perforator flap for contracture release. J Plast Reconstr Aesthet Surg 61:55-60, 2008.

46. Wong CH, Tan BK. Perforator-plus flaps or perforator-sparing flaps: different names, same concept. Plast Reconstr Surg 120:1746-1747, 2007.

47. Mehrotra S. Reply to Wong CH, Tan BK. Perforator-plus flaps or perforator-sparing flaps: different names, same concept. Plast Reconstr Surg 120:1748, 2007.

48. D'Arpa S. Reply to Mehrotra S. Perforator-plus flaps: a new concept in traditional flap design. Plast Reconstr Surg 120:2118-2119, 2007.

49. Mehrotra S. Perforator-plus flaps: a new concept in traditional flap design. Plast Reconstr Surg 119:590-598, 2007.

50. Sharma RK, Mehrotra S, Nanda V. The perforator "plus" flap: a simple nomenclature for locoregional perforator-based flaps. Plast Reconstr Surg 116:1838-1839, 2005.

51. Wong CH, Tan BK. Perforator-sparing transposition flaps for lower leg defects: anatomic study and clinical applications. Ann Plast Surg 58:614-621, 2007.

52. Nelson R, Lalonde DH. Treatment of the chronic pilonidal sinus wound with a local perforator-assisted transposition flap. Plast Reconstr Surg 122:47e-49e, 2008.

53. Vasile JV, Newman T, Greenspun DG, et al. Anatomic vascular imaging of perforator flaps for breast reconstruction: seeing is believing with magnetic resonance angiography. Plast Reconstr Surg 124(Suppl 4):S71, 2009.

54. Chen CM, Allen RJ. Breast reconstruction with the septocutaneous perforator flap: the next frontier. Plast Reconstr Surg 124(Suppl 2):S680, 2009.

55. Tuinder S, Chen CM, Massey MF, et al. Introducing the septocutaneous gluteal artery perforator flap: a simplified approach to microsurgical breast reconstruction. Plast Reconstr Surg 127:489-495, 2011.

56. Tuinder S, Van Der Hulst R, Lataster A, et al. Superior gluteal artery perforator flap based on septal perforators: preliminary study. Plast Reconstr Surg 122:146e-148e, 2008.

57. Lester M, Allen RJ, LoTempio MM. Septocutaneous deep inferior epigastric artery flap for breast reconstruction. Presented at the Twenty-fifth Annual Meeting of the American Society for Reconstructive Microsurgery, Maui, Hawaii, Jan 2009.

58. Massey MF, Spiegel AJ, Levine JL, et al; Group for the Advancement of Breast Reconstruction. Perforator flaps: recent experience, current trends, and future directions based on 3974 microsurgical breast reconstructions. Plast Reconstr Surg 124:737-751, 2009.

59. Woodburne RT, ed. Essentials of Human Anatomy, 4th ed. New York: Oxford University Press, New York, 1969, pp 15-17.

60. Woodburne RT, ed. Essentials of Human Anatomy, 4th ed. New York: Oxford University Press, 1969, p 366.

61. Woodburne RT, ed. Essentials of Human Anatomy, 4th ed. New York: Oxford University Press, 1969, p 11.

62. Dionyssiou DD, Grawanis A, Francis I, et al. Paramuscular and paraneural perforators in DIEAP flaps: radiographic findings and clinical application. Ann Plast Surg 63:610-615, 2009.

63. Hallock GG. Simplified nomenclature for compound flaps. Plast Reconstr Surg 105:1465-1470, 2000.

64. Hallock GG. Further clarification of the nomenclature for compound flaps (CME). Plast Reconstr Surg 117:151e-160e, 2006.

65. Hallock GG. The complete nomenclature for combined perforator flaps. Plast Reconstr Surg 127:1720-1729, 2011.

66. Huang WC, Chen HC, Wei FC, et al. Chimeric flap in clinical use. Clin Plast Surg 30:457-467, 2003.

67. Hallock GG. Branch-based conjoined perforator flaps. Plast Reconstr Surg 121:1642-1649, 2008.

68. Koshima I, Yamamoto Y, Moriguchi T, et al. Extended anterior thigh flaps for repair of massive cervical defects involving pharyngoesophagus and skin: an introduction to the "mosaic" flap principle. Ann Plast Surg 32:321-327, 1994.

69. Mathes SJ, Nahai F. Classification of the vascular anatomy of muscles: experimental and clinical correlation. Plast Reconstr Surg 67:177-187, 1981.

70. Taylor GI, Gianoutsos MP, Morris SF. The neurovascular territories of the skin and muscles: anatomic study and clinical implications. Plast Reconstr Surg 94:1-36, 1994.

71. Koshima I, Soeda S. Inferior epigastric artery skin flaps without rectus abdominis muscle. Br J Plast Surg 42:645-648, 1989.

72. Allen RJ, Treece P. Deep inferior epigastric perforator flap for breast reconstruction. Ann Plast Surg 32:32-38, 1994.

4

Anatomic Techniques

Maolin Tang
Daping Yang
Christopher R. Geddes
Steven F. Morris

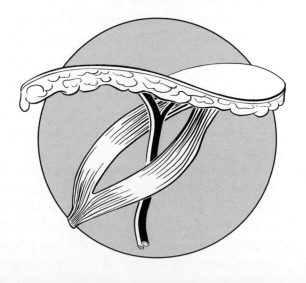

Anatomic research in one form or another has been conducted for more than 2000 years. The quest for an understanding of human anatomy dates from the time of Galen to modern times. In more recent history, the study of anatomy has continued to answer basic surgical questions. With respect to perforator flaps, the vascular anatomy of the skin has previously been studied, but not in the detail required to address certain questions about perforator flap harvest. Therefore further detailed analyses of the skin vasculature are required to fully elucidate the details important in perforator flap harvest.

Data on human vascular anatomy have traditionally been derived from time-consuming cadaver dissections. Vascular injection of a radiopaque medium is a rapid technique that allows anatomists to prepare anatomic specimens much faster and more efficiently than by dissection alone. This technique plays an important role in the laboratory study of microvascular anatomy. As we continuously seek to improve conventional surgery, this technique remains an indispensable tool in the search for new donor sites for tissue transfer. More recently, three-dimensional angiography using CT and specialized software have allowed anatomists to more fully digitally dissect the human body. This chapter reviews the evolution of the investigation of normal vascular anatomy of the human body by angiography and computer imaging techniques.

VASCULAR IMAGING
History of Angiography

Classical dissection techniques had long proved inadequate for demonstrating vascular anatomy. The discovery of x-rays proved to be a major advance in this field. The first postmortem angiographic study was performed only weeks after Roentgen's discovery of x-rays in 1895.[1] In 1896 Haschek and Lindenthal[2] injected the brachial artery of an amputated cadaver hand with a solution containing chalk. In 1923 Berberich and Hirsch[3] performed the first peripheral angiogram in a living subject, using strontium bromide as a contrast medium. Since then, many contrast media have been used in vascular research (Table 4-1).

The quest for improved angiographic resolution has stimulated efforts to use a variety of radiopaque materials, including mercury,[4] lead nitrate[5] and aluminum acetate,[6] lead oxide,[7,8] lead phosphate,[9] white lead,[10] barium sulfate,[11] and silver iodide.[12] To achieve effective perfusion and facilitate dissection of the injected specimens, some researchers combined angiographic injectate with a suspending medium such as starch,[6] agar,[9] gelatin,[13] and latex.[12] The suspending medium is a carrier as well as a stabilizer

Table 4-1 Historic Development of Contrast Media

Year	Researcher	Contrast Medium	Suspending Medium	Subject
1896	Haschek and Lindenthal	Chalk	N/A	Brachial artery
1923	Berberich and Hirsch	Strontium bromide	N/A	Clinical
1920s	Moniz*	Thorotrast	N/A	Clinical
1928	Horton	Mercury	N/A	Cadaver
1928	Moniz*	Thorotrast	N/A	Clinical
1934	Kellner	Lead nitrate Aluminum acetate	Starch	Cadaver
1936	Salmon	Lead oxide (Pb$_3$O$_4$)	N/A	Cadaver
1938	Schlesinger	Lead sulfate	Agar	Cadaver
1941	Olovson	White lead	Acacia	Cadaver
1950	Lindbom	Barium sulfate	Gelatin	Cadaver
1953	Trueta and Harrison	Barium sulfate Silver iodide	Latex	Cadaver
1957	Schlesinger	Barium sulfate	Gelatin	Cadaver
1961	Shehata	Lead nitrate	Starch	Cadaver
1969	Herman et al	Thorotrast	N/A	Dog and rat
1974	Shehata	Barium sulfate	Starch	Cadaver
1984	Cutting	Lead oxide (Pb$_3$O$_4$) Barium sulfate	Gelatin	Cadaver
1986	Rees and Taylor	Lead oxide (PbO)	Gelatin	Cadaver and animal

*In Herman PG, Ohba S, Mellins HZ. Blood microcirculation in the lymph node. Radiology 92:1073-1080, 1969. (*N/A*, Not applicable.)

and, when solidified, keeps the mixture a uniform and rubbery consistency. The homogeneous mixture facilitates dissection and provides much better detail on the angiogram. It enhances visualization of the small vessels in the tissues.

Thorotrast,[14] Microfil,[15] and iodinated Microfil are contrast media used in clinical angiography and animal and human cadaver vascular research. Although Microfil and iodinated Microfil are very expensive, they do perfuse efficiently and are well suited for radiography.[15] Thorotrast is a colloidal solution of thorium dioxide that was used as a radiographic contrast agent from the 1920s to the mid-1950s. It is retained by the reticuloendothelial system and has a biologic half-life of several hundred years. If used clinically, patients injected with this medium suffer a lifetime of exposure to internal radiation. Its use was discontinued when it was recognized that its radioactivity caused long-term deleterious effects.[16-19]

Some of the most striking contributions to our knowledge of detailed vascular anatomy were provided by Salmon[7] and Trueta and Harrison.[12] Salmon injected entire fresh cadavers with a preservative mixture that included lead oxide. Radiographs of

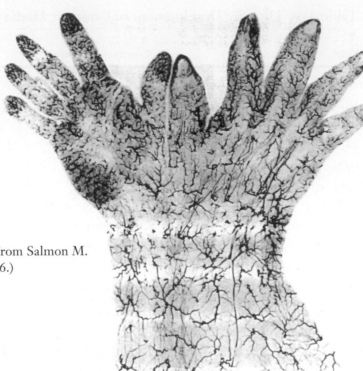

Fig. 4-1 Angiogram of the hand. (From Salmon M. Artères de la Peau. Paris: Masson, 1936.)

superb quality were obtained, not only of the entire cutaneous circulation, but also of every muscle in the body (Fig. 4-1). Trueta and Harrison's injectate was barium sulfate, silver iodide, and latex. This injection medium demonstrates the fine details of the vasculature and is characterized by high vascular perfusion, high radiopacity, and enhanced facility of dissection.

Until the mid-1980s, barium sulfate was generally accepted as the perfect contrast medium. Diener[1] devised postmortem intraosseous phlebography for evaluating venous thrombotic disease in the lower limbs. Barium sulfate had also been used to study arterial thrombosis, the microcirculation of peripheral nerves, lymph nodes, bones, the brain, and animal cutaneous microcirculation.[11-13,20-24] Cutting and colleagues[23] reported that the red lead (Pb_3O_4) injection technique was useful only for visualizing larger arteries, and barium sulfate was far superior to previous techniques in demonstrating details of the blood supply to the craniofacial skeleton.

In 1986 Rees and Taylor[25] modified Salmon's injection technique. They used the PbO form of lead oxide and combined it with gelatin to avoid staining surrounding tissues and to facilitate dissection. This technique provides radiographs of high quality both in contrast and detail. Since then, lead oxide has replaced barium sulfate as the ideal contrast medium for microangiography in plastic surgery research.

Angiography is a suitable method for studying peripheral arteries in the human body and yields excellent and clinically relevant results. However, with traditional plain film radiography, angiography has the major limitation of superimposition. That is, all three-dimensional anatomy is compressed into two dimensions. It can be difficult to determine three-dimensional position and the relationships of vessels to other structures. Stereoangiography and microtomography (micro-CT) or micro–magnetic

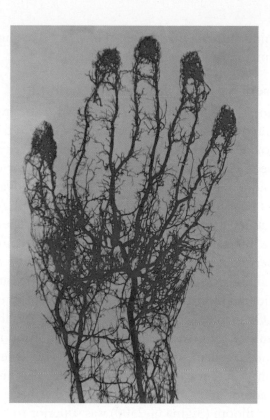

Fig. 4-2 Arterial cast of the hand.

resonance imaging (micro-MRI) can provide information concerning vessel position in three-dimensional space, the precise origin of vessels, and relationships of the vascular territories to each other and to other tissues.[15,26-29]

A variety of other injection staining techniques have been used in anatomic studies. Liquid media such as Berlin blue, merbromin, and India ink contain fine particles that, when injected, fill the capillaries. These liquid media are used to demonstrate the morphology of the microcirculation within organs and limbs. These agents stain the tissues and define a vascular territory, but can sometimes confuse the anatomic study. When any injection medium is overinjected into a vascular territory, it will exceed the "intraangiosomal volume and overflow into adjacent vascular territories via choke anastomotic vessels."[30]

Colored latex gels and ink-gelatin mixtures are excellent media for dissection. They combine perfect perfusion with a rubbery consistency. However, because they are not radiopaque, it is difficult to define the precise course of arteries and their interconnections.

Fluorescein dyes can be injected into vessels. Fluorescein clearly delineates various areas of vascular perfusion under ultraviolet light. These agents have been used to define the vascular territory of an injected artery. However, there is some overlap into adjacent vascular territories. Additionally, these agents stain the tissues, producing a tanned appearance under normal light.

Polyester resin and synthetic glass material such as acrylonitrile butradiene sturene and chlorinated polyvinyl chloride are excellent media for producing vascular corrosion casts (Fig. 4-2). When injected intravascularly, they produce high-quality specimens for scanning electron microscopy. However, these agents are not radiopaque, and injected specimens are unsuitable for dissection.

Current Vascular Injection Technique

Salmon[7] initially popularized the lead oxide injection technique in the 1930s. Rees and Taylor[25] revisited this work and improved the technique. They recommended the lead oxide–gelatin mixture for optimal cadaver angiographic study. This preparation has been used routinely since 1986. The quality of the angiography exceeds any other technique. However, this technique has disadvantages. Lead toxicity can potentially pose a health risk to researchers in this field.[31] Acute lead poisoning can lead to liver and kidney damage and encephalopathy.[32] Depending on the concentration of gelatin in the injectate, the injected vessels may be quite friable on dissection. Additionally, the perfusate may extravasate into surrounding tissues, creating stained areas that are not suitable for dissection or angiography. Because lead tends to precipitate out of the solution and form a sediment, it must be continuously stirred.

Over the past several years, we have modified the technique by decreasing the amount of lead oxide in the injectate solution to the minimum amount required to produce excellent angiograms. We have also tested the effects of using different types of gelatin, different concentrations of gelatin, varying temperatures and lead oxide dosages, and radiography.[33] We found that the pharmaceutical-grade gelatin with a gel strength of 300 Bloom (Sigma G-2500) was superior to household-grade gelatin.

The lead oxide that was used for preparing the angiograms in this book was a water-soluble orange powder available from chemical suppliers (CAS 1314-41-6, Carterchem Canada, Inc., Montreal, Quebec, Canada). Radiographic parameters such as kilovolts peak (kVp), milliamperes (mA), and seconds (s) were adjusted based on trial and error testing until angiograms with optimal exposure, contrast, and detail were obtained. The radiographs were taken from a standardized table-to-cassette height of 102 cm (40.8 inches).

The lead oxide–gelatin injection technique is an inexpensive angiographic tool characterized by excellent vascular perfusion, a high degree of radiopacity, ease of dissection of the vascular structures, and relatively simple, straightforward preparation. As a result, this technique has allowed very clear identification of each of the vascular perforators to the skin and the ability to relate these to the peripheral nerves and underlying muscular, fascial, and bony structures. The modifications that we have made to the technique appear to have improved the angiographic detail that can be obtained.[33] The industrial-strength gelatin yields a stronger and more viscous mixture, which is very useful as both a carrier and a stabilizer for the liquid lead oxide. It is easier to obtain a uniform solution. We have reduced the amount of lead oxide to 100 g/100 ml of gelatin solution, which reduces the toxicity. We have reduced the temperature of the preparation of the injectate to 40° C (104° F) to reduce the volatility of the lead oxide. It is important to maintain the gelatin concentration in injectate above 5%, or the solution will be too dilute to allow gel formation. Floating the cadaver in a 40° C water bath during injection improves the injection of blood vessels over pressure points and reduces the number of unfilled vessels.

Vascular Injection Technique and Radiography

Injection studies are carried out as soon as possible after the cadaver is available. The cadaver is warmed before it is injected with lead oxide. Measurements and photographs are taken. Bony landmarks are labeled with lead wire before digital photographs are taken. After the cadaver is injected through the femoral vessels, plain radiographs and a CT scan of the whole cadaver are obtained to plan a dissection approach. The overlapping vessels of a whole-cadaver radiograph create a confusing angiogram, with multiple injected vessels in various tissues. Therefore an unrolling technique is used in which the integument is removed and then spread out and radiographed to produce a two-dimensional image of the vascular supply to the tissue.

In our study, to show every arterial chain and the multiple perforators to the integument, different incisions were used in different cadavers or in different limbs of the cadaver. In general, each cadaver was divided into five anatomic regions: (1) head and neck, (2) upper extremity, (3) trunk, (4) perineum, and (5) lower extremity. Photographs were taken at each stage of the dissection, and dissection notes were recorded at each stage. The incisions were made along predetermined anatomic landmarks of the body, and the method used in each cadaver was recorded in the dissection notes. The integument was raised along the deep fascial planes and the site of emergence of cutaneous perforators from the deep fascia was identified with lead beads or surgical clips and noted. Other data collected included the type of perforator (musculocutaneous versus septocutaneous), the muscle of origin of the perforator, the main source vessel, pedicle length, and the diameter of the vessel at the deep fascial level.

Following dissection, the integument was unrolled and mounted on cardboard sheets to maintain its exact dimensions. Then the integument was radiographed. Finally, the muscle and bony structures were radiographed (Fig. 4-3). The lead oxide and gelatin injection technique provided excellent detail during both dissection and angiography (Fig. 4-4). In our original studies, individual radiographs were combined using Photoshop to prepare complete studies of the body (Fig. 4-5). This technique allows a visual overview of the vascular anatomy of the integument; however, it is difficult to use for specific flap planning.

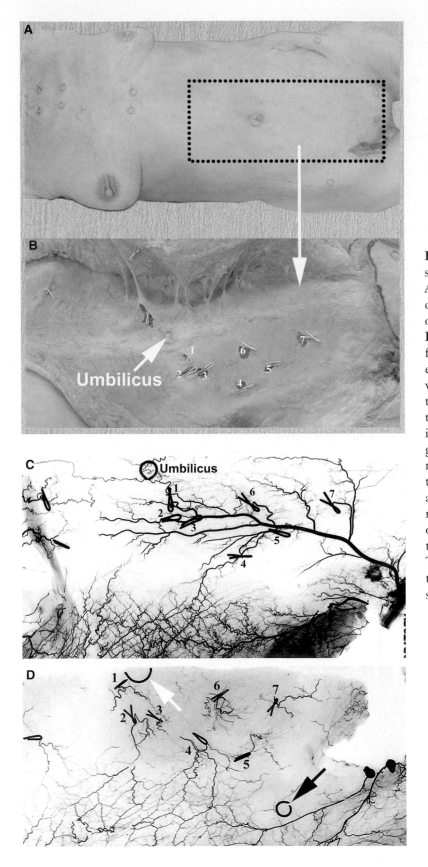

Fig. 4-3   Stages of data collection and source artery analysis of the muscles. **A,** The anterior trunk of a female cadaver is shown after injection with lead oxide through the right femoral artery. **B,** The integument has been elevated from the right side of the abdomen, and each perforator (1-7) has been marked with clips at the point of emergence from the deep fascia. **C,** This angiogram shows the abdominal wall after removal of the integument. Note the point of emergence of the perforators of the deep inferior epigastric artery (1-7), corresponding to perforators in Fig. 4-3, *B*. **D,** This angiogram of the integument, which was removed, shows the cutaneous territory of each musculocutaneous perforator of the deep inferior epigastric artery (1-7). The *white arrow* points to the umbilicus; the *black arrow* indicates the anterior superior iliac spine.

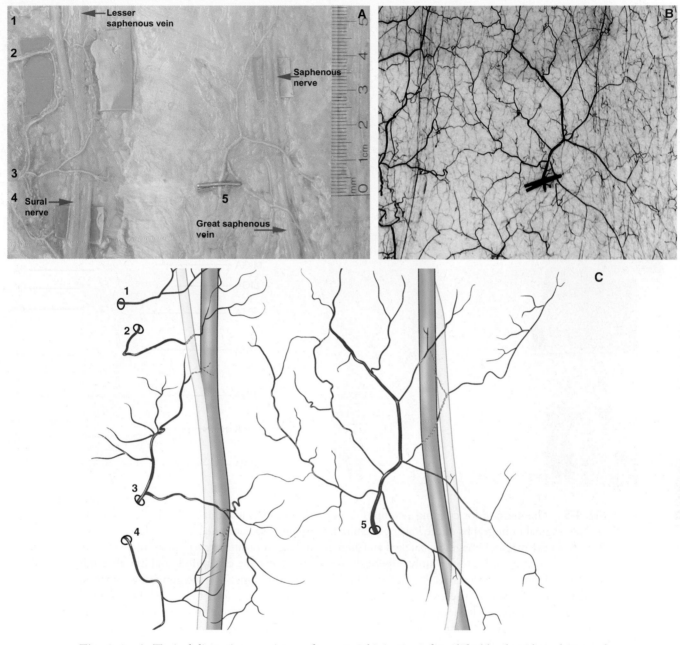

Fig. 4-4   A, Typical dissection specimen after arterial injection of modified lead oxide, gelatin, and water into a fresh whole cadaver. The image shows the medial and posterior aspects of the integument of the right leg with perforators *(1-5).* The great and small saphenous veins and the saphenous and sural nerves run adjacent to the perforators. **B,** This corresponding angiogram of the skin shows the details of the vascular anatomy noted in Fig. 4-4, *A.* Each perforating vessel to the skin is easily identifiable. **C,** This line drawing of the angiogram in Fig. 4-4, *B,* shows selected individual arterial perforators to the skin. Note the fine, reduced-caliber choke anastomotic vessels interconnecting the various perforators. The great and small saphenous veins *(blue)* and saphenous and sural nerves *(yellow)* are also depicted.

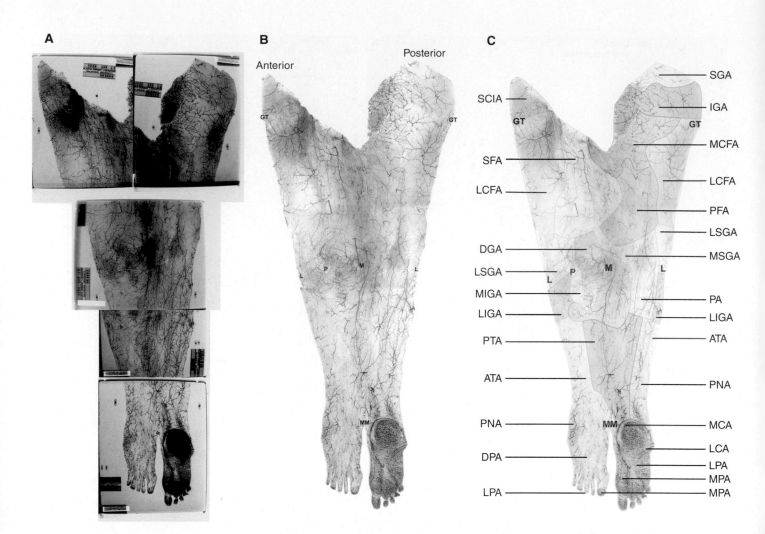

Fig. 4-5   The method for creating a composite angiogram using individual radiographs is shown. **A,** The original radiographs of the lower extremity integument are combined in one Photoshop file. **B,** Each of the original images is matched and aligned, and a composite angiogram is created of the integument of the entire lower limb. Superiorly, incisions followed a circumferential line through the inguinal ligament and across the iliac crest to the posterior midline. The integument was incised along the lateral aspect of the lower limb from the greater trochanter, along the lateral thigh, lateral epicondyle, and lateral malleolus, then along the lateral border of the foot, and finally bisecting the plantar and dorsal surfaces of the foot. **C,** Each territory of the artery was selected, and the *Fill* command was used to paint each one a different color. Using *Stroke Path* on the *Palette* menu, colored borders were placed around territories. The vascular territories of the integument are shown in different colors. (See Chapter 35 for anatomy of the lower extremity. See endpages for the names of vascular territories.) (*GT,* Greater trochanter; *L,* lateral epicondyle; *M,* medial epicondyle; *MM,* medial malleolus; *P,* patella.)

Table 4-2 Radiographic Settings of Various Tissues for Vascular Studies

Tissue	kVp	Tissue	kVp	Tissue	kVp
Integument		**Deep Tissue**		**Bone**	
<1.0 cm thick	44	Head	100-110	Skull	65-70
>1.0 cm thick	46	Neck	85	Spine	65
Muscle		Shoulder and arm	70-80	Scapula	50-55
<1.0 cm thick	44	Elbow and forearm	65	Rib	50
Latissimus dorsi	46	Hand and wrist	55-60	Humerus	60
Trapezius	46	Thorax	80-90	Hand	55-60
Quadriceps	50-55	Abdomen and pelvis	90-100	Pelvis	60
Gastrocnemius	50	Thigh and hip	75	Femur	65
Gluteus maximus	50-55	Knee and leg	70	Tibia	60
		Ankle and foot	65	Fibula	55

mA = 100 and sec = 3/20 for all images.

Radiographic analysis of the deep structures, including muscle and vascular trees, provides information on the source artery and pedicle length of each perforator. To facilitate the radiographic analysis and angiographic process, we developed a table specifying the settings used for each region, depending on the thickness, lead content, and density of tissues being examined (Table 4-2). Because of the limited size of the x-ray film, the integument of each region was radiographed as a series of overlapping angiograms. For each radiograph in a series, the same settings were used to facilitate the end-stage digital processing and combination of radiographic plates. By standardizing our radiographic techniques and settings, we were able to achieve consistent, reproducible results.

Three-Dimensional Anatomic Technique

The lead oxide–gelatin injection technique has allowed very clear identification of each of the vascular perforators to the skin, as well as their relationship to the peripheral nerves and underlying muscular, fascial, and bony structures. However, two-dimensional angiographic images can create confusing superimposed angiograms, which can be difficult to interpret for the purpose of assessing the three-dimensional position and relationship of vessels to other structures.[15,34] More recently, anatomic techniques have included a combination of vascular injection studies and three-dimensional CT to provide the most detailed illustrations of the vascular anatomy of the integument.[34-37]

We have further modified the lead oxide injection technique to optimize three-dimensional angiography and CT images. We combine angiography and Materialise's

Interactive Medical Image Control System (Mimics) (Materialise, Leuven, Belgium) to create a three-dimensional model of the anatomy of the area of interest.[34,37-39] The three-dimensional microvascular images prepared by whole body radiopaque medium injection and processed using the Mimics software package can be used to design a specific flap and trace the entire vascular supply from source vessel to the flap. After the cadaver vascular injection is completed, cadavers are imaged by a CT scanner and the data are transferred to a computer. Mimics interactively reads CT/MRI data in the DICOM format. Segmentation and editing tools allow the user to manipulate data to select the specific tissue type required (for example, bone, soft tissue, skin, or vessels) (Figs. 4-6 and 4-7). Once an area of interest is separated, it can be visualized in three dimensions. After visualization, a file can be made to interface with STL (standard triangulation language) and/or MedCAD data imported as STL files, or it can be visualized in three dimensions for design validation based on the anatomic geometry.[37-39] Surgeon can perform data analysis, plan and simulate surgical procedures, and make critical decisions on approaches to surgery using Mimics software. The degree of detail visible and the ability to select tissue types and regions of interest make this technique a powerful clinical, anatomic, and educational tool.

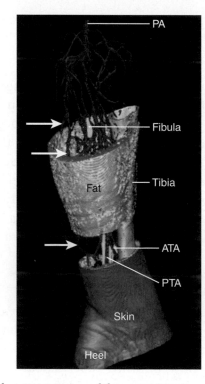

Fig. 4-6   Three-dimensional reconstruction of the posterior view of the leg from a female cadaver lead oxide angiographic injection specimen. The *white arrows* indicate the superficial sural arteries, and the *yellow arrow* points to the ascending branch of the peroneal artery perforator. *ATA,* Anterior tibial artery; *PA,* popliteal artery; *PTA,* posterior tibial artery. (From Tang M, Mao Y, Almutairi K, Morris SF. Plast Reconstr Surg 123:1729-1738, 2009).

The threshold of the data set was manipulated to obtain the best visual image of the vascular anatomy. To show different vascular density, the threshold unit can be adjusted—the lower the threshold, the higher the vascular density (see Fig. 4-7). Other structures such as bone have a density similar to that of the lead-filled arteries (see Fig. 4-7, *A*). Further manipulation physically and/or digitally removed these structures and improved the clarity of the blood vessels. After these procedures, a three-dimensional reconstruction of the vasculature is generated, which can be viewed stereoscopically.

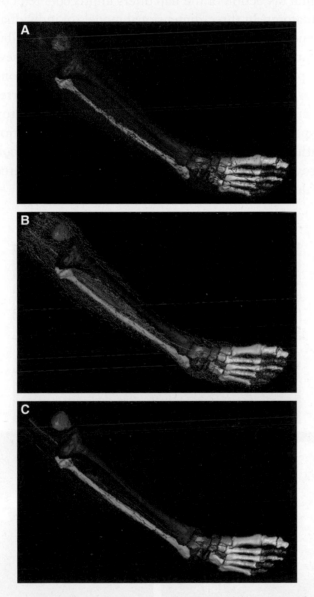

Fig. 4-7 This three-dimensional reconstruction of the leg and foot region from a human cadaver angiographic injection specimen shows the arterial and bony systems using Mimics software. The density of vessels changes with the threshold of the data set. **A**, 1000-3071 HU. **B**, 2000-3071 HU. **C**, 2500-3071 HU.

The same process was repeated for the three-dimensional reconstruction of overlying skin vascular perforators and underlying bone structure. This technique allows visualization of the details of the course of the arteries, their relationship to surrounding structures, and location.

Three-Dimensional Anatomy of Perforator Flaps

Individual perforator flaps can be studied using the three-dimensional CTA technique with Mimics. Digital dissection of the flap offers unprecedented control over the assessment of flap anatomy. In three-dimensional models of individual perforator flaps, it is possible to demonstrate the flap source artery, its course, distribution, and anastomoses with adjacent arteries (Fig. 4-8). Fig. 4-8, *A*, shows the framework of cutaneous perforators of the posterolateral leg. Fig. 4-8, *B*, shows the anastomosis between the deep inferior epigastric artery and superficial inferior epigastric artery. In Fig. 4-8, *C*, the detailed anatomy of the deep inferior epigastric artery perforators is seen through the fascia. A transparent image can be created to show the direction and location of source arteries within each layer of a perforator flap. Using the tools in Mimics, Dynamic Region Growing or Edit Mask in three dimensions, a source artery and each perforator can be delineated.

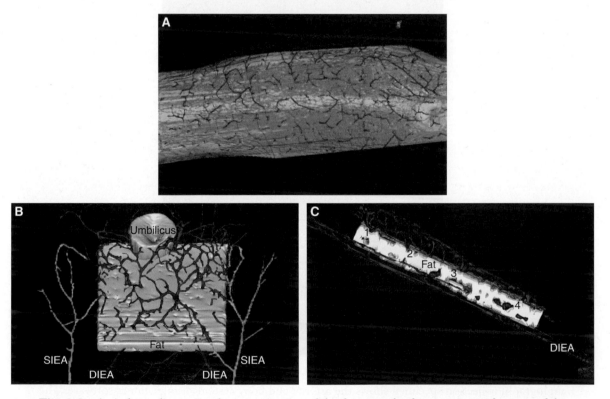

Fig. 4-8   A, A three-dimensional reconstruction of the framework of cutaneous perforators of the posterolateral leg. **B,** This three-dimensional angiogram shows the anastomosis of vessels around the umbilicus. The deep inferior epigastric artery *(DIEA)* and superficial inferior epigastric artery *(SIEA)* anastomose with each other in the periumbilical region. **C,** The deep inferior epigastric artery *(DIEA)* perforator passes through the fascia. *(1-4,* Perforators.)

There are several advantages of three-dimensional reconstruction by Mimics using a whole-cadaver radiographic medium-injection technique:

1. Flap design after whole body angiography and three-dimensional reconstruction is superior to individual flap dissection with isolated injection.
2. Three-dimensional visualization of vascular anatomy by whole body CTA produces a complete data set, so that layer-by-layer information exists to identify the location of an individual source artery with its course, direction, and anastomosis with other vessels. It is therefore very helpful for overall anatomic analysis.
3. This technique allows dissection of the cadaver after three-dimensional reconstruction to ascertain whether the vessels or other structures are correctly shown in the three-dimensional images.
4. After whole body angiographic injection, the arteries are marked by lead oxide in the series of CT images. The image capture, reorganization, and correlation with the microvasculature are therefore very straightforward using the Mimics process.

IMAGE PROCESSING
Digital Image

The cameras and recording media available for modern digital image processing applications are changing at a significant pace. Because most of the images in this chapter were produced using digital technology, we have included a short description of the applicable terminology and technology.

A digital image is represented in digital form as a set of discrete values taken at a regular grid of points called *picture elements*, or *pixels*. These values are transmitted or stored electronically, often in a compressed form. A pixel is one of the many tiny dots that make up the representation of a picture in a computer's memory. As the number of pixels used increases, the image more closely resembles the original. The number of pixels in an image is called the *resolution*. In computer programming, an image composed of pixels is known as a *bitmapped image* or a *raster image*. To obtain illustrations for publication, the pixels per inch of the original image from camera or scanner must be at least 300.

We used a Nikon Coolpix 5000 camera (Nikon, Melville, NY) and Perfection 636U (Epson, Long Beach, CA) scanner for digital image acquisitions. Nikon Coolpix 5000 is a 33× zoom digital camera that has a two thirds–inch type, charge-coupled device (CCD) with 5.0 effective megapixels image size of up to 2560 by 1920 pixels, which can be printed as large as A3 size (297 by 420 mm or 11 by 14 inches).

The Perfection 636U is a professional-quality scanner that can provide maximum hardware resolution of 600 by 2400 dots per inch (dpi). A pixel on the image is composed of several dots. Each 36-bit scan recognizes more then 68 billion colors for accurate color reproduction.

Preparation of Illustrations

Adobe Photoshop (Adobe, San Jose, CA) is a bitmap graphic editor that, with its comprehensive set of applications, including retouching, painting, drawing, and tools, assists with completing any image-editing task. With features such as the History Palette and Editable Layer Effects, we can experiment freely without sacrificing efficiency. We used Photoshop 7.0 to prepare many of the illustrations in this book.

To prepare composite figures consisting of many other figures, the original images are moved and opened in Photoshop. Next a new file is created, and all of the original files are replaced serially into this file (see Fig. 4-5, *A*).

Using the Editable Layers Effects feature, one can work on a single element without disturbing others. To rearrange elements, the order in the Layers Palette is shifted. The layers can be locked to prevent accidental changes, hidden to clearly view the element being worked on, and linked to move them as a group. Layers' opacity can determine to what degree it obscures or reveals the layer beneath it. The layer opacity option is very helpful for image matching and producing a combined-integument angiographic image of the body or a part of the body (see Fig. 4-5, *B*). Tools such as Lasso, Pen, and Convert Point may be used to select each territory of the artery, and the Fill command allows each one to be painted a different color. One can also choose Stroke Path from the Palette menu to paint a colored border around a territory (see Fig. 4-5, *C*). When the content of layers is finalized, the layers can be merged to create partial versions of the composite image. Merging layers also helps manage the size of image files.

The file format, image size, and color mode are then set according to the requirements for publication. For example, figures submitted for publication in the journal *Plastic and Reconstructive Surgery* must meet the following criteria:

- **Format**   Tag Image File Format (TIFF), Encapsulated PostScript (EPS), or PowerPoint (PPT)
- **Minimum width**   40 picas (that is, two landscapes or three portraits across), 30 picas (two portraits across), or 19 picas (for a figure that will be placed in one column). There are 12 points in a pica and 6 picas in an inch; therefore 30 picas equal 5 inches.
- **Color mode**   Cyan-magenta-yellow-black (CMYK) if they are produced digitally

The terms *TIFF, pica,* and *CMYK* represent a file format, unit of type size, and color model, respectively. Briefly, TIFF is a bitmap file format for images that is based on a simple 32-bit uncompressed image used to exchange images between application programs. CMYK is a color model in which all colors are described as a percentage mixture of the colors cyan, magenta, yellow, and black. HSB (hue, saturation, and brightness) and RGB (red, green, and blue) are also common color models.

Although all color and tonal corrections may be performed in either CMYK or RGB color modes, the mode should be carefully selected. Usually the RGB color mode is selected, because it has more advantages. Whenever possible, multiple conversions between modes should be avoided, because color values are rounded and lost with each conversion. If an image must be converted from one mode to another, most tonal and color corrections should be performed in RGB mode, and CMYK mode can be used for fine-tuning. Advantages of working in RGB mode include the following: (1) Performance is improved and memory is saved as a result of working with fewer channels; (2) Device independence is enhanced, because color spaces do not depend on ink; therefore corrections are preserved regardless of the monitor, computer, or output device used; and (3) More colors are preserved after adjustments, because the gamut of RGB spaces is much larger than that of CMYK spaces.

CONCLUSION

Although angiography can define the precise course of arteries and their interconnections with adjacent vessels, it has the major limitation of superimposition because all three-dimensional anatomy is compressed into two dimensions. Thus it can be difficult to determine three-dimensional positions and the relationships of vessels to each other or to other structures. The use of graphic editor software such as Photoshop helps delineate some of these relationships.

Preparing the anatomic information for this chapter has been an interesting exercise in using the best of old and new technologies. There is no substitute for the angiogram. Although we have modified and improved some older techniques, our work would still be familiar to past generations of anatomists. Modern computer-graphic technology and digital imaging help translate three-dimensional dissections into the two-dimensional pages of a book to enhance the reader's understanding of the material. The detailed three-dimensional anatomic information yielded by CTA with Mimics, however, provides a comprehensive anatomic understanding.

References

1. Diener L. Intraosseous phlebography of the lower limb. Postmortem investigation of thrombotic venous disease. Acta Radiol Diagn (Stockh) (Suppl 304):1-96, 1971.
2. Haschek E, Lindenthal OT. Ein beitrag zur praktischen verwertung der hotographie nach rontgen. Wien Klin Wchnschr 9:63-64, 1896.
3. Berberich J, Hirsch S. Die rontgenographische darstellung der arterien und venen im lebenden menschen. Klin Wchnschr 49:2226-2228, 1923.
4. Horton. A study of vessels of the extremities by injection of mercury. Proc Staff Meet Mayo Clin 38:33, 1928.
5. Shehata R. New modifications of Kellner's injection mass. Alexandria Med J 7:603-605, 1961.
6. Kellner CE. A new formula for injecting cadavers. Anat Rec 59:393, 1934.
7. Salmon M. Artères de la Peau. Paris: Masson, 1936.
   Salmon developed a lead oxide and gelatin radiopaque preservative mixture and injected it into cadavers. This mixture avoids staining surrounding tissues and facilitates dissection. It provides radiographs of superb quality, in both contrast and detail, and reveals the arterial framework of entire fresh human cadavers.
8. Taylor GI, Tempest MN, eds. Translation of Salmon M, ed. Artères de la Peau. London: Churchill Livingstone, 1988.
9. Schlesinger MJ. An injection plus dissection study of coronary artery occlusions and anastomoses. Am Heart J 15:528, 1938.
10. Olovson. Beitrag zur Kenntnis der verbindungen zwischen a. Iliaca interna und a. femoralis beim menschen. Acta Chir Scand (Suppl) Stockholm 67, 1941.

11. Epstein J. A method for visualizing the blood vessels of nerves and other tissues. Anat Rec 89:65-69, 1944.

12. Trueta J, Harrison MHM. The normal vascular anatomy of the femoral head in adult man. J Bone Joint Surg Br 35:442-461, 1953.

  The authors' injectate solution was barium sulfate, silver iodide, and latex. This injection medium is characterized by high vascular perfusion, high radiopacity, and high dissectibility, which demonstrates very fine details of the blood supply to the femoral head.

13. Lindbom A. Arteriosclerosis and arterial thrombosis in the lower limb; a roentgenological study. Acta Radiol 80(Suppl):1-80, 1950.

14. Herman PG, Ohba S, Mellins HZ. Blood microcirculation in the lymph node. Radiology 92:1073-1080, 1969.

15. Sedlmayr JC, Witmer LM. Rapid technique for imaging the blood vascular system using stereoangiography. Anat Rec 267:330-336, 2002.

16. Stanley RB Jr. Thorium-dioxide–induced pharyngeal hemorrhage. Am J Otolaryngol 4:437-441, 1983.

17. van Kaick G, Bahner ML, Liebermann D, et al. [Thorotrast-induced liver cancer: results of the German thorotrast study] Radiologe 39:643-651, 1999.

18. Travis LB, Hauptmann M, Gaul LK, et al. Site-specific cancer incidence and mortality after cerebral angiography with radioactive thorotrast. Radiat Res 160:691-706, 2003.

19. Krasinskas AM, Minda J, Saul SH, et al. Redistribution of thorotrast into a liver allograft several years following transplantation: a case report. Mod Pathol 17:117-120, 2004.

20. Schlesinger MJ. New radiopaque mass for vascular injection. Lab Invest 6:1-11, 1957.

21. Nobel W. Observations on the microcirculation of peripheral nerves. Bibl Anat 10:316-320, 1969.

22. Kormano M, Rijonen K. Microangiographic filling of the vascular system of the brain. Neuroradiology 5:83-86, 1973.

23. Cutting CB, McCarthy JG, Berenstein A. Blood supply of the upper craniofacial skeleton: the search for composite calvarial bone flaps. Plast Reconstr Surg 74:603-610, 1984.

24. Shehata R. Radio-opaque modification of Kellner's injection mass. Acta Anat (Basel) 87:461-466, 1974.

25. Rees MJ, Taylor GI. A simplified lead oxide cadaver injection technique. Plast Reconstr Surg 77:141-145, 1986.

  Rees and Taylor combined the PbO form of lead oxide with gelatin to avoid staining surrounding tissues and facilitate dissection. This technique provides radiographs of high quality in both contrast and detail.

26. Quinodoz P, Quinodoz M, Nussbaum JL, et al. Barium sulphate and soft-tissue radiology: allying the old and the new for the investigation of animal cutaneous microcirculation. Br J Plast Surg 55:664-667, 2002.

27. Lerman A, Ritman EL. Evaluation of microvascular anatomy by micro-CT. Herz 24:531-533, 1999.

28. Wan SY, Kiraly AP, Ritman EL, et al. Extraction of the hepatic vasculature in rats using 3-D micro-CT images. IEEE Trans Med Imaging 19:964-971, 2000.

29. Porcel MR, Kidd JG, Smith WE, et al. Altered myocardial microvascular 3D architecture in experimental hypercholesterolemia. Circulation 102:2028-2030, 2000.

30. Bergeron L, Tang M, Morris SF. A review of vascular injection techniques for the study of perforator flaps. Plast Reconstr Surg 117:2050-2057, 2006.

31. Maehara N. Experimental microcomputed tomography study of the 3D microangioarchitecture of tumors. Eur Radiol 13:1559-1565, 2003.

32. WHO Inorganic Health Criteria, EHC 165: Inorganic lead. Geneva: World Health Organization, 1995.

33. Tang M, Geddes CR, Yang D, et al. Modified lead oxide–gelatin injection technique for vascular studies. J Clin Anat 1:73-78, 2002.

34. Tang M, Yin Z, Morris SF. A pilot study on three-dimensional visualization of perforator flaps by using angiography in cadavers. Plast Reconstr Surg 122:429-437, 2008.

    The authors described an anatomic technique that combines angiography and Mimics software to create a three-dimensional model of the anatomy of the area of interest. The intricate vascular details captured by this technique clearly demonstrate the three-dimensional anatomy of the integument, bone, and soft tissue in a layer-by-layer transparent process. It is a powerful, quick, easy method of demonstrating cadaver vascular anatomy that may be useful in the design of surgical flaps.

35. Saint-Cyr M, Schaverien M, Arbique G, et al. Three- and four-dimensional computed tomographic angiography and venography for the investigation of the vascular anatomy and perfusion of perforator flaps. Plast Reconstr Surg 121:772-780, 2008.

36. Rozen WM, Phillips TJ, Ashton MW, et al. Preoperative imaging for DIEA perforator flaps: a comparative study of computed tomographic angiography and Doppler ultrasound. Plast Reconstr Surg 121:9-16, 2008.

37. Tang M, Mao Y, Almutairi K, Morris SF. Three-dimensional analysis of perforators of the posterior leg. Plast Reconstr Surg 123:1729-1738, 2009.

38. Lui KW, Hu S, Ahmad N, Tang M. Three-dimensional angiography of the superior gluteal artery and lumbar artery perforator flap. Plast Reconstr Surg 123:79-86, 2009.

39. Mei J, Yin Z, Zhang J, Tang M, et al. A mini pig model for visualization of perforator flap by using angiography and MIMICS. Surg Radiol Anat 32:477-484, 2009.

5

Instructional Models for Dissection Techniques of Perforator Flaps

Shuji Kayano
Geoffrey G. Hallock
David C. Rice
Masahiro Nakagawa

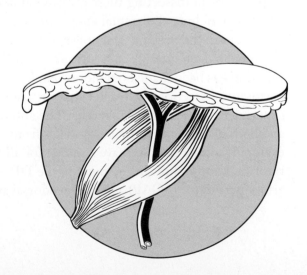

Since the publication of the first edition of this book in 2006,[1] the context of perforator flaps in reconstructive surgery has been transformed from being something of a curiosity to having an integral role in reconstruction. Not only has donor site morbidity been minimized compared with that of its conventional musculocutaneous flap counterpart, because by definition muscle is excluded, but also aesthetic and functional results may even be superior. Yet many surgeons still hesitate to adopt this concept, afraid that technical difficulties such as the tedious intramuscular dissection of the requisite perforators could lead to flap failure.

Perforator dissection requires skills similar to those needed for performing a microanastomosis, which are best learned by repetition using an animal model in the laboratory. Preclinical training in the techniques for harvesting a perforator flap is also best accomplished in the laboratory setting; however, appropriate perforator flap models have lagged somewhat behind clinical experience. Most investigators have studied the rat, because this animal is readily available worldwide, inexpensive, and anatomically reliable.[2-5] Okşar et al[3] showed that 75% of the abdominal skin of a rat will survive if based on only a single perforator of the rectus abdominis muscle. However, their studies were really examples of musculocutaneous flaps, because no intramuscular dissection of the perforator was required, as would be necessary in a "true" perforator flap, according to the definition of Wei et al.[6] For this reason, Hallock and Rice[2] went one step further in dissecting these abdominal perforators through the rectus abdominis muscle to include the cranial epigastric source vessels (CEVs), which, in the rat, are equivalent to the deep inferior epigastric vessels of the human, making this a true model of a human deep inferior epigastric artery perforator (DIEAP) flap. This more difficult variation has been made even more complex by Özkan et al[7] who further fine-tuned the perforator dissection itself, and kept only a short, small-caliber CEV pedicle to create a supermicrosurgical free flap model. The anteromedial thigh model of Rodríguez et al[8] and buttock and lateral thoracic models from Kayano et al[9] complement the preceding examples so that now we have a model for all four of the most commonly used perforator flap donor sites in the human: the DIEAP, anterolateral thigh, superior gluteal artery perforator (SGAP), and thoracodorsal artery perforator (TDAP) flaps (Fig. 5-1).

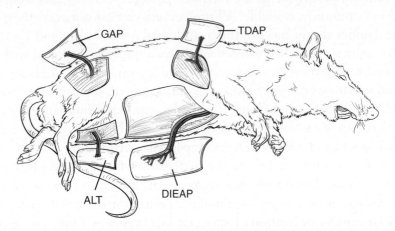

Fig. 5-1   Location of the four basic rat perforator flap models, named according to their human homolog. (*ALT*, Anterolateral thigh flap; *DIEAP*, deep inferior epigastric artery perforator flap; *GAP*, gluteal artery perforator flap; *TDAP*, thoracodorsal artery perforator flap.)

Table 5-1   Basic Rat Muscle Perforator Flap Models in Increasing Level of Difficulty

	Model	Source Artery	Region	Muscle Perforated
1	Anterolateral thigh flap	Common femoral	Medial thigh	Gracilis anterior and posterior
2	Gluteal artery perforator flap	Lateral circumflex femoral	Gluteal	Gluteus superficialis
3	Thoracodorsal artery perforator flap	Lateral thoracic	Lateral thoracic	Cutaneous trunci
4	Deep inferior epigastric artery perforator flap	Deep cranial epigastric	Abdomen	Rectus abdominis

TRAINING METHOD

Before one attempts live human dissections, it is reasonable to obtain sufficient skills in harvesting perforator flaps using a small animal model. At the Shizuoka Cancer Center in Japan, all plastic surgery residents are obliged to complete such a perforator flap training program using rats.[9] Models of the four most commonly used perforator flaps are listed in Table 5-1, according to increasing degree of difficulty. Residents must successfully complete each model before progressing to the next level of complexity.

Some generalized protocols are followed. Sprague-Dawley rats weighing 200 to 250 g are most commonly available. All projects are carried out according to national guidelines and under the auspices of the Institutional Animal Care and Use Committee (IACUC). All animals are administered a general anesthetic, induced with enflurane, and maintained with intramuscular ketamine, chlorpromazine, and glycopyrrolate.

To avoid variations caused by the size of the animal, topographic landmarks are used to mark the chosen flap. In each flap model, one skin boundary is first incised to allow the easiest flap retraction for identifying the desired perforator. Then the remaining skin boundaries can be incised to encompass the perforator.

Because of their diminutive size, the perforator artery is always isolated using an operating microscope. The necessary intramuscular dissection then proceeds carefully through the chosen muscle to the origin of the perforator from the source vessel, with cautious bipolar cautery or ligation of muscular side branches. Once the desired pedicle length is obtained, the dissection is completed. Use as a local or free flap requires the appropriate maneuvering and insetting.

After each surgical procedure, the rats are housed under temperature- and light-controlled laboratory conditions and fed standard rodent chow and water. Flap viability is determined by direct inspection, typically 1 week postoperatively, and is the means of assessing the adequacy of each trainee's work.

Anterolateral Thigh Flap Model[8]
Design (Fig. 5-2)
1. The rat is positioned supine with its limbs stretched outward.
2. A line is drawn along the groin crease, curving medially along the medial thigh.
3. Final boundaries of the flap are determined according to the location of the perforator entering the subcutaneous tissues of the anteromedial thigh.

Dissection
1. A groin incision is made, with retraction of the anteromedial thigh skin distally to expose the perforator, which is seen running within the anterior gracilis muscle.
2. Intramuscular dissection of the perforator is completed back to the common femoral vessel.
3. The remaining boundaries of the flap can be incised about the perforator to make an island flap.
4. The flap is then re-inset to allow evaluation for viability postoperatively.

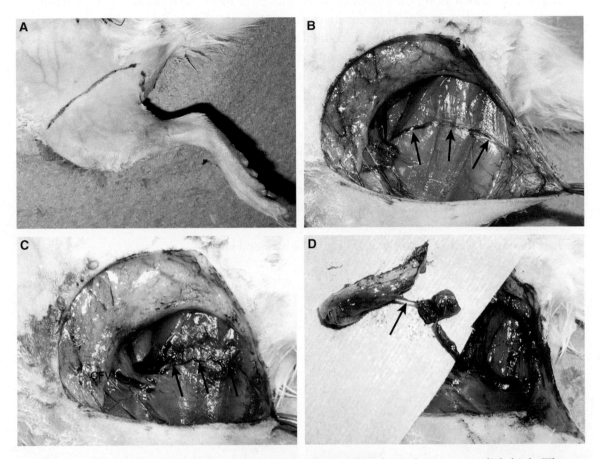

Fig. 5-2 Anterolateral thigh flap model. **A,** The flap is taken from the anteromedial thigh. The superior border is marked along the groin crease *(blue line),* curving medially along the posterior leg. **B,** The skin is incised, and the anteromedial thigh skin is retracted distally to expose the perforator *(arrows)* running over the anterior gracilis muscle. **C,** Intramuscular dissection of the perforator *(arrows)* is completed back to the common femoral vessel *(CFV).* **D,** The island anterolateral thigh flap is based on this solitary perforator *(arrow).*

Gluteal Artery Perforator Flap Model[9]

Design (Fig. 5-3)

1. The rat is positioned with the dorsal side up.
2. A line is drawn along the sulcus between the lower limb and gluteal region, starting adjacent to the anterior superior iliac spine (ASIS), to the midpoint of the tail.
3. A vertical line is drawn along the dorsal midline, beginning from the tail upward.
4. A nearly horizontal line is drawn from the ASIS to the midline.
5. A mirror image flap can be outlined on the contralateral side.

Dissection

1. The caudal border of the flap is incised down to the gluteal muscles.
2. The flap is raised from caudal to cephalad until the desired perforator is seen exiting from the gluteal muscle. These perforators have a relatively wide diameter compared with those in the deep inferior epigastric artery perforator model.
3. Intramuscular dissection is completed back to the source vessel to create an island flap based on a solitary perforator.
4. The flaps are inset to allow viability to be assessed later.

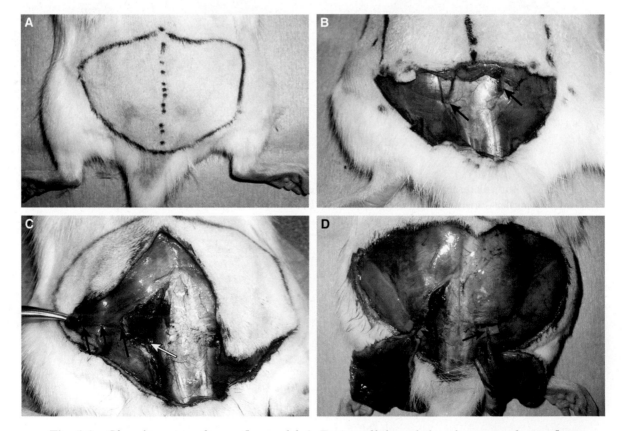

Fig. 5-3   Gluteal artery perforator flap model. **A,** Design of bilateral gluteal artery perforator flaps over the gluteal region. **B,** The caudal side of the flap is incised first and raised cephalad until perforators *(arrows)* are seen arising from the gluteal muscles. **C,** Intramuscular dissection of the left-side perforator *(black arrows)* has been completed to the source vessel *(white arrow).* **D,** The bilateral island perforator flaps are elevated, each on a solitary perforator *(arrows).*

Thoracodorsal Artery Perforator Flap Model[9]

Design (Fig. 5-4)

1. The rat is positioned laterally with the contralateral side down.
2. A line is drawn along the posterior axillary web from the upper limb onto the lateral thorax.
3. Subsequent boundaries of the flap are made as desired to ensure inclusion of the perforator, once it has been identified.

Dissection

1. An incision is made through the posterior axillary web to the level of the underlying cutaneous trunci muscle.
2. The thoracic skin is retracted dorsally to expose the perforator exiting the muscle.
3. The perforator is dissected back to the source vessel as desired.
4. The remaining boundaries of the flap are incised to create an island flap.
5. The flap is inset to allow viability to be assessed later.

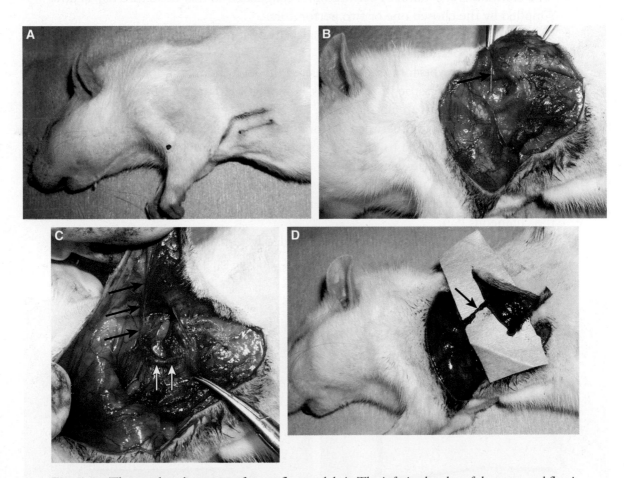

Fig. 5-4 Thoracodorsal artery perforator flap model. **A,** The inferior border of the proposed flap is marked in the lateral thoracic region. **B,** Dissection proceeds from ventral to dorsal until the perforator *(arrow)* is seen arising from the cutaneous trunci muscle. **C,** The intramuscular dissection of the perforator *(black arrows)* to the source vessel *(white arrows)* is completed. **D,** The remaining borders of the flap are incised to create an island flap based on a solitary perforator *(arrow).*

Deep Inferior Epigastric Artery Perforator Flap Model[2]
Design (Fig. 5-5)

1. The rat is positioned supine with its limbs stretched outward.
2. A rectangle is made, beginning with a line drawn from ASIS to ASIS as the inferior border.
3. A line parallel to the inferior border is drawn just inferior to the xiphoid and costal margin and will be the upper border of the rectangle.
4. Lines perpendicular to the ASIS are drawn to connect the parallel horizontal lines.

Dissection

1. Lateral and inferior flap borders are incised through the panniculus carnosus.
2. The flap is raised from lateral to medial, with minimal, sharp dissection through the loose areolar plane until a vertical array of rectus abdominis perforators is seen.
3. The largest one or two perforators are chosen over one hemiabdomen near the upper border of the flap.
4. The contralateral column of perforators is coagulated so that the entire flap is now supplied by the chosen one or two perforators.
5. To simplify perforator dissection, a small cuff of anterior rectus sheath is incised to encircle the perforator.
6. The perforator or perforators are dissected through the rectus abdominis muscle until the cranial epigastric vessels (CEVs, homologous to the deep inferior epigastric vessels in the human) are encountered.
7. The CEVs are dissected between perforators to join their common origin.
8. The CEVs are dissected toward the costal margin, staying lateral to the xiphoid, to lengthen the pedicle as needed.
9. The CEV distal to the last perforator is ligated to make this an island flap.
10. The rectus abdominis muscle and anterior rectus fascia are closed directly below the cutaneous flap.
11. The flap is inset onto the abdomen, if intended to remain as a local flap.

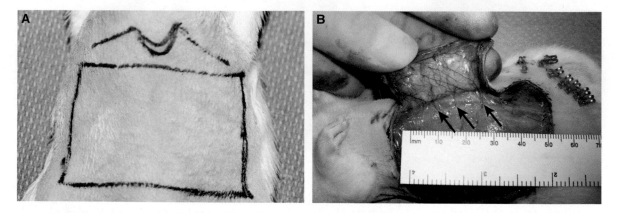

Fig. 5-5 Deep inferior epigastric artery perforator flap model. **A,** A rectangle is marked on the abdomen. **B,** The lateral border of the flap is retracted, and multiple perforators (*arrows*) can be seen arising in a vertical array through the anterior rectus sheath.

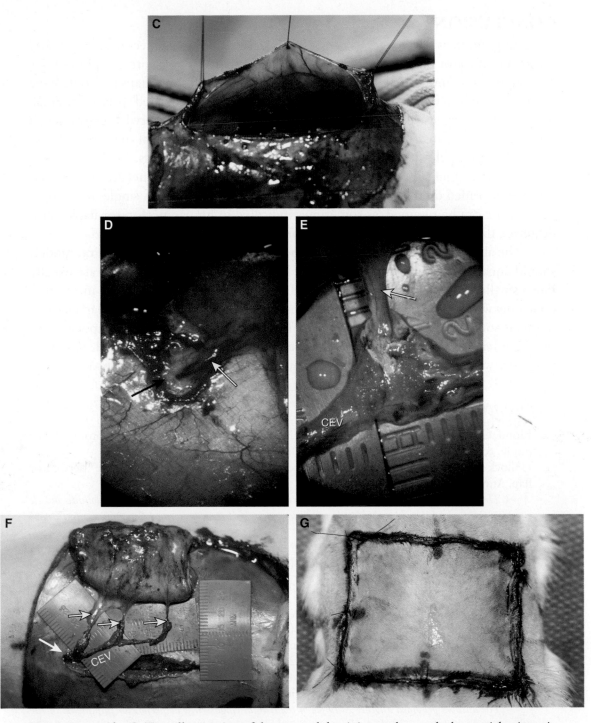

Fig. 5-5, cont'd   C, Transillumination of the rectus abdominis muscle reveals the cranial epigastric vessel running in the middle, near its undersurface (the head is to the right). **D,** A cuff of fascia *(black arrow)* around the perforator *(yellow arrow)* facilitates its handling. **E,** Intramuscular dissection of the perforator *(yellow arrow)* has been completed back to the cranial epigastric source vessel *(CEV)*. **F,** Three perforators *(yellow arrows)* have been retained with this flap, still attached to the cranial epigastric pedicle *(CEV)* near the xiphoid *(white arrow)*. **G,** The inset perforator flap is viable.

CONCLUSION

A training model is advantageous not only for learning how to dissect perforators and create a perforator flap, but also as a means for further research into the physiology, hemodynamics, and other biologic characteristics of perforator flaps.[10-15] Rats have been found to be a very useful model for perforator flaps, as dedicated space is minimal, maintenance inexpensive, and availability universal. Most microsurgery laboratories with the necessary fine instruments and operating microscopes essential to perform these procedures probably already have a vivarium to house these animals.

It is convenient that the four common perforator flaps that need to be learned can be performed on the same rat. Depending on the flap model, a single or multiple perforators can be retained, as sometimes indicated in human perforator flaps. With dexterity, the operating time should be approximately 1 hour per flap model.

The ability to successfully perform a perforator flap using any of these rat models should equate to a similar capability in the human, because rat perforators are usually much smaller and more difficult to dissect. In humans, these procedures are most often done only with loupe magnification. Trainees must remember that the vascular anatomy in rats is somewhat different than that in humans, so that a complete extrapolation of this experience is not possible. Details of these differences must be mastered separately, hopefully with the assistance of the remaining pertinent chapters in this text.

References

1. Blondeel PN, Morris SF, Hallock GG, Neligan PC, eds. Perforator Flaps: Anatomy, Technique, & Clinical Applications. St Louis: Quality Medical Publishing, 2006.

2. Hallock GG, Rice DC. Cranial epigastric perforator flap: a rat model of a "true" perforator flap. Ann Plast Surg 50:393-397, 2003.
    The actual intramuscular dissection of musculocutaneous perforators of the rectus abdominis muscle in a rat model clarified why this deep inferior epigastric artery perforator flap congener is a "true" perforator flap model.

3. Okşar HS, Coşkunfrat OK, Özgentaş HE. Perforator-based flap in rats: a new experimental model. Plast Reconstr Surg 108:125-131, 2001.

4. Coşkunfrat OK, İslamoğlu K, Özgentaş HE. Posterior thigh perforator-based flap: a new experimental model in rats. Ann Plast Surg 48:286-291, 2002.

5. Özkan Ö, Coşkunfrat OK, Özgentaş HE. A new experimental flap model: free muscle perforator flap. Ann Plast Surg 51:603-606, 2003.

6. Wei FC, Jain V, Suominen S, et al. Confusion among perforator flaps: what is a true perforator flap? Plast Reconstr Surg 107:874-876, 2001.

7. Özkan Ö, Koshima I, Gonda K. A supermicrosurgical flap model in the rat: a free true abdominal perforator flap with a short pedicle. Plast Reconstr Surg 117:479-485, 2006.
    The authors provided another example of the cranial epigastric true perforator flap model in the rat. They skeletonized the perforator and included only a short segment of the source vessel. The small-caliber pedicle of these, as free flaps, would be ideal for teaching supermicrosurgery skills.

8. Rodríguez A, Álvarez A, Aguirrezabalaga J, et al. The anteromedial thigh flap as a training model of a perforator flap in rat. J Reconstr Microsurg 23:251-255, 2007.

9. Kayano S, Nakagawa M, Nagamatsu S, et al. Why not perforator flap training models in rats? J Plast Reconstr Aesthet Surg 63:e134-e135, 2010.

    This correspondence extolled the virtues of perforator flap models in rats as an essential means for resident training in this concept. Two new rat flap models equivalent to the gluteal artery perforator or thoracodorsal artery perforator flap in humans were also introduced.

10. Hallock GG, Rice DC. Comparison of TRAM and DIEP flap physiology in a rat model. Plast Reconstr Surg 114:1179-1184, 2004.

11. Coşkunfrat OK, Okşar HS, Özgentaş HE. Effect of the delay phenomenon in the rat single-perforator-based abdominal skin flap model. Ann Plast Surg 45:42-47, 2000.

12. Hallock GG, Rice DC. Efficacy of venous supercharging of the deep inferior epigastric perforator flap in a rat model. Plast Reconstr Surg 116:551-555, 2005.

13. Demir A, Acar M, Yldz L, et al. The effect of twisting on perforator flap viability: an experimental study in rats. Ann Plast Surg 56:186-189, 2006.

14. Demirtas Y, Ayhan S, Findikcioglu K, et al. Selective percutaneous desiccation of the perforators with radiofrequency for strategic transfer of angiosomes in a sequential four-territory cutaneous island flap model. Plast Reconstr Surg 119:1695-1706, 2007.

15. Seyhan T, Deniz M, Borman H, et al. Comparison of two different vascular delay methods in a rat cranial epigastric perforator flap model. Ann Plast Surg 64:89-92, 2010.

6

Preoperative Planning

Jaume Masia
Carmen Navarro Coll
Juan A. Clavero Torrent
Phillip N. Blondeel

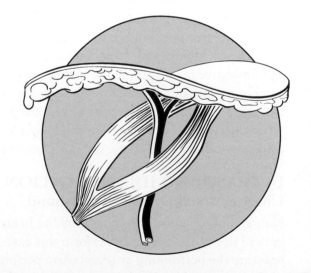

The Aim of Preoperative Imaging

The deep inferior epigastric artery perforator (DIEAP) flap has acquired wide popularity in breast reconstruction since it was first introduced in the 1990s. It provides fat and skin with characteristics that are very similar to those of normal breasts. Furthermore, donor site morbidity is minimized, because there is less injury to the rectus abdominis muscle.

A key point in breast reconstruction with a DIEAP flap is choosing the best supplying perforator, and several factors should be kept in mind when doing so. The ideal perforator vessel should have a large caliber, a short intramuscular course, the easiest dissection, a suitable location within the flap, and subcutaneous branching following the axial direction of the flap. After working with perforator flaps for almost 20 years, we can attest that perforator vessels vary greatly in location, intramuscular route, and distribution within the flap. We can find several different patterns. In some cases we may encounter a perforator with a very tedious intramuscular dissection, whereas others may have only a single perforator for the entire abdominal area.

Perforator vessels arising from their axial vessels are highly variable in number, location, caliber, and relationship with surrounding structures. Therefore a reliable method is needed to accurately locate and identify the dominant perforator before surgery. This can be achieved through preoperative anatomic images that provide information about vascularization of superficial tissues such as fat and skin. For example, for the lower abdomen, precise imaging can help us determine which hemiabdomen to raise, differentiate between superficial and deep epigastric vessels, and combine two or more perforator vessels when there is no dominant vessel. Precise imaging helps plan the operative technique, reduce operating time, and improve operative outcomes.[1] Without a preoperative investigation, the surgeon may not be aware of previous surgical damage, scar formation, or anatomic variants. Using preoperative imaging techniques to study the epigastric vessels, we have decreased the number of postoperative complications. An accurate preoperative evaluation with easy-to-interpret images of the vascular anatomy is extremely valuable for plastic surgeons, because it facilitates safer and faster procedures.

ULTRASOUND IDENTIFICATION
Unidirectional Doppler Ultrasound

Handheld Doppler ultrasonography has been in use since the early days of microsurgery in the 1970s. Surgeons perform this easy-to-use, relatively inexpensive technique to locate the perforating arteries before perforator flap elevation; it is the method most commonly employed to locate an individual vessel before surgery.[2] However, correlation between the audible volume of the signal and the diameter of the perforator vessel is poor and often imprecise. It offers only a limited amount of information and cannot distinguish perforator vessels from main axial vessels. Additionally, it does not provide any data on the perforator vessel's course, because the information is given as an acoustic signal. The number of false-positives is high, reaching 47% in one series. The value of Doppler sonography in this setting is therefore questionable. This technique may also be too sensitive, because even minuscule vessels that are not large enough to support a perforator flap can be selected for abdominal perforator surgery. If the perforator course from the exit point of the muscle fascia to the surface of the skin (through the subcutaneous fat) is not roughly perpendicular to the skin, Doppler localization of the perforator will be incorrect. Despite these drawbacks, handheld Doppler ultrasound remains useful in our daily practice and helps assess the course of the superficial epigastric vessels.

Color Doppler Imaging

Color Doppler imaging is performed with a color Doppler instrument, which presents gray-scale imaging in conjunction with color Doppler imaging. Gray-scale imaging provides anatomic information about muscles and bony landmarks. This diagnostic tool can help the surgeon locate main arterial and venous branches as well as perforators. Color Doppler imaging provides information about (1) the presence or absence of blood flow to allow localization of blood vessels, (2) the flow direction—toward or away from the probe, (3) the flow pattern—arterial or venous, and (4) the blood flow velocity. Doppler imaging is particularly useful for locating and qualitatively evaluating transmuscular perforator vessels, which are important for perforator flap reconstructive surgery.

Because most perforators lie in the subcutaneous tissue or subcutaneous fat layer, the ultrasound examination should be performed with a high-frequency linear-array probe. Usually a multifrequency (5 to 7.5 to 10 MHz) or broadband (5 to 10 MHz or 5 to 12 MHz) linear-array probe is used. Color Doppler settings are adjusted for maximal blood flow sensitivity. These settings include a low-wall filter (50 to 100 Hz), a pulse repetition frequency of 1000, maximum power, and the highest possible gain at a usable ratio of signal-to-background noise.

The position and flow of superficial vessels can be investigated with unidirectional Doppler flowmetry using a 5 or 8 MHz Doppler pencil probe. This is a handy, inexpensive, and operator-friendly probe that can be used intraoperatively. When looking for perforators, the area of interest is explored holding a Doppler probe perpendicular to the skin. When a Doppler signal is detected, the position of the probe is adjusted until the signal of maximum intensity is obtained. A perforator can be suspected in this location, running in the direction of the ultrasound beam.

Despite its ease of use, unidirectional Doppler flowmetry provides far less anatomic and hemodynamic information than a color Doppler instrument, and the number of false-positive and false-negative signals may be high. False-positive signals may be caused by interference from underlying axial vessels running superficially and parallel to the skin surface. Additionally, perforators can run parallel to and just above or below the deep fascia before piercing it. False-negative signals may be caused by imprecise execution, including using the wrong frequency, the applying excessive pressure over the perforator, and other factors that temporarily reduce blood flow, such as vasocon-striction and low blood pressure. A thicker panniculus requires a lower frequency (for example, 5 MHz), and thinner layers need a higher frequency (up to 10 MHz).

Color duplex imaging offers many advantages for perforator flap reconstruction. This procedure provides more qualitative and quantitative information than unidirectional Doppler flowmetry. Color Doppler investigation provides extremely accurate information about donor and recipient vessels. Deeper axial vessels can be identified, their three-dimensional course through the septum or muscle can be determined, and the position at which the perforator pierces the fascia and deep fascia can be localized precisely. The surgeon can intimately follow the course of the perforator either below or above the fascia. After the perforator has pierced the deep fascia, the exact size of the artery and vein and the number of branches above the deep fascia can be determined. With this technique, the direction of the flow of side branches can be visualized, an important consideration for flap design. Color Doppler investigation has a 100% positive predictive value and a very low number of false-negative results. Finally, color duplex imaging enhances the surgeon's ability to diagnose vascular diseases and predict vascular abnormalities following previous trauma surgery.

The most important advantage of preoperative color duplex imaging is that it saves time in the operating room. Information obtained preoperatively regarding vascular anatomy and physiology may reduce operating time by 30 to 60 minutes by allowing the surgeon to prepare a reliable plan. The surgeon feels more confident about the procedure. Unpleasant intraoperative surprises are avoided. Reduced expensive operating time compensates for the additional cost of the investigation. Postoperative complications such as fat necrosis and partial flap necrosis can be avoided by selecting the appropriate perforator preoperatively. Information about recipient vessels is as important as information about perforators, and this investigation provides both.

Color duplex imaging also has disadvantages. Compared with the conventional unidirectional Doppler modality, color duplex imaging is more time consuming and more expensive. The high cost of this technique may prohibit its use in other countries, depending on their health care system. Color duplex imaging requires a certain amount of experience to handle the device appropriately to obtain optimal data. The operator must have an exact knowledge of the three-dimensional vascular anatomy of the specific region. To enhance this knowledge, we encourage our colleagues to observe surgeries. The ability to appropriately interpret visual feedback and identify the most relevant anatomic structures is essential for the operator. Less-experienced surgeons can develop these skills by observing and interpreting duplex investigations and providing feedback regarding the surgical plan. It is impossible to obtain an exact measurement of vessel diameter and flow using color duplex imaging. Some operators record rough estimations of vessel caliber and flow velocity, whereas others use semiquantitative symbols such as +, ++, and +++.

Vessels are constantly influenced by nervous and humoral stimuli and are thus dynamic. For example, a patient's blood pressure affects blood flow within vessels. Therefore stress or relaxation experienced during a preoperative color duplex investigation may affect results. Because of these fluctuations, the surgeon should not look for vessels with a minimum size or flow velocity. Rather, the largest vessel in the area under consideration should be chosen for flap reconstruction.

Despite the advantages of preoperative color duplex investigation, not all patients are able to undergo this procedure for various reasons. The patient's resources may be limited. For some patients, the interval between the diagnosis and surgery is too short. This may be true for trauma patients and some patients undergoing primary breast reconstruction.

MULTIDETECTOR-ROW COMPUTED TOMOGRAPHY

Since the beginning of this century, technical developments in multidetector-row helical computed tomography (MDCT) have dramatically changed the use of CT angiography in assessing vascular pathologies.[5,6] The simultaneous acquisition of multiple, thin collimated slices in combination with enhanced gantry rotation speed offers thin-slice coverage of extended volumes with extremely high spatial resolution. MDCT has proved very useful not only in evaluating the aorta and peripheral arteries, but also as a promising noninvasive technique for detecting, visualizing, and characterizing stenotic coronary artery disease. It is helpful in evaluating the coronary vessels for luminal size, patency, and sites of occlusions.[7,8] From this application emerged the idea of studying perforator vessels with MDCT, a more reliable method for precisely localizing the most suitable vessels.[5-9]

MDCT enables rapid scanning of large areas of interest (such as an entire abdomen) and produces images of excellent quality with very thin sections and low-artifact rating. Images obtained using MDCT have extremely good resolution, which facilitates visualization of perforators. This emerging technology has greatly enhanced our ability to study the lower abdominal wall.

In 2002 we started using the Sixteen Multidetector-Row Helical CT (Aquilion 16; Toshiba Medical Systems, Tokyo, Japan). Currently, our MDCT studies are performed using a 64 or 320 detector-row CT scanner (Toshiba Medical Systems) (Fig. 6-1). This is a special CT system equipped with a multiple-row detector array that has improved the volume coverage speed of the scanner. We use the following parameters: 120 kVp, 80 to 120 mAs (0.4 sec gantry rotation period), detector configuration 64 by 0.5 mm, 54 mm table travel per rotation, 512 by 512 matrix, and a 180 by 240 mm field of view. All scanning is performed during IV administration of 100 ml of nonionic iodinated contrast medium with a concentration of 300 mg L/ml (Xenetix 300 [iobitridol]; Guerbet, Paris, France). The contrast material is mechanically injected (Missouri XD 2001; Ulrich GmbH, Ulm, Germany) at a rate of 4 ml/sec through an 18-gauge IV catheter inserted into an antecubital vein.

The patient is positioned on a CT table exactly as he or she will be positioned for surgery. Axial and perforator vessels of both the donor and the recipient area can be investigated by MDCT. Sections are obtained from 5 cm above the umbilicus to the lesser trochanter of the hip while the patient's breath is held for approximately 10 to 12 seconds. Acquisition takes about 3 to 4 seconds. Some centers scan down from the

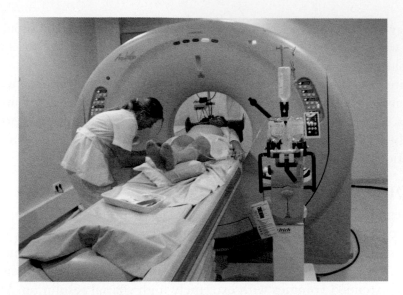

Fig. 6-1   Multidetector-Row Helical CT Aquilon 16 (Toshiba Medical Systems).

clavicle to include the internal mammary artery and vein. The entire procedure takes less than 10 minutes and is therefore very well tolerated by the patient. The volumetric data acquired are then used to reconstruct images with a slice width of 1 mm and a reconstruction interval of 0.8 mm. The resulting complete set of reconstructed images is automatically transferred to a computer workstation (Vitrea version 4.0.1, Vital Images, Plymouth, MN), which generates the reformatted images in multiple planes (coronal, axial, sagittal, and oblique) and three-dimensional volume-rendered images. This system allows measurements to be taken so that different planes of space can be automatically correlated. Data can be stored on a pen drive (e-Film Medical, Toronto, Ontario, Canada) that is easy to use and manage on a standard computer and can be viewed as often as needed.[10]

We validated the technique in the study conducted in 2003 and published in 2006. We raise the flaps while simultaneously identifying and inspecting all perforators. This allows us to compare the intraoperative findings with previous MDCT results to study the validity of the anatomic information from MDCT. When we compared MDCT results with intraoperative findings, neither false-positive nor false-negative results were obtained.

This technique also facilitates visualization of certain perforator variants, such as paramuscular or extramuscular variants, as described previously in anatomic cadaveric studies[11] (Fig. 6-2). Before preoperative studies with imaging techniques were performed, these paramuscular perforators were difficult to identify in the operating room because of their medial location, and a more lateral perforator was usually selected. Paramuscular perforators have a medial location and, typically, an extramuscular course, making them easier to dissect. With their excellent caliber, they are likely the ideal perforator.[10]

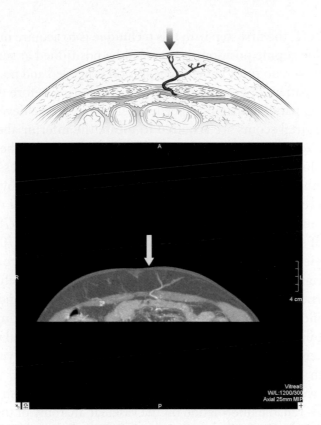

Fig. 6-2 Axial MDCT image of a medially located paramuscular perforator branching to both the ipsilateral and contralateral side. The *arrow* indicates the point where the perforator arises from the fascia.

NONCONTRAST MRI

In 2005 we began to investigate MRI for abdominal perforator mapping, because this technique does not require radiation. Over the following 3 years, we worked with several MRI applications, all of which needed a contrast injection to obtain a good-quality image of the perforator vessels.

During our investigation our attention was drawn to methods used to study renal tumors with noncontrast MRI. This technique allowed good visualization of the vessels, without contrast. We began to consider the possibility of using the same sequence for preoperative perforator mapping of the abdominal wall in women undergoing breast reconstruction with a DIEAP flap after mastectomy.

We then started working with Toshiba engineers to improve the image acquisition sequence. We switched to a new MR angiography technique of fresh blood imaging (FBI) with a Toshiba ZGV Vantage ATLAS 1.5 T system with an ultrashort bore (Toshiba Medical Systems). This technique accurately locates the dominant perforator, providing good definition of its intramuscular course and excellent evaluation of the superficial inferior epigastric system. We were also able to define the perforator branching within the subcutaneous abdominal tissue and evaluate the vascular connections between the superficial and the deep inferior epigastric vessels.

As with MDCT, the first step with this technique is to acquire multiplanar images with patients in the supine position, as they will be positioned at surgery. In contrast with MDCT, however, no prior patient preparation is needed and no contrast medium is required, so the patient does not require 6 hours of fasting before image acquisition. We use high-speed parallel imaging (speeder technology) to achieve accelerated scan times. Initially, sagittal scouts are acquired to locate the inferior abdominal wall and delimit the study zone. A sequence phase 3D+5_FSfbi is used in the anterior coronal plane with the following parameters: TR:2694, TE:80, slice thickness 1.5 mm, number of slices: 50, number of acquisition: one, 512 by 512 matrix, 380 by 380 mm field of view, TI:160, and resp + ECG gate. A sequence phase 3D+5_FSfbi is then performed in the axial plane with the following parameters: TR:2900, TE:78, slice thickness 3 mm, number of slices: 56, number of acquisition: one, 704 by 704 matrix, 380 by 380 mm field of view, TI:160, and resp + ECG gate. The anterior coronal plane phase includes only the anterior abdominal wall, from a plane immediately below the pubis to the xiphoid process of the sternum. The axial plane phase includes the area from the infrapubic zone to 3 cm above the umbilicus. The acquisition time ranges from 10 to 20 minutes. Multiplanar formatted images and three-dimensional volume-rendered images are regenerated on a Vitrea computer workstation (Vitrea version 4.0.1.; Vital Images, Plymouth, MN).

In the study we conducted between 2007 and 2009,[13] we demonstrated that noncontrast MRI provides reliable information on the vascular anatomy of the abdominal wall. Imaging results were compared with the intraoperative clinical findings in all patients. Preoperative MRI without contrast showed no false-positive or false-negative results.

PREOPERATIVE PERFORATOR SELECTION AND LOCALIZATION

The images obtained are usually interpreted by both the radiologist and the plastic surgeon who will harvest the flap. The team chooses the perforator considered the most suitable according to the following criteria: largest caliber, arborization, best location, shortest intramuscular course, and intraflap axiality. A nearby fixed anatomic point (bony prominences, umbilicus, fixed creases) is used as a reference to give coordinates on an x,y axis. For the abdomen, the location of perforator selected corresponds to a pair of x,y coordinates based on an axial system centered on the umbilicus, and the flap can be raised based on the dominant perforator. The surgeon is given three types of image: axial, sagittal, and coronal. The axial views and sagittal reconstructions are helpful for assessing the perforator's dependence on the main trunk or any direct branch of the deep inferior epigastric artery and for delimiting its origin on the fascia and its distribution through subcutaneous fat and skin. Rendered reconstructions allow us to mark on the patient's skin the exact point where the perforator vessel emerges through the fascia of the rectus abdominis muscle.

Image Assessment
Axial View

In the axial view, we study the course of the deep inferior epigastric artery, from its origin, through the muscle, to 5 cm cranial to the umbilicus. The two or three best

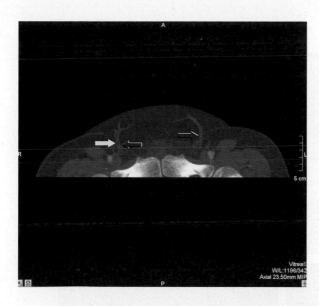

Fig. 6-3 Axial MDCT image of the superficial inferior epigastric vessels arising from the femoral artery and vein. The *yellow arrow* indicates the right superficial inferior epigastric artery and the *magenta arrows* indicate the bilateral superficial veins.

perforators are typically identified on each side of the abdomen, marked with an arrow, and classified according to their external caliber into three categories (small, medium, and large). At the suprafascial level we assess the perforator branching in the subcutaneous tissue. We evaluate the intramuscular course of the deep inferior epigastric artery and define its relationship to the tendinous intersections and the number of branches. We also study the superficial epigastric system and note the caliber of the artery at its origin. In our experience, a vessel size of 0.6 mm or larger can potentially be used for raising an SIEA flap if it has a medial distribution on the abdomen (Fig. 6-3). When we choose the best perforator in the imaging technique, we look for the point where it pierces the fascia in the axial view and mark an arrow on the skin at this level. From there on, the arrow will appear in all views. A coordinate x,y axis is drawn on the umbilicus, and the exit of the perforating vessel in relation to the umbilicus is measured. First, we measure the distance from the midline to the perforator in the axial view, and this is given the value x.

Sagittal View

We evaluate the sagittal view to double check the quality of the chosen perforators and to place them in three planes. The second measurement, from the umbilicus level to the exit of the perforator, is recorded. This will be the y value. We also assess the interconnections between the superficial and deep systems.

Three-Dimensional View

A three-dimensional reconstruction of the abdomen is undertaken to precisely locate the points on the skin surface where the three best perforators emerge from the fascia of the rectus abdominis muscle. Using a virtual coordinate system with the umbilicus at the center, all information is transferred to a data form sheet so that the perforators are mapped in a format that allows us to transpose their position preoperatively onto the patient's abdominal skin. By transferring these values from the computer to paper, we locate the exact point where we will find the perforator when raising the flap (Fig. 6-4).

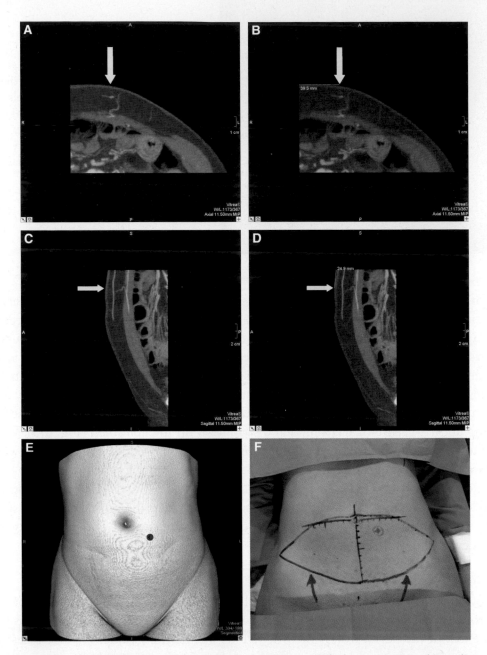

Fig. 6-4   **A,** Axial MDCT image of the chosen perforator. (The *arrows* in **A** and **B** indicate the point at which the perforator arises from the muscle.) **B,** We measure the distance from the midline to the perforator in the axial view, and this is assigned the value *x*. **C,** Sagittal MDCT image of the chosen perforator. The *arrow* indicates the point where the perforator arises from the muscle. **D,** The second measurement is taken in the sagittal view, from the level of the umbilicus to the perforator's exit. This will be the *y* value. **E,** MDCT three-dimensional reconstruction for the same patient. The *purple dot* is where the perforator pierces the fascia. **F,** Preoperative markings. The *green marking* indicates where the dominant perforator pierces the fascia; *red arrows* indicate the direction of flow by the inferior epigastric vessels.

Coronal View

Before completing the study with the radiologist, we like to review the coronal cuts to visualize the subcutaneous distribution pattern of the superficial inferior epigastric arterial system and assess the connections between the superficial and deep systems (Fig. 6-5).

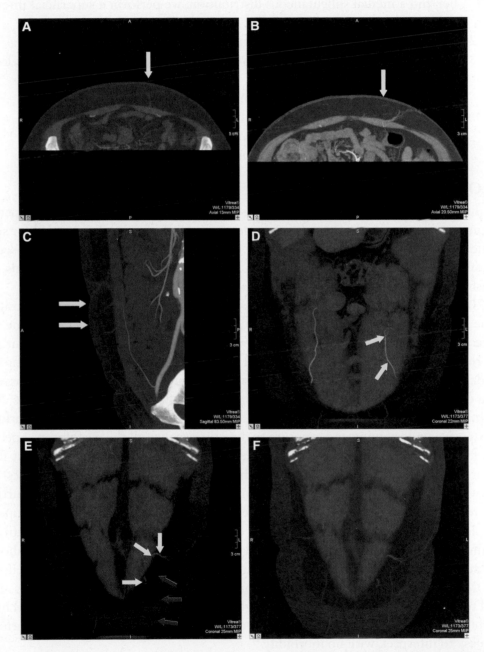

Fig. 6-5 MDCT imaging. **A** and **B,** Axial images of two perforators at different levels in the same patient. The *arrow* indicates the point where the perforators arise from the muscle. **C,** This sagittal view MDCT image shows the deep inferior epigastric system and the intramuscular course of two dominant perforators *(arrows)* branching to the surface and connecting with the superficial system. **D,** Coronal image of the deep epigastric vessels and the exit of the two main perforators *(arrows)*. **E,** Coronal image showing connections of the deep *(yellow arrows)* and superficial *(magenta arrows)* systems. **F,** Coronal image of the abdominal vascular network (superficial layer).

After surgery we always compare the results from the intraoperative findings with the MDCT or the MR images to improve our preoperative decision making for selecting perforators. Our preferred order for selecting the perforator is based on the following considerations:

1. Our first preference is a good superficial system. If the artery has a good caliber and a medial subcutaneous distribution, we perform a superficial inferior epigastric artery flap.
2. Our second option is a good paramuscular perforator if available.
3. If neither of these criteria is valid, we choose an intramuscular perforator, looking for:
   • A direct branch from the deep inferior epigastric vessels
   • A short intramuscular course
   • Location as central as possible within the flap
   • Flap axiality and subcutaneous branching

CHOOSING A TECHNIQUE

Raising a perforator flap requires meticulous dissection of the perforator vessels, sparing the muscle structure with its segmentary motor nerves. Special skill is needed for such surgical dissection, and the intraoperative time is considerable. Because the vascular anatomy of the vascular tree in the human body varies greatly among individuals, establishing a vascular map of each patient before surgery facilitates dissection.

Improving our preoperative planning by identifying the three-dimensional position of the largest perforator included in the flap allows us to reduce both operating time and surgeon stress. The benefits of a shorter operating time thus extend to the patient and also reduce costs and conserve resources. The intraoperative decision of selecting the perforator with the best caliber and position becomes much easier, because the surgeon has a clear overview of all perforators nourishing the flap before the procedure. As a result, valuable time is saved during surgery, because it is no longer necessary to perform an extensive undermining and exposure to directly visualize all the perforators. Specifically for the lower abdominal wall, preoperative planning ensures that any highest-flow perforators that may be on the midline of the abdomen (the pararectal perforators) are not overlooked. Previously the surgeon might have been reluctant to dissect further and would have either settled for a lateral perforator or a TRAM conversion. Preoperative planning also allows us to preserve the contralateral side of the abdomen until the dominant perforator has been selected and completely dissected. The surgeon should be assured that the flap always contains the abdominal perforator with maximal flow.

Many techniques have been used to preoperatively map perforating vessels. The ideal technique should have a low cost, high availability and reproducibility, and high reliability in selecting the dominant perforator. In addition, it should be fast to perform and easy to interpret, with no morbidity.[14]

Since 2003 MDCT has proved highly reliable in preoperative planning of abdominal free flap breast reconstruction, demonstrating excellent results and significantly reduced operative time and complications.[1,12,15,16] Unlike the handheld Doppler and color duplex Doppler ultrasound, it provides anatomic images that are easy to interpret, not only by the radiologist but also by the plastic surgeon. It offers information on the caliber, location, and course of any perforating vessel,[17] specifically between the deep fascia and the skin. Here, resolution of duplex Doppler imaging is too low and only two-dimensional. With the recent development of MDCT, a considerable number of thin-sliced CT images are obtained in a short time. With the 64 and 320 multidetector-row helical CT we can obtain slices with an interval of 0.8 mm. Intravenous contrast medium can be injected at high velocities, and excellent images of the vasculature are obtained. The increased spatial resolution offered by MDCT provides highly accurate multiplanar and three-dimensional reconstructed images. The data are stored on a CD or pen drive, which can easily be used and managed with a standard computer and reviewed as often as necessary. This technique is easily reproducible and fast to perform, thereby minimizing patient discomfort and health care costs as compared with color Doppler imaging. In addition, it provides unique and valuable information for surgical planning.

The main drawbacks of CT are unnecessary radiation to the patient and potential systemic allergic reactions to the intravenous contrast medium. Although patients are exposed to radiation, the effective dose is 5.6 mSv, which is less than that for an opaque enema or conventional abdominal CT scan. The average dose of radiation during exposure is 321 $mGy.cm^2$, which is less than reference doses used for exploring the pelvis and abdomen (570 and 780 $mGy.cm^2$, respectively), approved by the European Union in the document "European Guidelines on Quality Criteria for Computed Tomography."

To avoid the limitations of MDCT, we investigated MRI for preoperative perforator mapping. In 2008 the new image acquisition sequence, obtained with noncontrast 1.5T MR angiography using the fresh blood imaging (FBI) technique, provided a further notable improvement. We could see the perforating vessel's intramuscular course, its anatomic relationship with the surrounding structures, and its branching within the flap in a way that no other technique has allowed so far. Noncontrast 1.5T MRI has proved highly valuable in abdominal perforator mapping. It accurately depicts abdominal wall microcirculation, enabling us to choose the appropriate dominant perforator. According to our intraoperative findings, it provides 100% reliability in selecting the most suitable perforator, as does MDCT. Acquisition time ranges from 10 to 20 minutes. Although this is longer than the acquisition time with MDCT, we consider it acceptable, because patients are not irradiated and intravenous contrast is not needed.

By using imaging techniques to decide preoperatively which perforators are most suitable, we can reduce the amount of stress for the surgeon, who can now proceed directly to the chosen perforator with confidence and ligate the other perforators safely without wasting time. The amount of time saved in the operating room can be balanced against the extra cost of the investigation. These techniques (MRI and CT) also allow us to plan an optimal design for the flap size to include the best vascularized tissue supplied by the dominant perforator (Fig. 6-6). In our 2006 study[1] in which we validated MDCT, fat necrosis and partial flap loss were reduced, because the surgeon was able to choose the optimally vascularized region of abdominal tissue supplied by the dominant perforator. The information provided by this technique is extremely valuable for patients who have had previous surgery in the abdominal area, such as liposuction or a hysterectomy. The high sensitivity, specificity, and the 100% positive predictive value

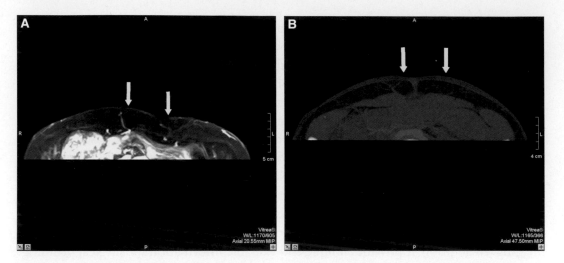

Fig. 6-6 Axial image with two different imaging techniques: **A,** Noncontrast MRI and **B,** MDTC. The *arrows* indicate where the bilateral perforators arise from the muscle.

of this noninvasive and easy-to-interpret preoperative mapping technique have made it a highly promising diagnostic tool for planning DIEAP flaps.

Considerable discussion remains about which technique is best for preoperative study—MDCT or noncontrast MRI. The answer depends on the facilities and logistics of each center, but if the same information is obtained with both techniques, we should use the one with least morbidity. MDCT is mainly indicated in two situations: (1) when it is applicable for oncologic staging and perforator vessel identification and (2) when an extensive CT investigation of large parts of the body is necessary to rule out morphologic abnormalities.

PLANNING PERFORATOR FLAPS AFTER IDENTIFYING THE DOMINANT PERFORATOR

Meticulous preoperative planning is the key to successful reconstructive procedures, including perforator flap surgery. Before beginning surgery, the recipient site is evaluated. Tissues to be replaced are defined and the requirements of the perforator flap delineated. These requirements can follow either the musculocutaneous flap or free-style free flap principles. Following the principles of musculocutaneous flap planning, a perforator flap is designed after the main perforator vessel is selected. The dimensions of the perforator flap are positioned over the vessel. Alternatively, following the free-style free flap principle, a skin flap is selected for its properties (for example, thickness or pliability of tissue over a certain area of the body). After choosing the skin paddle, vessels that provide dominant vascularization of the area are found. Probably the most important difference between these two principles is that for musculocutaneous flaps, the surgeon needs to be willing to adjust the preoperative plan intraoperatively.

Evaluating the Recipient Site

Regardless of the cause of the defect, preoperative evaluation is essential for perforator flap reconstruction. In 80% of reconstructive procedures, it is necessary to cover vital structures with skin and subcutaneous tissue. If the surgeon's philosophy is to replace "like with like," perforator flaps are required in most patients. Before marking the flap at the donor site, the recipient site is carefully examined. The exact area of the required skin paddle, thickness of the subcutaneous layer, and total flap volume are determined. If a large flap is planned, closure of the donor site is also considered. In cases requiring two-dimensional resurfacing (for example, the extremities), the skin surface area of the flap is the most important priority. In other cases (for example, three-dimensional reconstruction of a breast), flap volume and consistency are the most important considerations.

Occasionally, more complex reconstructions need to be offered. Flaps combining different types of tissues such as bone, muscle, nerve, and fascia can often be designed at the donor site, based on one source vessel. Large source vessels with multiple branches such as the thoracodorsal artery, the lateral circumflex femoral artery, and the variable arterial tree in the groin area may be the source of a limitless number of tissue combinations. In contrast to the traditional osteomusculocutaneous flaps and others, the perforator flap principle has an important advantage. Although the same tissues may be harvested, the skin flap is separated from the surrounding tissues based on its own perforator supply to allow a more flexible reconstruction. Bone, nerve, fascia, and muscle are positioned to provide functional, dynamic reconstructions or skeletal support. After completing the deep reconstructions, skin cover is achieved in an orientation that ensures the ideal contour.

Methods of Flap Selection

Basing a Flap on a Known Perforator

During the past few decades, traditional musculocutaneous and fasciocutaneous flaps have been designed over large, well-defined source vessels. Although the size of the defect and the type of tissues required help determine the flap, the preference and experience of each surgeon play a pivotal role in flap selection. These principles can also be applied to perforator flaps; rather than selecting a specific source vessel, the most favorable perforator vessel on which a flap can be designed is chosen. The perforator is centered beneath the skin flap. Following Taylor's angiosome principle,[18] only one adjacent territory should be included to ensure adequate vascularization of the entire flap. We now know from accumulated clinical experience that, in some areas of the body, more than two adjacent territories can be safely included. Both the anatomic features of the vascular tree and the flow physiology of the flap help explain this principle. The choke vessels that open after sympathetic denervation and Poiseuille's law applied to the impedance of flow in tubular structures determine whether a large flap will survive. Therefore systemic blood pressure is probably the most important determinant of vascularity of the entire flap. Although antegrade flow of arterial blood is important to the survival of a perforator flap, venous pressure also plays a major role in maintaining sufficient tissue oxygenation. Pressures acting on the venous system must be appropriate to allow deoxygenated blood to return to the source vein through the perforator complex.

In addition to identifying the main perforator that will be incorporated as the flap pedicle, adjacent perforators that will eventually be transected at the level of the deep fascia must also be identified. If the perforators surrounding the dominant pedicle of the flap are identified and localized adequately preoperatively or intraoperatively, the viable boundaries of the flap are better defined and a safer flap can be harvested. Doppler sonography and duplex Doppler imaging can help accomplish these goals.

Free Choice of the Skin Island

In contrast to basing a flap on a perforator identified preoperatively, the skin island can be selected and the appropriate feeder pedicle located afterward. Essentially, this is the basis of free-style free perforator flap surgery. A specific donor or source artery does not limit the surgeon. Soft tissue criteria such as type, texture, and thickness of the flap skin and subcutaneous tissue take precedence over the flap pedicle. After the location and dimensions of the flap are determined and a specific donor site is selected, the surgeon looks for appropriate nutrient vessels.

Although this method of perforator flap reconstruction provides the surgeon with liberty in the choice of tissue, there are disadvantages to this technique. A certain level of expertise is required to handle the ultrasound sonography or duplex Doppler probe. Perforators may be large or small septocutaneous or musculocutaneous vessels, or even a more superficial system such as the superficial inferior epigastric artery. Excellent knowledge of possible variations in dominance of the superficial and deep systems and the likely number, size, and location of different perforators to a specific skin area is requisite. The surgeon should be able and willing to occasionally deal with very small vessels that need ultradelicate dissection techniques and supermicrosurgery.

The choice of perforator flap planning need not be as clearly dichotomized as described here. The surgeon can apply either or both of these principles with one flap. For example, the surgeon may select a skin flap with which he or she has experience and augment this flap with a free-style free flap to achieve specific modifications, or to be more creative in flap design.

Intraoperative Changes and Decision Making

Another major difference between performing traditional free flaps and free perforator flaps is the ability to change the preoperative plan during flap harvest. Despite the results of preoperative ultrasound sonography or duplex Doppler scanning to determine the size, flow, three-dimensional course, and arborization of the perforator vessel, flap vessels are dynamic. At any point in time, these vessels are undergoing a continuous dynamic equilibrium influenced by many physiologic factors, including nervous and humoral stimuli. Preoperative ultrasound provides a static picture of that dynamic status. Therefore vessels that appeared small preoperatively may be larger intraoperatively as the result of vasospasm in the preoperative phase. Correlating and comparing the preoperative ultrasound data with the intraoperative findings regarding the perforator vessels is essential to selecting the most suitable perforator. When selecting the dominant perforator, absolute dimensions of the vessel are one of many factors that must be evaluated. Minimal vessel diameters must be respected; however, the proportionate size of the perforator vessels relative to the overall flap size is also important. An arterial perforator 1 mm in diameter is considered a large vessel in a small flap harvested from the distal extremities, but would be considered a small vessel on which to base a DIEAP or a SGAP flap. For this reason, it is not vital to select a perforator of a certain diameter. It is more important to obtain an accurate preoperative image of the different perforators that provides information about their location and size. If a superficial system is suspected to be present, it needs to be compared with the deep system. In certain areas of the trunk, the superficial system is clearly dominant over the deep system. This information should be recorded preoperatively to avoid intraoperative surprises or embarrassment.

Planning the "Great Four" Flaps

DEEP INFERIOR EPIGASTRIC ARTERY PERFORATOR FLAP

The preoperative color Doppler ultrasound examination, MDCT, or MRI for a deep inferior epigastric perforator flap has different aims: it evaluates the presence and caliber of the internal mammary vessels and the deep inferior epigastric arteries; it locates and evaluates the caliber of the inferior epigastric transmuscular perforator vessels and its branches after piercing the deep fascia; it informs the surgeon about anatomic conditions that could be a contraindication for operation, or that the surgeon should at least be aware of, before starting the operation.

Duplex Doppler Ultrasound

The patient is placed in the supine position and the following steps are performed:
1. Measurement of the blood velocity in and the diameter of the internal mammary arteries
2. Measurement of the diameter of the internal mammary veins
3. Measurement of the blood velocity in and the diameter of the inferior epigastric arteries
4. Localization of the tendinous intersections of the rectus abdominis muscle
5. Localization of the perforator arteries
6. Evaluation of the presence of perforating venae comitantes
7. Evaluation of the number of the main side branches of the perforating arteries

Internal Mammary Artery and Vein

The internal mammary artery is visualized on a parasagittal parasternal cross section in the third intercostal space. Color Doppler examination shows the artery, which originates from the ipsilateral subclavian artery, flowing in a caudad direction. Pulsed Doppler reveals a low resistance flow pattern with high diastolic forward flow. The Doppler curve allows measurement of the peak systolic velocity (cm/sec). The diameter of the artery (mm) can be measured on a gray-scale longitudinal cross section of the artery, which shows the artery walls. Color Doppler visualization of the left internal mammary artery may be slightly disturbed by tissue vibrations from heart contractions. A narrow internal mammary artery with reduced arterial flow, an aberrant course of the artery, or the absence of the internal mammary artery is of clinical interest and should be reported.

The internal mammary vein or veins are visualized on a parasagittal and transverse cross section in the third intercostal space. Color Doppler examination shows the flow in the vein to be directed to the ipsilateral subclavian vein. There is usually one vein, located on the medial aspect of the internal mammary artery. Less frequently, one vein is visualized along the lateral side of the artery, or the artery is accompanied by two veins, one on each side. Because the walls of the veins are hardly visible on the gray-scale image, the vein diameter is estimated by measuring its diameter (mm) on a color-encoded image, on a transverse cross section. The diameter of the right internal mammary vein is usually the largest one. As with the left internal mammary artery, color Doppler visualization of the left internal mammary vein may be disturbed by tissue vibrations from heart contractions. Absence of venous flow along the internal mammary artery suggests internal mammary vein thrombosis. Inversion of flow direction, with flow running caudad, should raise suspicion of an occlusive subclavian vein thrombosis. This can be caused by infusion thrombophlebitis or the presence of an intravenous device (for example, a Port-A-Cath for chemotherapy).

Intercostal arteries and veins may be visualized when looking for the internal mammary vessels. When the internal mammary vessels cannot be visualized in the third intercostal space, they should be looked for in the second or fourth intercostal space.

Deep Inferior Epigastric Artery

The deep inferior epigastric artery is a side branch of the common femoral artery. With color Doppler imaging, the artery can be traced from its origin on the anteromedial aspect of the common femoral artery, to its course in the posterior rectus abdominis fascia. The blood flows cranially, away from the groin. Pulsed Doppler reveals a high resistance vessel. On the Doppler curve, peak systolic velocity is measured (cm/sec). The diameter of the artery is measured on a gray-scale longitudinal cross section of the artery. The artery is usually accompanied by one or two veins that flow in the opposite direction. From the dorsal aspect of the rectus abdominis muscle, one or more side branches of the deep inferior epigastric artery perforate through the fascia. They can be visualized within the muscle. When the diameters and/or blood flow velocities of the right and left deep inferior epigastric arteries differ considerably, particularly in a patient with a surgical scar on the pelvic wall, one should suspect an arterial interruption, with collateral arterial blood supply.

Tendinous Intersections of the Rectus Abdominis Muscle

The rectus abdominis muscle consists of different muscle bodies joined together by tendinous intersections that course transversely. On a parasagittal cross section of the abdominal wall, the rectus abdominis muscle presents as a striated area. The tendinous intersections and the muscle bodies are not sharply delineated from each other. The muscle bodies are slightly larger and less echogenic than the tendinous intersections. The tendinous intersections can be distinguished on parasagittal and transverse cross sections. The position of the tendinous intersections relative to the umbilicus is marked on the registration form. The tendinous intersections near the umbilicus are of greatest interest, because often large perforators pass through this anatomic landmark.

Between the right and the left rectus abdominis muscle lies the linea alba. In diastasis, the right and left rectus abdominis muscle are separated from each other. A dense fibrous fascia can be visualized between the medial borders of both muscles, delineating the subcutaneous fat layer from the abdominal cavity. If an important diastasis is present, all perforators will have shifted laterally. The medial perforators might be mistaken for the lateral ones, and therefore the search for perforators should be continued more laterally than usual.

The Grid

A grid is drawn on the patient's abdominal wall. The center of the grid is the umbilicus. The grid extends laterally 10 cm on each side, cranially 2 cm and caudally 8 cm. A complete 1 cm grid can be drawn, with transverse and parasagittal bars, or the grid may be drawn more arbitrarily (for example, only the transverse bars are drawn at 1, 2, or 3 cm intervals, with distance markers on the transverse bars). The grid drawn on the patient's abdominal wall corresponds with a 1 cm grid drawn on the patient's registration form.

Transmuscular Perforators

The transmuscular perforators have a much smaller diameter than the intramuscular axial branches. Therefore they should be looked for with low color settings. Perforators running perpendicular to the anterior rectus abdominis fascia are easily detected with color Doppler, because they run in the direction of the ultrasound beams. However, many perforators run oblique to the anterior fascia, or may even run for a short distance through the fascia, parallel to the skin. In these cases the perforating artery may hardly be distinguished because of a weak Doppler signal. Therefore steering the color box is essential, and the perforating artery and the exit point should be visualized under different angles to obtain the best signals.

The area of interest at the exact point where the artery perforates the anterior rectus abdominis muscle fascia can be evaluated in two ways. One can follow the intramuscular branches of the deep inferior epigastric artery. Where the branches are in close contact with the anterior fascia, a special search for perforating arteries is performed. Usually an exit point through the anterior muscle fascia is seen on the gray-scale image as a less echogenic interruption of the strongly echogenic fascia. The second way consists of looking for the arteries within the subcutaneous fat layer, and following each artery to its origin.

We usually search for perforating arteries on transverse cross sections of the abdominal wall, with a slight cranial angulation of the probe. Every part of the rectus abdominis muscle that lies within the grid should be examined. When an artery is visualized perforating the anterior fascia, a meticulous search is undertaken for branches in the direct neighborhood. Because not all branches run in a transverse plane, sometimes the probe should be turned around its axis over 90 degrees to make a parasagittal cross section through the exit point.

The exact diameter of the perforating artery at the exit point through the muscle fascia can hardly be measured, even with high-frequency transducers. However, the color image of the artery gives a good qualitative estimation of the arterial caliber in that area.

Within the subcutaneous fat layer, some arterial branches can be seen running in the direction of the skin, while others run back to the anterior fascia, without perforating it. The color Doppler examination of the inferior epigastric transmuscular perforator vessels may be disturbed by color artifacts from bowel movements. These disturbances occur predominantly on the left side.

Evaluating a Perforating Artery

Initially we try to locate the exact exit point of the perforator through the muscle fascia and let it correspond with a point on the grid drawn on the patient's abdominal wall. This position is drawn on the registration form. The exit point through the muscle fascia is a fixed zone within the anterior rectus abdominis fascia. In patients with a very thick or lax panniculus adiposus, and/or a very lax skin, pressure with the scan head on the abdominal wall may disturb the correlation between the anatomy and the grid drawn on the patient's abdominal wall. Reconstructive surgeons should be aware of this discordance.

We qualitatively estimate the caliber of the perforating artery at the exit point in the anterior rectus abdominis fascia on the color Doppler image. We then try to count the number of (main) side branches of each perforating artery within the subcutaneous fat layer. This provides an idea about the mass of fatty tissue supplied by the perforating artery. The course of arterial branches running away over a long distance from the exit point is indicated on the registration form. Finally, the presence of venae comitantes, as well as a qualitative estimation of their importance, is registered on the form.

In our opinion, arterial blood flow velocity at the exit point is a less reliable parameter. Blood flow velocity measurements depend on the vessel diameter, which can be reduced at the exit point if fascia is tight. Furthermore, the tortuosity of the artery at the exit point precludes the exact angle correction and exact blood flow velocity measurements.

Evaluating Perforating Veins and Veins in the Subcutaneous Fat Layer

Venae comitantes can be visualized within the subcutaneous fat layer, and even at the exit point through the muscle fascia. They can be distinguished from the arteries by a nonpulsatile flow pattern and an opposite flow direction. Both parameters can be estimated from color Doppler images and Doppler flow curves. However, some veins are not accompanied by an artery. Larger veins are well visualized, but smaller veins may be difficult, or even impossible, to see. When looking for veins, gentle pressure should be applied; heavy pressure can compress vessels and preclude visualization on color images. Perforating veins are qualitatively evaluated and marked on the patients' registration form as follows: (+) represents a small vein with low flow velocity, (++) a vein of medium interest, and (+++) a large vein with persistent high flow velocity.

Pitfalls

The presence of relatively large arteries in the subcutaneous fat layer that run mainly in the direction of the anterior rectus abdominis fascia (or even perforate the anterior fascia in an opposite direction) should elevate suspicion of collateral arterial circulation. In cases of interruption of the deep inferior epigastric artery by trauma or surgery, blood may be supplied to the subcutaneous fat layer by collateral arteries. Usually these are branches from arteries lying outside (lateral to) the grid drawn on the patient's abdominal wall. They are found by tracing the artery with opposite flow direction to its origin.

The presence of large veins flowing in the same direction as the perforating arteries and/or large veins crossing the linea alba to the opposite side should increase suspicion of an outflow obstruction of the deep inferior epigastric vein. The veins with opposite flow direction can be traced to their end. They may be the landmarks of an old and fairly well compensated occlusive deep venous thrombosis of a common femoral or iliac vein or even of the inferior vena cava. It is a contraindication for a deep inferior epigastric perforator flap breast reconstruction.

Both conditions should be suspected based on the patient's history and physical examination. Vessel abnormalities should be suspected in patients with history of abdominal or pelvic surgery, deep venous thrombosis of the lower extremities or pelvic thrombosis, the presence of surgical scars on the abdominal or pelvic wall, a swollen leg, or subcutaneous collateral veins in the groin and on the pelvic wall.

Multidetector-Row Computed Tomography and Magnetic Resonance Imaging

MDCT and MRI have constituted a major advance in the preoperative mapping of perforator flaps. Compared with ultrasound techniques, MDCT and MRI provide a clearer view of the intramuscular part of the perforator and the three-dimensional structure of branching between the deep fascia and the skin. This helps define adjacent vascular territories more precisely and reduces the possibility of vascular compromise in peripheral areas of our flaps. It becomes much easier to compare different perforators and determine their relative importance. Depending on the number and direction of branches, the relative size of the vessel, the location within the flap, and the anticipated length and difficulty of intramuscular dissection, the most dominant perforator or perforators can be chosen. The additional information that MRDC and MRI provide compared with ultrasound techniques results in less operative time and fewer postoperative complications. MDCT and MRI are currently considered the gold standard for preoperative study of abdominal perforators.

The main advantages of MDCT and MRI for the abdominal area can be summarized as follows:

- High sensitivity and high specificity
- Good three-dimensional evaluation of quality, course, and location of perforators
- Easy interpretation and good reproducibility by the radiologist and plastic surgeon
- Easy storage of data on a pen drive, simplifying reproducibility
- Reduced operating time and complications
- Good patient tolerance
- Reduced surgeon's stress

SUPERIOR GLUTEAL ARTERY PERFORATOR FLAP
Ultrasound Techniques

To locate the superior or inferior gluteal artery perforators, the patient is placed in a prone position. The region of interest is delineated on the skin of the patient's gluteal area. The position of the suprapiriform foramen (foramen ischiadicum majus) is marked at the cranial third of a line connecting the posterior superior iliac spine and the apex of the greater trochanter of the femur (see Chapters 33 and 34). The position of the piriformis muscle is located by connecting the middle of a line between the posterior superior iliac spine and the coccyx with the superior edge of the greater trochanter of the femur. The main perforators of the superior gluteal artery should be looked for above the piriformis muscle, distal and laterodistal to the perforating point of the superior gluteal artery. Usually, the perforators lie on a line parallel to the line that connects the posterior superior iliac spine and the apex of the greater trochanter of the femur. Perforators of the inferior gluteal artery originate from in between the pirifomis muscle and the tuber ischiadicum and fan out laterally and caudally toward the infragluteal crease.

The relatively constant anatomy of the branches of the superior gluteal artery and the presence of a low number of large perforators (one to six per flap) traveling through a thick muscle and crossing the muscle fascia almost perpendicularly, make it easy to locate the exit point of the perforators at the level of the superficial muscle fascia with unidirectional Doppler flowmetry. This can be performed preoperatively and intraoperatively.

Gray-scale ultrasound in conjunction with color Doppler imaging provides more anatomic and hemodynamic information about the perforators. This technique should be performed preoperatively. On gray-scale ultrasound examination, the suprapiriform foramen, as well as the gluteus maximus and the gluteus medius muscles, can be distinguished. The superior gluteal artery is a side branch of the internal iliac artery. It is visualized with color Doppler imaging as it leaves the pelvis through the suprapiriform foramen and runs between the gluteus maximus and the gluteus medius muscle. The position of the perforators is marked with dots on the patient's skin. A grid is drawn using the most superior point of the intergluteal crease and the posterior iliac spine.

A qualitative evaluation of the perforators is reported on the patient's registration form. It is based on the blood flow velocity, measured by pulsed Doppler, and on the caliber of the artery on the color Doppler image.

Multidetector-Row Computed Tomography and Magnetic Resonance Imaging

The gluteal and lumbar perforator flaps, similar to abdominal area flaps, have considerable adipose tissue thickness in a large anatomic area. This type of flap therefore is easy to study using MDCT and MRI. Visualization is excellent; these techniques help visualize the perforator above the fascia and its axiality inside the subcutaneous tissue (Fig. 6-7). The grid with coordinates for the perforators is often positioned vertically over the midline and horizontally through the posterior iliac spine or posterior crest of the pelvis.

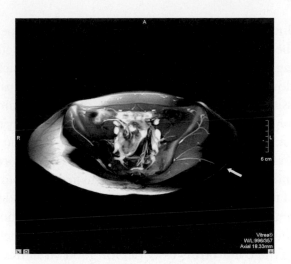

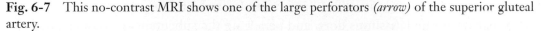

Fig. 6-7 This no-contrast MRI shows one of the large perforators *(arrow)* of the superior gluteal artery.

During imaging, the patient must be positioned as on the day of surgery. Whether to place the patient in the prone or lateral decubitus position for this flap is the surgeon's preference.

Although excellent images can be obtained from this area, MDCT and MRI may not be one's first choice for several reasons. The thickness of the subcutaneous fat layer often makes it very difficult to mark the exact position of the perforator on the skin. Fixed landmarks are far from the perforators; the posterior iliac spine and the posterior ridge of the pelvis are often located much more cranially. Tissue laxity and the curved buttock shape make retrieval of the coordinates difficult. In contrast to the abdominal system, there is no superficial system present, and the total number of large perforators is limited in the areas of the superior gluteal artery and inferior gluteal artery. Because they course relatively perpendicular to the skin, these few large perforators always easily found by unidirectional Doppler or color duplex Doppler. One need not look for a separate vein, because the perforating arteries are always accompanied by two large veins. Once the patient is positioned on the operating table, the surgeon reconfirms the location of the perforators by handheld Doppler to eliminate any confusion about shifting of the soft tissues over fixed bony structures.

In patients with extensive trauma, liposuction, infections (for example, Fournier's disease), or any other condition possibly causing extensive scarring or damage to the perforators, MDCT and MRI are clearly beneficial in demonstrating vessel patency.

THORACODORSAL ARTERY PERFORATOR FLAP
Ultrasound Techniques

To locate the thoracodorsal artery perforators, the patient is placed in the lateral decubitus position, with maximum elevation of the arm on the side of interest. Because a high number of false-positive signals have been documented with unidirectional Doppler flowmetry, gray-scale ultrasound in conjunction with color Doppler imaging is the method of choice.

A gray-scale ultrasound examination of the axillary region is performed to visualize the muscles of the thoracic wall. The serratus anterior muscle is delineated along its inner side by the strong reflections of the aerated lung and ribs, which can be recognized by the acoustic shadow behind them. The outer side of the serratus anterior is partially covered by the latissimus dorsi. The lateral border of the latissimus dorsi, which is of particular interest for this investigation, is visualized in the axillary region and followed in a caudad direction. This border is marked with a dotted line on the patient's skin.

The thoracodorsal artery is 1 to 2 cm medial to the lateral border of the latissimus dorsi. This artery and the vena comitans can be visualized on color Doppler imaging. It is a side branch of the subscapular artery, which by itself is a side branch of the axillary artery. The thoracodorsal artery runs parallel to the lateral border of the scapula, between the latissimus dorsi and serratus anterior muscles. As the artery runs parallel to the skin, steering the color box is essential for good visualization. Usually one to three perforators can be visualized originating from the thoracodorsal artery. Most of them perforate the latissimus dorsi and penetrate the subcutaneous tissue. They run perpendicular to the skin. Sometimes the perforating artery runs along the outer side of the latissimus dorsi. Some perforators may be accompanied by a vein.

The position of the perforating arteries is marked on the patient's skin. A grid can be used, starting from the posterior axillary crease and centered on the anterior border of the latissimus dorsi muscle. Most perforators are found 3 to 15 cm distal to the posterior axillary crease and 1 to 6 cm posterior to the anterior border of the latissimus dorsi muscle.

A qualitative evaluation of the perforators is reported on the patient's registration form. It is based on the blood flow velocity, measured by pulsed Doppler, and on the caliber of the artery on the color Doppler image.

Multidetector-Row Computed Tomography and Magnetic Resonance Imaging

For any preoperative planning technique, including MDCT and MRI, the most important problem is that there are no fixed anatomic structures in the area that can serve as a reference for placing a grid on the skin and providing cutaneous coordinates for the perforators. Another major limitation of preoperative mapping for thoracodorsal axis flaps is the difficulty of studying patients in the same position that they will be placed for surgery. This means that MDCT and MRI are not the most suitable techniques for planning flaps in this area. Additionally, the caliber of the perforators is often smaller than in other areas of the body, the subcutaneous fat layer is often thin in nonobese patients and perforators often run oblique through the subcutaneous fat. Because of these factors, MDCT and MRI are not ideal means of visualizing perforators in this area. As with gluteal flaps, however, MDCT and MRI have a clear benefit when anatomic anomalies or prior soft tissue damage and scarring are expected. Duplex Doppler ultrasound remains the technique of choice in routine cases.

THE ANTEROLATERAL THIGH FLAP

MDCT and MRI have the same shortcomings for the anterolateral thigh flap as those described previously for the TDAP flap. The limited adipose tissue thickness and considerable thickness of the muscular fascia make it difficult to visualize the perforator at the

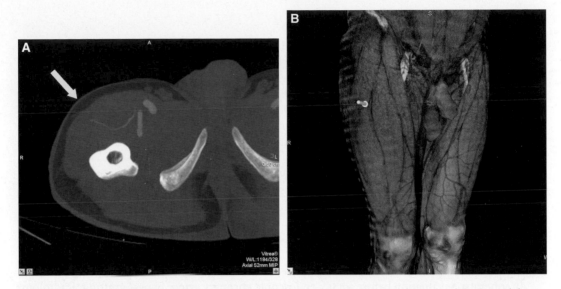

Fig. 6-8 A, Axial MDCT image of a septal perforator of the descending branch of the lateral femoral circumflex artery. The *arrow* indicates the point where the perforator arises from the fascia. **B,** A three-dimensional reconstruction. The *marker* indicates the exit point of the perforator.

suprafascial level, resulting in a considerable number of false-negatives. Unidirectional Doppler yields numerous false-positive signals, because the probe cannot distinguish between the oblique course of perforators above the fascia and smaller axial vessels just below the fascia. Duplex Doppler ultrasound investigation provides the most exact imaging but is very time consuming and highly operator dependent. A reference grid can be drawn on the skin over a vertical line connecting the anterior superior iliac spine and the lateral border of the patella and a horizontal line at the halfway point of the vertical line. Most large perforators are located in a circle with a 5 cm radius centered on the intersection of these two lines (Fig. 6-8).

Considering the difficulty of interpreting the preoperative imaging and the low complexity of dissecting this flap, imaging techniques are used when an additional study of the lower limb vascular axis is required. MDCT or MRI is performed rather than conventional arteriography.

Other Perforator Flaps
All investigations presented in this chapter can be used for any flap in the body. MDCT and MRI can be used to examine any area, but these techniques are not as beneficial for smaller and more peripheral vessels. Areas with thin layers of subcutaneous fat lend themselves well to the use of unidirectional, handheld Doppler, specifically in the distal parts of the extremities, where very little anatomic vaiation is present. More central areas, where it is hard to distinguish between the axial vessel and perforator vessels because their proximity, can be better examined with duplex Doppler ultrasound. MDCT and MRI are preferred in areas with large vessels with a lot of anatomic variability, and in areas where the normal anatomy has been disturbed by (previous) trauma, surgery, infections, or congenital anomalies. Technologic availability and logistics as well as cost and other financial implications need to be considered when choosing the right investigation.

References

1. Masia J, Clavero JA, Larrañaga JR, et al. Multidetector-row computed tomography in the planning of abdominal perforator flaps. J Plast Reconstr Aesthet Surg 59:594-599, 2006.

   The authors described a new method for the preoperative study of abdominal perforator flaps. They validated the technique in a study comparing the CT images with intraoperative findings. Neither false-positives nor false-negatives were encountered. They also describe the main advantages of MDCT, such as reduced operating time and complications and concluded that MDCT provides valuable preoperative images and information about the perforators and main vessels of the inferior abdominal wall.

2. Giunta RE, Geisweid A, Feller AM. The value of preoperative Doppler sonography for planning free perforator flaps. Plast Reconstr Surg 105:2381-2386, 2000.

3. Blondeel PN, Beyens G, Verhaeghe R, et al. Doppler flowmetry in the planning of perforator flaps. Br J Plast Surg 51:202-209, 1998.

4. Hallock GC. Doppler sonography and color duplex imaging for planning a perforator flap. Clin Past Surg 30:347-357, 2003.

5. Herzog C, Dogan S, Diebold T, et al. Multi-detector row CT versus coronary angiography: preoperative evaluation before totally endoscopic coronary artery bypass grafting. Radiology 229:200-208, 2003.

6. Lawler LP, Fishman EK. Multi-detector row computed tomography of the aorta and peripheral arteries. Cardiol Clin 21:607-629, 2003.

7. Ropers D, Baum U, Pohle K, et al. Detection of coronary artery stenoses with thin-slice multidetector row spiral computed tomography and multiplanar reconstruction. Circulation 107:664-777, 2003.

8. Wintersperger BJ, Nikolaou K, Becker CR. Multidetector-row CT angiography of the aorta and visceral arteries. Semin Ultrasound CT MR 25:25-40, 2004.

9. Nikolaou K, Becker CR, Muders M. Multidetector-row computed tomography and magnetic resonance imaging of atherosclerotic lesions in human ex vivo coronary arteries. Atherosclerosis 174:243-252, 2004.

10. Clavero JA, Masia J, Larrañaga J, et al. MDCT in the preoperative planning of abdominal perforator surgery for postmastectomy breast reconstruction. AJR Am J Roentgenol 191:670-676, 2008.

    This study evaluated the utility of MDCT in planning abdominal perforator surgery for breast reconstruction in 126 patients who had undergone mastectomy and were reconstructed with deep inferior epigastric perforator flaps. This article was written not only for plastic surgeons, but also for radiologists to explain the importance and applications of MDCT. The authors described the technique and radiologic characteristics. MDCT facilitates accurate identification of the most suitable dominant perforator vessel, making surgical perforator flap procedures for breast reconstruction faster and safer.

11. Vandervoort M, Vranckx JJ, Fabre B. Perforator topography of the deep inferior epigastric perforator flap in 100 cases of breast reconstruction. Plast Reconstr Surg 109:1912-1918, 2002.

12. Masia J, Larrañaga J, Clavero JA, et al. The value of the multidetector row computed tomography for the preoperative planning of deep inferior epigastric artery perforator flap: our experience in 162 cases. Ann Plast Surg 60:29-36, 2008.

13. Masia J, Kosuotic D, Cervelli D, Clavero JA, et al. In search of the ideal method in perforator mapping: noncontrast magnetic resonance imaging. J Reconstr Microsurg 26:29-35, 2010.

    The authors discussed the drawbacks of MDCT in abdominal wall free flap reconstruction, and presented their good results obtained with noncontrast MRI. They validated the technique, comparing the images with the operative findings. They also emphasized the advantages of nonradiation for the patient, such as eliminating the need for intravenous medium, which is required for MDCT.

14. Mathes DW, Neligan PC. Preoperative imaging techniques for perforator selection in abdomen-based microsurgical breast reconstruction. Clin Plast Surg 37:581-591, 2010.

    In this review article the authors described different techniques for preoperative study in microsurgical breast reconstruction. They emphasized the advantages of imaging techniques over classical techniques and concluded that CTA seems to be the gold standard for preoperative evaluation, but MRI is increasingly achieving better results. They also provided an in-depth review of recent publications associated with imaging techniques.

15. Hijjawi JB, Blondeel PN. Advancing deep inferior epigastric artery perforator flap breast reconstruction through multidetector row computed tomography: an evolution in preoperative imaging. J Reconstr Microsurg 26:11-20, 2010.

16. Hamdi M, Van Landuyt K, Hedent EV, et al. Advances in autogenous breast reconstruction. The role of preoperative perforator mapping. Ann Plast Surg 58:18-26, 2007.

17. Rozen WM, Ashton MW, Grinsell D, et al. Establishing the case for CT angiography in the preoperative imaging of abdominal wall perforators. Microsurgery 28:306-313, 2008.

18. Taylor GI, Palmer JH. The vascular territories (angiosomes) of the body: experimental study and clinical applications. Br J Plast Surg 40:113-141, 1987.

7

Technical Aspects of Perforator Flap Dissection

Phillip N. Blondeel

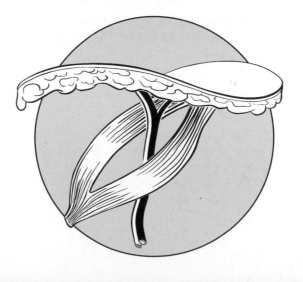

The principal advantage of perforator flaps is that they spare deeper structures and thus limit functional morbidity.[1-7] The size of the skin paddle that can be raised is, to a certain extent, related to the size of the perforator. Inclusion of muscle has no influence on flap perfusion, and it should be spared whenever possible.[8] The possible disadvantages of perforator flaps lie in specific technical demands that most surgeons were not used to until recently. In the hands of surgeons with a limited experience in the field of perforator flap surgery, this procedure may result in increase operative time. Professor Fu-Chan Wei likes to compare performing perforator flap surgery with eating with chopsticks. In Western cultures, this adjustment may be very difficult, whereas small children in Oriental cultures use them very fluently at a very young age. It is a matter of becoming accustomed through experience. Dissecting a perforator flap requires meticulous attention to detail and a high degree of flexibility of the operative plan, depending on the position, size, and presence of perforating vessels. However, the somewhat unpredictable nature of the vessels can be partly addressed by accurate preoperative imaging.

Harvesting a perforator flap differs from harvesting a more traditional skin or musculocutaneous flap essentially in the way the nourishing vascular pedicle is dissected. Following the definition of true muscle perforators, the vessels need to be dissected from between the muscle fibers while creating the least possible damage to this muscle, its secondary blood supply, and the motor innervation. These simple principles and techniques of perforator flap dissection can be applied to all perforator flaps, regardless of their location in the body, provided the surgeon has an intimate knowledge of the regional anatomy. The preoperative identification of perforating vessels, the intraoperative approach, and the surgical tools and techniques are the same for every flap. For preoperative identification of the dominant perforator, refer to Chapter 6. A more challenging way to identify the main perforator is with the principles of the free-style free flap (see Chapter 72). This chapter will explain the basic surgical technique for approaching and dissecting the vessels through the muscle down to the axial vessels.

CHOOSING THE RIGHT PERFORATOR
Flap Planning

Accurate preoperative planning is an essential component of perforator flap surgery. This begins with delineating the anatomic defect to replace "like with like." Both the dimensions and constituent parts of the defect need to be considered. This includes the surface area of the skin paddle, the thickness and consistency of the subcutaneous layer, the total flap volume, and any specialized structures. If a complex reconstruction is necessary, the flap may need to incorporate specific anatomic components such as bone, fascia, muscle, and nerve. A perforator flap in these circumstances allows the skin flap to be mobilized from the other constituents to provide flexibility in its placement. In this instance, the bone, muscle, and other components can be placed to facilitate a functional reconstruction, with the skin paddle draped to provide optimal contour. These are called *chimeric flaps.*[9]

Having determined what needs to be replaced, the surgeon must consider the most appropriate donor site and method of flap transfer (pedicle or free). For practical purposes, it is also preferable to select a flap that does not require position changes and facilitates a two-team approach.

Although the technical aspects of flap dissection are similar for pedicle and free flaps, there are essential differences in flap planning and raising. The epicenter of a free perforator flap must lie at the level of the feeding vessel to ensure adequate tissue perfusion to all zones.

Local perforator flaps offer limited flap movement around the perforator, which represents the pivot point of rotation. The extent of flap movement depends on the tissue elasticity, skin island design, and perforator vessel length. The latter can be increased by following the perforator into the fascia or muscle. Several studies have shown that longer pedicles are less sensitive to twisting forces, because the length of a vessel is inversely proportion to the critical angle of twisting.[10-14] Flaps that include only one perforator are likely to have greater flap mobility and can be mobilized in a propeller fashion, with a maximum of 180 degrees counterclockwise or clockwise, without compromising perfusion. Flaps with multiple perforators are more suitable to rotation or advancement maneuvers, depending on the number of vessels preserved. If more than one perforator is included, then the vessels must be in proximity to each other and dissected for a sufficient distance.

The position of the perforator selected is dependent on the planned movement of the flap. In a propeller flap, the perforator closest to the defect is chosen to allow the flap to pivot on the vessel and thus increase the potential coverage of the defect.[15,16] For advancement, transposition, and rotation flaps, the perforator or perforators farthest from the defect are selected, because this provides the longest possible pedicle, thereby giving the flap a large arc of motion. Regardless of the type of flap movement, any stretching of the perforator vessels should be avoided to minimize the risk of vascular complication.

Perforator flaps can also be based on a known, named perforator (in a similar manner to standard musculocutaneous or fasciocutaneous flaps), or they can be designed free-style on a random, unnamed perforator of sufficient caliber.[17]

Free-style flaps can be considered a form of reverse planning. The required characteristics of the skin flap determine its anatomic location, and the perforating vessels are selected as a secondary consideration. The benefits of this method lie in its flexibility in assuring that the most suitable flap is raised with regard to skin thickness, texture, and quality. However, the surgeon must be competent in locating perforators with an ultrasound/duplex Doppler probe and direct intraoperative visualization, and possess an excellent anatomic knowledge of the region. These flaps can be technically demanding and often require dissection and anastomosis of vessels considerably smaller than standard perforator flaps.

Imaging

When designing a perforator flap, the main question that concerns us is: How much tissue, skin, and subcutaneous fat can be harvested on one particular perforator? Regardless of whether one believes in the angiosome principle or considers vascularization to occur through a subcutaneous vascular plexus influenced by flow physiology, the toughest challenge remains the same—accurately predicting the territory of viable tissue. This is as relevant in free flaps as it is in flaps based on axial vessels. The most accurate indicator is preoperative localization of the most dominant source of blood influx by duplex Doppler or CT imaging. Often absolute vessel caliber is less important than relative size compared with surrounding perforators. A 1 mm artery in a thin patient may be a sizeable vessel able to vascularize a large territory, possibly comparable to a 2 to 3 mm perforating artery in an obese patient.

In addition to defining the safe flap territory, these techniques provide some reassurance to the surgeon by preventing intraoperative surprises and can considerably reduce operative time and costs, which, to some degree, helps offset the cost of the procedure. More recently, MR angiography has shown to be promising in perforator imaging. Not only does it produce accurate and detailed images, it does so without exposure to radiation, unlike CT imaging.[18]

Many have stopped using color duplex Doppler because of its main disadvantages: lack of anatomic detail and operator dependence. It requires a detailed knowledge of three-dimensional vascular anatomy, as well as expertise in handling the devise. Although it provides dynamic information about blood flow, this may lead to a false sense of security. It is essential to look for vessels with a minimum size and select the largest perforator in the region of interest. This is necessary because of the constant humeral and nervous stimuli that affect microcirculation and cause fluctuations in vessel flow. As a result, flow rates do not always correlate with the size of the perforator.

Multidetector-row helical CT is a recent innovation that rapidly delineates an anatomic area of interest to provide excellent resolution and low-artifact rating. The scanning is performed in conjunction with intravenous contrast medium and allows evaluation of the donor and recipient vessels. Information collected includes the exact location and intramuscular course of vessels from their origin, caliber of perforators, and identification of the dominant vessel. The relative dominance of deep and superficial systems is delineated, removing the element of surprise and allowing the surgeon to consider options preoperatively. Not only can this modality be used to select suitable patients preoperatively, but operative times are reduced by 21%, with obvious cost benefits.[19] More details on preoperative planning and imaging are given in Chapter 6.

ANATOMY AND SKIN MARKINGS
Anatomy of the Donor Area

Once the dominant perforator is identified in the area where the skin and fat flap will be harvested, familiarity with the underlying anatomy of fascia, muscle, septi, nerves, and axial vessels is essential. Because we harvest flaps from all over the body, a good reconstructive surgeon needs to have a decent understanding of soft tissue anatomy of the entire body. Of specific importance is the relationship of the axial vessels and its perforators to underlying muscles. Perforators can have a purely septal course, a purely intramuscular course, or can partially run in the muscle and later in the septum, or vice versa. The type of perforator will determine the type and difficulty of the dissection technique. Septal perforators are very easy to separate from the surrounding tissues; however, intramuscular dissection can sometimes be tedious and will certainly take more time.

It must be determined whether muscle fibers need to be preserved. For example, saving the integrity of the entire rectus muscle in a deep inferior epigastric artery perforator (DIEAP) flap dissection helps maintain global function of the muscle, including that of motor nerves, which traverse the muscle obliquely and must be preserved. On the other hand, sacrificing a few muscle fibers during dissection of the perforators of a gracilis perforator flap or an anterolateral thigh flap, which are partially intramuscular and septal, will not interfere with muscle strength and function.

The length of the perforator must be estimated before designing the flap. Often muscle perforators with a long oblique course through the muscle are longer than septal perforators with a course perpendicular to the skin. CT angiography scans and duplex Doppler investigations can provide this information preoperatively so that one can not only design the size and surface of the flap, but also calculate the amount of displacement for a pedicle flap. If a part of the axial vessels is harvested along with the perforator or perforators, flap movement can be increased, or, for free flaps, the length of the pedicle can be increased.

Finally, if there is a need to harvest a flap composed of different soft tissue components or even bone, a good knowledge of the vascular anatomy is required. Specifically, the axilla and groin are areas where composed flaps can be harvested with multiple skin islands, muscle flaps (to fill dead space), and bony components. However, vascular branching is often variable and requires intraoperative decisions. A good preoperative vascular evaluation can be of substantial help.

Skin Markings

Free Flaps

The size of the skin paddle and the volume of the free flap need to be determined by examining the needs of the recipient site. Resurfacing large limb defects requires large and thin flaps, such as a thoracodorsal artery perforator (TDAP), whereas voluminous reconstructions such as breast reconstructions mainly need bulk from a thick subcutaneous fat layer, as provided by a DIEAP or superior gluteal artery perforator (SGAP) flap. The free perforator flap is preferentially centered over the dominant perforator. With a centrally located perforator, equal distribution of blood flow is ensured and the risk for fat necrosis is decreased.

After the position of the perforator flap is determined, consideration is given to the optimal location of the skin incisions, including the following:
- The position of the incision in relation to the normal skin creases and body folds (inframammary crease, axilla, groin, and subgluteal fold)
- The position of the final scar, including coverage by underwear or bathing apparel
- The ability to close the donor defect, depending on the elasticity of the skin and tension lines
- Cultural preferences (for example, scars in the buttock area are more difficult to accept for South American women than for European women)
- Personal preferences that need to be discussed individually with each patient

Finally, an additional incision may be needed to expose the axial vessels of the donor pedicle. The edges of large flaps are slightly undermined and additional incisions can be avoided. Smaller flaps with a long pedicle, such as a small TDAP, may require a longer incision or a second separate incision in the axilla.

Pedicle Flaps

For pedicle perforator flaps the design of the skin island depends on the amount of movement needed to cover the defect with the flap. For perforator flaps with a short perforator that runs perpendicular to the skin and only allows rotation and no advancement, the pivot point of the flap is the point where the perforator pierces the deep fascia. The skin paddle is often larger than the defect itself, because not only the defect needs to be filled but also (1) a certain amount of tissue needs to be left around the entry point of the perforator in the flap and (2) the distance needs to be bridged between the pivot point and the closest edge of the defect.

Flaps with a long perforator vessel with a long, oblique course through the muscle have not only a higher mobility, but also the combined potential of rotation and advancement at the same time. The pivot point of the flap is where the perforator dissection ends—at the point where it enters the axial vessels—or, if a part of the axial vessels is harvested, the point where this dissection ends. In these cases, smaller, more dedicated flaps can be harvested and tailored to the defect at the recipient site.

The position where the perforator enters the flap is often eccentric in pure rotation flaps or propeller flaps, whereas it can be more centered for perforator flaps with longer pedicles. Though one perforator can vascularize large surfaces even when the perforator enters the flap near its border, it still is not possible to predict in all cases with absolute certainty whether the blood circulation will be reliable in the most distal part of the flap. Anatomic variations and variable perforator vessel size need to be taken into account. A conservative approach is advised for surgeons with limited experience with certain flaps.

As with free flaps, several other factors need to be considered when designing the flap and skin incisions: normal skin lines and creases, the position of the final scar, the amount of tension on skin edges, cultural preferences, and the alternatives in case of dissection failure or flap loss.

CT angiography or duplex Doppler investigation can provide a certain amount of information, but the final pedicle perforator flap can often only be designed after visually localizing the perforator and evaluating its mobility. The primary goal of a pedicle flap is thus exposure of the dominant perforator before committing to a complete flap skin incision. If the perforator is localized close to the defect, this can be done by undermining and lifting the wound edges.

If exposure is not sufficient, an additional incision is made on one of the edges of the planned pedicle flap. It is always safe to place this additional incision on the common incision line of the scheduled perforator flap and a backup flap. This backup flap can be any type of traditional pedicle random-pattern flap that can close the same defect. In many cases, certain parts of the incision lines coincide (Figs. 7-1 through 7-3). If the perforator is exposed through this incision, the plan can be modified, because no commitments have been made yet. If the perforator is not of a decent caliber or if a mishap occurs while dissecting the perforator vessel, one can still change the plan and perform the reconstruction with the more traditional flap. For flaps that cross the midline, an alternative is to assess the perforators of the contralateral side and harvest the same flap. If, however, the perforator vessel dissection was performed flawlessly, the exact entry point of the vessel into the flap and the perforator length will be known, allowing calculation of perfect flap dimensions and movement.

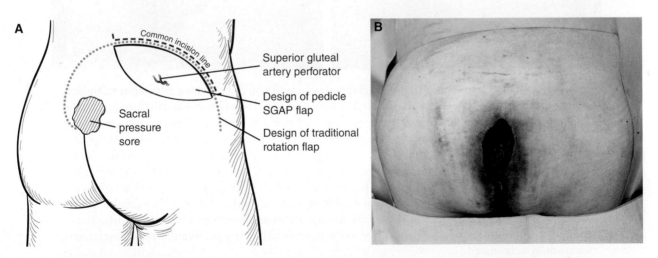

Fig. 7-1 **A,** SGAP design for a paraplegic man with a sacral pressure sore. The dominant perforator was located (by CT angiography or Doppler), and the design of the flap was adjusted so that the superior border coincided with the incision of a random-pattern fasciocutaneous rotation flap. The perforator vessels were retrieved and dissected through this common incision line *(red).* **B,** A typical sacral pressure sore.

Continued

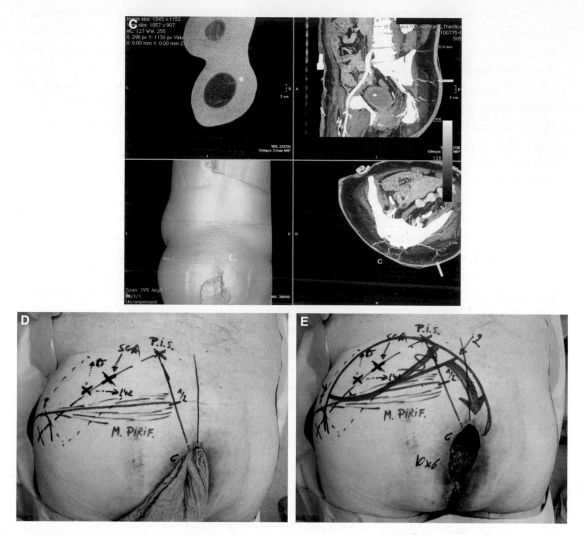

Fig. 7-1, cont'd C, Preoperative CT angiography showed a large branching perforator of the left superior gluteal artery *(yellow mark top left and yellow arrows)*. Its position was calculated from the midline and a horizontal line running through the posterior iliac spine. **D,** Preoperative landmarks, together with the position of the most dominant perforator (*x* to the left) and the superior gluteal artery (*x* to the right), were identified by CT angiography. For preoperative markings of the SGAP, see Chapter 33. **E,** Relative to the mobility of the perforator and the distance from the defect, a temporary flap design was drawn. The upper border is a large half circle *(upper red line)* that represents an incision of a large random-pattern rotation flap that can be used *(red arrow)* if no suitable perforators are found or the perforator vessels are damaged during dissection. The lower border *(lower red line)* is an indication of where the lower incision needs to be once perforator vessel dissection is successfully terminated.

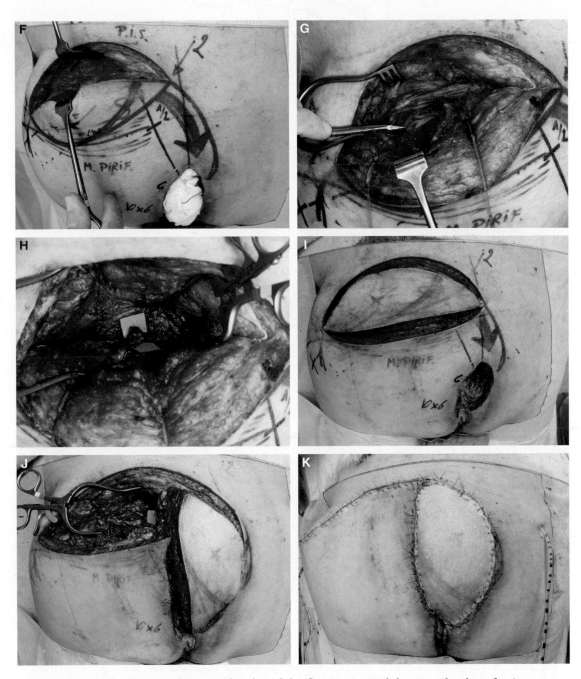

Fig. 7-1, cont'd   F, Only the upper border of the flap was incised down to the deep fascia over a distance that allowed easy access to the perforators. **G,** Partially prefascial, and once closer to the perforator, subfascial undermining was performed until the perforator was identified. **H,** A 5 cm long perforator was freed down to pregluteal fascia. **I,** After reevaluating the mobility of the perforator (in this case, 2 by 5 cm medial advancement with a 90-degree rotation), the distance to the most distal point of the defect was measured and the length of the flap determined. Then the lower incision of the flap was made. **J,** The skin bridge between the donor and recipient site was opened and the flap moved in place. **K,** The final result after closure. (*C,* Coccyx; *M. Pirif.,* musculus piriformis; *P.I.S.,* posterior iliac spine; *SGA,* superior gluteal artery; *T,* trochanter.)

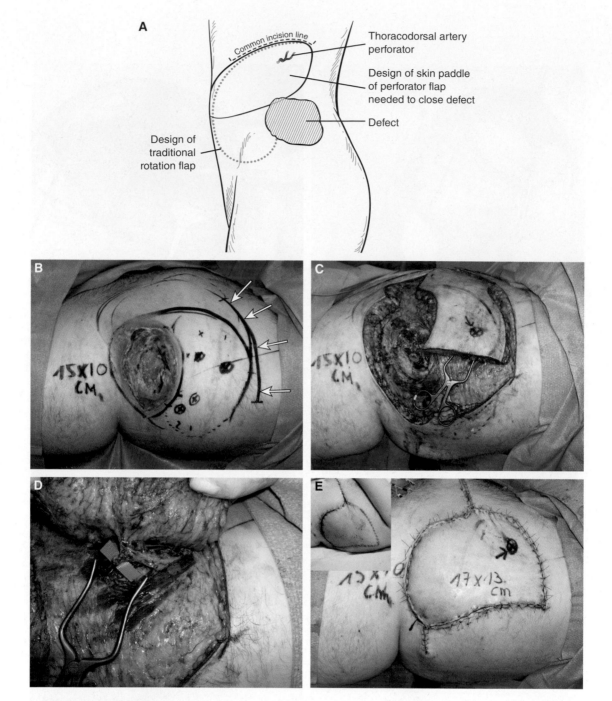

Fig. 7-2   A, An intended lateral intercostal artery perforator (LICAP) flap, extended anteriorly, following the corresponding dermatome, was planned for a 42-year-old man with spina bifida and a chronic pressure sore over the left iliac crest. Many of these flaps can be vascularized by either the intercostal or thoracodorsal perforators. In this case a TDAP flap was used instead of the planned LICAP flap. The upper border of a randomized rotation flap extending anteriorly was made to coincide in a common incision line *(red).* The perforators, localized by duplex Doppler, could be explored through the upper border of the defect or through the common incision line. **B,** The patient is in right lateral decubitus position. Several lateral intercostal and thoracodorsal perforators were identified. The common incision line is indicated with *white arrows.* **C,** The main thoracodorsal perforator was identified and the flap design adjusted and circumscribed. **D,** Two perforators close to each other were freed on the anterior branch of thoracodorsal vessels. **E,** The flap, rotated in place, covered the entire defect. (The inset shows the result after 2 weeks.)

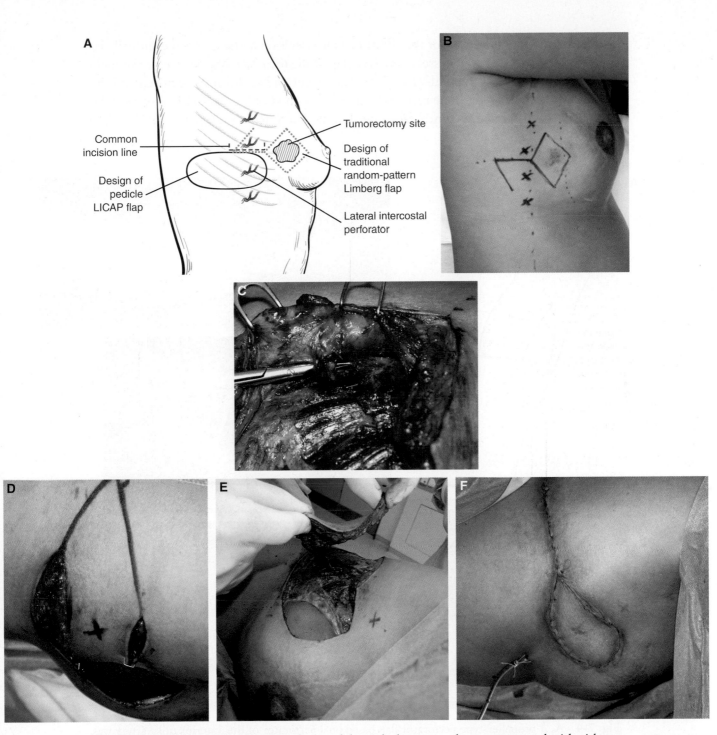

Fig. 7-3 **A,** This lesion in the lateral part of the right breast can be reconstructed with either a traditional Limberg (Dufourmentel) flap or a small lateral intercostal artery perforator (LICAP) propeller flap. The common incision line of both flaps *(red line)* lies between two lateral intercostal perforators to allow exploration of both the cranial and caudal perforator. **B,** This 31-year-old woman had breast cancer recurrence after skin-sparing mastectomy and implant reconstruction. **C,** After the lesion was resected and the horizontal common incision line opened, the caudal perforator was freed from between the serratus anterior muscle strips. An artery, two veins, and a sensory nerve were identified. **D,** The skin incision was adjusted to a horizontal flap following the skin lines. **E,** The flap was isolated on its perforator. Some dissection between the strips of the muscle provided additional length for gentle rotation of the perforator. **F,** The inset flap and donor scar are shown at the end of the procedure.

Another good position for the additional incision is on a line that can eventually be incised to expose recipient vessels for a free flap, if the local perforators are not suitable or the local perforator flap fails (Fig. 7-4). After a suitable perforator is chosen and the flap movement calculated, the rest of the flap is designed or adjusted. Flaps can still be lengthened or widened if only a short incision has been made on one side of the flap.

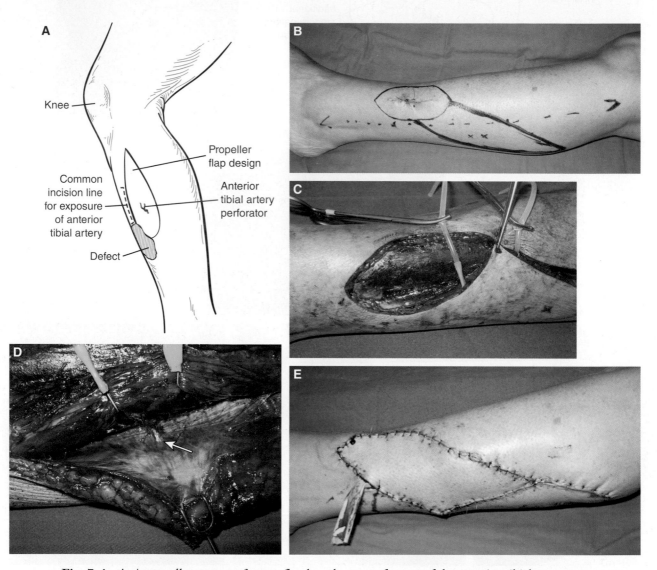

Fig. 7-4 **A,** A propeller-type perforator flap based on a perforator of the anterior tibial artery was planned for a patient with a melanoma lesion on the distal anterolateral surface of the left lower leg. The anterior incision *(red line)* can be used as the common incision line for either exploring the perforators or eventually approaching the anterior tibial vessels if no convenient perforator can be found. **B,** Positive-section margins of the lesion required wide resection. With a handheld Doppler, two perforators *(x)* were localized and the skin incisions were provisionally drawn. **C,** The patient is shown after resection, the anterior incision, and undermining of the anterocaudal part of the flap. **D,** A decent perforator was identified *(arrow)* and will be further freed to allow rotation. **E,** The flap was rotated 180 degrees to cover the defect, and the donor area was closed primarily.

OPERATIVE TECHNIQUE
Perforator Flap Dissection

Perforator flaps differ from traditional free flaps in both allowing and demanding flexibility of decision making. As previously discussed, perforating vessels are dynamic structures whose flow is in constant flux because of varying humeral and neural stimulation. Directly visualizing these perforators allows assessment of caliber not afforded by static preoperative imaging. One must assess vessel diameters, particularly in relation to flap dimensions. Although a small flap from the extremities would be well perfused by a perforator of 1 mm caliber, it would be insufficient for a DIEAP or SGAP flap. The surgeon must consider not only the main perforating vessel, but also adjacent perforators. Delineating these additional vessels preoperatively and intraoperatively helps establish viable boundaries of the flap and potentially avoid flap necrosis.

Incision and Approach of the Perforator

The surgeon begins by incising the edge of the skin flap. Initially only one skin edge is incised so that the skin paddle can be altered according to the feeding vessel selected. When mobilizing the flap and approaching the main pedicle itself, a number of additional subcutaneous vessels more than 0.5 mm in diameter should be preserved. These can be dissected to a reasonable length for anastomosis in case they are required later to augment arterial or venous flow. The flap can be beveled as necessary to provide additional tissue, minimizing the skin paddle and donor site defect.

The dissection proceeds at either the suprafascial or subfascial level, depending on the flap being raised and surgeon's preference. Small vessels can be identified within the flap as the dissection proceeds, and these are followed until they converge on the vessel of origin. Loupe magnification assists in identifying vessels. Several intraoperative factors indicate the caliber of the perforator encountered. These are the size of the converging branches, whether they have any visible pulsation, and the extent of the facial opening traversed by the perforator. Larger fascial openings tend to be associated with larger perforators, even if this is not immediately apparent because of vessel spasm. It is crucial to approach the vessels in a blood-free environment, because this helps identify converging prefascial branches. Furthermore, the relative transparency of subcutaneous fat facilitates visualizing the approximate location of the perforator in advance (Fig. 7-5), thus avoiding inadvertent damage. Blood-free, clean dissection

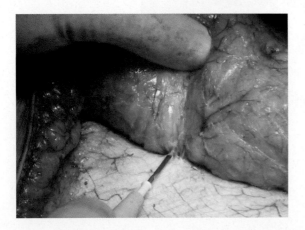

Fig. 7-5 A slit in the deep fascia and a blue hue shining through the subcutaneous fat indicate the location of the perforator at the cautery tip.

can be achieved by separating the tissue with low-current electrocautery and a wide spatula tip. It is essential to preserve all perforating vessels until a more dominant vessel is encountered. This avoids the inadvertent transection of a dominant perforator that would compromise perfusion. If more than one perforator is to be included in the flap, then the perforators can be approached from different directions for simultaneous dissection and identification. The inclusion of multiple perforators must not sacrifice muscle or divide important motor nerves, which would negate the advantages of raising a perforator flap. If it is essential to divide a motor nerve, then it must be surgically repaired. It is at this stage in flap dissection that accurate preoperative imaging allows speedier vessel dissection and sacrifice of nondominant vessels before reaching the predetermined dominant perforator.

Deep Fascia

Once the perforator has been identified and approached in the prefascial plane, further undermining should be performed between the subcutaneous fat and deep fascia for a distance of 2 to 4 cm around the perforator (Fig. 7-6). It is crucial to perform this step before opening the deep fascia, because once the fascia has been breached the dissection becomes increasingly difficult. In addition, it provides an easily visible safety zone around the perforator. This helps avoid potential damage to the vessel when the remaining flap is lifted off the deep fascia in the final phase of dissection.

Once a clear, circumferential view of the perforator has been established, it is necessary to open the deep fascia and follow the vessel through its intramuscular course. This is considerably easier if the fascial opening is large. The collagenous cuff around the perforator is cut and opened with specially designed fine scissors (Blondeel scissors; S&T AG, Neuhausen, Switzerland) until the loose connective tissue around the

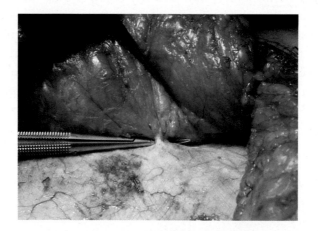

Fig. 7-6 Lifting fat off the deep fascia about 2 cm behind and around the perforator makes dissection easier.

perforator is encountered (Fig. 7-7). The loose connective tissue allows the perforator to glide between the muscle fibers and tendinous inscriptions of the rectus abdominis muscle when it moves and contracts. Dissection close to the vessels and within this loose connective tissue facilitates liberation of the vessels in a bloodless environment. Small fascial openings often adhere closely to the perforator. In this situation it may be necessary to incise the deep fascia lateral to the perforator, identify the immediate intramuscular course, and then leave a cuff of fascia around the vessel. The perforator may be seen running obliquely under the fascia before diving into the muscle. Therefore diligence is required to avoid inadvertent damage to the vessel.

In certain flaps, such as the SGAP flap, perforators may be approached from underneath the deep fascia. In such situations, a safe and slow approach to the perforator is hampered by the presence of thick epimysia that need to be cut throughout their entire length (Fig. 7-8). In a subfascial approach, the perforator can easily be identified

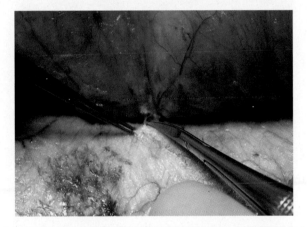

Fig. 7-7 Incising the collagenous cuff around the vessels exposes the gap in the deep fascia and frees the perforator.

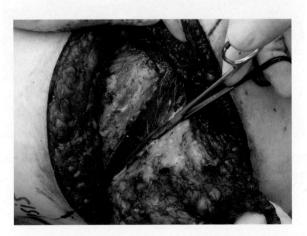

Fig. 7-8 In a subfascial approach, muscular epimysia is easily lifted and cut with tenotomy scissors.

because of the transparency of the epimysia (Fig. 7-9). The same subfascial approach is performed for septal perforator flaps. The approach over the muscle is easy, and identifying the septum is very simple. Perforators shine through at different levels, and the size of the artery and veins can be evaluated (Fig. 7-10).

After identifying the main perforator below the deep fascia just before it enters muscle or septum, circumferential dissection around the perforator is performed, as above the fascia. This space is avascular and filled with loose collagenous tissue, so dissection advances very easy. Here, it is also important to release the remaining attachments of the deep fascia to the perivascular tissue cuff, freeing the perforator entirely above the muscle (Fig. 7-11).

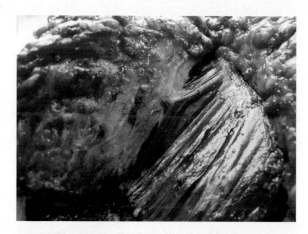

Fig. 7-9   The transparency of the epimysia facilitates localizing small and large vessels.

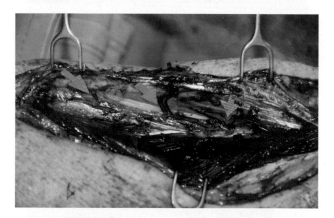

Fig. 7-10   A septal perforator is easy to identify in its septum by a subfascial approach. Different perforators (*green arrows*) can be evaluated for location and size.

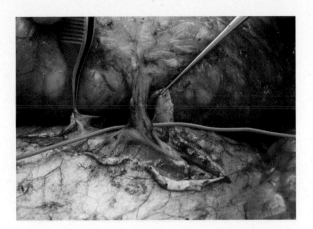

Fig. 7-11 Splitting the deep fascia in the direction of the muscle fibers above and below the perforator and an easy subfascial circumferential release complete a swift and easy dissection of the narrowest part of the perforator.

Intramuscular Dissection

Once the initial fascial incision is made above and below the perforator and following the direction of the muscle fibers, the fascia can be opened further for better exposure. This can be done in any direction, but is preferentially performed in the same direction as the underlying muscle fibers and toward, or over, the main supplying deep vessels. It is crucial to incise the deep fascia as much as necessary to gain wide exposure of the vessels in the surgical field. Opening the fascia leaves no donor site morbidity (provided proper resuturing is performed), whereas inadequate exposure risks damaging the vessel. At the point where the perforator enters the muscle, the muscle fibers are split in both directions by blunt dissection (Fig. 7-12). The loose connective tissue cuff around the vessels guides the path through the muscle and indicates where the muscle fibers need to be split. In a first phase, the muscle fibers on top of the perforator and the axial vessels are split to expose the course of the pedicle through the muscle. This so-called

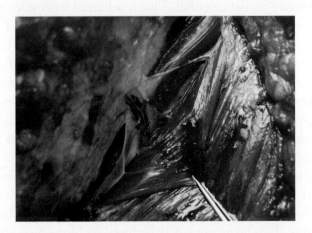

Fig. 7-12 The first step of intramuscular dissection is splitting the muscle in the direction of the muscle fibers.

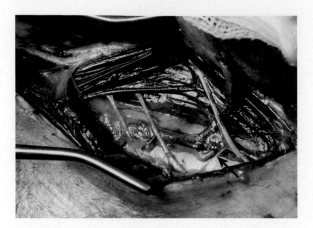

Fig. 7-13   All tissues running over the perforator are dissected off the vessels while the back side is still adherent (deroofing). Motor nerves almost always run anterior to the lateral branch of the deep inferior epigastric artery and need to be preserved. Recurrent branches of the intercostal motor nerves *(arrow)* can often be seen innervating the lateral part of the rectus abdominis muscle.

deroofing process allows fast visual inspection of the pedicle to confirm its patency and valid vessel size, allows early and quick adjustments to the intraoperative surgical strategy, but, of most importance, provides wide exposure and thus good visualization of the entire pedicle (Fig. 7-13).

Intramuscular dissection requires meticulous technique to identify the main vessels and ligate any side branches. Accidental rupture, damage, or division of these branches results in bleeding, which obscures the operative view and risks damage to the vessels when attempting hemostasis. It is therefore essential to maintain a bloodless field at all times. Hemostasis should be secured with bipolar cautery or by clipping larger vessels, while constantly irrigating with warm saline to ensure an adequate view of the vessel. Every side branch should be coagulated, ligated, or clipped at least 1 to 2 mm away from the perforator to avoid damage to the vessel and allow hemostasis to be resecured if needed.

Adequate exposure is also essential. This is achieved with self-retaining retractors or elastic retractor hooks (Lone Star Medical Products, Houston, TX). These consist of a metal hook attached to a length of elastic. The hook retracts the tissue while tension is maintained by securing the elastic to a drape or skin staple. These allow surgical instrumentation within the operative field to be kept to a minimum and free the surgical assistant for diathermy and irrigation. The perforator is always kept under direct vision to ensure that there is no tension on the vessel during flap manipulations and that it does not become desiccated. Securing the flap to the patient with staples or sutures should help prevent such inadvertent damage.

Direct handling of the vessels is avoided, and, when the perforators are completely freed from the surrounding tissue, the direction of dissection is always away from the vessel itself. The dissection plane is at the level of the loose connective tissue layer that surrounds the vessels. This layer can easily be freed by blunt dissection, and any resistance encountered is indicative of a side branch. The instruments used for dissection are the surgeon's preference. We use bipolar diathermy forceps and dissection scissors, such as Blondeel dissection scissors (S&T AG). The ring handle configuration of these scissors makes them suitable for preparing fine structures. The additional round handle and spring instrument configuration of the curved blades are extremely useful for fine trimming and dissection work. Once the larger, deeper vessel is reached, dissection proceeds until sufficient caliber and length are achieved.

The Main Pedicle

Nerves are often encountered at the level of the deeper vessels, just under or within the deeper part of the muscle. Depending on the region of dissection, nerves can be sensory, motor, or both. Adequate anatomic knowledge and nerve stimulators can help differentiate among these different fibers. Sensory nerves to the flap can be reanastomosed to recipient sensory nerves. The length of the donor nerve can be increased as necessary by retrograde dissection. Motor nerves are dissected off vessels over an adequate length to allow easy dissection of the vessels underneath. These nerves are always accompanied by one or more vascular side branches that need to be clipped. Occasionally it is necessary to divide the motor nerve. In such circumstances, a quick reanastomosis can be performed with two 9-0 nylon stitches in the perineurium. This is carried out once the flap has been harvested or moved.

In a free perforator flap, the main vessel is dissected until an adequate pedicle length has been achieved for easy anastomosis. It is equally important to reach a donor vessel diameter that is suitable in size for the recipient vessels. Good interaction between the two teams harvesting the flap and preparing the recipient site saves valuable operative time and permits simultaneous identification and characterization of recipient vessels. Often one artery and two venae comitantes are included in the pedicle. The smallest vena comitans is immediately ligated at the end of the dissection of the pedicle to redirect and precondition flow into the larger vein. The vein is preferentially transected immediately downstream of a branch interconnecting both venae comitantes, the so-called H-connectors. Although multiple H-connectors exist over the entire pedicle, anastomosis at this site allows easy flow over the anastomosis. A good anastomosis of one vein is preferred over linking two veins to ensure appropriate venous flow.

Pedicle perforator flaps are planned as rotation, advancement, or transposition flaps. They may include one or more perforating vessels. However, flaps that include only one perforator offer increased freedom of movement without vascular compromise.[17]

Once the feeding vessel is identified, vessel dissection continues for as long as necessary to allow tension-free positioning of the flap in the recipient defect. Tracing the perforator to its original source vessel is not always necessary once sufficient flap mobility is obtained. The aim is to obtain a degree of redundancy in the vessels when the flap is in the recipient site, which will ensure there is no tension on the perforator, even when subjected to postoperative swelling or hematoma.

Rotation Flap

With a rotation flap, the dominant perforator acts as a pivot point. The flap is designed in the fashion of a propeller blade. The longest part of the flap turns approximately 180 degrees into the defect. The perforator is often dissected over a short distance but long enough to ensure turning of the flap will not cause torsion of the vessel to the extent that it compromises perfusion. To sufficiently liberate the pedicle, the distance between the end of the dissection and the entry point in the flap needs to be slightly shortened. This allows the vein to gently turn around the artery.

Advancement Flap

An advancement flap is simply slid in one direction, parallel to the direction of the muscle fibers. Dissection can proceed down to the axial vessels, which occasionally also require mobilization. An oblique course of the vessels to the skin surface is needed to allow flap movement. The longer the perforator, the more the movement of the flap. Any design of skin island is acceptable, provided the limits of viability are respected.

Transposition Flap

For further displacements, a longer leash is necessary. Movements of displacement, advancement, and rotation are performed simultaneously. Sufficient slack of the pedicle is needed, without causing kinking of the pedicle. It is essential to plan accurately and take exact measurements before making skin incisions. The size of the skin island is determined by the limits of blood flow to the periphery of the flap. Therefore a perforator located in the center of the flap is preferred. It is also important to avoid subcutaneous tunneling of flaps in areas of dense subcutaneous tissues such as the sacral and gluteal areas. This may compromise perfusion, resulting in fat necrosis or, in the worst case, flap loss.

Recipient Vessel Selection and Preparation

Ideal recipient vessels are nontraumatized, nonscarred, nonirradiated, disease-free vessels (at least one artery and one vein) with sufficient length for easy microanastomosis and a diameter that corresponds to the donor vessels. Traumatized or irradiated vessels are difficult to expose and can result in considerable risk of iatrogenic trauma and higher rates of thrombosis and flap failure. For some conventional free flaps, an interposition graft may be required to lengthen the flap pedicle and allow anastomosis out to the zone of injury. Unfortunately, many studies have shown such grafts to increase the rate of flap failure.[20-23]

Unlike conventional free flaps, perforator flaps have consistently longer vascular pedicles, which give them increased flexibility for anastomosis to most recipient vessels. Thus a perforator flap can ensure that the most appropriate recipient vessels are selected, maximizing the chance of flap success. The only limitation is the size of the flap vessels, which may necessitate an end to side anastomosis, the use of perforator recipient vessels, or anastomosis to the side branch of a large recipient vessel. In the field of supermicrosurgery, perforator-to-perforator anastomosis eliminates the need to dissect the flap vessels down to the larger axial vessels. Not only does this increase the ease of dissection, but vessels are more compatible in size. Though this may seem like an obvious progression, smaller vessel diameters increase the risk of thrombosis and flap failure.[24-26]

Preparing the recipient vessels requires the same meticulous technique as flap raising. Hemostasis must be controlled by vascular clips or bipolar coagulation and aided by irrigation. Perivascular hematoma has been shown to cause vasospasm and flow disturbances, as well as prolonged vessel wall ischemia with resultant increased inflammatory response.[27]

Exposure should be wide to facilitate dissection and prevent compression of the pedicle against adjacent structures. Most of the vessel dissection is carried out under loupe magnification, with the final stages sometimes requiring an operating microscope, especially for perforator-to-perforator anastomosis. The key aspect of vessel dissection is to advance the perivascular plane between the vessel and its vascular sheath. Once the sheath is divided, it can be retracted by gentle pulling and then removed. The vessel is then sharply divided and the adventitia trimmed. It is important to facilitate the anastomosis as much as possible by preparing the field adequately. A green or blue background is placed behind the vessel to be anastomosed, keeping all other structures out of the way. Continuous low negative-pressure microsuction can be secured under the background by a small drain held with staples. Skin retraction is achieved with the self-retaining retractors mentioned previously. The flap is secured atraumatically in a suitable position by wrapping it in saline-soaked gauze and stapling the gauze to the skin around the recipient site. All these maneuvers free the assistant to help with vessel preparation. Irrigation is performed with normal saline or heparin solution (5000 to 50,000 U in 500 ml lactated Ringer solution),[28,29] as long as the intima is exposed. Either the artery or the vein can be repaired first, and the sequence is often determined by vessel position rather than an optimal order. Vessels located in deeper planes or furthest away from the surgeon's hands are sutured first. Two venous anastomoses may seem to be an obvious option if there is any doubt about venous outflow. However, caution should be exercised, because this potentially reduces the venous outflow in each vessel and can lead to sludging and thrombosis.[30]

(AVOIDING) COMPLICATIONS AND LIMITATIONS

With all promising techniques, there is a specific learning curve[31]; the perforator flap is by no means an exception. This learning curve is composed of three main elements.[32] The first is the surgical technique itself, which is experience dependent. In inexperienced hands, the dissection of small vessels through muscle can be difficult, tedious, and time consuming. However, once a surgeon has reached the plateau of their learning curve, it has been shown that the mean time for a DIEAP can be significantly less than for a transverse rectus abdominis musculocutaneous flap.[33] Good preoperative planning with the aid of CT angiography, operating in a bloodless field, and creating wide exposure are the key elements for a complication-free and swift operation. The presence of two operating teams obviously reduces operative time significantly.

The second element of the learning curve is the experience and organization of the operating staff. It is essential to have a strong support team, in both the theater and wards, with good clinical experience who can ensure smooth running of the surgery and follow-up. The best way to maximize flap salvage is through early detection of postoperative problems in blood circulation by staff members, and prompt reexploration of the vessels. Most flaps are lost because surgeons wait and observe too long. When there is doubt, the patient is returned to the operating room and the flap explored.

The third component of the learning curve is also referred to as the *pendulum effect*. Introducing a new technique results in much excitement and enthusiasm. The surgeon may be inclined to apply the technique excessively, even in cases that would be better served with an alternate procedure. After gaining personal insight into the difficulties of the procedure, the pendulum swings back to the neutral position, and the surgeon uses the flap when indications are optimal.

Preoperative imaging aids greatly in predicting problems and can allow modification of the surgical plan to avoid these pitfalls. Even with this reassurance, surgeons should avoid completely circumscribing the flap until they have localized the main perforator and ensured that the flap is centered on this vessel. With a limited incision technique the flap design can be modified, converted to a conventional musculocutaneous technique, or even abandoned and directly closed without unnecessary sacrifice of tissue.

The key to success in perforator surgery is to anticipate potential problems and save any anastomosable vessels as a lifeboat if needed. For example, if venous or arterial compromise becomes evident with a single perforator or a superficial vascular system, then additionally prepared vessels can be anastomosed to other recipient vessels to augment blood flow. The size of the perforator selected is of extreme significance and is closely correlated to the size of the flap it perfuses. For large flaps, such as a DIEAP or SGAP flap, the size of the perforating vena comitans should be at least 1 mm. The artery can be much smaller than the vein, but it needs to deliver sufficient antegrade blood flow and retrograde venous return. It is very hard to give advice about the absolute size and diameter of the vessels. Large, thick flaps need and mostly have large perforators. Small, thin flaps can survive perfectly well on a very small pedicle. Perforators in the same anatomic area can vary in size from one patient to another, depending on body habitus. Patients with a higher body mass index tend to have larger perforators. An ideal patient is one who has lost a significant amount of weight, because the size of the perforators is maintained after weight reduction. So instead of looking for absolute figures for diameters, one should look for relative sizes and compare different perforators in the same area. The largest of these perforators is most often dominant. The dominant perforator can always be harvested with an additional perforator localized close to, or within, the same epimysium.

It is important to make the dissection as simple as possible. Perforators can course through the septum or have a short or protracted intramuscular course. If there are similar-sized perforators, then those requiring the simplest dissection should be selected. In addition, the surgeon should consider the proximity of motor nerves. Crossover or adherence of these nerves to the perforator can also make the dissection more tedious.

When the flap has been dissected, the surgeon should avoid transecting secondary perforators until the dominant vessel has been dissected to its origin and the flap is ready for anastomosis. The flap should be constantly secured to the patient and attention paid to the perforator to ensure that it is not placed under any tension. Strict adherence to these guidelines should prevent accidental damage, but, should this occur, the flap can be raised on a contralateral perforator or as a musculocutaneous flap.

The success rate of perforator flaps is directly related to the experience of the microsurgeon. The small size of the pedicle, combined with the absence of a muscular cuff to protect the vessels, makes the anastomosis more vulnerable to injury. Vessel dissection often results in vasospasm. However, the mechanical effect of adventitial stripping often causes compensatory vasodilation by interrupting the sympathetic supply and mechanically thinning the walls. Unless the vessels are abnormal (for example, perivascular fibrosis), it is highly unlikely that vascular spasm will persist to the extent it causes permanent flap damage. If this spasm lasts 30 minutes or longer, then papaverine (opium alkaloid acting through smooth muscle) can help alleviate the problem. If arterial input to the flap is still insufficient after the patient's physiologic status is optimized (flow is predominantly influenced by the mean arterial blood pressure), it is most likely the result of an inadequate anastomosis, flap dissection error, or arterial problems proximal to the anastomosis. The surgeon should ensure that there is flow in the proximal feeding artery and that there is no kinking, twisting, or tension. The site of clamp application should be examined for damage to the vessel wall. If the proximal flow is adequate, then the anastomosis should be inspected and resected completely. The flap should be thoroughly washed with urokinase (600,000 IU in 100 ml NaCl 0.9%), streptokinase, or plasminogen activator.[34-36] Direct injection of these agents into the artery, with the venous outflow left open to drain in the operating field, prevents systemic side effects of an intravenous infusion and allows toxins to be washed out of the vein. If the vessel is heavily thrombosed, it should not be used and another flap or recipient site vessel should be explored. Interposition grafts may be necessary.

The venous system is more fragile than the arterial side because of thinner walls and low flow conditions. This makes veins more sensitive than arteries to kinking or torsion. Venous insufficiency of a perforator flap can be caused by inadequate drainage of the vena comitans, sometimes seen when the superficial system is dominant and the perforators are of a small caliber. In such an event the following options are available to the surgeon[32]:

- The superficial veins preserved during dissection can be used. If an adequate length of vein has already been preserved as a lifeboat, this can be anastomosed directly to the recipient vessels or to an additional recipient vessel to augment flow. If the length of the vessel is inadequate, then an interposition graft is an option. We prefer arterial interposition grafts over vein grafts, because they are stiffer and maintain patency of the vein, resulting in less vascular impedance to flow.
- A second arterial/venous perforator can be anastomosed to a side branch of the main vascular pedicle.
- A superficial vein on the ipsilateral side can be attached to the main vascular pedicle. This can be performed in an end-to-side fashion or end-to-end with a side branch and may require an interposition graft.
- An anastomosis across the midline of the flap can be added, between the two deep systems.
- A superficial vein can be anastomosed to an additional vein at the recipient site.

The no-flow phenomenon occurs when tissue fails to perfuse adequately, despite a patent arterial anastomosis. There is a progressive obstruction to blood flow with increasing ischemic time, which is thought to result from cellular swelling, leakage of intravascular fluid, and intravascular aggregation and stagnation, with sludging and thrombus formation. One other factor that could influence the no-flow phenomenon is microemboli that form following a microvascular anastomosis. The fate of these emboli remains unclear, but they may be responsible for flap ischemia.[37]

References

1. Blondeel N, Boeckx WD, Vanderstraeten GG, et al. The fate of the oblique abdominal muscles after free TRAM flap surgery. Br J Plast Surg 50:315-321, 1997.
2. Blondeel N, Vanderstraeten GG, Monstrey SJ, et al. The donor site morbidity of free DIEP flaps and free TRAM flaps for breast reconstruction. Br J Plast Surg 50:322-330, 1997.

    The free DIEAP flap provides the advantages of autologous breast reconstruction with lower abdominal tissue and limits the late postoperative weakness of the lower abdominal wall. Surgical damage to the rectus abdominis and oblique muscles is minimal. The main disadvantage of this procedure is the added surgical time.
3. Futter CM, Webster MH, Hagen S, et al. A retrospective comparison of abdominal muscle strength following breast reconstruction with a free TRAM or DIEP flap. Br J Plast Surg 53:578-583, 2000.
4. Futter CM, Weiler-Mithoff E, Hagen S, et al. Do pre-operative abdominal exercises prevent post-operative donor site complications for women undergoing DIEP flap breast reconstruction? A two-centre, prospective randomised controlled trial. Br J Plast Surg 56:674-683, 2003.
5. Hamdi M, Decorte T, Demuynck M, et al. Shoulder function after harvesting a thoracodorsal artery perforator flap. Plast Reconstr Surg 122:1111-1117; discussion 1118-1119, 2008.
6. Nahabedian MY, Dooley W, Singh N, et al. Contour abnormalities of the abdomen after breast reconstruction with abdominal flaps: the role of muscle preservation. Plast Reconstr Surg 109:91-101, 2002.
7. Nahabedian MY, Manson PN. Contour abnormalities of the abdomen after transverse rectus abdominis muscle flap breast reconstruction: a multifactorial analysis. Plast Reconstr Surg 109:81-87; discussion 88-90, 2002.
8. Angrigiani C, Grilli D, Siebert J. Latissimus dorsi musculocutaneous flap without muscle. Plast Reconstr Surg 96:1608-1614, 1995.
9. Hallock GG. Further clarification of the nomenclature for compound flaps. Plast Reconstr Surg 117:151e-160e, 2006.
10. Bilgin SS, Topalan M, Ip WY, et al. Effect of torsion on microvenous anastomotic patency in a rat model and early thrombolytic phenomenon. Microsurgery 23:381-386, 2003.
11. Demir A, Acar M, Yldz L, et al. The effect of twisting on perforator flap viability: an experimental study in rats. Ann Plast Surg 56:186-189, 2006.
12. Salgarello M, Lahoud P, Selvaggi G, et al. The effect of twisting on microanastomotic patency of arteries and veins in a rat model. Ann Plast Surg 47:643-646, 2001.
13. Selvaggi G, Anicic S, Formaggia L. Mathematical explanation of the buckling of the vessels after twisting of the microanastomosis. Microsurgery 26:524-528, 2006.

    The authors studied the phenomenon of "buckling" of the femoral artery and vein on an experimental rat model. They calculated the critical twisting angle that induces buckling: Maintaining a constant length of dissection of 25 mm, a minimum twisting angle of 360 degrees (plus 161 degrees or 105 degrees, respectively, for the femoral artery or vein) was required for the buckling phenomenon, with the appearance of two wave-like deformations of the vessel wall and decreased section area.
14. Topalan M, Bilgin SS, Ip WY, et al. Effect of torsion on microarterial anastomosis patency. Microsurgery 23:56-59, 2003.
15. Hallock GG. The propeller flap version of the adductor muscle perforator flap for coverage of ischial or trochanteric pressure sores. Ann Plast Surg 56:540-542, 2006.
16. Hyakusoku H, Yamamoto T, Fumiiri M. The propeller flap method. Br J Plast Surg 44:53-54, 1991.

    The authors reported a method of elevating and rotating a flap, similar to a propeller, for releasing scar contractures in the cubital and axillary regions. This flap may be applied in other areas.

17. Bravo FG, Schwarze HP. Free-style local perforator flaps: concept and classification system. J Plast Reconstr Aesthet Surg 62:602-608; discussion 609, 2009.

18. Alonso-Burgos A, Garcia-Tutor E, Bastarrika G, et al. Preoperative planning of DIEP and SGAP flaps: preliminary experience with magnetic resonance angiography using 3-tesla equipment and blood-pool contrast medium. J Plast Reconstr Aesthet Surg 63:298-304, 2010.

19. Uppal RS, Casaer B, Van Landuyt K, et al. The efficacy of preoperative mapping of perforators in reducing operative times and complications in perforator flap breast reconstruction. J Plast Reconstr Aesthet Surg 62:859-864, 2009.

20. Bayramicli M, Tetik C, Sonmez A, et al. Reliability of primary vein grafts in lower extremity free tissue transfers. Ann Plast Surg 48:21-29, 2002.

21. Miller MJ, Schusterman MA, Reece GP, et al. Interposition vein grafting in head and neck reconstructive microsurgery. J Reconstr Microsurg 9:245-251; discussion 251-242, 1993.

22. Suominen S, Asko-Seljavaara S. Free flap failures. 16:396-399, 1995.
    A retrospective analysis of 75 consecutive free flap patients was performed to better understand factors associated with free flap failure or immediate vascular complications. Preoperative infection of the recipient site or prolonged operation time correlated with flap failure. The use of a vein graft or long perioperative ischemia correlated with immediate vascular complications. Many factors often given as reasons for failure (age, body mass, history of cardiovascular disease, smoking, or previous irradiation of the recipient site) were not significant in this study.

23. Yazar S. Selection of recipient vessels in microsurgical free tissue reconstruction of head and neck defects. Microsurgery 27:588-594, 2007.

24. Haywood RM, Raurell A, Perks AG, et al. Autologous free tissue breast reconstruction using the internal mammary perforators as recipient vessels. Br J Plast Surg 56:689-691, 2003.

25. Hong JP. The use of supermicrosurgery in lower extremity reconstruction: the next step in evolution. Plast Reconstr Surg 123:230-235, 2009.
    Supermicrosurgery in lower extremity reconstruction expands the number of possible recipient pedicles. With perforator-to-perforator anastomosis, securing the recipient vessel and elevating the flap are less time consuming, and the risk for major vessel injury is minimized. Flap survival is acceptable; however, the learning curve is steep.

26. Munhoz AM, Ishida LH, Montag E, et al. Perforator flap breast reconstruction using internal mammary perforator branches as a recipient site: an anatomical and clinical analysis. Plast Reconstr Surg 114:62-68, 2004.
    The internal mammary perforator branch is studied as a recipient site for free flap breast reconstruction. The main advantages of using this vessel include spared internal mammary vessels for a possible future cardiac surgery, prevention of thoracic deformities, and reduced operative time by limited dissection. The main disadvantages include limited surgical exposure, caliber incompatibility, and technical difficulties.

27. Bayramicli M, Yilmaz B, San T, et al. Effects of hematoma on the short-term fate of experimental microvenous autografts. J Reconstr Microsurg 14:575-586, 1998.

28. Li X, Cooley BC, Gould JS. Influence of topical heparin on stasis-induced thrombosis of microvascular anastomoses. Microsurgery 13:72-75, 1992.

29. Rumbolo PM, Cooley BC, Hanel DP, et al. Comparison of the influence of intralumenal irrigation solutions on free flap survival. Microsurgery 13:45-47, 1992.

30. Futran ND, Stack BC Jr. Single versus dual venous drainage of the radial forearm free flap. Am J Otolaryngol 17:112-117, 1996.

31. Blackwell KE, Brown MT, Gonzalez D. Overcoming the learning curve in microvascular head and neck reconstruction. Arch Otolaryngol Head Neck Surg 123:1332-1335, 1997.

32. Blondeel PN, Morris SF, Neligan P, Hallock GG. Perforator Flaps: Anatomy, Techniques, & Clinical Applications, 1st ed. St Louis: Quality Medical Publishing, 2006.

33. Kaplan JL, Allen RJ. Cost-based comparison between perforator flaps and TRAM flaps for breast reconstruction. Plast Reconstr Surg 105:943-948, 2000.
34. Panchapakesan V, Addison P, Beausang E, et al. Role of thrombolysis in free-flap salvage. J Reconstr Microsurg 19:523-530, 2003.

    An algorithm for using thrombolytics to manage failing free flaps was presented, based on the authors' own results and other published results.
35. Serletti JM, Moran SL, Orlando GS, et al. Urokinase protocol for free-flap salvage following prolonged venous thrombosis. Plast Reconstr Surg 102:1947-1953, 1998.

    The authors established a protocol for administering urokinase for postoperative venous thrombosis.
36. Yii NW, Evans GR, Miller MJ, et al. Thrombolytic therapy: what is its role in free flap salvage? Ann Plast Surg 46:601-604, 2001.
37. Wang WZ, Tsai TM, Anderson GL. Late-preconditioning protection is evident in the microcirculation of denervated skeletal muscle. J Orthop Res 17:571-577, 1999.

8

Avoiding Complications

Phillip N. Blondeel
Peter C. Neligan

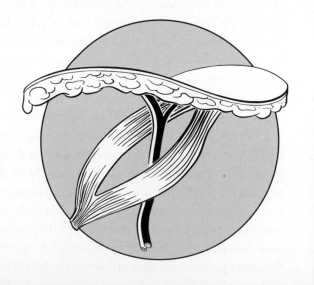

As with all emerging procedures, there is a learning curve with perforator flap surgery. The learning curve is self-explanatory; it only stands to reason that there are new things to learn. The curve is shortened by gaining knowledge of the procedure from those who have already made the mistakes. This is our reason for writing this chapter—so that you can learn from our mistakes and add these procedures to your reconstructive armamentarium. There is also a pendulum effect associated with new techniques that is intrinsically part of the learning curve, though less self-evident. When a new procedure is introduced, it is overly applied. Caught in the zeal and excitement of the new technique, the surgeon tends to apply it in cases where other procedures might better serve the patient. After gaining experience, the surgeon uses the procedure for the most appropriate situations (the pendulum swings back toward the center point).

The angiosome principle[1] and the theory that no more than two choke vessels can be exceeded to ensure adequate flap vascularization provided a clear basis for designing new flaps. The only variable that a surgeon cannot control is the size of the angiosome. Some more recent studies have demonstrated that the unpredictable orientation and course of the deep inferior epigastric artery perforators indicate that the blood supply of abdominal perforator flaps, raised without clear knowledge of their unique vascular anatomy, may often be more random than axial. This is not consistent with the angiosome theory.[2] Depending on the donor area, this variability may be limited, and surgeons have empirically determined the safe limits of flaps such as the latissimus dorsi flap. With perforator flaps we are moving one echelon lower, or, stated another way, one branch higher on the vascular tree during dissection. We are working with perforator vessels and not axial vessels. Clinical experience, at least initially, may play less of a role in decision making at this level. In some areas of the body the location and size of the perforators are well known. The intercostal perforators are such an example. In other areas the number, position, and size of the angiosomes can be very variable. The abdominal wall is an example of this situation. Because the size of the angiosome is the only determining factor for predicting a safe perforator flap harvest, visualizing and delineating the position and size of the angiosome would be ideal. It would provide a clear indication of which perforator or perforators are dominant and need to be included in the flap. Currently such an investigation is not widely available, but real-time perfusion imaging is gaining popularity and promises to help enhance our understanding of flow dynamics and the relationship of flow dynamics to anatomy. Additionally, our understanding of the exact parameters that influence the physiology of flow is inadequate. This is another important factor that can determine survival or ischemia of areas farther away from the feeding perforator. Specifically, if the subdermal plexus were vascularized by a random network instead of by angiosomes, knowledge of flow physiology would play a crucial role in tissue survival. Duplex Doppler[3,4] and CT angiography[5] are currently the best tools available for evaluating vascular trees arising from the axial vessels and nourishing the skin after piercing the muscle and deep fascia. Both techniques help determine the exact position of different perforators and estimate their size and flow. By plotting the different perforators, the flap, including perforators, can be roughly mapped and safe flap borders can be estimated and marked (see Chapter 6). Recently, indocyanine green (ICG), a fluorescent dye, and near-infrared angiography have been used to obtain real-time video images of perfusion and facilitate the decision-making process when choosing the most appropriate perforator or perforators to perfuse a given flap.[6] In the United States this system is known as the *SPY System.* It was developed by the Novadaq Corporation (Bonita Springs, FL) and is marketed by LifeCell Corporation (Branchburg, NJ). The process involves intravenous injection of ICG. The SPY System emits near-infrared light under which ICG fluoresces. The SPY camera then records, in real time, the territory supplied by a given perforator by noting the extent of fluorescence. Microscope-integrated ICG near-infrared videoangiography (ICGA) is another new technique in which the near-infrared light source and fluorescence-capturing technology are incorporated in the microscope and can assess flow across anastomoses in real time,[7] which is the beauty of this system. I (P.C.N.) have adopted this in my practice. When performing a DIEAP flap, for example, all potential perforators are isolated (using the guidelines outlined previously). The best perforator is chosen, and the others are clamped with Acland clamps. ICG is then injected and perfusion assessed. On most occasions the ICG merely confirms that perfusion by the given perforator will be sufficient to sustain the flap. However, on several occasions the predicted perforator has proved to be insufficient, and the operative plan has been changed as a consequence. This technology can also evaluate the viability of mastectomy flaps. Complications from poor perfusion in the flaps can be reduced with this technique.[8]

After perforating muscle and deep fascia, muscle perforators give off branches destined to perfuse the dermal plexus and provide a connection between the deep and superficial systems. In some areas such as the buttock, the superficial system is virtually absent. In most areas of the body the superficial venous drainage system is dominant, as in the lower arm. Other areas include a dominant superficial arterial system such as the superficial circumflex iliac vessels. Some areas have a variable balance of dominance between the deep and superficial systems. The lower abdominal wall is a very specific example where, in most cases, the superficial epigastric artery and vein are dominant to the deep system. A comparable example is the variable balance between the cutaneous branch of the thoracodorsal vessels and the deep perforators of the latissimus dorsi muscle. Determining the dominance of either the superficial or the deep system preoperatively will avoid major problems of flap perfusion. Often intraoperative direct visualization of different vascular pedicles to the same skin island may be necessary, in addition to the information gained by CT scanning or ultrasound investigations, even if it is somewhat time consuming.[9] ICGA can be of great assistance in making these decisions. Insufficient knowledge of the vascular anatomy may lead to erroneous transection of vascular pedicles that later prove to be dominant. In general, the free-style free flap principle needs to be followed (see Chapter 72). Basically, this means that any vessel encountered while incising the borders of the flap that is considered to be anastomosable (larger than 0.5 mm) needs to be isolated and preserved with some length. If later during the dissection arterial inflow or venous outflow is insufficient with either one single perforator or the superficial system, additional vessels can be anastomosed to other recipient vessels to increase blood flow. In the future it is likely that ICGA or some similar technology will become routine. These vessels act as lifeboats that might be extremely important in specific cases. Obviously, the smaller the planned skin island, the lower the number of available (but necessary) anastomosable vessels, and the more difficult it will be to place the skin island on top of a specific perforator. Alternatively, small skin flaps rarely have problems with inadequate blood flow and fat necrosis. The larger the skin flap, the greater the chance to include large superficial or deep vessels.

We can never prepare for the unexpected, but we can anticipate potential problems and take appropriate measures to avoid them. Dissecting perforator flaps is demanding, but also extremely safe. In most cases, a flap ultimately relies on a single perforator, though we generally start with more than one. The deep inferior epigastric artery perforator (DIEAP) flap is a perfect example. The rationale for using this flap over the transverse rectus abdominis musculocutaneous (TRAM) flap is that there is no muscle or fascial excision, and the perforator supplying the flap is dissected out from the muscle. In this way we are able to harvest the same tissue that a TRAM flap provides, while minimizing donor morbidity.[10,11] The reason it is so safe to raise a flap, and so safe to teach one, is that dissection can begin on one side while the other side remains intact. If the perforator is damaged during dissection, it is a simple matter either to find an appropriate perforator on the other side or convert to a TRAM flap on the other side. We recommend evaluating the perforators on one side and, presuming an appropriate one is found, proceeding with its dissection while all the perforators on the other side are still intact. This also makes the DIEAP flap a very safe one for learning dissection. The safety net of the contralateral, intact perforators alleviates some of the stress involved while learning the technique.

Though we generally think of perforator flaps as free flaps, many of these can be applied as pedicle flaps, making these convenient for teaching and learning. For example, the SGAP flap is frequently used for breast reconstruction, but can also be used as a pedicle flap in the ischial and sacral regions.[12,13] Similarly, the anterolateral thigh flap (lateral circumflex femoral artery perforator–vastus lateralis or LCFAP-*vl*) can be used as a pedicle flap in the groin and perineum.[14-17] Using these flaps as local pedicle flaps that provide excellent local tissue for closing defects is a good way to gain familiarity with flap dissection.

GOLDEN RULES FOR PREVENTING COMPLICATIONS WITH PERFORATOR FLAPS
Map the Perforators

Locating perforators and estimating perforator size preoperatively are essential steps in flap design and help avoid partial flap necrosis and/or fat necrosis. The goal is to identify the most dominant perforator relative to the surrounding and/or contralateral perforators. Not only is the size of the perforator at the level of the deep fascia relevant for estimating flap size and location, but also the number and direction of its branches between the skin and the deep fascia (Fig. 8-1). Once the dominant perforator is identified, the flap margins are drawn according to the position of the main perforator (Fig. 8-2). See Chapters 6 and 7 for further details on preoperative planning of perforator flaps.

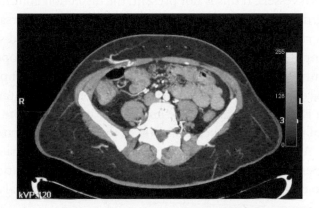

Fig. 8-1   CT angiography of the lower abdomen showing the tortuous course through the rectus abdominis muscle, lateral bending of the perforator vessels after piercing the deep fascia, and clear branching of the perforator below the skin. This perforator had the largest size compared with any other perforator in the lower abdomen.

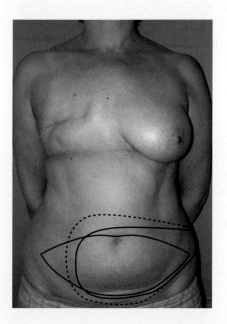

Fig. 8-2   Design of a DIEAP flap on top of the main perforator (+). In contrast to the design of a TRAM flap over the midline *(blue line)*, the skin paddle *(black line)* is positioned more lateral with the main perforator as its center point. More tissue can be included by extending the flap more laterally (up to the midaxillary line) or beveling cranially *(dotted line)*.

Identify the Main Perforator With a Limited Incision

We recommend avoiding a full-thickness skin and fat incision down to the fascia at the full circumference of the skin island. By making an incision on only one side of the skin island, lifting the flap, and localizing the main perforator, as defined preoperatively, the surgeon can modify the design of the flap later. With a handheld unidirectional Doppler device the main perforator can be localized in a different position than expected preoperatively, or additional larger perforators may be found. With a limited incision on one side the design can be changed intraoperatively, or a conventional technique such as a musculocutaneous flap can be used, as discussed previously with the DIEAP flap.

Another example of the importance of a limited incision is the dissection of thoracodorsal artery perforator (TDAP) flaps. By making an incision at the level of the anterior border of the latissimus dorsi muscle, the surgeon can first look for the cutaneous branch of the thoracodorsal vessels. If this is not present, the dissection continues over the edge of the anterior border for the dominant perforator of the thoracodorsal vessels. Because these perforators run somewhat obliquely through the muscle and subcutaneous fat, unidirectional Doppler can provide erroneous information. Intraoperative visualization can help identify the exact position of the main perforator. Duplex Doppler, CT angiography, and contrast medium–free MRI provide only momentary imaging of the perforator, which is physiologically active and can be in either a contracted or relaxed state at the time of imaging. Visual comparison of the largest perforator will help make the final decision. And if one has the luxury of access to ICGA, decision making is even easier. Once the perforator is identified, the size, shape, and orientation of the flap can still be changed to ensure perfect vascularization of the skin island (also see Chapter 7).

Preserve Each Perforator Until a Larger One Is Encountered

This philosophy is very simple. After lifting up the border of the flap in a prefascial or subfascial plane, the dissection continues until the first perforator in the preferred vascular territory is reached. If the perforator is considered to be large enough to sufficiently nourish the flap, it is preserved and dissection continues until a second perforator is encountered (Fig. 8-3). The smallest perforator is then transected, and dissection continues until the next perforator is found. Again, the smaller of the two is ligated.

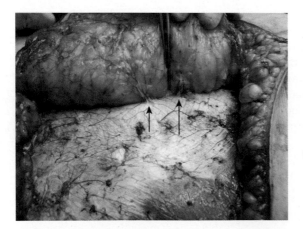

Fig. 8-3 Lateral prefascial approach to perforators of the deep inferior epigastric artery of the left abdominal wall. First a small lateral perforator is identified *(small arrow)*. By moving more medially, going around the first perforator, a second more medial and larger perforator *(large arrow)* is visualized. The first one can then be sacrificed.

This continues until the largest perforator of the flap is identified. If two or more perforators are preferred, these can be left intact before making a final decision on transecting perforators. This principle is extremely important if no preoperative information is available, because it ensures sufficient safety and easy decision making. Obviously, if preoperative imaging has been performed, one can proceed directly to the main perforator and avoid wasting time[18] dissecting other perforators.

Select the Best Perforator

The size of the perforator is extremely important. Poiseuille's law is elementary in understanding the relationship between the diameter of the perforator artery and vein and the flow rate within the vessels (Fig. 8-4). The viscosity and length of the vessels do not undergo significant changes. Blood pressure will be the only significant factor influencing flow in a denervated flap in the postoperative phase. Choosing a perforator artery with twice the diameter of a smaller, neighboring perforator will increase flow by a factor of 16. A 19% increase in radius will double the intraluminal flow. This means that the flow in a single 2 mm perforator artery is eight times higher than in two neighboring perforator arteries of 1 mm. This demonstrates that it is crucial to identify and harvest the most dominant perforator in relation to its surrounding perforators.

Although there is a critical minimum size for perforator vessels, there is no absolute size that can be handled. The larger the surface and volume of the flap, the larger the perforator needs to be. In general, the size of the vena comitans of the perforator needs to be at least 1 mm in large perforator flaps such as the DIEAP and superior gluteal artery perforator (SGAP) flaps. Although the artery can be much smaller, it should be sufficiently large to guarantee adequate antegrade blood flow and retrograde venous return. In general, if the largest perforator is selected from a dominant deep system, adequate vascularization is guaranteed up to the angiosome across the second choke vessel. Localizing the perforators is at least as important as their size. The harvested perforator should be one closest to the middle point of the skin flap, or the skin paddle

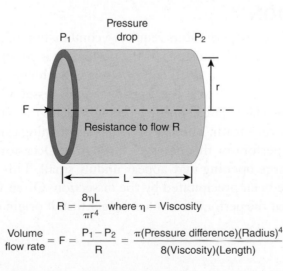

$$R = \frac{8\eta L}{\pi r^4} \quad \text{where } \eta = \text{Viscosity}$$

$$\frac{\text{Volume}}{\text{flow rate}} = F = \frac{P_1 - P_2}{R} = \frac{\pi (\text{Pressure difference})(\text{Radius})^4}{8(\text{Viscosity})(\text{Length})}$$

Fig. 8-4 Poiseuille's law. (*F*, Flow; *P*, pressure; *r*, radius; *R*, resistance to flow.)

should be positioned on top of the main perforator. Maintaining a normal to slightly higher mean blood pressure postoperatively is another important point to ensure ubiquitous blood flow in the flap.

Consider the Easiest Dissection

The length and type of intramuscular dissection to be performed after the deep fascia has been opened is important. Some perforators have a long and tortuous course through the muscle, and their dissection is long and tedious. If other perforators of similar size are available with a shorter intramuscular course, these might be preferred. Typical examples are the medial and lateral perforators of the rectus abdominis muscle. Lateral perforators that run through tendinous inscriptions have a very short and easy dissection before entering the dominant lateral branch of the deep inferior epigastric vessels. Medial perforators have a long course through the muscle and often run obliquely distally and laterally to finally reach the medial branch or a dominant central branch of the deep inferior epigastric vessels. Also, the proximity and involvement of motor nerves need to be considered when dissecting perforator flaps. For example, dissecting inferior gluteal perforators can be tedious because of crossover or adherence of motor nerves to the perforators. This is much less likely in the dissection of perforators of the superior gluteal artery.

Transect Other Perforators After the Entire Pedicle Is Dissected

Although several perforators may be identified while dissecting fat from the deep fascia, it is recommended not to cut all of them until the entire pedicle is dissected. If a mistake is made during dissection of the intramuscular and submuscular part of the vascular pedicle, one can still rely on other perforators and other pedicles to guarantee adequate blood flow to the flap. The specific example of a unilateral DIEAP flap has already been explained. If an accident occurs and blood vessels are accidentally damaged, the same flap can still be harvested on a contralateral perforator, or, in case of uncertainty, even as a musculocutaneous flap.

FLAP DISSECTION

The technique of dissecting perforators requires a combination of patience, gentleness, and meticulous attention to hemostasis. If the perforator is passing through fascia, it is perfectly reasonable to take a small cuff of fascia with the perforator if this seems the easiest way to proceed. Often it is easier to take the vessel without fascia. This is particularly true when a large fascial opening accommodates the perforator, as we often see in the anterior rectus sheath. The size of the fascial opening can also provide a clue as to the size of the perforator that emerges through it. Occasionally, the perforator passing through a large opening may appear unduly small. This is often because of spasm that may have been precipitated by the dissection. Often when fascia is cut it becomes apparent that the perforator is much bigger than it originally appeared. When cutting fascia, regardless of the flap being dissected, it is important to realize that the perforator may run obliquely under fascia before diving into the muscle, and it is very easy to damage the perforator in this situation. For this reason, the exact location of the perforator should always be known before cutting fascia.

The first glimpse of the perforator often gives the best clue about its actual size. It is not uncommon to come across what appears to be a reasonable perforator only to have it contract during dissection and look much less impressive. In this case the original impression is usually correct. It is sometimes useful to irrigate the flap pedicle with papaverine when dissection is complete to produce vasorelaxation before ultimate pedicle ligation and flap transfer.

Once intramuscular dissection has begun, hemostasis becomes very important for visualizing the perforator. Any blood staining makes it very difficult to see clearly. Hemostasis can be ensured with bipolar cautery or clipping. For smaller vessels, clipping is probably excessive and bipolar coagulation is safe and effective. Dissection is generally carried out with a combination of blunt spreading and sharp dissection. However, the emphasis is on blunt dissection.

Surgeons use different instruments, depending on personal preference. Some prefer a combination of fine artery forceps and fine dissecting scissors, whereas others use an elevator such as a Freer or a Howarth to tease the tissue away from the perforator so that the small branches can be seen and managed. The McCabe facial nerve dissector (Specialty Surgical Instrumentation, Nashville, TN) is a very nice instrument for dissecting around perforators. The Blondeel scissors (S&T AG, Neuhausen, Switzerland) have been specially developed for perforator vessel dissection and are particularly handy for combining cutting (in two different ways) and blunt dissection (Fig. 8-5).

Be careful about dividing major branches! It is often obvious which is the main pedicle; in this situation the decision is easy. However, the course of the main pedicle is not always so apparent. In this situation, knowledge of the anatomy is critical before making an irrevocable move.

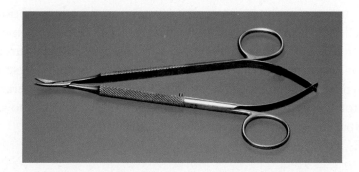

Fig. 8-5 Blondeel scissors (S&T AG, Neuhausen, Switzerland).

Good visibility and good assistance are important. Retraction is important so that the surgeon can see the operative field. However, the small branches arising from the perforator are very delicate, and a gentle touch is essential. For this reason some people depend on instrumentation. Orthostatic retraction is extremely useful. One such device is the DuraHook (Weck Closure Systems, Research Triangle Park, NC). This device looks like a fishhook. It is attached to an elastic band. The hook is invaluable for gently retracting muscle to facilitate perforator dissection. This also allows the assistant to help clip and cauterize vessels.

MANAGING INTRAOPERATIVE COMPLICATIONS

Perforator flap dissections may present several problems for surgeons, which can be categorized into four main groups. First, the anatomy of angiosomes within the flap and of the vascular pedicle is variable. Second, the choice of recipient vessels must be appropriate. Next, intraoperative and postoperative microsurgical problems such as thrombosis of the vascular pedicle at the site of the anastomosis must be corrected. Although these are very similar to problems that arise in conventional free flap surgery, the low-flow conditions will necessitate specific measures. Finally, rare complications can occur. All these are discussed below.

Variable Vascular Anatomy
Variable Vascular Anatomy of the Vascular Pedicle

An agonizing question that enters any surgeon's mind is: What if no suitable perforators are found during the dissection? Although it is possible, this is an exceptional situation. Vascularization of the skin flap has to come from somewhere—if it is not from the deep system, there has to be a dominant superficial system.[19] Likewise, if there is no dominant superficial system present, the vascularization has to come from the deep perforators. The skin paddle obviously has to be placed on top of one of these perforators.

Some solutions are available. If the dissection has started on one side of the flap only, the contralateral side can be explored for perforators. If several rows of perforators are available, as in the DIEAP flap, one can advance through the most lateral row and up to the medial row of perforators. If perforators still cannot be found or only several smaller ones are available, a muscle-sparing procedure is an option. Sometimes two or tree smaller perforators can be found and dissected, but with some muscle fibers interposed. In this case, the muscle fibers can be transected and resutured. This is also true for specific motor nerves that run between the perforators. These motor nerves can be transected and microsurgically reanastomosed. To avoid postoperative functional problems, the total amount of muscle transected is limited. The key to safe dissection is the stepwise pattern of dissection and decision making.

Anatomic Variability of the Vascular System Within the Flap

Adequate blood flow throughout the entire flap depends on not only physiologic parameters but also anatomic properties. Flow through a free flap completely detached from the body is almost completely dependent on arterial blood pressure and the size of the perforating artery. The perforating artery and vein are the bottleneck for flow through a flap. Arterial blood pressure also determines the antegrade flow within the capillary network and therefore the venous return. Maintaining adequate blood pressure after completing vascular anastomosis is extremely important and may determine the amount of tissue that will survive in the early postoperative phase.

Regardless of arterial blood pressure, there has to be an adequate tubular system through which blood flows throughout the flap. From clinical experience we have found that venous congestion of the entire DIEAP flap[20] or venous congestion in zone IV of DIEAP flaps is observed from time to time. To explain these phenomena, anatomic injection studies were performed to evaluate the venous anatomy of DIEAP flaps. The inconsistent venous drainage of zone IV was explained by variable venous crossovers over the midline of the lower abdominal skin flap. Large connecting branches between both superficial epigastric veins were found in only 18% of cases. Both superficial epigastric veins were indirectly linked by multiple smaller perforating vein branches in 32%, and no significant connections were found in half of the cases. Additionally, an inverse relationship was discovered between the diameter of the superficial epigastric vein and the venae comitantes of the perforators, leading to the philosophy of dominance of either the superficial or the deep systems. For these reasons, zone IV was considered nonreliable and is discarded in all cases. Specifically, if lateral perforators have been used, zone IV needs to be resected. In some cases in which medial perforators enter the flap at the midline, zone IV can be preserved. Similar to the DIEAP flap, other perforator flaps need to be evaluated for their dominant venous drainage and their vascular anatomy within the flap. It is important to design the flap on top of the main perforator. For example, for the DIEAP flap, if a lateral perforator is dominant, the flap should be designed more laterally, even partially over the iliac crest to include more lateral tissue. This maneuver can be safely carried out to the midaxillary line.

Diffuse venous insufficiency of a perforator flap can result from a dissection error or because of insufficient drainage of the vena comitans of the perforator. This phenomenon is specifically seen in flaps with a dominant superficial venous drainage system and small-caliber perforators. Diffuse venous insufficiency is hardly ever seen in flaps without a superficial drainage system, such as gluteal perforator flaps. The solution for this problem is obvious: the superficial system has to be used to drain the flap. With the systematic use of CT angiography before DIEAP flap surgery, unexpected partial or total venous flap congestion is very rarely observed. Furthermore, ICGA may help detect these issues before they become a clinical problem.

Perforator flaps in the extremities often have decent-sized superficial veins. Similarly, flaps of the torso, such as the DIEAP and TAP flaps (see Chapter 11), often have decent-sized superficial veins that can be used for additional venous drainage. When

Box 8-1   Ways to Augment Venous Drainage in Flaps

- Direct arterial interposition grafts are placed between the superficial vein and recipient vein.
- A second perforator is anastomosed to a side branch of the main vascular pedicle of the flap (both artery and vein).
- The superficial vein is connected to the main vascular pedicle of the deep system with or without an arterial interposition graft (as an end-to-side anastomosis or end-to-end anastomosis to the side branch).
- After two different perforators are dissected, each with its own deep axial vessels (eventually across the midline), both deep systems are anastomosed together at the level of the main pedicles.
- A superficial vein is anastomosed to a second recipient vein (for example, the cephalic vein) or a perforator at the recipient site.

harvesting the flap, these veins can be left with some length to avoid later use of vascular grafts. To bridge draining veins of inadequate length, we prefer an arterial interposition graft. Arterial grafts are more rigid and have less vascular impedance to low-flow conditions in perforator flaps. Therefore these vessels are less likely to collapse and kink after inset. Other ways to augment the venous drainage of flaps are listed in Box 8-1.

Choice of Recipient Vessels

One of the main advantages of perforator flaps is that there is always an adequate pedicle length available. The point where the vascular pedicle needs to be transected is determined by comparing the diameter of the donor vessels and recipient vessels. Although sufficient pedicle length allows easy flap shaping, the correct choice of recipient vessels (internal mammary artery, thoracodorsal vessels, or others) is important in maximizing the survival rate of perforator flaps. Large axial vessels at the recipient site always provide sufficient inflow and outflow. However, perforator flaps have smaller-sized vessels, and it may not always be necessary to sacrifice large axial vessels or perform more difficult end-to-side anastomosis. Anastomoses can easily be made on side branches of these axial vessels or even on perforating vessels. A typical example is the more frequent use of internal mammary artery perforating arteries and veins to hook up DIEAP and SIEAP flaps. In the head and neck region, several smaller side branches are available that can be used to connect often smaller flaps for reconstructing the head and neck area. In the field of supermicrosurgery, the perforating vessels of the flap electively do not need to be dissected all the way down to the axial vessels, and a direct connection can be made between the perforator vessels of the flap and a perforator vessel at the recipient site. Nevertheless, one has to remember that the smaller the vessel anastomosis, the higher the risk of vascular thrombosis. Therefore the success rate will be directly related to the experience of the microsurgeon. Very small microsurgical anastomoses cannot be recommended to inexperienced microsurgeons but can be performed with high levels of success after a few years of microsurgical experience.

Postanastomotic Problems

Although vascular microanastomosis is very similar to conventional free flap surgery, some specific issues relate to perforator flap surgery. Low-flow conditions rule in a perforator flap and, therefore, at the level of the microvascular anastomosis. Moreover, the vascular pedicle is not protected by a muscular cuff. This makes it more vulnerable to injury. Arterial spasm and dissection errors are most frequently observed in cases of flap ischemia. Vascular spasm that occurs during flap dissection can be disregarded. Once the anastomosis is made, the pedicle should be given some time in a warm and moist environment to return to its normal diameter. If spasm persists 30 minutes or later after anastomosis, extravascular papaverine can help alleviate the problem. Unless specific extravascular conditions such as perivascular scar formation or vascular diseases are present, vascular spasm is almost never a permanent problem. If no pulsations are found at the point where the perforator enters the subcutaneous fat, a dissection error is most likely. Usually a clip on a side branch or a tie-off has been positioned too close to the main pedicle and is compressing the artery. The artery itself is rigid enough to avoid kinking.

Venous drainage is more prone to problems than the arterial side because of the low-flow conditions and the thinner vascular wall. Insufficient flow and pressure within the lumen of the vena comitans will make this vessel more susceptible to kinking and torsion. Compression by bony or tendinous eminences should be avoided. From clinical experience, the low-flow condition at the anastomosis site will not lead to a higher thrombosis rate. Based on their multicentered study, Khouri et al[21] recommend visual inspection of the vascular pedicle just before performing final closure to prevent many problems of kinking and torsion.

Once thrombosis occurs after microanastomosis, reexploration is performed as soon as possible, and the causes of insufficient flow are investigated. Regardless of the location of the thrombosis, the flap will always be rinsed with 600,000 IU of urokinase, streptokinase, or tissue plasminogen activator (tPa).[22,23] This can be administered as an injection or drip according to Serletti et al.[22,24] Although they recommend performing a new venous anastomosis before injecting urokinase, we will first inject the thrombolysing agent and leave the vein open for the period of the thrombolysis.[23] This helps prevent bleeding disorders in the rest of the body but also rinses out all toxins from the free flap while it is excluded from the general circulation. Heavily thrombosed veins are never used, and it is advisable to immediately use the larger superficial veins if they are available. If thrombosis is noted in the recipient vessels, the flap can be repositioned and other recipient vessels can be used. Sometimes it is sufficient to recruit a vein from a distance, such as the cephalic or jugular vein in cases of breast reconstruction.

Vascular grafts can be used as an interposition for either veins or arteries. Although arterial interposition grafts are preferred for bypassing veins, in some cases a combined arteriovenous graft can be harvested from vessels in the groin area. A typical example is the remainder of the deep inferior epigastric artery and vein if the vascular pedicle has been transected at the lateral border of the rectus muscle. This often provides a combined arterial venous graft of 3 to 6 cm that is suitable for both arterial and venous bypass.

Rare Problems

Dissection errors can occur at any time with any kind of flap. The technique of perforator flap dissection is often regarded as more difficult than conventional free flap dissection. Although more care is needed in handling the vascular pedicle, dissection itself is not more difficult. It is a different kind of dissection that follows different rules than conventional free flap surgery. By adhering to the following few simple rules, most dissection errors can be avoided:

- Pedicle dissection should stay in a plane that is very close to the vessels themselves. Around the perforator and the deeper axial vessels is a loose connective tissue layer that can easily be freed from the surrounding tissues by blunt dissection. Blunt dissection is the key to successfully harvesting the perforator flap pedicle. If resistance to blunt dissection is encountered, it is either because of a side branch or a nerve crossing over.
- A bloodless field is necessary in all types of dissections. Even the smallest amount of blood will turn the surrounding tissues into a dark red background with very little contrast, making it impossible to distinguish the different anatomic structures. Even the slightest bleeding needs to be controlled with bipolar coagulation. Regular rinsing with a plain saline solution facilitates the dissection.
- Wide exposure is elemental in the dissection. Too often surgeons like to pursue the course of the perforator and do not spend enough time obtaining a decent view of the perforator itself. Splitting the muscle in the direction of the muscle fibers and providing wide exposure with orthostatic retractors greatly facilitates dissection.
- Every side branch, small and large, should be coagulated, ligated, or clipped at a distance of about 1 to 2 mm from the main vessels, even if this means additional dissection of the side branch in the muscle over that length. By ligating at this distance, one always has a second chance if the side branches start bleeding or if the clip comes off.

Rarely the vascular pedicle cannot be used because of an erroneous design or unexpected scarring around the pedicle and/or vascular disease (atherosclerosis). If the guidelines presented previously are followed, other perforators will be present and another pedicle can be dissected. Unexpected vascular disease affecting the total vascular tree is difficult to work with. Specific situations and conditions must be evaluated and medical treatment provided. Rare and unexpected coagulopathy is also extremely uncommon, very hard to treat, and often leads to major problems.

Finally, we offer a word of caution about reexploration and pedicle manipulation. Because perforator vessels are not protected by a muscle cuff, and because they are so delicate, they are extremely easy to damage. If a perforator flap pedicle must be explored after flap inset, an understanding of the ease with which these pedicles can be avulsed is critical. One particularly dangerous situation occurs with the DIEAP flap following skin-sparing mastectomy when the flap has to be delivered from the pocket before the pedicle can be evaluated. Extreme care is required, and it can be difficult to see the pedicle if it is encased in hematoma. Gentleness combined with copious irrigation with warm saline solution helps ensure safe pedicle exploration.

CONCLUSION

Complications with perforator flaps are rare, and the incidence is comparable with other types of free flap surgery. With a better understanding of the vascular anatomy of each flap, several solutions are available for salvaging flaps. The type of dissection necessary to successfully harvest a perforator flap is different from that required for conventional free flap surgery. The learning curve is steep, and adequate training in this area is absolutely necessary.

References

1. Taylor GI, Palmer JH. The vascular territories (angiosomes) of the body: experimental study and clinical applications. Br J Plast Surg 40:113-141, 1987.

   The autors investigated the blood supply to the skin and underlying tissues by ink injection studies, dissection, perforator mapping, and radiographic analysis of fresh cadavers and isolated limbs. The results were correlated with previous regional studies. The blood supply was shown to be a continuous three-dimensional network of vessels in all tissue layers. The angiosomes defined the tissues available for composite transfer.

2. Tregaskiss AP, Goodwin AN, Acland RD. The cutaneous arteries of the anterior abdominal wall: a three-dimensional study. Plast Reconstr Surg 120:442-450, 2007.

   The authors examined the vascular anatomy of the abdominal integument to determine why vascular complications occur and how they may be prevented. The unpredictable orientation and course of DIEA perforators indicated that the blood supply of abdominal perforator flaps, raised without clear knowledge of their unique vascular anatomy, may often be more random than axial. This may account for much of the ischemia-related morbidity observed with DIEAP-based perforator flaps. The superior epigastric artery perforators should be preserved adjacent to the costal margin during abdominoplasty to improve abdominal wall perfusion and reduce donor site morbidity.

3. Blondeel PN, Beyens G, Verhaeghe R, et al. Doppler flowmetry in the planning of perforator flaps. Br J Plast Surg 51:202-209, 1998.

4. Cheng MH, Chen HC, Santamaria E, et al. Preoperative ultrasound Doppler study and clinical correlation of free posterior interosseous flap. Changgeng Yi Xue Za Zhi 20:258-264, 1997.

5. Tregaskiss AP, Goodwin AN, Bright LD, et al. Three-dimensional CT angiography: a new technique for imaging microvascular anatomy. Clin Anat 20:116-123, 2007.

   A new technique for both qualitative and quantitative assessment of the microvasculature in three dimensions was presented. The finest vessel caliber reliably represented was 0.4 mm internal diameter.

6. Betz CS, Zhorzel S, Schachenmayr H, et al. Endoscopic measurements of free-flap perfusion in the head and neck region using red-excited Indocyanine Green: preliminary results. J Plast Reconstr Aesthet Surg 62:1602-1608, 2009.

7. Holm C, Dornseifer U, Sturtz G, et al. Sensitivity and specificity of ICG angiography in free flap reexploration. J Reconstr Microsurg 26:311-316, 2010.

8. De Lorenzi F, Yamaguchi S, Petit JY, et al. Evaluation of skin perfusion after nipple-sparing mastectomy by indocyanine green dye. Preliminary results. J Exp Clin Cancer Res 24:347-354, 2005.

9. Blondeel PN, Landuyt KV, Monstrey S. Surgical-technical aspects of the free DIEP flap for breast reconstruction. Oper Tech Plast Reconstr Surg 6:27-37, 1999.

10. Blondeel N, Vanderstraeten GG, Monstrey SJ, et al. The donor site morbidity of free DIEP flaps and free TRAM flaps for breast reconstruction. Br J Plast Surg 50:322-330, 1997.

    The free DIEAP flap provides the advantages of autologous breast reconstruction with lower abdominal tissue and limits the late postoperative weakness of the lower abdominal wall. Surgical damage to the rectus abdominis and oblique muscles is minimal. The main disadvantage of this procedure is the added surgical time.

11. Nahabedian MY, Dooley W, Singh N, et al. Contour abnormalities of the abdomen after breast reconstruction with abdominal flaps: the role of muscle preservation. Plast Reconstr Surg 109:91-101, 2002.

12. Blondeel PN, Van Landuyt K, Hamdi M, et al. Soft tissue reconstruction with the superior gluteal artery perforator flap. Clin Plast Surg 30:371-382, 2003.

13. Verpaele AM, Blondeel PN, Van Landuyt K, et al. The superior gluteal artery perforator flap: an additional tool in the treatment of sacral pressure sores. Br J Plast Surg 52:385-391, 1999.

14. Terashi H, Hashimoto H, Shibuya H, et al. Use of groin flap and anterolateral thigh adipofascial flap of tensor fascia lata for reconstruction of a wide lower abdominal wall defect. Ann Plast Surg 35:320-321, 1995.

15. Tiguemounine J, Picard A, Fassio E, et al. [Uterine liposarcoma invading abdominal wall and inguinal region. Immediate reconstruction using a pedicled anterolateral thigh flap] Ann Chir Plast Esthet 48:180-186, 2003.

    The authors presented a case using the anterolateral thigh flap as a pedicle flap to reconstruct the abdominal wall and to cover the inguinal region following resection of a voluminous tumor of the womb that invaded the abdominal wall, the femoral vessels, and the skin. The flap included a large fascial paddle nourishing a skin island and a little muscle paddle containing the perforator vessel.

16. Huang LY, Lin H, Liu YT, et al. Anterolateral thigh vastus lateralis myocutaneous flap for vulvar reconstruction after radical vulvectomy: a preliminary experience. Gynecol Oncol 78:391-393, 2000.

    The anterolateral thigh vastus lateralis myocutaneous flap was performed in a 75-year-old patient who underwent radical vulvectomy with bilateral inguinal lymphadenectomy for locally advanced squamous cell carcinoma of the vulva.

17. Luo S, Raffoul W, Piaget F, et al. Anterolateral thigh fasciocutaneous flap in the difficult perineogenital reconstruction. Plast Reconstr Surg 105:171-173, 2000.

    A pedicle anterolateral thigh fasciocutaneous flap was used to cover a complicated perineogenital defect after bilateral gracilis myocutaneous flap for perineal reconstruction. The indications and advantages of this approach were discussed.

18. Uppal RS, Casaer B, Van Landuyt K, et al. The efficacy of preoperative mapping of perforators in reducing operative times and complications in perforator flap breast reconstruction. J Plast Reconstr Aesthet Surg 62:859-864, 2008.

    The effects of preoperative perforator mapping on various aspects of perforator flap reconstruction were examined, including operative times, ischemia time, flap reexploration rate, complications, and inpatient length of stay.

19. Rozen WM, Grinsell D, Koshima I, et al. Dominance between angiosome and perforator territories: a new anatomical model for the design of perforator flaps. J Reconstr Microsurg 26:539-545, 2010.

20. Blondeel PN, Arnstein M, Verstraete K, et al. Venous congestion and blood flow in free transverse rectus abdominis myocutaneous and deep inferior epigastric perforator flaps. Plast Reconstr Surg 106:1295-1299, 2000.

21. Khouri RK, Cooley BC, Kunselman AR, et al. A prospective study of microvascular free-flap surgery and outcome. Plast Reconstr Surg 102:711-721, 1998.

22. Serletti JM, Moran SL, Orlando GS, et al. Urokinase protocol for free-flap salvage following prolonged venous thrombosis. Plast Reconstr Surg 102:1947-1953, 1998.

23. Panchapakesan V, Addison P, Beausang E, et al. The role of thrombolysis in free flap salvage. J Reconstr Microsurg 19:523-530, 2003.

24. Serletti JM, Moran SL, Orlando GS, et al. Urokinase protocol for free-flap salvage following prolonged venous thrombosis. Plast Reconstr Surg 102:1947-1953, 1998.

9

Perforator Flaps in Children

Koenraad Van Landuyt
Colin M. Morrison

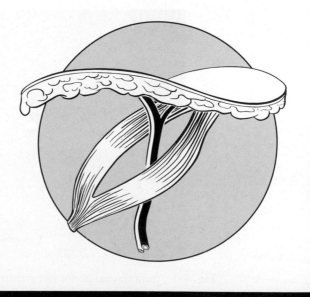

In pediatric patients, surgeons are frequently confronted with large, soft tissue defects from trauma, burns, disease (meningococcal septicemia), or oncologic resection. Most of these cases call for skin and soft tissue coverage rather than a functional reconstruction. Many surgeons still hesitate to perform perforator flaps in children because of the concern of the high failure rate related to the small diameter of children's perforator vessels.[1] There are, however, many benefits. These include minimizing donor site morbidity and the aesthetic, functional, and psychological advantages.[2]

The first cases of free flap reconstruction in children primarily dealt with the technical feasibility of the procedure, the principal concern being the size of the vessels and the tendency for spasm and anastomotic occlusion. Potential donor sites were scarce, and tissue with direct cutaneous vessels was chosen, such as the groin flap.[3-5]

It soon became apparent that the relative size of the donor and recipient vessels was larger in children than in adults; however, the absolute size could still be rather disappointing (Fig. 9-1). As a result, with the advent of free muscle and myocutaneous transfer, reconstructive surgeons opted for more anatomically reliable and larger pedicles at the cost of donor site morbidity. Therefore the latissimus dorsi flap with its consistent and large thoracodorsal pedicle was used even if only soft tissue coverage was required.[6-8]

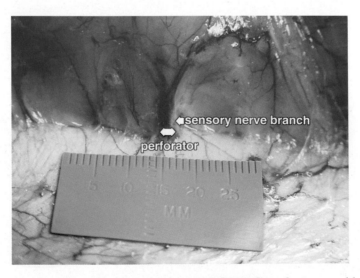

Fig. 9-1   Suprafascial perforator size in a DIEAP flap of a 4-year-old girl.

Free flap surgery in the pediatric population continued to gain acceptance, with success rates approaching those of adults. This has also been the case with perforator flaps. After an initial period where they were performed more as a platform for displaying technical prowess than as a clinical advantage, perforator flaps achieved wider popularity, essentially because of their versatility and reduced donor site morbidity, broadening the repertoire of pediatric reconstructive surgery.

The question should no longer be whether or not free tissue transfer can be safely performed in children, but rather which flap will optimally fill the defect and result in the fewest donor site problems.[9] Perforator flaps provide large skin islands based on well-established vascular anatomy of the underlying muscle flaps and offer the least donor site morbidity, with long, reliable pedicles.

The deep inferior epigastric artery perforator (DIEAP) flap potentially provides the largest skin area; however, even in children the adipose layer can be relatively thick. This can subsequently be easily corrected with tumescent liposculpture. Because the abdominal wall musculature is left innervated and functionally intact, there are no contraindications to augmenting the size of the DIEAP flap by harvesting a bilateral pedicle utilizing zone IV. Alternatively, the contralateral superficial epigastric vein can be recruited to enhance venous outflow. A further advantage of the DIEAP flap is the relatively inconspicuous donor site scar (Fig. 9-2, *A*).

The thoracodorsal artery perforator (TDAP) flap is based on thinner skin of the lateral thoracic wall. The scar, though partially hidden by the upper limb, can be quite conspicuous (Fig. 9-2, *B*). This donor site does, however, prevent the contour defor-

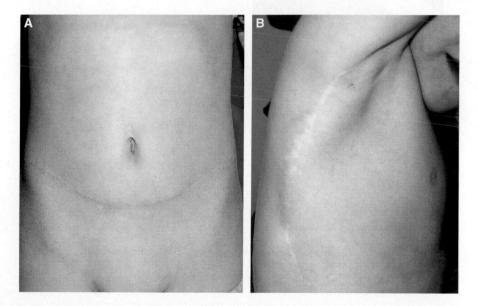

Fig. 9-2 Donor site scars in children. **A,** This 5-year-old child is shown 1 year after a DIEAP flap. **B,** This TDAP flap was raised when the child was 6 months old. He is shown at 4 years of age.

mity associated with harvesting a myocutaneous flap. For patients in whom the lack of sufficient skin is critical, such as those with widespread meningococcal septicemia, the TDAP flap offers the second largest skin paddle available and still allows primary closure of the donor site. In addition, the TDAP flap can be raised as a compound flap, increasing both its size and versatility. Harvesting specialized tissue on the same pedicle is also possible, depending on individual requirements (Fig. 9-3).

The DIEAP and TDAP flaps rely on easily identifiable, sizeable, and anatomically consistent pedicles. Releasing the perforator adds to the ultimate length of the pedicle, which is a marked benefit if the anastomosis is to be performed outside the zone of injury. Finally, both of these flaps lend themselves to reinnervation through coaptation of the intercostal branches, providing sensate flaps.

Recently children have also been found to have well-developed perforators supplying the anterolateral thigh (ALT) flap. This flap can therefore be harvested safely and reliably in children, increasing our reconstructive armamentarium.[10]

In our experience, the dissection time, complications, and outcomes with free perforator flaps in the pediatric age group are comparable to those of adults. As a result of the additional advantage of reduced donor site morbidity, perforator flaps have become our preferred option for covering the various soft tissue defects encountered in children.

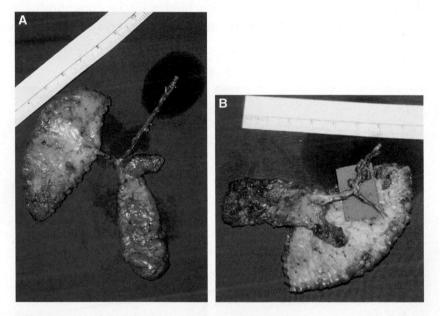

Fig. 9-3 **A** and **B,** Bilateral compound TDAP flap from a 6-month-old boy.

References

1. Kim SE, Rhyou IH, Suh BG, et al. Use of thoracodorsal artery perforator flap for soft tissue reconstruction in children. Ann Plast Surg 56:451-454, 2006.

    Many reconstructive surgeons still hesitate to perform perforator flaps in children. The main concern is the perceived high failure rate related to the small diameter of children's perforator vessels. The authors presented four consecutive cases of successful transfer of a TDAP flap in children.

2. Van Landuyt K, Hamdi M, Blondeel P, et al. Free perforator flaps in children. Plast Reconstr Surg 116:159-169, 2005.

    A series of 23 consecutive free perforator flaps performed in 20 children was presented. Their ages ranged from premature (born at 28 weeks) to 16 years (mean age 7 years 5 months). Three children presented with upper limb defects; the remaining 17 children sustained major soft tissue defects of the lower limb. Flaps used in this series included nine DIEAP flaps, seven TDAP flaps, and seven compound (chimera) TDAP flaps. All flaps but one were successful.

3. Harii K, Ohmori K. Free groin flaps in children. Plast Reconstr Surg 55:588-592, 1975.

    The authors presented two successful transfers of free groin flaps to the lower legs of children, reporting that this method could be safely applied and could often take the place of distant pedicle flap transfers in children.

4. Ohmori K, Harii K, Sekiguchi J, et al. The youngest free groin flap yet? Br J Plast Surg 30:273-276, 1977.

    A successful free groin flap transfer to the arm in a 3-month-old baby was described. The vessels were large enough for microvascular anastomosis. The authors stated that there is no minimum age restriction for free flap transfer.

5. Van Beek AL, Wavak PW, Zook EG. Microvascular surgery in young children. Plast Reconstr Surg 63:457-462, 1979.

    A series of eight children, all less than 6 years of age, was presented, demonstrating the feasibility of primary microvascular replantation or reconstruction of amputated or devascularized parts in this age group. The function and appearance obtained were excellent, and the potential for growth was maintained. Fortunately, the vessels were larger in these young children than one would expect.

6. Banic A, Wulff K. Latissimus dorsi free flaps for total repair of extensive lower leg injuries in children. Plast Reconstr Surg 79:769-775, 1987.

    A well-established belief is that with crushed and contaminated wounds, closure should be delayed. An emergency procedure involving very thorough debridement, complete reconstruction of all injured tissues, and cover by a latissimus dorsi free flap in the same operation was evaluated in 15 children with severe lower limb injuries. The authors reported that the procedure is superior to the established method, because it requires only one stage. It is, in some cases, a limb-saving procedure.

7. Yu ZJ. The use of bilateral latissimus dorsi myocutaneous flaps to cover large soft tissue defects in the lower limbs of children. J Reconstr Microsurg 4:83-88, 1988.

    Large soft tissue lower leg defects in children, especially those around joints, can cause severe secondary and progressive deformity that may interfere with growth of the affected limb. If function is to be restored and possible amputation prevented, repair procedures are necessary. Eight children with such defects, ranging from 6 to 9 years of age, were treated successfully with bilateral latissimus dorsi myocutaneous flaps. All the flaps survived, and both the functional recovery and cosmetic improvement of the repaired limbs were satisfactory.

8. Parry SW, Toth BA, Elliott LF, et al. Microvascular free-tissue transfer in children. Plast Reconstr Surg 81:838-840, 1988.

    Twenty-two microvascular free tissue transfers in children were reviewed. Ages ranged from 2 to 14 years; the success rate was 96%. The results indicate that microvascular free tissue transfer can be accomplished safely and expeditiously in children. Care should be taken in preoperative and postoperative planning, especially with regard to immobilization.

9. Arnez ZM, Hanel DP. Free tissue transfer for reconstruction of traumatic limb injuries in children. Microsurgery 12:207-215, 1991.

Free tissue transfer was used for reconstructing soft tissue defects in 94 children. Of the 127 procedures performed, the latissimus dorsi, scapular skin, lateral arm skin, rectus abdominis, and gracilis were used most often. The microsurgical success rate was 96%. Microsurgical failures were successfully corrected, and in all cases the limbs were salvaged. Other than decreased vessel size and avoiding continuous suture lines in children, there is little difference in technique or outcome of free tissue transfer between children and adults.

10. Gharb BB, Salgado CJ, Moran SL, et al. Free anterolateral thigh flap in pediatric patients. Ann Plast Surg 66:143-147, 2011.

The authors described their clinical experience with the ALT flap in the pediatric population. Twenty patients with an average age of 9.5 years underwent free ALT flap reconstruction. All flaps were commonly raised on two perforators. There were no complete flap losses. Hypertrophic scars developed in four patients. Secondary procedures included flap debulking (five) and Z-plasties (two).

PART II

Regional Flaps:
Anatomy and Surgical Technique

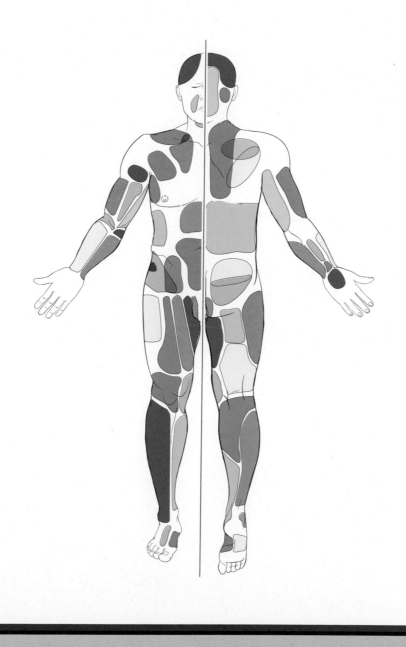

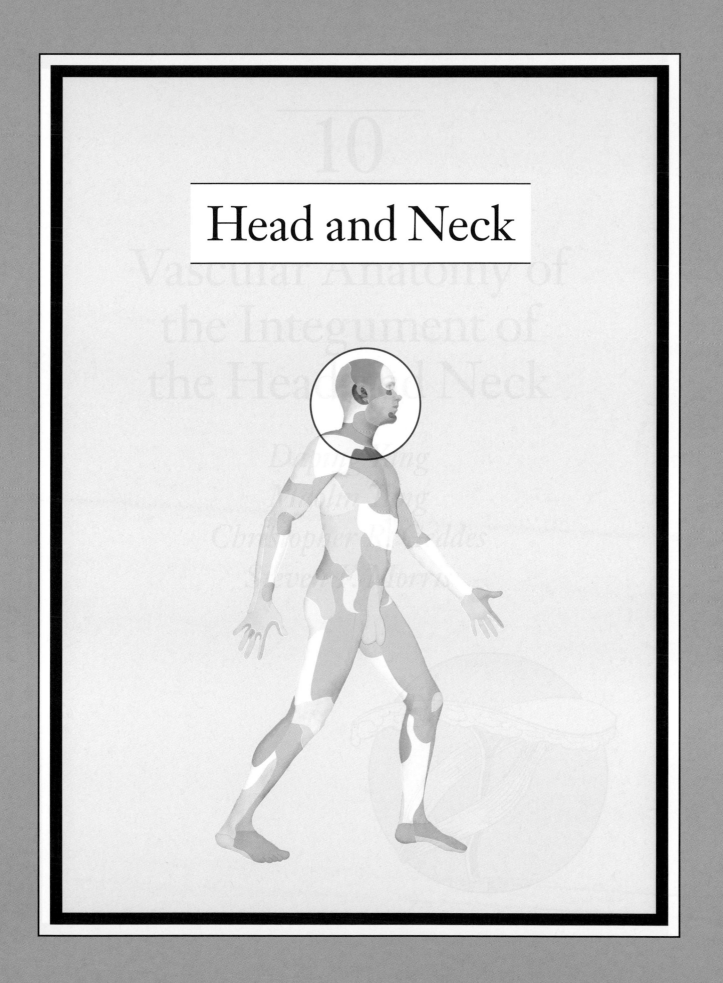

Head and Neck

10

Vascular Anatomy of
the Integument of
the Head and Neck

Daniel Jung

Ian Taylor

Christopher Geddes

Steven Morris

OVERVIEW
The Head

The skin of the head and neck is richly vascularized by numerous septocutaneous and musculocutaneous vessels that extensively anastomose. The head skin is supplied primarily by septocutaneous vessels because of the rigidity of the skull and facial bones. Branches of the external carotid system (Fig. 10-1) supply most of the head skin, except for a mask-shaped area that surrounds the eyes, and cover the central forehead and upper two thirds of the nose. Arteries to the area around the eyes arise from the ophthalmic branch of the internal carotid system (Fig. 10-2). The largest branches—the dorsal nasal, supratrochlear, and supraorbital arteries—emerge from the concavity of the inner canthus. Their branches radiate to supply the eyelids, central forehead, and dorsum of the nose. There is a rich midline network of vessels in the forehead and nose provided by branches of the internal carotid system, which link the facial and superficial temporal arteries of either side as an arcade.[1-4]

The branches of the external carotid system are well known. They pierce the deep fascia along a curved loop around the base of the skull (occipital, posterior auricular, and superficial temporal arteries), along the lower border of the mandible (facial and submental arteries), from the groove in front of the parotid gland (buccal arteries), and from the foramina in the maxilla and mandible (infraorbital and mental arteries). The latter three arteries, by comparison, are relatively small and derive from the internal maxillary branch of the external carotid system (Figs. 10-3 through 10-5).

The cutaneous perforators radiate from fixed points, either from bony foramina or from sites where the deep fascia is attached to bone. They radiate from concavities and grooves, especially around the base of the skull, orbital margins, lower border of the mandible, nasolabial grooves, and preauricular and postauricular regions. Branches of the cutaneous perforators converge on the convexities of the ears, nose, lips, chin, and apex of the skull. They connect with their opposite artery horizontally across the midline, and vertically to adjacent vessels to form a series of vascular arches. Most of the connections between vessels to the skin are reduced-caliber choke anastomotic arteries, but frequently they are true anastomoses with no change in caliber between vascular territories. The latter pattern is particularly well developed in the scalp (see Fig. 10-5). This gives rise to the excellent vascular supply for cutaneous perforator flaps.

Text continued on p. 196

Head and Neck

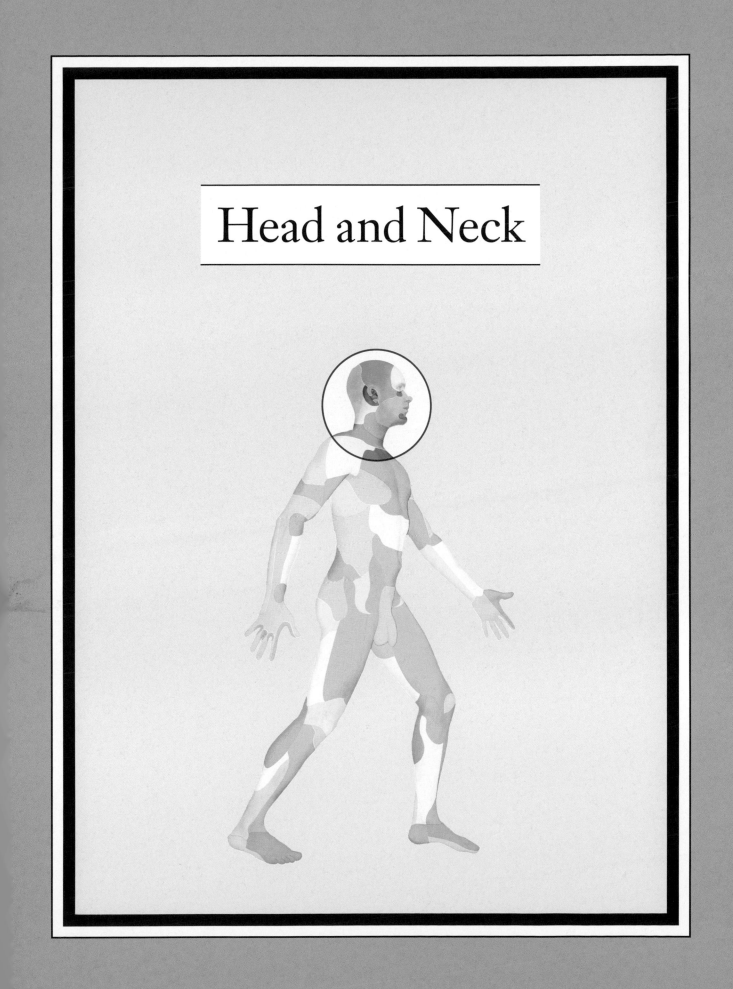

Head and Neck

10

Vascular Anatomy of the Integument of the Head and Neck

Daping Yang
Maolin Tang
Christopher R. Geddes
Steven F. Morris

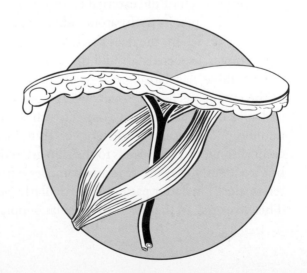

OVERVIEW
The Head

The skin of the head and neck is richly vascularized by numerous septocutaneous and musculocutaneous vessels that extensively anastomose. The head skin is supplied primarily by septocutaneous vessels because of the rigidity of the skull and facial bones. Branches of the external carotid system (Fig. 10-1) supply most of the head skin, except for a mask-shaped area that surrounds the eyes, and cover the central forehead and upper two thirds of the nose. Arteries to the area around the eyes arise from the ophthalmic branch of the internal carotid system (Fig. 10-2). The largest branches—the dorsal nasal, supratrochlear, and supraorbital arteries—emerge from the concavity of the inner canthus. Their branches radiate to supply the eyelids, central forehead, and dorsum of the nose. There is a rich midline network of vessels in the forehead and nose provided by branches of the internal carotid system, which link the facial and superficial temporal arteries of either side as an arcade.[1-4]

The branches of the external carotid system are well known. They pierce the deep fascia along a curved loop around the base of the skull (occipital, posterior auricular, and superficial temporal arteries), along the lower border of the mandible (facial and submental arteries), from the groove in front of the parotid gland (buccal arteries), and from the foramina in the maxilla and mandible (infraorbital and mental arteries). The latter three arteries, by comparison, are relatively small and derive from the internal maxillary branch of the external carotid system (Figs. 10-3 through 10-5).

The cutaneous perforators radiate from fixed points, either from bony foramina or from sites where the deep fascia is attached to bone. They radiate from concavities and grooves, especially around the base of the skull, orbital margins, lower border of the mandible, nasolabial grooves, and preauricular and postauricular regions. Branches of the cutaneous perforators converge on the convexities of the ears, nose, lips, chin, and apex of the skull. They connect with their opposite artery horizontally across the midline, and vertically to adjacent vessels to form a series of vascular arches. Most of the connections between vessels to the skin are reduced-caliber choke anastomotic arteries, but frequently they are true anastomoses with no change in caliber between vascular territories. The latter pattern is particularly well developed in the scalp (see Fig. 10-5). This gives rise to the excellent vascular supply for cutaneous perforator flaps.

Text continued on p. 196

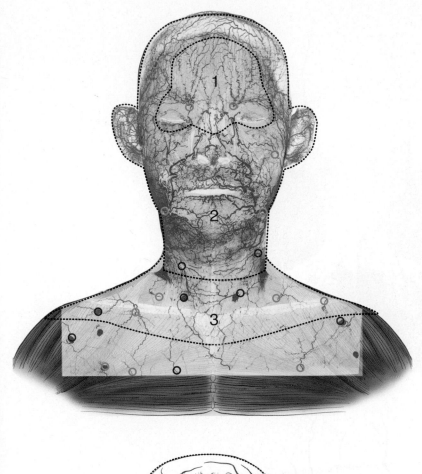

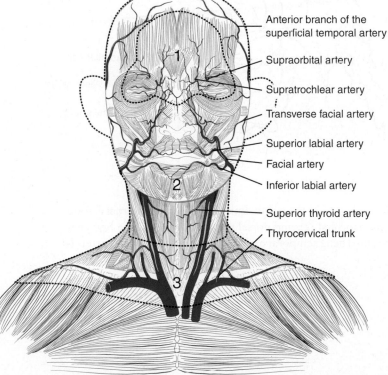

Fig. 10-1   An angiogram of the integument of the head and neck from a human cadaver (anterior view) injected with lead oxide and gelatin. *Red circles* demonstrate musculocutaneous perforators; *blue circles* show septocutaneous perforators. (*1,* Vascular territories of the ophthalmic branch of the internal carotid system; *2,* vascular territories of the external carotid system; *3,* vascular territories of the subclavian system.)

Anterior branch of the superficial temporal artery

Supraorbital artery

Supratrochlear artery

Transverse facial artery

Superior labial artery

Facial artery

Inferior labial artery

Superior thyroid artery

Thyrocervical trunk

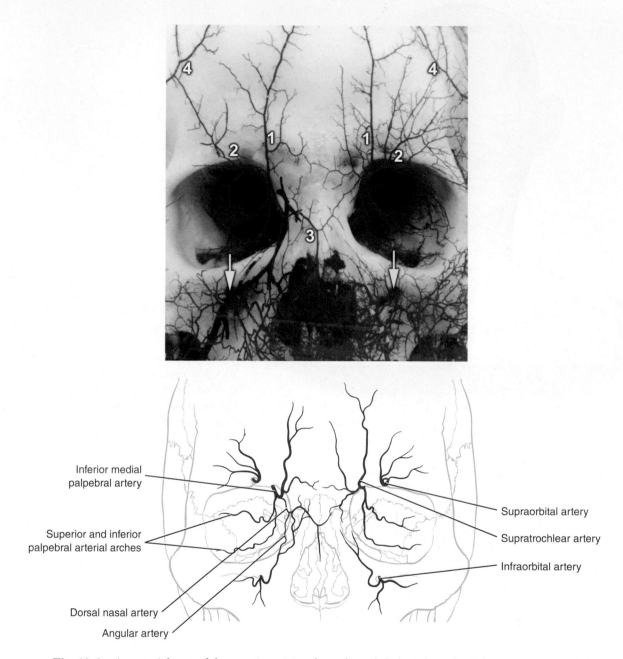

Fig. 10-2   An arterial cast of the arteries arising from the ophthalmic branch of the internal carotid artery, including the supratrochlear *(1)*, supraorbital *(2)*, and dorsal nasal *(3)* arteries. The branches link the facial and frontal branch of the superficial temporal arteries *(4)*. The infraorbital arteries *(arrows)* arise from the maxillary artery.

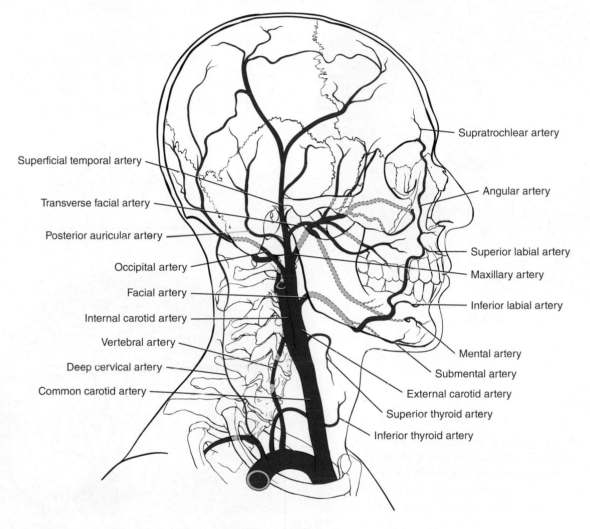

Fig. 10-3 The principal branches from the external carotid artery.

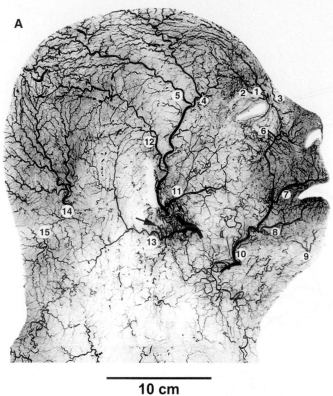

10 cm

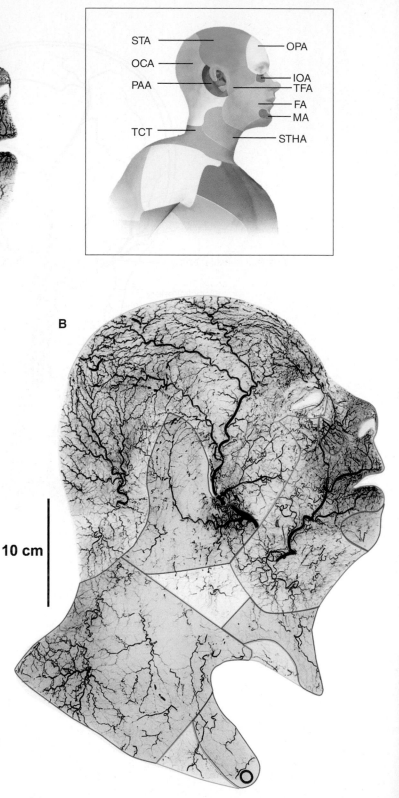

Fig. 10-4 An angiogram of the integument of the head and neck (lateral view). **A,** The principal branches to the integument are numbered as follows: *1,* supratrochlear artery; *2,* supraorbital artery; *3,* dorsal nasal artery; *4,* frontal branch of the superficial temporal artery *(STA); 5,* parietal branch of the superficial temporal artery; *6,* infraorbital arteries *(IOA); 7,* superior labial artery; *8,* inferior labial artery; *9,* mental artery *(MA); 10,* facial artery *(FA); 11,* transverse facial artery *(TFA); 12,* superior auricular artery; *13,* posterior auricular artery *(PAA); 14,* occipital artery *(OCA);* and *15,* the descending branch of the occipital artery. **B,** The vascular territories of the integument are shown in different colors. The *black circle* represents the acromion. *(OPA,* Ophthalmic artery; *STHA,* superior thyroid artery; *TCT,* thyrocervical trunk.)

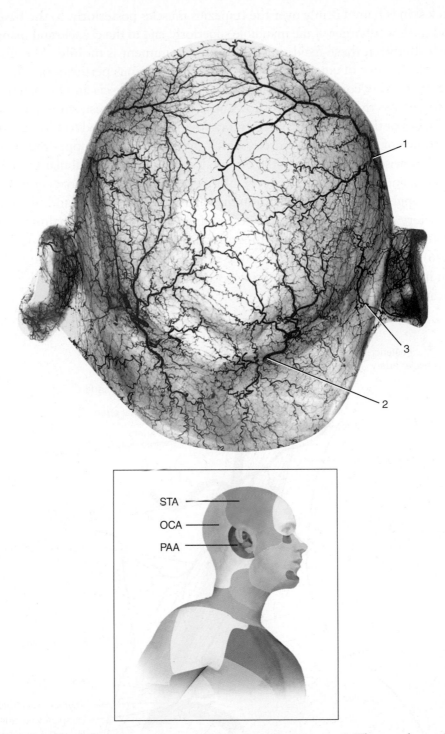

Fig. 10-5 An angiogram of the integument of the scalp region (top view). The vascular territories of the scalp are shown in different colors. There are true anastomoses between the *1,* superficial temporal arteries *(STA), 2,* occipital arteries *(OCA),* and *3,* posterior auricular artery *(PAA).*

The Neck

The neck skin is bound firmly over the trapezius muscles posteriorly, to the base of the skull and the lower border of the mandible superiorly, and to the clavicle and manubrium inferiorly. Between these fixed skin zones the integument is mobile. The fixed skin zones mark the sites of emergence of the musculocutaneous perforators. The origins of these vessels vary considerably. They pierce the cervical fascia and branch to form a rich plexus across the neck that overflows onto the adjacent chest, shoulder, and back. The branches of these cutaneous perforators are intimately related to the undersurface and substance of the platysma muscle, which they perforate to supply the subdermal plexus. They arise superiorly from the occipital artery, the submandibular branch of the facial artery, and the submental artery; inferiorly from the transverse cervical and/or the suprascapular artery; anteriorly from the superior thyroid artery and the transverse cervical artery; and posteriorly from a descending branch of the ophthalmic artery and direct cutaneous perforators of the muscular branches of transverse cervical arteries (Fig. 10-6). These vessels emerge from the surface of the trapezius muscle and from a position in front of the muscle's anterior border to form a rich anastomosis across the midline anteriorly.

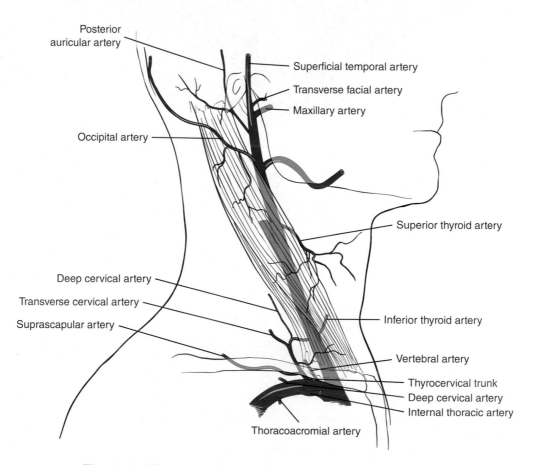

Fig. 10-6   The arteries that supply the sternocleidomastoid muscle.

PERFORATORS WITH SOURCE VESSELS

The head and neck area makes up about 10% of total body surface area and has a mean of 25 perforators (larger than 0.5 mm). The inferior boundary of the head and neck region is marked by a line joining the suprasternal notch to the angle of the acromion along the superior border of the clavicle (anterior boundary), and a line joining the angle of the acromion through the spinous process of the seventh cervical vertebra (posterior boundary).

The vascular anatomy of the integument of the head and neck can be analyzed as four subregions: the scalp, face, neck, and nuchal areas. The scalp comprises the frontal, temporoparietal, occipital, and auricular regions. The face includes the periorbital, nasal, zygomatic, oral, mental, and buccal regions. The neck includes the anterior triangle, sternocleidomastoid region, and posterior triangle. The nuchal region is bound laterally by the anterior border of the trapezius muscle and superiorly by the superior nuchal line.

The vascular supply to the integument of the head and neck is from the terminal cutaneous vessels of 10 source arteries, which are the vascular territories in this region. These arteries are listed in Table 10-1, which summarizes our results for the cutaneous vascular territories of the head and neck region. The primary blood supply to the integument of the face and scalp is from large cutaneous branches of the external and internal carotid arteries (see Fig. 10-6). The large caliber and superficial nature of the

Table 10-1 Summary of Quantitative Data for the Cutaneous Vascular Territories of the Head and Neck Region

Name of Vascular Territory	Number (>0.5 mm)	Superficial Length (mm)	Diameter (mm)	Total Area (cm²)	Area/Perforator (cm²)	Area of Region (%)	Ratio (MC/SC)
Superficial temporal artery	1 (± 1)	131 (± 44)	1.3 (± 0.6)	154 (± 39)	154 (± 39)	18 (± 5)	0:1
Ophthalmic artery	3 (± 1)	38 (± 17)	0.7 (± 0.1)	43 (± 14)	14 (± 7)	5 (± 1)	1:3
Occipital artery	3 (± 2)	62 (± 35)	1.3 (± 0.7)	128 (± 59)	43 (± 19)	15 (± 7)	0:1
Posterior auricular artery	1 (± 1)	64 (± 13)	0.9 (± 0.2)	49 (± 31)	49 (± 31)	6 (± 4)	0:1
Infraorbital artery	1 (± 1)	23 (± 4)	0.8 (± 0.1)	8 (± 5)	8 (± 5)	1 (± 1)	0:1
Transverse facial artery	1 (± 1)	40 (± 21)	1.0 (± 0.3)	23 (± 14)	23 (± 14)	3 (± 2)	0:1
Facial artery	1 (± 1)	86 (± 35)	1.1 (± 0.4)	110 (± 43)	110 (± 43)	13 (± 5)	0:1
Mental artery	1 (± 1)	13 (± 4)	0.8 (± 0.3)	11 (± 1)	11 (± 1)	1 (± 1)	0:1
Thyrocervical trunk	6 (± 2)	24 (± 23)	0.6 (± 0.2)	258 (± 162)	43 (± 33)	31 (± 19)	4:3
Superior thyroid artery	2 (± 1)	33 (± 9)	0.7 (± 0.2)	25 (± 10)	14 (± 5)	3 (± 1)	1:1

All values are means ± standard deviation (SD) for the number, diameter, length, and area calculated in our series (n = 10). The total area of each vascular territory, in addition to the average area supplied by a single perforator within that territory, was calculated from digital angiograms using Scion Image for Windows (Scion Corporation, Frederick, MD).
MC, Musculocutaneous; *SC*, septocutaneous.

vessels in this region can be attributed to the overlay of the facial and scalp skin on the bony skeleton of the head and face. In contrast, the longitudinal muscle structure of the neck allows smaller, more numerous musculocutaneous perforators to supply the skin in this region. Perforators from the internal and external carotid arteries and from the branches of the thyrocervical trunk supply the integument of the neck. Perforators in the neck region have been described as suitable donor sites for perforator flap harvest. Fig. 10-1 shows an angiogram of the vascular territories of the integument of the head and neck region.

The Scalp

The scalp region includes the frontal, temporoparietal, and occipital areas. The integument of this region is characteristically thin with large superficial vessels that traverse long, tortuous paths. These arteries form a network of true anastomoses with adjacent territories and with arteries from the contralateral side. Perforators and branches of four main vascular territories are presented: (1) superficial temporal artery, (2) occipital artery, (3) ophthalmic artery, and (4) posterior auricular artery (see Figs. 10-4 and 10-5).

Superficial Temporal Artery

The superficial temporal artery, with an external diameter (D) of 2.5 to 3.2 mm, is the smaller of the two terminal branches of the external carotid artery. The superficial temporal artery originates posterior to the ramus of the mandible in the parotid region of the face, and courses superiorly across the root of the zygomatic process of the temporal bone. The vessel lies anterior to the auriculotemporal nerve and the superficial temporal vein. Before reaching the skin, the superficial temporal artery gives branches to the face (transverse facial artery) and temporalis muscle (middle temporal branch), and a series of branches to the auricle. Its main trunk courses only a short distance (approximately 6.7 cm) before splitting into anterior (D = 1.8 mm) and posterior (D = 2.1 mm) branches. The anterior branch gives rise to two primary rami: the zygomaticoorbital (D = 0.9 mm) and frontal (D = 1.1 mm) branches. The zygomaticoorbital artery courses superior to the zygomatic arch and anastomoses with the lacrimal and palpebral branches of the ophthalmic artery. The frontal branch supplies the anterosuperior region of the scalp and anastomoses with its contralateral branches and with the supraorbital and supratrochlear arteries. The posterior branch divides further into the auricular (D = 0.9 mm) and parietal (D = 1.3 mm) arteries. The auricular artery descends posterior to the auricle and anastomoses with the posterior auricular and occipital arteries. The parietal branch ascends superiorly in the direction of the main trunk of the superficial temporal artery, following the coronal suture. The superficial vein accompanies this terminal branch of the superficial temporal artery. The parietal branch anastomoses with its contralateral branch and with the frontal and occipital arteries.

In our study, the area of skin supplied by the superficial temporal artery was 154 cm². This area equals approximately 47% of the surface area of the scalp and approximately 18% of the total head and neck region. The large diameter, superficial course, and predictable branching of the superficial temporal artery make it suitable for skin flap harvest. The superficial temporal vessels are large and consistent and provide an excellent basis for a variety of flap designs in this region.

Ophthalmic Artery

The ophthalmic artery is a terminal branch of the internal carotid artery that exits the cranial vault through the optic canal. It sends branches to the eye and lacrimal gland before branching into the supraorbital artery and its terminal branches, the supratrochlear and dorsal nasal arteries. The territory of the ophthalmic artery includes the skin of the forehead and dorsum of the nose. In addition, the ophthalmic artery sends off the medial palpebral arteries (superior and inferior arches) that course posterior to the lacrimal sac and enter the eyelids. Each palpebral arch courses alongside the tarsal plate and anastomoses laterally with the lacrimal artery and branches of the zygomaticoorbital artery. The lacrimal artery did not supply any significant perforators to the skin in our dissections. The inferior palpebral arch anastomosed inferiorly with tiny branches of the facial and transverse facial arteries.

The supraorbital and supratrochlear arteries are well known as the vascular basis of pedicle forehead flaps for nasal reconstruction.

Occipital Artery

The occipital artery is the second of the dorsal branches of the external carotid artery (opposite the facial artery). It courses deep to the posterior belly of the digastric muscle, medial to the mastoid process, and deep to the sternocleidomastoid, splenius capitis, and longissimus capitis muscles before piercing the deep fascia between the sternocleidomastoid and trapezius muscles. The occipital artery has several branches that supply the skin of the scalp. First, the occipital artery sends a small branch to the posterior aspect of the ear that anastomoses with the posterior auricular artery. Second, terminal occipital branches (D = 1.3 mm) emerge approximately 5 cm lateral to the external occipital protuberance and course superiorly with the greater and lesser occipital nerves. Finally, descending branches from the occipital artery supply the muscles of the superior nuchal region and send musculocutaneous perforators through the trapezius muscle to supply the overlying skin.

The average area supplied by the occipital artery is 128.1 cm², which is equal to approximately 39% of the scalp and 15% of the integument of the head and neck. The terminal occipital branches of the occipital artery provide the vascular basis of well-defined skin flaps.

Posterior Auricular Artery

The posterior auricular artery (D = 1.1 mm) is a dorsal branch of the external carotid artery that commonly originates at the superior border of the digastric and stylohyoid muscles. It ascends posteriorly, following the styloid process between the mastoid process and the cartilage of the ear. The vessel pierces the deep fascia after branching into occipital and auricular branches. The occipital branch supplies the skin of the scalp opposite the ear. The auricular branch passes behind the small auricularis posterior muscle and supplies the skin of the cranial surface of the auricle. The auricular branch of the posterior auricular artery has very prominent anastomoses with auricular branches of the superficial temporal artery within the auricle. The dense vascularity of the auricle is easily seen in Figs. 10-1 and 10-5.

A previously unreported cutaneous branch of the posterior auricular artery was seen in two of our dissection specimens. This branch (D = 0.7 mm) originated 1.5 cm from the external carotid artery and coursed inferiorly in a semicircular pattern around the inferior margin of the mandible toward the submandibular triangle. It had a true anastomosis with a branch of similar caliber of the facial artery. The posterior auricular artery supplied an average area of 9 cm². The vessel's cutaneous perforators commonly emerged from the deep fascia as two distinct perforators.

The Face

The integument of the face has a high density of large cutaneous arteries (see Figs. 10-1 and 10-4). Most of the region is supplied by direct septocutaneous perforators. Some musculocutaneous perforators reach the skin through small facial muscles. The integument of the face includes many specialized areas, including the periorbital, nasal, zygomatic, oral, mental, and buccal regions. The arterial supply to the face is through branches of the external carotid artery, primarily the facial artery. The cutaneous perforators of four dominant vascular territories are presented: the infraorbital artery, transverse facial artery, facial artery, and mental artery (see Figs. 10-2 and 10-4).

Infraorbital Artery

The infraorbital artery is a terminal branch of the maxillary artery that emerges from the infraorbital foramen, accompanying the infraorbital nerve. Along most of its course and on exiting the foramen, this small artery (D = 1.0 mm) follows the distribution of the nerve and supplies several muscles of facial expression. The mean cutaneous territory of the infraorbital artery is only 8 cm² and is located 2 cm inferior to the orbit and 4 cm lateral to the alar cartilage of the nose. The infraorbital artery anastomoses with the facial, transverse facial, and ophthalmic arteries. In one specimen, it was observed that a branch from the infraorbital artery supplied the lateral nose in the absence of prominent lateral nasal branches from the facial artery.

Transverse Facial Artery

The transverse facial artery is a branch of the superficial temporal artery, which arises at the level of the tragus deep to the parotid gland. A significant transverse facial artery (D = 1.0 mm) was present in 85% of our dissections. In most cases, this artery coursed to the skin as a single trunk, and its average number of perforators was 1.3. When absent, the territory of the transverse facial artery was supplied by an ascending branch (D = 0.8 mm) of the facial artery beginning 2 cm above the inferior mandibular border. The transverse facial artery supplies the parotid gland and the superficial head of the masseter muscle before reaching the skin. The vessel passes through the superficial musculoaponeurotic system (SMAS) and contributes branches to the SMAS on its way to the dense subdermal plexus, forming a continuous anastomotic network. The major cutaneous anastomoses of the vessel include the zygomaticoorbital branch of the superficial temporal artery superiorly, the infraorbital and ophthalmic territories anteriorly, and the facial and angular arteries inferiorly. When the transverse facial artery perforator is transected during a face lift in the clinical setting, the vascular territory of the transverse facial artery is supplied by these adjacent vascular territories through the subdermal plexus. The average area supplied by the transverse facial artery was 23 cm². The vascular territory of the transverse facial artery extends superiorly to the zygomatic arch, anteriorly to the lateral canthus and over the malar eminence, inferiorly to 2 cm above the mandibular border, and posteriorly to 2 cm anterior to the ear.

No perforator flaps from this vessel have been described for face reconstruction. However, the transverse facial artery perforator supplies a large portion of the lateral face-lift flap following rhytidectomy. The face-lift flap of the lateral cheek is located directly over the SMAS.

Facial Artery

The facial artery originates from the external carotid artery, opposite the occipital artery, and slightly superior to the greater horn of the hyoid bone. It is the principal artery to the skin of the facial region and has an average diameter of 2.1 mm at its origin. The facial artery is the major arterial supply to the integument of the face; it also supplies the tonsils, submandibular gland, and many muscles of the facial region. The facial artery courses deep to the posterior belly of the digastric muscle and through the submandibular triangle, where it reaches the inferior border of the mandible and pierces the fascia near the anterior border of the masseter muscle. At this point, the facial artery sends a submental artery branch to the neck. Also at this point, the facial muscle gives off a premasseteric branch, which ascends along the anterior border of the masseter to anastomose with the transverse facial artery superiorly. The main trunk of the facial artery continues toward the angle of the mouth, where it gives off the inferior and superior labial arteries. Between the angle of the mouth and the medial canthus, the facial artery traverses superficial to, deep to, or through the levator labii superioris and the levator labii superioris alaque nasi muscles. As the facial artery approaches the medial canthus, it becomes the angular artery and sends lateral nasal branches to the nose. Finally, the angular artery anastomoses with multiple branches of the ophthalmic and infraorbital arteries.

The area supplied by the facial artery (Fig. 10-7) in our series was 109.7 cm². The facial artery branches are the (1) submental, (2) premasseteric, (3) lateral nasal, (4) inferior labial, (5) superior labial arteries, and (6) the lateral nasal artery. The facial artery and its branches provide the basis for a wide variety of potential perforator flaps for facial reconstruction.

Mental Artery

The mental artery is a branch from the maxillary artery that reaches the skin through the mental foramen of the mandible. This artery (D = 0.8 mm) courses with the mandibular branch of the trigeminal nerve and reaches the skin below the second premolar tooth. Branches of the mental artery anastomose with the facial, inferior labial, and submental arteries. The average size of the territory supplied was 11 cm².

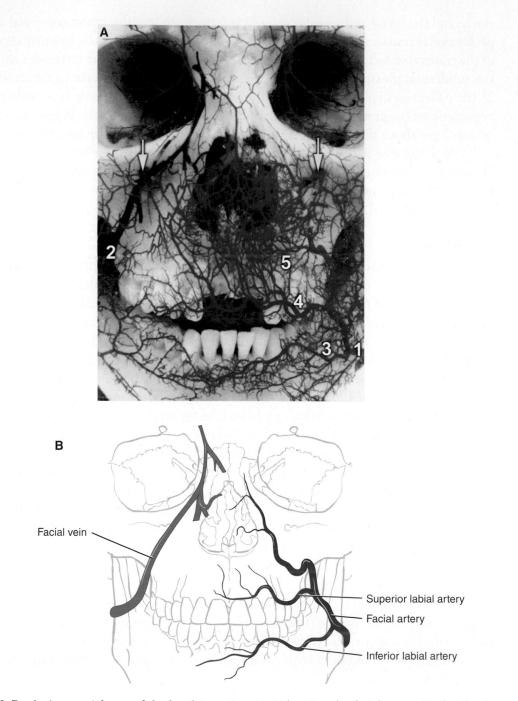

Fig. 10-7 **A,** An arterial cast of the head (anterior view) showing the facial artery *(1)*, facial vein *(2)*, inferior labial artery *(3)*, superior labial artery *(4)*, and lateral nasal artery *(5)*. *Arrows* mark the infraorbital arteries. **B,** The facial artery and vein vascular supply to the midface.

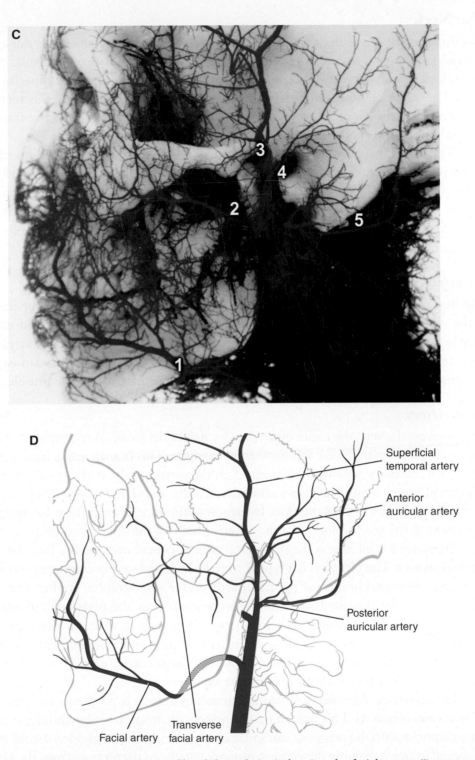

Fig. 10-7, cont'd C, An arterial cast of head (lateral view) showing the facial artery *(1)*, transverse facial artery *(2)*, superficial temporal artery *(3)*, anterior auricular artery *(4)*, and posterior auricular arteries *(5)*. **D,** Branches of the external carotid.

The Neck

The integument of the neck is supplied by both small septocutaneous and musculocutaneous perforators from the external carotid artery and thyrocervical trunk. Several musculocutaneous perforators emerge from the sternocleidomastoid muscles of the neck. These vessels were smaller (D = 0.5 to 1.0 mm) and had cutaneous territories supplying an average of 27 cm². Larger septocutaneous arteries from the transverse cervical artery and submental artery supply the largest area of the neck.

The vascular supply of the neck is enhanced by the platysma muscle. This remnant of the panniculus carnosus layer is supplied through the same cutaneous perforators that reach the skin. The neck is divided into the anterior triangle, sternocleidomastoid region, and posterior triangle. The vascular territories supplying the neck include the occipital artery, facial artery, thyrocervical trunk, and superior thyroid artery (see Figs. 10-6 and 10-8).

Occipital Artery

The first major branch of the occipital artery is a muscular branch to the superior part of the sternocleidomastoid muscle. This artery also pierces the sternocleidomastoid muscle as a musculocutaneous perforator to supply the skin of the superolateral neck. The sternocleidomastoid branch of the occipital artery sends one to three musculocutaneous perforators (D = 0.8 mm) through the superior portion of the muscle.

Facial Artery

The submental artery, the major cutaneous branch of the facial artery, supplies the territory over the submandibular and submental triangles. This branch arises from the facial artery as it leaves the submandibular gland on the surface of the mylohyoid muscle. The submental artery sends branches to muscles, glands, and skin in the central submental region on its course toward the chin. Its largest perforating branch (D = 0.6 mm) arises from behind the medial border of the anterior belly of the digastric muscle.

Of particular interest is the submental artery's contribution to the vascular supply of the platysma. The platysma is a type II muscle. Its blood supply comes predominantly from the submental branch of the facial artery. Our angiographic studies of the neck with and without the platysma clearly demonstrate how the platysma enhances the vascular supply to the integument. Inclusion of this muscle in perforator flaps of this region greatly improves skin paddle vascularity without functional deficits. Inferiorly, the submental artery perforators anastomose with large cutaneous perforators from the superior thyroid artery within the platysma muscle.

In two of our dissections, a second cutaneous branch from the facial artery (D = 0.5 mm) was observed. This branch passed posteriorly from the submandibular triangle to anastomose with the posterior auricular artery over the sternocleidomastoid muscle. However, in our remaining dissections, musculocutaneous perforators from the occipital artery supplied this territory through the sternocleidomastoid muscle.

Thyrocervical Trunk

The branches of the thyrocervical trunk (Fig. 10-8) were highly variable in our dissection specimens. For this reason, we included the areas supplied by its major branches

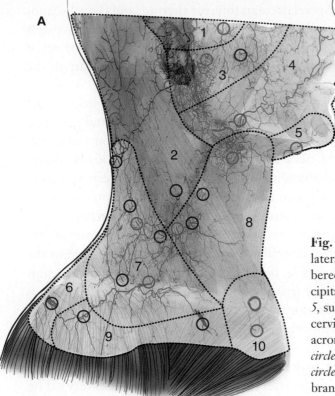

Fig. 10-8 A, An angiogram of the integument of the lateral aspect of the neck, with vascular territories numbered as follows: *1,* superficial temporal artery; *2,* occipital artery; *3,* transverse facial artery; *4,* facial artery; *5,* submental artery; *6,* suprascapular artery; *7,* transverse cervical artery; *8,* superior thyroid artery; *9,* thoracoacromial artery; and *10,* anterior intercostal artery.) *Red circles* demonstrate musculocutaneous perforators; *blue circles* indicate septocutaneous perforators. **B,** Principal branches to the integument.

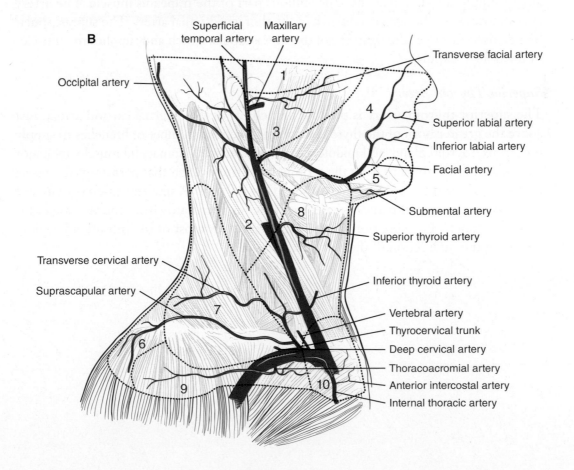

(transverse cervical, suprascapular, supraclavicular, inferior thyroid, and dorsal scapular arteries) under a single vascular territory. It is probable that some of these vessels originated independently, or from separate trunks, of the subclavian axis. However, it can be safely assumed that the origins of these rami are within close proximity to the first part of the subclavian artery.

The vascular territory of the thyrocervical trunk was the largest territory in the head and neck. It supplied approximately 30% of the total surface area, and gave rise to approximately six significant perforator vessels. The primary distribution of the thyrocervical trunk's branches to the neck came from musculocutaneous branches (D = 0.5 mm) through the sternocleidomastoid muscle inferiorly, insignificant branches of the inferior thyroid artery anteriorly, and from two or three large septocutaneous perforators (D = 0.8 mm) laterally that emanated from the posterior triangle.

The transverse cervical artery provides the primary blood supply to the integument of the inferior, anterior neck. It courses laterally deep to the omohyoid muscle to the lateral border of the levator scapulae muscle, before entering the nuchal region to supply the trapezius muscle. In the posterior triangle, the transverse cervical artery always sent at least one septocutaneous perforator through the supraclavicular triangle. This artery also sent two or three perforators via the occipital triangle, before the anterior border of trapezius muscle.

The supraclavicular perforator may arise from the suprascapular artery or as an independent branch of the subclavian artery (as the supraclavicular artery). The suprascapular artery lies deep to the transverse cervical artery and courses more laterally to supply the skin over the supraspinous part of the trapezius muscle. The artery anastomoses with the acromial branch of the thoracoacromial artery. The suprascapular branch descends over the ligament of the suprascapular notch and supplies the muscles of the dorsal scapula.

Superior Thyroid Artery

The superior thyroid artery is the first branch off of the external carotid artery, just above the greater horn of the thyroid cartilage. It sends a number of branches to supply the larynx, thyroid gland, and middle part of the sternocleidomastoid muscle. Its major cutaneous perforators are from the terminal anterior branch that perforates the fascia in front of the sternocleidomastoid muscle (D = 0.9 mm). A smaller musculocutaneous perforator often accompanies this septocutaneous perforator from the sternocleidomastoid branch. The superior thyroid artery supplies most of the infrahyoid region, including the midsection of the platysma muscle.

Nuchal Region

The nuchal region is bound laterally by the anterior border of the trapezius muscle, superiorly by the superior nuchal line, and inferiorly by a horizontal line through the spine of the seventh cervical vertebra. The territory was supplied by an average of four perforators, each greater than 0.5 mm in diameter. These perforators were either septocutaneous or musculocutaneous perforators from the occipital artery or thyro-cervical trunk. Some authors have reported that perforators from the deep cervical artery contributed to this system; however, we were unable to identify any significant perforators (larger than 0.5 mm) from this vessel. The vascular territories of the nuchal region include the occipital artery and thyrocervical trunk (Fig. 10-9).

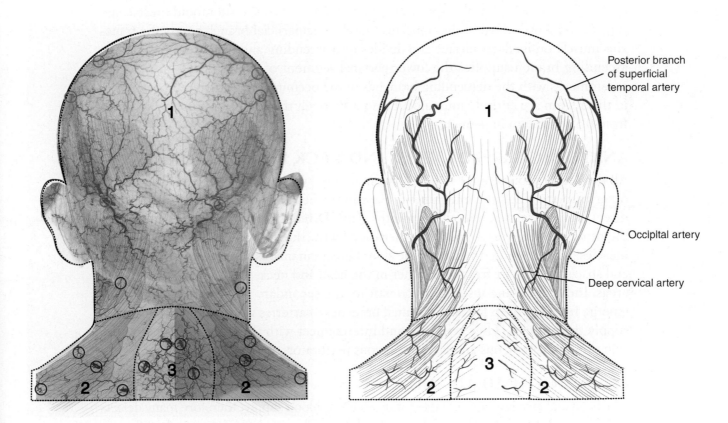

Fig. 10-9 An angiogram of the integument of the head and neck (posterior view). The vascular territories of the head and neck are shown, including the following vascular territories: *1*, external carotid arterial system, *2*, subclavian arterial system, and *3*, vascular territories of the posterior intercostal arteries. *Red circles* demonstrate musculocutaneous perforators; *blue circles* indicate septocutaneous perforators.

Occipital Artery

On emerging from between the sternocleidomastoid and trapezius muscles, the occipital artery gives off several descending branches that course inferiorly along the semispinalis muscle. These branches supply the upper segment of the trapezius muscle and anastomose intramuscularly with branches of the transverse cervical artery. More commonly, multiple musculocutaneous perforators (D = 0.5 mm) supplied the upper nuchal region. In a few specimens, the area was supplied by a single septocutaneous branch (D = 0.8) from the occipital artery.

Thyrocervical Trunk

After reaching the lateral border of the levator scapulae muscle, the transverse cervical artery divides into two muscular branches that supply the trapezius muscle.[1] The descending branch (dorsal scapular artery) courses deep to the rhomboid muscle and supplies the lower third of the trapezius muscle. A superficial branch enters the trapezius muscle on its deep surface and divides into ascending and descending rami. The ascending branch supplies the lower cervical segment of the trapezius muscle and anastomoses with the descending branches of the occipital artery. Arterial perforators in this region are entirely musculocutaneous through the trapezius muscle and range from 0.5 to 1.0 mm in diameter.

ANATOMIC BASIS OF HEAD AND NECK PERFORATOR FLAPS

All perforators course either directly from a source vessel or indirectly through some other tissue to reach the integument. Flaps in the head and neck may be divided into direct and indirect cutaneous perforator flaps. Direct cutaneous arteries constitute the primary cutaneous supply. Whether they follow the intermuscular septa or pierce muscles, their main destination is the skin. Direct cutaneous arteries are usually large and spaced well apart from each other in the head and neck, especially in mobile skin areas. Indirect cutaneous arteries constitute the secondary cutaneous supply. They emerge from the deep fascia as terminal branches of arteries whose main purpose is to supply the muscles. They reinforce and interconnect with the primary supply to the skin (musculocutaneous and fasciocutaneous perforators).[2-6]

FLAPS IN THE HEAD AND FACE

The head and face region is notable for its excellent blood supply; therefore many defects may be reconstructed with perforator island flaps. There are two groups of perforator flaps based on identifiable vascular anatomy: direct and indirect.[6]

Direct Perforator Flaps

Direct perforator flaps are based on vessels of the direct cutaneous system. Although modifications in detail are numerous, they are all variations of basic patterns supported by the supratrochlear and/or supraorbital artery, superficial temporal artery, occipital artery, posterior auricular artery, and facial artery.

Forehead Flap

A forehead flap can be designed based on the supraorbital, supratrochlear, and superficial temporal arteries for nasal reconstruction.

Paramedian Forehead Flap Based on the Supratrochlear and/or Supraorbital Arteries

This is the most useful flap in nasal reconstruction. Originally called the *midline forehead flap*, it was based on both the supratrochlear and supraorbital arteries. Presently, it is generally based on only one of these vessels. McCarthy et al[7] demonstrated sufficient collateral flow from the internal angular vessels to sustain the flap, even when the supratrochlear vessels had been ligated. Millard[8] has developed a seagull-shaped or cruciform flap for nasal reconstruction based on these vessels. With this design, transverse extensions are created on the standard paramedian flap.[4]

Forehead Flap Based on the Superficial Temporal Artery

Forehead flaps that are based on the frontal branch of the superficial temporal artery can be used for facial or nasal reconstruction with the full width of the forehead. The vascular anatomy of forehead flaps has shown that the dynamic territory of the forehead flap is made up of four anatomic territories: (1) the frontal branch of the superficial temporal artery, (2 and 3) two supratrochlear arteries, and (4) the contralateral frontal branch of the superficial temporal vessels. All of these arteries anastomose extensively through large-diameter branches, which readily allow the separate anatomic territories to link up with adequate vascularity. The flap can be raised primarily on a broad pedicle containing one superficial temporal artery and its accompanying veins. It extends across the width of the forehead and reaches from the eyebrows to the normal position of the frontal hairline. A flap approximately 30 cm long may survive without a delay procedure.[4]

Scalp Flap

Many versatile scalp flaps are available, including those designed on the named branches to the scalp. The vascular anatomy of the scalp has several important features related to scalp flaps. The scalp arteries course close to the surface of the galea (deep fascia) and send numerous radiating branches to the subdermal plexus. There is a rich network of vessels with numerous ipsilateral and contralateral anastomoses. Because of these extensive anastomoses, dynamic and potential territories may greatly exceed anatomic ones. This fact is well demonstrated by the temporoparietooccipital flap. These flaps are based on the posteriorly directed branches of the superficial temporal artery. This artery can support various forms of hair-bearing flaps, generally used for reconstructing the frontal hairline. Unilateral or bilateral flaps can be transposed to the frontal region, depending on the degree of baldness. A further modification for the treatment of occipital baldness involves creating an occipitoparietotemporal flap on an occipital artery pedicle.

Retroauricular Flap

The skin in the retroauricular mastoid area is considered to be an ideal donor site for facial reconstruction because of its good color and texture match to the face, ideal thickness, great vascularity, and concealed donor site deformity.[4] The blood supply to the cranial aspect of the auricle and the mastoid region is derived from the posterior auricular and superficial temporal arteries. The vascular territory of the retroauricular flap depends to a large extent on the relative distribution of the superficial temporal and posterior auricular arteries, as well as the vascular communication between them. Various flaps have been designed to move retroauricular skin on a pedicle containing branches of the superficial temporal artery. In general, there are two kinds of retroauricular flaps based on either the posterior auricular artery or the superficial temporal artery. The anatomic vascular basis of the retroauricular flap based on the superficial temporal artery depends on two sets of anastomoses. First, on the cranial surface of the auricle, auricular anastomoses exist between auricular branches derived from the superficial temporal artery and the posterior auricular artery. Second, in the scalp superior to the ear, scalp anastomoses occur between the parietal branch and the terminal branches of the posterior auricular artery (Fig. 10-10).

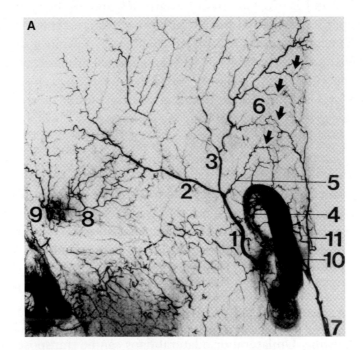

Fig. 10-10   A, An angiogram of the scalp before retroauricular flap elevation. Superior to the ear there are scalp anastomoses *(arrows)* between the parietal branch of the superficial temporal artery and the terminal branches of the posterior auricular artery.

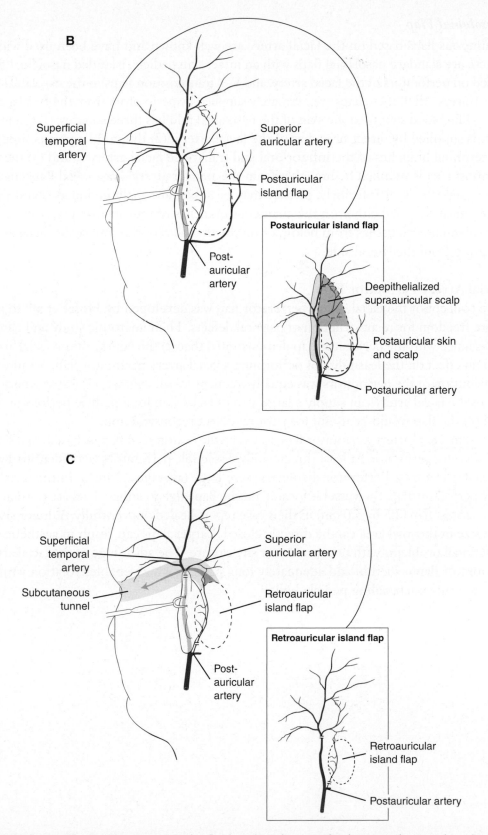

Fig. 10-10, cont'd **B,** The retroauricular flap based on the superficial temporal artery, described by Guyuron.[9] **C,** The retroauricular flap based on the supraorbital artery used by Song et al.[10]

Nasolabial Flap

Numerous flaps based on the facial artery are well known and have been used widely. These are standard nasolabial flaps with an intact skin pedicle, islanded nasolabial flaps based on perforators of the facial artery, and V-Y transposition flaps in the nasolabial and cheek areas. All of these flaps are ultimately supplied by perforators from the facial artery.

The blood supply to the skin of the nasolabial fold has three sources: (1) the lower part is supplied by direct branches of the facial artery; (2) the middle part is supplied by terminal branches of the infraorbital and transverse facial arteries; and (3) the uppermost part is supplied by branches from the angular artery. Nasolabial flaps may be based superiorly or inferiorly, or they may be subcutaneously pedicled island flaps. They must be based either on the cutaneous branches of the facial artery, penetrating the subcutaneous tissues from below, or on the branches of the transverse facial artery entering from the lateral side.

Facial Artery Perforator Flap

The concept of the facial artery perforator flap was developed by Hofer et al[11] to gain more freedom for reconstruction of perioral defects. Their anatomic study and clinical experience with the perforator flap demonstrated that (1) the course of the facial artery had no effect on the feasibility of performing a facial artery perforator flap, because the distribution of the perforators was equally frequent for all courses; (2) a single perforator of the facial artery can supply a large area of facial skin for a pedicle perforator flap; and (3) the flap would be useful for perioral defect reconstruction.[12]

The facial artery perforator flap, as a versatile customized flap, is based on a single facial artery perforator. At least three readily dissectible perforators were identified with every facial artery. Perforator diameters were large (average 1.2 mm). In the facial artery perforator flap, the vessel is located on the flap edge to enhance its arc of rotation. The largest flap (2.5 by 5.0 cm) in their case report healed uneventfully. A donor site of this size in the jowl area can be directly closed. Larger flaps can result in aesthetic and functional problems with primary donor site closure. The advantage of the facial artery perforator flap is its thin and adequately long pedicle, which enables rotation without cosmetically unappealing pedicle bulk.[11]

Face-Lift Flap

Although no perforator flaps for reconstruction have been described based on the transverse facial artery, its perforators supply a large portion of the lateral face-lift flap that is elevated during rhytidectomy. The face-lift flap of the lateral cheek is located directly over the SMAS. Clinical studies suggest that the incidence of skin slough is higher in subcutaneous face-lift dissections, because this vessel is at risk of transection during elevation of the flap, or with elevation of the superficial muscular aponeurotic system (SMAS) during rhytidectomy. Several studies have compared the arterial blood supply of the lateral face-lift flap when the flap is elevated either above or below the SMAS to better understand whether the SMAS contributes to the flap's vascularity.[12-15] Whetzel and Stevenson[13] concluded that the SMAS was an avascular layer, with perfusion of the lateral face-lift flap unaffected by supra-SMAS or sub-SMAS flap dissection. When the transverse facial artery perforator is transected during a face lift, the vascular territory of the transverse facial artery is supplied by adjacent vascular territories, primarily the facial artery. The recent anatomic study by Schaverien et al[15] suggests that the composite face-lift flap (sub-SMAS) in the preauricular region receives better perfusion, compared with a subcutaneous-plane dissection. The lateral face-lift flap is supplied predominantly by the transverse facial artery perforator, and its ligation reduces perfusion, which may have relevance in patients with vascular compromise.[15]

Indirect Perforator Flaps

There are few true musculocutaneous flaps on the face, because the skin is rarely supplied by perforators from the underlying muscles. Rather, the vessels on the face give off branches to muscles and separate branches to the skin. Flaps combining muscle and skin around the mouth can be based on the superior and inferior labial arteries. The superior labial artery was found within the orbicularis oris in approximately one fifth of specimens, and between the mucosa and the orbicularis oris in about four fifths. The inferior labial artery was found within the orbicularis oris in 13%, and between the mucosa and the orbicularis oris in 87%. The superior labial artery is found within 10 mm of the free margin of the upper lip. This artery varies in its course, up to 15 mm from the free margin of the lower lip. A variety of local lip flaps can be designed based on the vascular anatomy of the perioral arterial anatomy. A composite flap from the lower lip supplied by the inferior labial artery can be used to safely restore combined defects of the upper lip and nose, or partial defects of the lower lip.

FLAPS IN THE NECK

Similar to flaps in the head and face, flaps in the neck may be considered either direct or indirect perforator flaps. The platysma lies in the superficial fascia and might be considered as having blood supplied by direct cutaneous arteries. However, platysma musculocutaneous flaps are considered to be indirect perforator flaps.

Direct Perforator Flaps

Submental Artery Perforator Flap

Ideal flaps for facial reconstruction should be thin and pliable with sufficient mobility. The submental flap meets these criteria. Both clinical and anatomic evaluations have validated that one or two reliable perforators are present in the unilateral submental territory originating from the submental artery. The submental artery arises from the facial artery and runs over the mylohyoid and inferior to the mandible (Fig. 10-11).[16] It continues either superficial or deep to the anterior belly of the digastric muscle. The submental artery supplies the skin of almost the entire submental region of the neck, and a variable area across the midline. The submental artery perforator flap (see Chapter 14) has a long vascular pedicle and is useful in facial and intraoral reconstructions. The submental flap has become a reliable option for reconstructing facial defects. It has an excellent skin color match and a wide arc of rotation, extending to the lower two thirds of the homolateral face if needed. The submental flap is also versatile; it can be used as a cutaneous, musculofascial (cervicofascial and platysma), or osteocutaneous flap. Three-dimensional angiographic images of the vascular anatomy of the submental artery are shown in Fig. 10-12.[16]

Supraclavicular Artery Flap

The supraclavicular artery is a cutaneous perforator that arises from either the suprascapular artery or the superficial branch of the transverse cervical artery. The artery runs deep or lateral to the posterior belly of the omohyoid bone and reaches the deep fascia just posterior to the middle third of the clavicle. The supraclavicular artery rapidly divides into many small branches that enter the supraclavicular fat pad, the platysma muscle, and skin over the base of the posterior triangle of the neck. The vessels pass directly laterally toward the acromioclavicular joint and anastomose with cutaneous branches of the posterior circumflex humeral artery, especially the posterior perforator at the level of the deep fascia.

The supraclavicular artery flap can be safely elevated on the supraclavicular artery. The extent to which this territory can be extended down the upper arm is uncertain and depends on the variable nature of the anastomoses with the perforators from the posterior circumflex humeral artery. The cervicohumeral flap includes the supraclavicular artery and also the musculocutaneous perforators through the lateral part of the trapezius muscle. The territory extends to the midpoint of the upper arm.

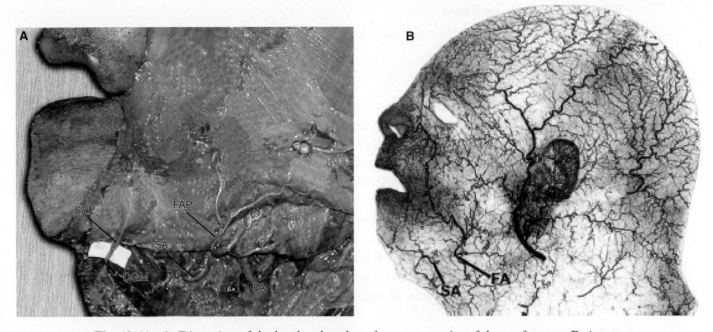

Fig. 10-11 A, Dissection of the head and neck, and sources arteries of the perforators; **B,** An angiogram of the integument of the head and neck. (*DGM,* Digastric muscle; *FA,* facial artery; *FAP,* facial artery perforator; *SA,* submental artery; *SAP,* submental artery perforator.) (Reprinted from Journal of Plastic, Reconstructive and Aesthetic Surgery, Volume 64, Tang M, Ding M, Almutairi K, Morris SF, Three dimensional angiography of the submental artery perforator flap, pages 608-613, Copyright 2011, with permission from Elsevier.)

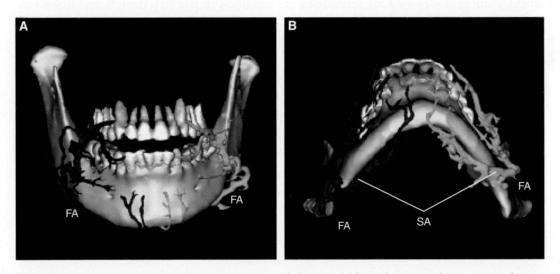

Fig. 10-12 Three dimensional-reconstruction of the mandible and surrounding arteries from a cadaver angiographic injection specimen. **A,** Anterior view. **B,** Inferior view. (*FA,* Facial artery; *SA,* submental artery.) (Reprinted from Journal of Plastic, Reconstructive and Aesthetic Surgery, Volume 64, Tang M, Ding M, Almutairi K, Morris SF, Three dimensional angiography of the submental artery perforator flap, pages 608-613, Copyright 2011, with permission from Elsevier.)

Musculocutaneous Flaps

Musculocutaneous flaps in the neck may be based on the platysma, sternomastoid, and trapezius muscles.

Platysma

The platysma muscle is vascularized by branches of the facial, superior thyroid, transverse cervical, and subclavian arteries. These branches form a plexus in and beneath the muscle from which the skin is supplied. The principal blood supply to the muscle comes from the submental branch of the facial artery superiorly, and the superior thyroid and transverse cervical arteries inferiorly. These vessels form a rich network within the platysma muscle and in the subdermal plexus. The pattern of supply is responsible for the versatility of the platysma musculocutaneous flap. The muscle has been used as a pedicle carrier for an island of skin situated in the lower lateral neck over the posterior triangle. As a further development, the flap has been reversed, with the skin island superior and the vascular pedicle inferior. The cutaneous paddle is usually designed as an ellipse over the lower or upper part of the muscle.

Sternomastoid

There are two potential musculocutaneous flaps based on the sternomastoid muscle. They are based on either the superior or inferior end of the muscle and pedicled around the opposite end. These flaps are rather unreliable because of (1) the small size and tenuous nature of the musculocutaneous perforators from the surface of the muscle to the overlying skin and (2) the poor anastomoses within the muscle. The musculocutaneous flap based superiorly with the skin paddle is notoriously unpredictable. In these circumstances, three or four territories are included in the flap design and linked by reduced-caliber choke vessels.

Trapezius

There are three different musculocutaneous flaps based on the trapezius muscle: (1) the upper trapezius musculocutaneous flap based on a branch of the occipital artery, (2) the lateral trapezius musculocutaneous flap based on the superficial branch of the transverse cervical artery, and (3) the lower trapezius musculocutaneous flap based on the dorsal scapular artery or on the deep branch of the transverse cervical artery.[1] The vascular anatomy of the lower trapezius musculocutaneous flap has been studied in great detail. This flap has become the first choice for resurfacing a wide variety of neck and lateral skull defects.

FLAP OPTIONS

The anatomic information outlined in this chapter provides some concepts to aid in the design of flaps. Because of our advanced knowledge of the branches derived from the source arteries of each angiosome, many new cutaneous perforator and musculocutaneous flaps from the head and neck have been designed for island and distant transfer.

With careful planning, large vascular territories can be captured in succession from adjacent vascular territories to provide very long flaps. For example, the extended forehead flap, which is based on the superficial temporal artery, captures two adjacent territories on the supraorbital and supratrochlear arteries. If the flap is extended beyond the midline to the opposite side, it borrows the contralateral territory of the superficial temporal artery. The long flap may consist of four substantial territories: (1) the frontal branch of the superficial temporal artery, (2 and 3) two supratrochlear arteries, and (4) the contralateral frontal branch of the superficial temporal vessels.

The submental and retroauricular regions provide additional options for flap reconstruction in the facial region. Compared with the conventional nasal, glabellar, or forehead flap, these regions have the common advantages of excellent color and texture match to facial skin, with a well-hidden donor site. Both the submental and postauricular flaps are elevated as thin skin flaps, ideal for facial resurfacing and oral lining in the midfacial region.

The Reverse Submental Perforator-Based Flap

Martin et al[17] introduced the submental island flap based on the submental artery to reconstruct orofacial defects. The flap has the advantages of a long pedicle, a wide range of applications, and well-concealed donor scars. They also described the reverse submental island flap as a distally based flap. Sterne et al[18] recommended a separate venous anastomosis in a reverse-flow manner against the consistent valve in the facial vein. Kim et al[19] have presented their anatomic study on the reverse submental perforator–based island flap. (This information is presented in detail in Chapter 14.) In brief, considering these anatomic data, the reversed flap including the superficial vein can reach the oral cavity and the root of the nose without tension, and it can be used successfully to reconstruct the middle and lower face.

Retroauricular Flap Based on the Upper Auricular Branch of the Superficial Temporal Artery

Guyuron[9] developed a one-stage retroauricular island flap based on the superficial temporal artery. Song et al[10] reported on another type of one-stage retroauricular island flap based on the superior auricular artery of the superficial temporal artery. The results of our study provide the anatomic basis for better understanding of the vascular territory of the flaps. Our radiographs show that the vascular territory of the flaps consists of three anatomic territories and two sets of anastomoses between them. The flap developed by Guyuron[9] consists of three vascular territories: (1) the superficial temporal artery, (2) the superior auricular artery of the superficial temporal artery, and (3) the posterior auricular artery. The vascular basis of the flap described by Song et al[10] depends on the supraorbital artery, the superior auricular artery of the superficial temporal artery, and the posterior auricular artery. These vessels anastomose extensively to allow three anatomic territories to survive in a pedicle or free flap.

The angiographic study showed that another kind of retroauricular flap can be developed.[20] Our radiographs showed that the upper auricular branch of the superficial temporal artery is constant, with a larger diameter and a longer pedicle, and it communicates with the posterior auricular artery at the cranial aspect of the auricle. Furthermore, a composite retroauricular flap combined with an ascending helical flap based on the upper auricular branch of the superficial temporal artery as a reverse-flow island flap can be transferred to repair complicated nasal defects. The vascular basis of this flap relies on anastomoses between the frontal branch of the superficial temporal artery and the supraorbital artery, and between the upper auricular branch and the posterior auricular artery. The reverse-flow blood supply comes from the supraorbital artery through the frontal branch of the superficial temporal artery and the upper auricular branch into the posterior auricular artery (Fig. 10-13).[20]

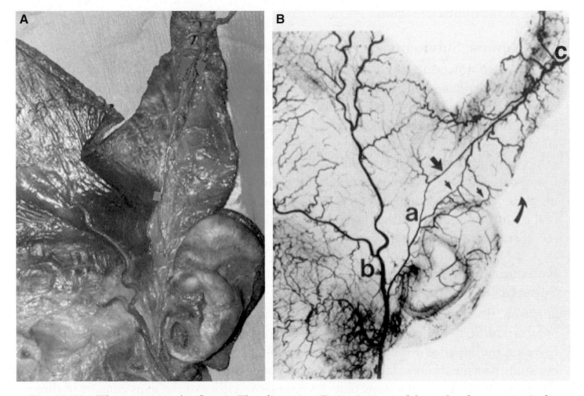

Fig. 10-13   The retroauricular flap. **A,** Flap dissection. **B,** Angiogram of the scalp after retroauricular flap elevation based on the upper auricular branch *(a)* from the superficial temporal artery *(b)*. On the cranial surface of the auricle, auricular anastomoses exist between the upper auricular branch of the superficial temporal artery and the posterior auricular artery *(c)*. (From Yang D, Morris SF. Vascular basis of the retroauricular flap. Ann Plast Surg 40:28-33, 1998.)

References

1. Yang D, Morris SF. Trapezius muscle: anatomic basis for flap design. Ann Plast Surg 41:52-57, 1998.

2. McCraw JB, Arnold PG, eds. McCraw and Arnold's Atlas of Muscle and Musculocutaneous Flaps. Norfolk, VA: Hampton Press, 1986.

3. Mathes SJ, Nahai F. General principles. In Mathes SJ, Nahai F, eds. Reconstructive Surgery: Principles, Anatomy, & Technique. St Louis: Elsevier Health Science, 1997.

4. Cormack GC, Lamberty BG, eds. The Arterial Anatomy of Skin Flaps. London: Churchill Livingstone, 1986.

5. Taylor GI, Gianoutsos MP, Morris SF. The neurovascular territories of the skin and muscles: anatomic study and clinical implications. Plast Reconstr Surg 94:1-36, 1994.

    In this anatomic study, the authors analyzed neurovascular relationships in the skin and underlying muscles in seven fresh human cadavers and nine animals. Either the arterial or the venous system was injected with a radiopaque lead oxide mixture. The results were presented, with special emphasis on the design of long axial skin flaps placed along neurovascular systems and their relationship with the current design of skin flaps. The muscles were classified according to their extrinsic and intrinsic neurovascular supplies, and suggestions were made as to how they may or may not be subdivided into functional units for local and distant transfer.

6. Hallock GG. Direct and indirect perforator flaps: the history and the controversy. Plast Reconstr Surg 111:855-865, 2003.

    The vascular supply to the fascial plexus is considered the most important factor in ensuring the reliability of skin-bearing flaps. The deep fascial perforators to this plexus have numerous origins, and have led to confusing terminology intended to encompass all possible flap options. A brief review of the history of the evolution of cutaneous flaps provides insight essential in understanding a simple proposal for their classification.

7. McCarthy JG, Lorenc ZP, Cutting C, et al. The median forehead flap revisited: the blood supply. Plast Reconstr Surg 76:866-869, 1985.

8. Millard DR Jr. Reconstructive rhinoplasty for the lower half of a nose. Plast Reconstr Surg 53:133-139, 1974.

9. Guyuron B. Retroauricular island flap for eye socket reconstruction. Plast Reconstr Surg 76:527-530, 1985.

    An island flap based on superficial temporal vessels was used successfully in eight patients to reconstruct missing or contracted eye sockets. Flap anatomy was discussed.

10. Song R, Song Y, Qi K, et al. The superior auricular artery and retroauricular artery island flaps. Plast Reconstr Surg 98:657-667, 1996.

11. Hofer SOP, Posch NA, Smit X. The facial artery perforator flap for reconstruction of perioral defects. Plast Reconstr Surg 115:996-1003, 2005.

12. Schuster RH, Gamble WB, Hamra ST, et al. A comparison of flap vascular anatomy in three rhytidectomy techniques. Plast Reconstr Surg 95:683-690, 1995.

13. Whetzel TP, Stevenson TR. The contribution of the SMAS to the blood supply in the lateral face lift flap. Plast Reconstr Surg 100:1011-1018, 1997.

14. Houseman ND, Taylor GI, Pan WR. The angiosomes of the head and neck: anatomic study and clinical applications. Plast Reconstr Surg 105:2287-2313, 2000.

15. Schaverien MV, Pessa JE, Saint-Cyr M, et al. The arterial and venous anatomies of the lateral face lift flap and the SMAS. Plast Reconstr Surg 123:1581-1587, 2009.

16. Tang M, Ding M, Almutairi K, Morris SF. Three dimensional angiography of the submental artery perforator flap. J Plast Reconstr Aesthet Surg 64:608-613, 2011.

17. Martin D, Pascal JF, Baudet J, et al. The submental island flap: a new donor site. Anatomy and clinical applications as a free or pedicled flap. Plast Reconstr Surg 92:867-873, 1993.

This paper presented a new island flap based on the submental artery. This flap has an excellent skin color match and a wide arc of rotation. It can extend to the homolateral face, except for a part of the forehead and the whole oral cavity.

18. Sterne GD, Januszkiewicz JS, Hall PN, et al. The submental island flap. Br J Plast Surg 49:85-89, 1996.

19. Kim JT, Kim SK, Koshima I, et al. An anatomic study and clinical applications of the reversed submental perforator-based island flap. Plast Reconstr Surg 109:2204-2210, 2002.

20. Yang D, Morris SF. Vascular basis of the retroauricular flap. Ann Plast Surg 40:28-33, 1998.

The aims of this study were to investigate the vascular communication between the superficial temporal artery (STA) and the posterior auricular artery (PAA) and to determine the vascular territory of various retroauricular flaps for flap design. The findings provided anatomic information and guidance for designing reliable flaps.

11

Temporoparietal Artery Perforator Flap

Willy Boeckx

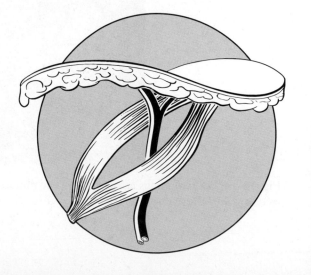

The temporoparietal artery perforator (TAP) flap is the thinnest, most pliable free flap in the body[1] (Fig. 11-1). A TAP flap averaging 12 by 17 cm provides a sufficiently large area for many types of reconstruction.[2] This flap can be used as a hair-bearing skin flap,[3] gliding tissue,[4,5] or as a carrier for neovascularization.[6] The TAP flap has a short pedicle with small vessels, adapts to a variety of shapes and sizes,[7] and leaves an almost inconspicuous donor site scar.[8] These characteristics make the TAP flap an ideal tool for reconstructing superficial defects, or for covering bone and joints. This flap can also be used for enveloping tendon reconstructions,[5] filling cavities in the face, providing a vascular carrier, and covering bony elements[9] without adding bulk. The TAP flap has demonstrated resistance to friction and has a high degree of durability, especially when covered with a split-thickness skin graft. It is highly resistant to infection and has been useful in traumatic cases.[2]

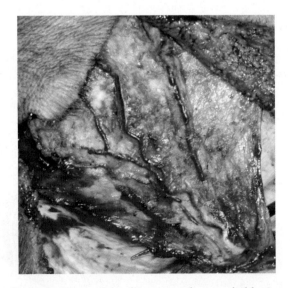

Fig. 11-1   The temporalis fascia is one of the thinnest and most pliable tissues of the body, vascularized by a dense vascular network.

ANATOMY

A rich vascular network in the temporoparietal fascia allows dissection of a flap as large as 17 by 12 cm (see Fig. 11-16). The scalp in the temporoparietal region consists of five layers: skin and subcutis, temporoparietal fascia, loose areolar tissue, deep temporal fascia, and temporalis muscle[8] (Fig. 11-2). The temporoparietal fascia is located between the skin and subcutaneous tissue and the temporalis muscle fascia.[10] It lies below the superior temporal line, above the zygoma, and is the superior extension of the superficial musculoaponeurotic system (SMAS), as described by Mitz and Peyronie.[11]

Above the superior temporal line, the temporoparietal fascia extends into the galea aponeurotica. Deep to the temporoparietal fascia and below the temporal line is a layer of loose areolar tissue,[1,12] which is superficial to the temporalis muscle fascia. Above the temporal line, the temporalis muscle fascia and the periosteum come together to continue as the pericranium[13] of the most superior part of the scalp. The temporoparietal fascia is continuous with the SMAS[1,12] inferiorly, the galea aponeurotica cranially, the frontalis muscle anteriorly, and the occipitalis muscle posteriorly.

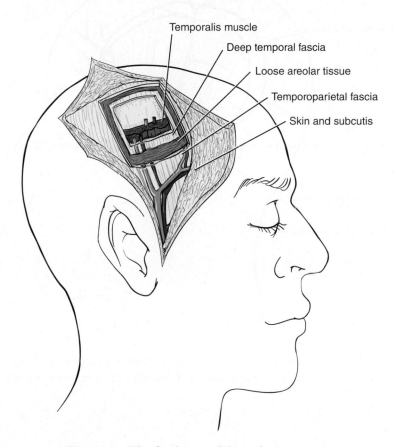

Fig. 11-2 The five layers of the scalp.

The TAP flap covers the temporal fossa, which is filled by the temporalis muscle and its overlying deep temporal fascia (Fig. 11-3). The temporal fossa is bounded by the upper border of the zygoma, the supramastoid crest, and the superior and inferior temporal lines, which extend from the posteroinferior angle of the parietal bone. The floor of the temporal fossa is composed of the temporal bone, parietal bone, frontal bone, and greater wing of the sphenoid. The pterion is the junctional point of these bones. Just above the zygomatic arch, the superficial temporoparietal fascia is loosely attached to subdermal fibrofatty tissue immediately deep to the hair follicles. At the vertex of the skull, the fascia is more closely attached to the scalp by multiple septa and blood vessels.

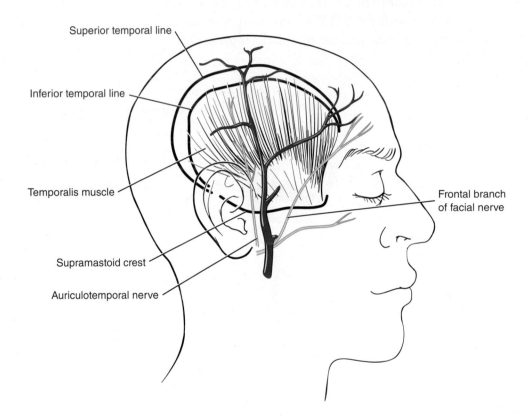

Fig. 11-3 The bony landmarks of temporal fascia are the supramastoid crest and the superior and inferior temporal lines. The temporal fossa is filled with the temporalis muscle and its overlying deep temporal fascia.

Arterial Anatomy

The superficial temporal artery and vein supply the temporoparietal fascia flap.[1] The artery originates from the external carotid artery, posterior to the vertical ramus of the mandible. This vessel passes through the parotid gland and courses over the zygomatic process of the temporal bone, anterior and deep to the superficial temporal vein (Fig. 11-4).

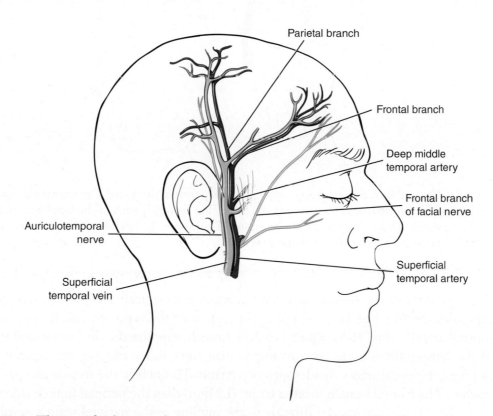

Parietal branch

Frontal branch

Deep middle temporal artery

Frontal branch of facial nerve

Superficial temporal artery

Auriculotemporal nerve

Superficial temporal vein

Fig. 11-4   The superficial temporal artery gives a frontal branch overlying deep fascia, and a parietal branch. The deep middle temporal artery supplies the deep temporal fascia. The frontal branch of the facial nerve lies on a line that extends from 0.5 cm below the tragus to 1.5 cm above the lateral eyebrow. The auriculotemporal nerve lies posterior to the temporal vessels. The superficial temporal artery lies anterior and deep to the vein.

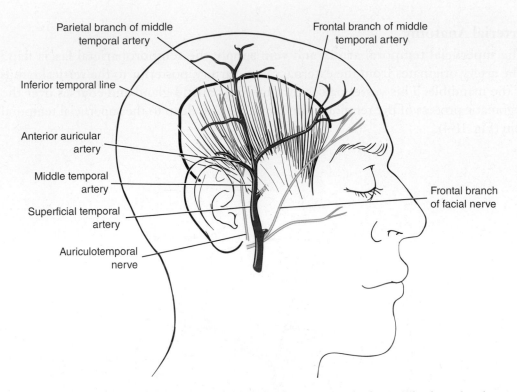

Parietal branch of middle
temporal artery

Frontal branch of middle
temporal artery

Inferior temporal line

Anterior auricular
artery

Middle temporal
artery

Superficial temporal
artery

Auriculotemporal
nerve

Frontal branch
of facial nerve

Fig. 11-5 The middle temporal artery supplies the deep temporalis fascia. The frontal and parietal branches supply the superficial temporoparietal fascia. The frontal branch of the facial nerve lies on a line that extends from 0.5 cm below the tragus to 1.5 cm above the lateral eyebrow. The auriculo-temporal nerve lies posterior to the temporal vessels.

More distally, the superficial temporal artery runs superficially on the superficial temporal fascia (see Fig. 11-2). At the upper margin of the zygomatic arch, the middle temporal artery[12] (Fig. 11-5), which is a deep branch, supplies the deep temporal fascia and the temporalis muscle. Two to four centimeters above the zygomatic arch, the superficial temporal artery divides into two terminal branches: the frontal and parietal branches. The frontal branch is often larger (1.2 mm) than the parietal branch (1.1 mm). The parietal branch continues directly to the midline of the parietal scalp toward the vertex. Posteriorly this branch anastomoses with branches of the occipital artery. The frontal branch runs toward the frontalis muscle, forehead skin, and frontal scalp. Above the zygoma, the superficial temporal artery has a diameter of 1.8 to 2.7 mm. Several branches supply the temporalis fascia and end in the subdermal and pilar plexuses of the skin[14] and hair follicles. The length of the vessel from its origin at the external carotid artery to the superior border of the zygomatic arch is 4 cm. The length of the pedicle in clinical cases is usually 2 to 3 cm when measured from the tragus distally. Within the flap, the diameter of the artery gradually diminishes as it extends distally, and ranges in size between the transverse fascial artery and the frontal branch of the superficial temporal artery. The deep branch of the temporal artery is the deep middle temporal artery.[1] This branch enters the temporalis muscle immediately superior to the zygomatic arch, branching from the posterior surface of the superficial temporal artery. The middle temporal artery supplies the temporalis muscle fascia and can be raised on a single vascular pedicle with the temporoparietal fascia (Fig. 11-6).

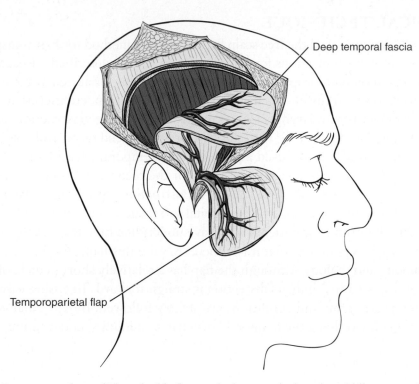

Fig. 11-6 On one vascular pedicle, a double flap can be harvested when the middle temporal artery is preserved on the posterior surface of the temporoparietal artery. The TAP flap and the deep temporal fascia are nourished by a combined vascular pedicle.

Venous Anatomy

The superficial temporal vein drains into the external jugular vein and is usually posterior and superficial to the artery,[12,15,16] subjacent to the hair follicles and subdermal fat (see Fig. 11-4). The vein terminates at the retromandibular vein, which drains into the external jugular vein. The middle temporal vein runs parallel to the middle temporal artery. The diameter of the vein at the level of the zygoma is 2.1 to 3.3 mm.

Facial Nerve

The facial nerve, with its temporal branch, crosses the zygomatic arch obliquely. This nerve is deep to the superficial temporal fascia and supplies the frontalis muscle. The facial nerve can be damaged when the vascular pedicle is dissected below the tragus. The frontal branch of the facial nerve lays in a line extending from 0.5 cm below the tragus to 1.5 cm above the lateral eyebrow (see Fig. 11-3). The nerve is vulnerable in this region, because the superficial temporal fascia is very thin in this inferior area.[1,5]

Auriculotemporal Nerve

The sensory branch of the mandibular branch (V_3) of the trigeminal nerve lies in the superficial temporal fascia posterior to the vessels just in front of the tragus (see Fig. 11-5). The sensory branch innervates the temporal region, external meatus, temporomandibular joint, auricle, and tympanic membrane. If this nerve is damaged, only sensory function is lost and no gustatory sweating (Frey syndrome) occurs.

SURGICAL TECHNIQUE

Harii et al[17] first described the free scalp flap in 1974 as a method for hair transplantation. Subsequently, many indications for this free flap have been described.* Recently, Collar et al[23] reported on temporoparietal fascia reconstructions for auricular reconstruction, hair-bearing tissue transfer, facial soft tissue augmentation, cutaneous and mucosal oncologic defect repair, laryngectomy salvage, skull base reconstruction, and orbital reconstruction. Hocaoglu et al[24] used this flap for lower eyelid reconstruction in pediatric patients, and Altindas et al[25] used a prefabricated temporal island flap for eye socket reconstruction that included a strip of scalp for the reconstruction of the lid margins and eyelashes. It allows stable eye socket reconstruction with natural-looking eyelids, eyelashes, and lid margins. Also, the periorbital soft tissue volume can be adjusted, which is especially important for patients who have undergone radiation therapy. However, most investigators point out that it is difficult to raise this flap, and that the dissection can be bloody and tedious. Although the flap has a relatively short pedicle of 3 cm and the vessel size is 1.5 to 2 mm, its dissection is straightforward. To ensure ease of dissection, some precautions and conditions are strictly followed. In particular, a Y-shaped incision is made overlying the temporal fascia flap to minimize undermining (Fig. 11-7).

*References 1, 3-5, 7, 14, 18-22.

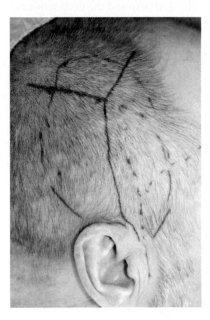

Fig. 11-7   To minimize skin flap undermining, a Y-shaped incision is outlined on the scalp with the vertical incision posterior to the parietal branch of the temporoparietal artery.

Free Flap Dissection

The incision to expose the TAP flap is made 1 to 2 cm behind the parietal branch of the superficial artery (Fig. 11-8). The incision runs in front of the tragus and almost vertically to the vertex. Precise identification of the artery can easily be performed with a Doppler probe. Making the incision 1 to 2 cm behind the vessel minimizes the risk of damaging it when searching just below the hair follicles. The incision is started 1 cm above the upper pole of the ear. Using pure cut unipolar cautery to make the skin incision and the spray coagulation mode to control dermal bleeding, a dry field can be obtained. Keeping the field dry greatly facilitates further dissection and identification of the outer layer of the superficial temporoparietal fascia. Bipolar coagulation can be used to occlude slightly larger vessels with a diameter of 0.2 to 0.4 mm. The incision is deepened to the temporoparietal fascia for a length of 2 to 3 cm. The anterior skin flap is lifted with a Miller-Senn retractor (Fig. 11-9). Retractors can also improve hemostasis in the wound. With increased traction, the cutaneous and subcutaneous veins collapse. Gradual release of the Senn-Miller retractor reopens the veins, which can then be co-

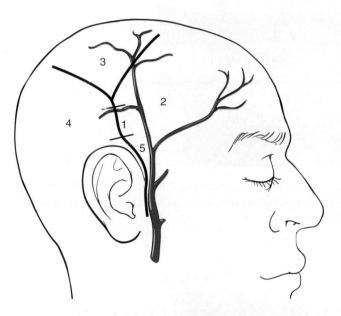

Fig. 11-8 The skin incision for free flap dissection starts 1.5 cm behind the parietal branch (*1*), well above the upper pole of the ear. The flap is developed anteriorly (*2*), superiorly (*3*), and posteriorly (*4*). Finally, the vascular pedicle is identified (*5*). If necessary, the pedicle is extended in front of the ear and tragus.

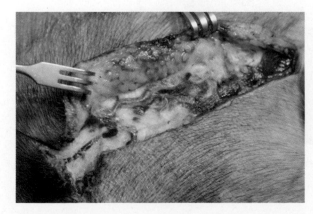

Fig. 11-9 The anterior skin is lifted from the underlying temporoparietal fascia. The temporoparietal vessels lie very superficial on this fascia and can be damaged when the skin incision overlies the vessels.

agulated with bipolar cautery. When the exact plane of cleavage is found just below the hair follicles, the temporoparietal fascia is dissected anteriorly (Fig. 11-10). The incision is extended downward to the zygomatic arch or 1 cm below it. Cranially the incision is extended 6 cm above the auricle, and then divided into a Y-shaped incision to further expose the most cranial part of the temporoparietal fascia flap (see Figs. 11-7 and 11-8).

By following this dissection technique, a flap length of 12 to 14 cm can be achieved. The anterior skin flap can be further developed. Although the dissection can be done according to the surgeon's preference, I find it helpful in this part of the operation to use bipolar scissors. These can be used as bipolar forceps or as a cutting electrocautery instrument, allowing easy coagulation of the 0.2 to 0.4 mm vascular perforators from the temporal parietal fascia to the skin (Fig. 11-11).

The venous network in the subcutaneous tissue is especially rich and must be coagulated at numerous places. A plane is dissected between the temporoparietal fascia

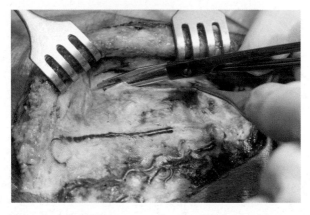

Fig. 11-10   The overlying skin and subcutis are dissected free from the temporoparietal fascia for approximately 5 to 6 cm in front of the vessels. The terminal vascular branches are clipped, because venous congestion can occur after revascularization.

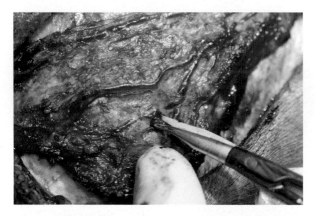

Fig. 11-11   The emerging superficial skin vessels are carefully coagulated with bipolar scissors, which act as a bipolar coagulation forceps.

and the subcutaneous tissue, lifting the skin flaps off the fascia (Fig. 11-12). The normal dissection time for this flap is approximately 45 minutes. When the cranial and anterior parts of the flap are dissected free, Miller-Senn retractors are used to free the posterior skin flap from the fascia (Fig. 11-13). Here the skin and subcutaneous tissue are thicker, and the fascia is more adherent to them. Larger venous branches extend in the direction of the occipital vessels. The width of the flap can be from 6 to 10 cm and can be extended to 12 cm. However, in this situation care must be taken not to damage the frontal branch of the facial nerve. This nerve crosses the zygomatic arch in an oblique manner and lies deep to the superficial temporal fascia, supplying the frontalis muscle. It lies approximately 1 cm behind the zygomatic process of the frontal bone. The frontal branch can be traced along a line running from 0.5 cm below the tragus to 1.5 cm above the lateral eyebrow. When the full length and width of the flap is freed from the overlying skin, the temporoparietal fascia can be incised anteriorly, starting in the middle and

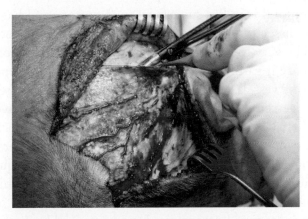

Fig. 11-12   After complete development of the anterior flap surface, the anterior, cranial, and posterior margins are incised and the posterior surface is accessed.

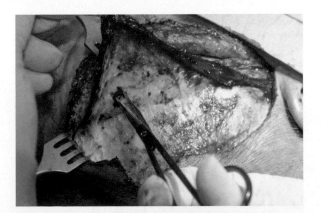

Fig. 11-13   Bipolar coagulation with bipolar scissors is performed. The deep surface of the temporoparietal fascia is much smoother than the superficial surface, and in most instances will be placed superficially in the recipient bed.

extending both cranially and caudally. Small hemoclips are used to occlude the arterial and venous branches connecting to the anterior auricular artery and occipital artery. After transecting the posterior extension of the temporoparietal fascia, the fan-shaped flap is tapered down to its pedicle, where the flap becomes narrow (1.5 to 2 cm). The posterior surface of the temporoparietal fascia is easily dissected free from the loose areolar tissue covering the temporalis muscle fascia. The middle temporal artery arises from the posterior surface of the superficial temporal artery at the level of the zygomatic arch (see Fig. 11-6). This vessel has to be clipped very precisely. This clipping is best done when the main proximal pedicle of the flap has been dissected out. If required, the temporalis muscle fascia can be harvested together with the temporoparietal fascia (see Fig. 11-6). It is essential to preserve the middle temporal artery and vein, which are found at the level of the zygomatic arch, so that it is possible to cover even larger defects with this flap.

Dissection of the Vascular Pedicle

The superficial temporal vein lies superficial to the artery and has a diameter of 1.5 to 3.2 mm. Careful dissection of the vein should be performed over a length of up to 2 cm (Fig. 11-14). The very tortuous course of the superficial temporal artery must be recognized to prepare it carefully down to the tragus, and to prepare a pedicle 3 to 4 cm long. Because the vessels lie superficial to the fascia, careful dissection of the fascia behind the vessels is essential (Fig. 11-15). Care must be taken to avoid damaging the frontal branch of the facial nerve in front of the vessels. If the superficial temporal artery becomes spastic, it is irrigated with papaverine. If the spasm persists, the final part of pedicle dissection can be performed using the microscope. Adequate magnification allows an appreciation of the delicacy of the vessels; the especially thin-walled vein can be dissected free more precisely.

When the flap is ready to be transferred, medium-sized hemoclips are used to clip the pedicle (Fig. 11-16). The posterior surface of the fascia is much smoother than the anterior surface. Almost no bleeding occurs on the posterior surface. However, on the

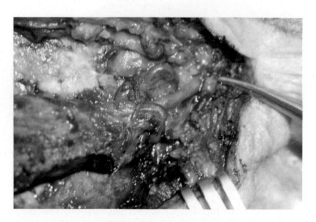

Fig. 11-14 The superficial temporal artery and vein are separated to facilitate microvascular anastomosis. The very tortuous course of the artery must be dissected free from surrounding fibrous bands, thereby lengthening the pedicle to avoid kinking the anastomosis.

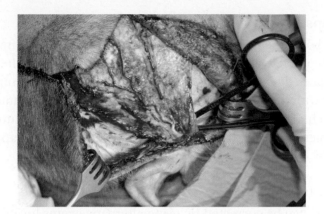

Fig. 11-15   When the entire flap is elevated except for the distal attachment, the pedicle is carefully isolated to prevent spasm during the dissection and to enhance hemostasis.

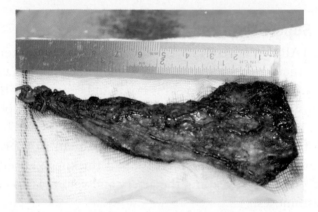

Fig. 11-16   When the flap is completely free its average size can be 12 by 8 cm. If required, the flap can be extended up to 17 by 12 cm, but the edges may be less viable.

anterior surface of the fascia, an average of 10 to 15 perforating bleeding points have to be coagulated with bipolar forceps or bipolar scissors. This surface contains more loose connective tissue than the posterior surface, which is more fibrous. We turn the fascia over in the recipient site so that the posterior surface becomes superficial. The auriculotemporal branch of the trigeminal nerve lies superficially in the temporal fascia behind the vessels, just in front of the tragus (see Fig. 11-5). If this sensory nerve is removed together with the flap, sensation is lost to the anterior auricle, temporal region, and external meatus.

MODIFICATIONS
Tissue Expansion

A tissue expander can be introduced behind the fascia to extend the size of the superficial temporal fascia. This procedure increases the venous network, and care must be taken to ensure that sufficient centripetal venous drainage is developed before raising the flap. Therefore expansion should be done slowly, because rapid expansion may occlude the venous drainage in the most prominent area of the expanded flap.[21]

Combined Flaps

For vascularized bone, the outer table or even the full-thickness temporoparietal bone can be included in the flap at its superior edge. The outer table of the temporoparietal bone at the superior edge of the temporal fossa in the area of the temporal line may be elevated together with the fascia as vascularized bone. Vascular communications between the parietal branch of the superficial temporal artery and periosteum are sufficient to nourish this segment of bone. It is important to include the galea aponeurotica when bone is harvested.

Alternative Venous Sources

Venous anomalies may be corrected by using alternative veins located behind the ear, or at the cranial end of the flap. Searching for the vein with the biggest diameter at the edges of the flap can correct this problem.

PITFALLS
Absence of the Superficial Temporal Vein

Dissection of the TAP flap is generally straightforward. One potential pitfall is the absence of the superficial temporal vein. Occasionally the vein lies up to 3 cm behind the temporal artery. Therefore, if the vein is not found centrally in the pedicle, it may be located more posteriorly,[5,16] very close to the tragus and upper pole of the ear. On one occasion we did not find a draining vein near the anterior pedicle; however, a large draining vein was found close to the vertex. In this patient we were able to fold the flap, thereby decreasing its length and increasing its thickness. Distal venous drainage could be reflected proximally, keeping the artery and vein next to each other for the microvascular anastomoses.

Alopecia

When the incision is started behind the vessels, there is an area of approximately 4 by 2 cm where we can progressively identify the outer surface of the fascia and find the proper plane of cleavage, decreasing the risk of alopecia. If the dissection is carried out too superficially, hair follicles may be damaged, resulting in alopecia. This complication occurs most commonly in an area approximately 0.5 to 1 cm in front of and behind the incision line, and may require scar revision in a later procedure.

INDICATIONS
Thin Cover for Tendons and Bones

The temporoparietal fascia free flap is the thinnest flap available in the body. Maximal dimensions are approximately 10 by 18 cm. This is my flap of choice for covering the calcaneus, Achilles tendon, dorsum of the foot, and inner and outer ankle region. Covering the extensor tendons with this flap provides a gliding tissue for the tendons.[2,3] Additionally, tendon grafts can be covered on both sides by temporoparietal fascia free flaps. This flap is a good choice for reconstructing dorsal hand injuries where extensor tendons have been crushed, or where a capsulotomy of metacarpophalangeal joints must be performed. Hand and wrist joints can also be reconstructed with this flap.

Fasciocutaneous Flap

As a fasciocutaneous perforator flap, the TAP flap can be used for eyebrow reconstruction, for example, in burn victims (Fig. 11-17). When an eyebrow is completely missing[3] as the result of a full-thickness burn injury of the forehead, and the ipsilateral forehead has been damaged severely, a contralateral free microvascular temporoparietal fasciocutaneous flap can be transplanted. Care must be taken to outline the hair-bearing skin exactly on top of the parietal branch of the superficial temporal artery and to ensure

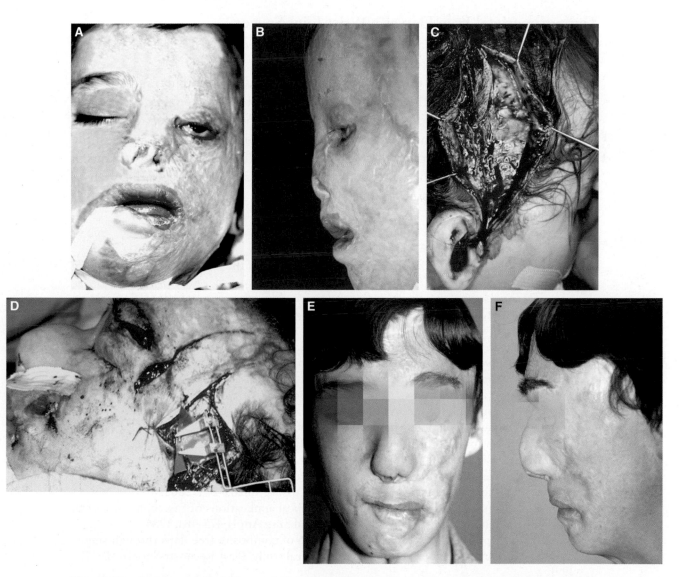

Fig. 11-17 A, After a full-thickness facial burn, this patient's eyebrow was destroyed down to the bone. **B,** The eyebrow could not be reconstructed with ipsilateral hair-bearing skin. **C,** The contralateral temporoparietal fasciocutaneous flap was dissected free on a long vascular pedicle. **D,** The microvascular anastomosis was performed with the contralateral vessels using 10-0 nylon sutures. **E,** Complete symmetry of the reconstructed eyebrow was achieved. **F,** The direction of the hairs on the reconstructed eyebrow was normal.

that the direction of the hair shafts is appropriate. The transplanted eyebrow has to be symmetrical with the opposite eyebrow. After identifying the superficial temporal vessels (see Figs. 11-4 and 11-5), the flap is dissected free on its vascular pedicle.

The vessels are transected before the tragus. After tunneling through the temporal skin, the pedicle is rerouted from the reconstructed eyebrow to the superficial temporal vessels just in front of the ear. Arterial and venous microsurgical anastomoses with 10-0 nylon are performed to revascularize the reconstructed eyebrow. Good symmetry of the reconstructed eyebrow can be achieved.

Temporoparietal Free Flap as a Wrist Joint Spacer

The temporoparietal free flap has been successfully used as a vascularized spacer in patients with severe rheumatoid arthritis of the wrist.[4]

Further indications for the TAP flap in hand surgery are found in traumatic cases where complete absence of the dorsal skin and extensor tendons requires reconstruction of all extensor tendons. To achieve good gliding of the reconstructed tendons and optimal revascularization, the extensor tendons are placed between two layers of the TAP flap. When covered with a full-sheet skin graft, aesthetically pleasing contour of the dorsum of the hand can be achieved, with optimal revascularization of the extensor tendons and good gliding tissue around the tendons.

References

1. Kaplan IB, Gilbert DA, Terzis JK. The vascularized fascia of the scalp. J Reconstr Microsurg 5:7-16, 1989.

   The fascial layers of the temporal and occipital regions of the scalp were examined in 11 fresh cadavers. In the temporal region, three independently vascularized layers were isolated, all of which could be elevated on a single superficial temporal artery, but separated to remain independently vascularized from specific branches of this parent trunk. In the occipital area, the occipital vessels could be dissected to yield a long pedicle for an independent fascial territory that could be transposed locally or elevated as a free flap and that will, in all likelihood, carry vascularized occipital bone. As yet unrealized uses of these ultrathin vascularized tissues remain boundless. Three representative cases were presented.

2. Boeckx WD, van den Hof B, van Holder C, et al. Changes in donor site selection in lower limb free flap reconstruction. Microsurgery 17:380-385, 1986.

3. De Lorenzi F, van der Hulst RR, Boeckx WD. Free flaps in burn reconstruction. Burns 27:603-612, 2001.

4. Boeckx WD, De Lorenzi F, van der Hulst RR, et al. Free fascia temporalis interpositioning as a treatment for wrist ankylosis. J Reconstr Microsurg 18:269-274, 2002.

5. Upton J, Rogers C, Durham-Smith G, et al. Clinical applications of free temporoparietal flaps in hand tendon cover reconstruction. J Hand Surg Am 11:475-483, 1986.

6. Khouri RK, Upton J, Shaw WW. Prefabrication of composite free flaps through staged microvascular transfer: an experimental and clinical study. Plast Reconstr Surg 87:108-115, 1991.

7. Brent B, Byrd HS. Secondary ear reconstruction with cartilage grafts covered by axial, random, and free flaps of temporoparietal fascia. Plast Reconstr Surg 72:141-151, 1983.

8. Cheney ML, Varvares MA, Nadol JB Jr. The temporoparietal fascia free flap in head and neck reconstruction. Arch Otolaryngol Head Neck Surg 119:618-623, 1993.

   The technique for the temporoparietal fascia flap in head and neck reconstruction was described. The advantages and applications were presented with case reports. Donor site morbidity was discussed, and the details of flap harvesting were reviewed.

9. Musolas A, Colombini E, Michelena J. Vascularized full thickness parietal bone grafts in maxillofacial reconstruction: the role of the galea and superficial temporal vessels. Plast Reconstr Surg 87:261-267, 1991.

Based on the studies of Cutting et al, Psillakis et al, and Casanova et al, the authors developed the full-thickness galeoparietal bone flap, which was applied initially for mandibular reconstruction but was of great use for all maxillofacial reconstructions. The four cases were presented. Some technical details, the surgery, results, and possible sequelae or complications were also discussed.

10. Tolhurst DE, Carstens MH, Greco RJ, et al. The surgical anatomy of the scalp. Plast Reconstr Surg 87:603-612, 1991.

11. Mitz V, Peyronie M. The superficial musculoaponeurotic system (SMAS) in the parotid and cheek area. Plast Reconstr Surg 58:80-88, 1976.

The authors investigated the superficial musculoaponeurotic system (SMAS) in the parotid and cheek areas by anatomic dissections, radiographs, and histologic sections. This paper helped in our understanding of this anatomic structure and helped establish its place in facial surgery.

12. Abul-Hassan HS, Ascher GV, Acland RD. Surgical anatomy and blood supply of the fascial layers of the temporal region. Plast Reconstr Surg 77:17-24, 1986.

13. Cormack GC, Lamberty BGH. Posterior auricular artery fasciocutaneous free flap. In Cormack GC, Lamberty BGH, eds. The Arterial Anatomy of Skin Flaps. Edinburgh: Churchill Livingstone, 1986.

14. Antonyshyn O, Gruss JS, Birt BD. Versatility of temporal muscle and fascial flaps. Br J Plast Surg 41:118-131, 1988.

The muscle and superficial fascia of the temporal area differ in their physical characteristics, vascular supply, and clinical applications. Both can be employed independently or simultaneously as regional flaps for reconstructing a variety of complex craniofacial defects. The paper reviewed the anatomy, surgical technique, and utilization of temporal flaps.

15. Casanova R, Cavalcante D, Grotting JC, et al. Anatomic basis for vascularized outer-table calvarial bone flaps. Plast Reconstr Surg 78:300-308, 1986.

16. Upton J. Surgical anatomy and blood supply of the fascial layers of the temporal region (discussion). Plast Reconstr Surg 77:25-28, 1986.

17. Harii K, Ohmori K, Ohmori S. Hair transplantation with free scalp flaps. Plast Reconstr Surg 53:410-417, 1974.

18. De Lorenzi F, van der Hulst RR, Boeckx WD. Nostril reconstruction with ear helix free flap. Eur J Plast Surg 24:253-255, 2001.

19. McCarthy J, Cutting CB, Shaw WW. Vascularized calvarial flaps. Clin Plast Surg 14:37-47, 1987.

20. Chowdary RP. Use of temporoparietal fascia free flap in digital reconstruction. Ann Plast Surg 23:543-546, 1989.

21. De Lorenzi F, van der Hulst RR, Boeckx W. Horseshoe expanded scapular flap shows no venous congestion. Br J Plast Surg 54:604-609, 2001.

22. Brent B, Upton J, Acland RD, et al. Experience with the temporoparietal fascial free flap. Plast Reconstr Surg 76:177-188, 1985.

23. Collar RM, Zopf D, Brown D, et al. The versatility of the temporoparietal fascia flap in head and neck reconstruction. J Plast Reconstr Aesthet Surg 65:141-148, 2012.

24. Hocaoglu E, Ozden BC, Aydin H. Lower eyelid reconstruction in a paediatric face: a one-stage aesthetic approach using the versatile temporoparietal fascia flap. J Plast Reconstr Aesthet Surg. 2012 Mar 27. [Epub ahead of print]

25. Altindas M, Yucel A, Ozturk G, et al. The prefabricated temporal island flap for eyelid and eye socket reconstruction in total orbital exenteration patients: a new method. Ann Plast Surg 65:177-182, 2010.

12

Facial Artery Perforator Flap

Stefan O.P. Hofer

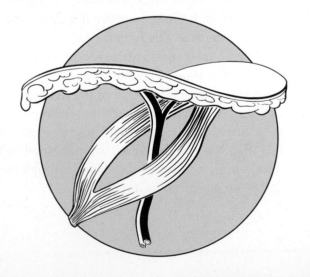

The nasolabial fold area is a source of skin that can be used for reconstructive purposes. There is a large amount of skin available in this area, because skin laxity increases in the jowl region as one ages. This skin is supplied by perforating branches from the facial artery and has traditionally been used for nasolabial flaps based inferiorly or superiorly.[1-5] The inferior or superior base of a nasolabial flap contains the skin bridge and subcutaneous tissue down to the facial artery. This makes the nasolabial flap somewhat bulky at times, necessitating a second stage of pedicle division. The flap was initially refined as an island flap. In this fashion, a second stage of skin pedicle division could be avoided, although the fuller base could still require debulking. The latest refinement in the application of nasolabial skin for reconstructive purposes was the introduction of the facial artery perforator (FAP) flap concept.[6] Individual perforators from the facial artery could supply sufficient blood flow to sustain the overlying skin. This was the basis for multiple perforator flaps in other areas of the body. The advantage of the FAP flap is that it is performed in one stage. A second stage is not needed to divide the pedicle or correct bulkiness around the pivot point of the flap. This flap is most suitable for perioral defects where the facial aesthetic unit principle[7] of reconstructive surgery can be applied.

ANATOMY

The facial artery is the fourth branch of the external carotid artery and follows a tortuous course through the submandibular gland, around the anterior surface of the mandible, and onto the face. Once on the face it has an oblique course toward the nasal alar base, where it connects or continues as the angular branch. The total length of the facial artery between the anterior mandible and the nasal alar rim has been shown to be on average 176.6 mm (range 140 to 225 mm).[6] The actual length of the facial artery is longer than the straight distance between these two points because of its very tortuous course. The facial artery and facial vein do not run closely together. This means that, in general, the FAP flap has a well-defined arterial blood supply but often no single venous outflow. The venous outflow of the flap is through the periarterial tissue, and the FAP should not be skeletonized to its core.

The cadaver study that was the basis for the initial description of this flap provides some basic anatomic information that is very helpful for planning and executing this flap.[6] Three points about these perforators are essential. First, the surgeon should know how many perforators branch from the facial artery to be confident that there will be a perforator close to a potential defect. Second, knowing the length of the perforator helps determine the possible arc of rotation of this flap. Finally, knowing the diameter of these perforators helps the surgeon estimate the skin size that can be perfused. In this study, multiple FAPs were identified and dissected to their origin at the facial artery (Fig. 12-1).

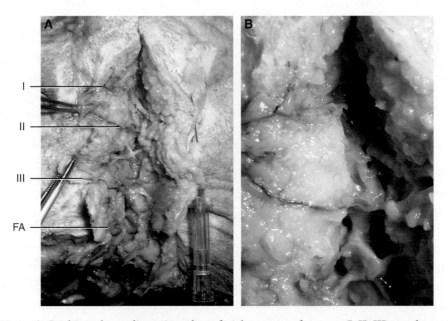

Fig. 12-1 **A,** In this cadaver dissection, three facial artery perforators *(I, II, III)* are shown branching from the facial artery *(FA)* in a medially reflected deepithelialized facial skin flap. **B,** Two facial artery perforators branch from the facial artery and extend toward the facial skin. (From Hofer SO, Posch NA, Smit X. The facial artery perforator flap for reconstruction of perioral defects. Plast Reconstr Surg 115:996-1003, 2005.)

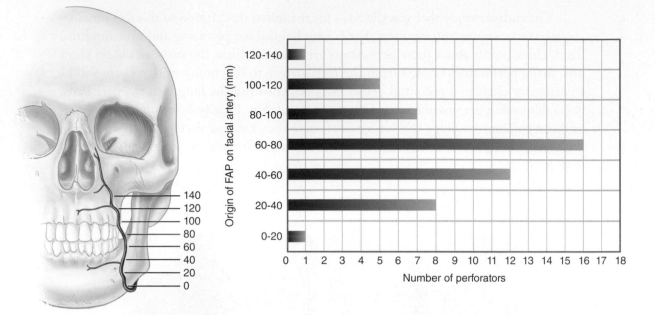

Fig. 12-2   Distribution of perforators over the course of the facial artery. The bars represent the cumulative number of facial artery perforators in consecutive 20 mm (2 cm) sections of facial arteries. The distribution of perforators between 2 and 10 cm is even closer than the bar graph suggests because of the tortuous course of the facial artery, as depicted in the illustration of the face. (Adapted from Hofer SO, Posch NA, Smit X. The facial artery perforator flap for reconstruction of perioral defects. Plast Reconstr Surg 115:996-1003, 2005.)

The average number of facial artery perforators was 5.7 per facial artery (range 3 to 9) (Fig. 12-2). The arc of rotation for a possible FAP flap, as derived by the length of the facial artery perforator from its origin to the skin, ranged from 13 to 51 mm (average 25.2 mm). Finally, the diameter of the facial artery perforators, measured at their origin from the facial artery, ranged from 0.6 to 1.8 mm (average 1.2 mm). Vessels of similar diameter in the lower extremity have been reported to supply skin paddles of 5 by 10 cm, which is larger than any skin area that could be harvested in the face, while still being able to close the donor site primarily.[8,9]

SURGICAL TECHNIQUE
Surface Landmarks

The surface landmarks of the FAP flap are governed by the course of the facial artery. Because this flap is, in essence, a freestyle flap, no fixed exterior surface markings are available. The surface area most suitable for designing the flap is the jowl area. This area gains significant laxity over the course of one's life and is one of the major zones of concern in individuals seeking facial rejuvenation procedures. To reliably plan the surgery, the course of the facial artery is mapped on the facial skin with the help of a handheld Doppler device. This is important to know exactly where to expect to find the facial artery perforators. In general, it is not possible to detect individual facial artery perforators, because the background noise of the facial artery is too loud. On occasion it may be possible to detect a slight crescendo at the level of a perforator.

Flap Dissection

The flap is dissected in the style of a freestyle flap, because the exact location of the perforator that will provide the best range for the arc of rotation is not known beforehand. Flap dissection can start in one of two ways. The flap can be raised after a perforator is identified through the wound edge, or it can be raised by making an incision at one side of a proposed flap through which a suitable perforator is identified. In general, the first method is best for the FAP flap, because this is a local pedicle perforator flap and the exact and optimal position of the perforator is crucial for its arc of rotation. Searching for a perforator through an incision of a proposed flap works better for a freestyle free flap, where the position of the perforator as it enters the flap is important but of lesser concern.

Before dissection begins, the defect is carefully evaluated. In some cases, the defect can be adapted before planning the flap to make it adhere to the principles of facial aesthetic reconstruction. The reconstructive requirements for the defect are then marked on a foil template that will be used at the donor site once the adequate perforator has been identified. Dissection is performed with 2.5× loupe magnification. Through the wound edge or through a separate incision, meticulous dissection is carried out to identify facial artery perforators. The plane of dissection is above the facial mimetic musculature so that these muscles are preserved. Once a perforator of sufficient caliber in a suitable position has been identified, the template is used to mark the skin (Fig. 12-3). Before cutting the flap, it must be confirmed that the selected perforator will provide the desired arc of rotation. The flap is raised in the plane superior to the facial musculature. The pedicle is dissected only to the level where tensionless rotation of the flap is possible. In general, venous outflow is from the cuff of fibrofatty tissue that is left with the facial artery perforator, because the facial artery and vein run separately from each other. In rare cases these vessels run close together, and a readily identifiable artery and vein can be incorporated in the pedicle. Once the flap and pedicle are raised, rotation over 180 degrees is possible without any concern for blood supply. The flap is inset and sutured without tension and usually has a classic blue shimmer of congestion, similar to that of a forehead flap. This will make the flap swell in the postoperative phase, which is an additional reason to inset this flap without undue tension. Fig. 12-3 presents a clinical example of FAP flap dissection.

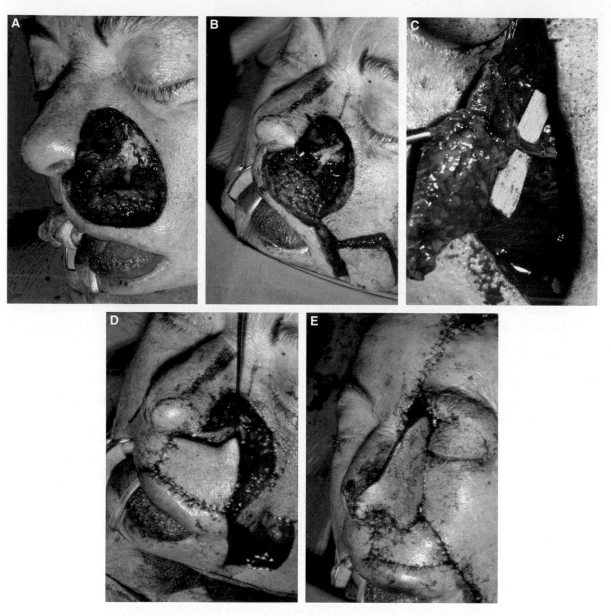

Fig. 12-3   A, This patient had a defect of the upper perioral region, cheek, and left nasal ala and tip after sweat gland carcinoma resection. **B,** The FAP flap was designed and cut in the jowl area. **C,** Example of an FAP with a vena comitans in a different patient. **D,** The FAP flap was dissected from the left jowl area and rotated into the defect. **E,** The patient is shown intraoperatively, after FAP flap, cheek advancement, and nasal ala and hemitip reconstruction.

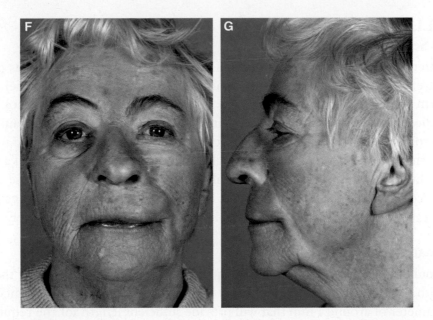

Fig. 12-3, cont'd   F and **G,** The patient is shown 2 years after reconstruction and 66 Gy of radiation therapy. (From Hofer SO, Posch NA, Smit X. The facial artery perforator flap for reconstruction of perioral defects. Plast Reconstr Surg 115:996-1003, 2005.)

Neighboring Anatomic Structures

The flap is raised above the facial musculature to prevent facial nerve weakness following ablative surgery. Care should be taken to avoid harvesting flaps that are too large, because this could distort the perioral area and possibly lead to functional complications. The facial aesthetic unit principles of scar placement should be followed. According to the governing principle, scars are best camouflaged if they are positioned at the transition of convex and concave surfaces where light and shadow blend.

MODIFICATIONS

The FAP flap is best suited for perioral reconstructions, because the facial aesthetic unit principles can be followed in this region. The flap can be designed with an inferior- or superior-based pedicle. A different application for the superior-based pedicle flap is the lower eyelid region and nose, which can be confidently reached with a sufficient perforator.

The edges of the flap can be thinned conservatively to make to achieve a better fit. The area around the perforator entering the flap should not be further dissected. Flaps of up to 2.5 by 5 cm can be harvested if the donor site can be closed without distortion.

PITFALLS
Patient Selection

Poor patient selection can result in increased postoperative complications or even flap failure. The FAP flap should only be used if the donor site has sufficient laxity to perform primary closure without undue distortion of the local area. Smoking is a contraindication for this flap procedure, as it is for forehead flaps. It is the main reason for compromised flap circulation. Relative contraindications for this flap are previous radiation therapy and neck dissection, which generally results in a cut facial artery in the neck, but should not prevent successful application of this flap, because there is extensive collateral circulation in the face. Wound-healing complications can occur in both of these situations. This should be discussed with the patient preoperatively.

Inadequate Planning

Time should be taken to plan the flap adequately by marking the course of the facial artery with a handheld Doppler device. An appropriate perforator is identified—one with a diameter of around 1 mm that will provide sufficient length for the required arc of rotation for flap inset without undue tension.

Dissection

Dissection should be above the facial musculature to avoid weakening facial expression. Thinning efforts should stay well away from the perforator.

Intraoperative Salvage

A facial artery perforator is generally present. If, during dissection, there is doubt whether the perforator will be able to sustain the designed flap, one has the option of using a standard nasolabial flap. This can only be done if the skin incision at the pedicle end is saved until last. I have never needed to use this flap. It requires some experience and confidence when first starting to rely on these perforators.

CONCLUSION

The FAP flap is a valuable addition to the facial reconstructive armamentarium. It provides a reconstructive option allowing one to replace like with like. The vicinity of the aesthetically pleasing donor site supplies good color and texture match. Harvesting the FAP flap leaves no donor site morbidity, because the level of dissection is above the facial musculature and outside of the course of the facial nerve. The pedicle is readily available with a good arc of rotation. Furthermore, it provides a thin pedicle, which allows the FAP flap to be performed in one stage.

References

1. Whetzel TP, Mathes SJ. Arterial anatomy of the face: an analysis of vascular territories and perforating cutaneous vessels. Plast Reconstr Surg 89:591-603, 1992.
2. Park C, Lineaweaver WC, Buncke HJ. New perioral arterial flaps: anatomic study and clinical application. Plast Reconstr Surg 94:268-276, 1994.
3. Feinendegen DL, Langer M, Gault D. A combined V-Y advancement turnover flap for simultaneous perialar and alar reconstruction. Br J Plast Surg 53:248-250, 2000.
4. Pribaz JJ, Meara JG, Wright S, et al. Lip and vermillion reconstruction with the facial artery musculomucosal flap. Plast Reconstr Surg 105:864-872, 2000.
5. Lazaridis N, Zouloumis L, Venetis G, et al. The inferiorly and superiorly based nasolabial flap for reconstruction of moderate-sized oronasal defects. J Oromaxillofac Surg 56:1255-1259, 1998.
6. Hofer SO, Posch NA, Smit X. The facial artery perforator flap for reconstruction of perioral defects. Plast Reconstr Surg 115:996-1003, 2005.

    The authors introduced the FAP flap. Cadaver dissections were performed to illustrate the feasibility of the concept. Clinical cases were presented to show the successful application. This flap is excellent for perioral reconstruction, because the donor site in the jowl area is readily available, and the flap allows a reliable free-style flap technique that can be applied as a one-stage reconstruction.

7. Menick FJ. Artistry in aesthetic surgery. Aesthetic perception and the subunit principle. Clin Plast Surg 14:723-735, 1987.

    The visual process of seeing and the psychology of perception were examined. The authors derived a method of facial reconstruction that emphasizes restoring subunits so that expected contours and landmarks are maintained.

8. Koshima I, Nanba Y, Tsutsui T, et al. Perforator flaps in lower extremity reconstruction. Handchir Microchir Plast Chir 34:251-256, 2002.
9. Koshima I, Nanba Y, Takahashi Y, et al. Future of supramicrosurgery as it relates to breast reconstruction: free paraumbilical perforator adiposal flap. Semin Plast Surg 16:93-99, 2002.

13

Facial Artery Musculomucosal Flap

Stephen M. Warren
Julian J. Pribaz

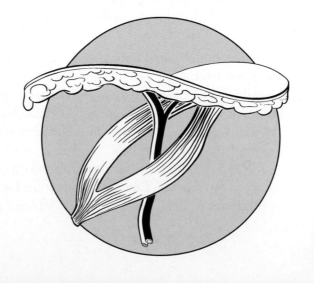

The facial artery musculomucosal (FAMM) flap is principally an amalgamation of the nasolabial and buccal mucosal flaps. The pedicle FAMM flap, however, exceeds the versatility, mobility, and functional applications of its predecessors. The flap can be reliably based superiorly (retrograde flow) or inferiorly (antegrade flow) to reconstruct a wide variety of oronasal mucosal defects. Whereas the groundwork for this flap was established more than 2500 years ago, the modern FAMM flap is little more than a decade old.

The nasolabial flap was first described in the Sushruta Samhitá in 600 BC.[1] This treatise, based on the lectures and teachings of the surgeon-king Lord Devadas, described the use of cheek flaps for reconstructive rhinoplasty. By the fourth century, Vagbhat, an Indian physician, had compiled a medical primer that included a compendium of local cutaneous facial flaps.[2] These ancient Indian surgical procedures were introduced in Greece and Arabia by Buddhist missionaries during the Middle Ages.[3] At the Persian hospital of Gondi-Sapor (sixth to tenth century), Hindu, Greek, and Arab surgical principles were unified, and a new school of thought moved west.[3] By the middle of the Industrial Revolution, Thiersch[4] (1868) was routinely using superiorly based nasolabial flaps for nasal reconstruction. Rosenthal[5] (1916) and Esser[6] (1918) developed an inferiorly based nasolabial flap for two-stage repairs of posttraumatic orocutaneous fistulas. Schuchardt[7] and others[8-11] learned that nasolabial flaps could be pedicled on branches of the facial artery. This led to the implementation of tunneled nasolabial flaps for intraoral/intranasal reconstruction. In the late 1960s and early 1970s, Georgiade et al[12] and Elliot[13] were regularly using one-stage operations to repair anterior palate, nasal septum, columella, and upper lip defects. Based on this work, Rose[14] described the first one-stage arterialized nasolabial skin island flap for floor of mouth reconstruction. The nasolabial flap solved many mucocutaneous problems, but it required a skin incision and was a poor functional and aesthetic match for oronasal mucosa. Moreover, surgeons had to divide distal branches of the facial nerve and perioral musculature to transpose and inset the nasolabial flap.

Although the buccal mucosal flap evolved in parallel with the nasolabial flap, its history is far shorter. The random-pattern buccal mucosal flap was initially described by Filiberti[15] in 1965. Later that year, Tipton[16] passed random buccal flaps based in the superior labial sulcus through the piriform aperture to close large nasal septal perforations. Both Jackson[17] and Kaplan[18] used buccal transposition flaps to repair secondary palatal fistulas and cover the raw nasal surface of cleft-repaired levator slings. Maeda et al[19] made modifications to improve the vascularity of mucosal flaps. They described a T-shaped musculomucosal flap that included a small amount of buccinator, allowing the surgeon to lengthen the palate, repair velopharyngeal incompetence, and line the oral/nasal surfaces of soft palate pushback flaps. Bozola et al[20] created the first axial-pattern musculomucosal flap based on the buccal artery. Bozola's success was an important technical accomplishment that increased pedicle length and reliability. Using this technique, Rayner[21] extended buccal musculomucosal flaps to reconstruct the midface, orbits, and conjunctiva. Carstens et al[22] refined Bozola's technique by adding a nasolabial incision to dissect the buccinator and raise a musculomucosal island pedicle flap based on the facial artery. They successfully reconstructed the palate and floor of mouth and built up the alveolar ridge; however, they struggled with large donor site defects, buccal fat pad herniation, and cheek tethering.

In 1992 Pribaz et al[23] combined the principles of the nasolabial and buccal flaps to create the FAMM flap. The FAMM flap is an axial flap based on the facial artery as it courses through the cheek lateral to the buccinator muscle, but medial to most of the muscles of facial expression. It consists of mucosa, submucosa, a small amount of buccinator muscle, the facial artery, and venous plexuses. Based on its relatively long pedicle and robust blood supply, the FAMM flap can be used to reconstruct the hard and soft palate, alveolus, nasal septal/antral lining, upper/lower lip and vermilion, floor of mouth, tonsillar fossa, cheek, maxillary antrum, and orbit. Compared with nasolabial and buccal flaps, the pedicle FAMM flap has tremendous versatility, mobility, and functional applications.

ANATOMY

FAMM flap dissection is fast and straightforward, but the anatomy is complex. The cheek is a multilayered structure containing more than a half-dozen muscles, intricate overlapping motor and sensory neural networks, two dominant arterial systems, and an interwoven plexus of veins. The parotid gland lies between the mastoid process and the ramus of the mandible; Stensen's duct travels anteromedially piercing the buccinator just opposite the second upper molar. The FAMM flap lies just anterior to Stensen's duct and includes mucosa, submucosa, a small amount of buccinator, facial artery, and, as stated above, venous plexuses.

Muscles

The buccinator is a thin, quadrilateral muscle that forms the deepest lamina of the perioral musculature. It is covered by submucosa and mucosa medially and the masseter, ramus of the mandible, buccal fat pad, facial artery and vein, and buccopharyngeal fascia

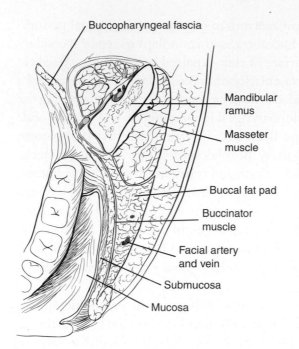

Buccopharyngeal fascia

Mandibular ramus

Masseter muscle

Buccal fat pad

Buccinator muscle

Facial artery and vein

Submucosa

Mucosa

Fig. 13-1 Cross section of the cheek depicting the relationship of the mucosa, submucosa, buccinator muscle, masseter, ramus of the mandible, buccal fat pad, facial artery and vein, and buccopharyngeal fascia laterally.

laterally (Fig. 13-1). The buccinator originates from the alveolar processes of the maxilla and mandible, the pterygomandibular raphe, and the pterygomaxillary ligament. The muscle converges anteriorly to insert on the modiolus. Muscle fibers originating from the ligament and raphe decussate at the modiolus, whereas those originating from the alveolar processes pass directly into the nearest lip without crossing. The buccinator forms part of the pharyngeal-buccal-orbicularis sphincter muscular system that is essential for whistling, sucking, and propelling food during mastication. Other muscles of the cheek (for example, levator anguli oris, zygomaticus minor; zygomaticus major, risorius, depressor anguli oris, and depressor labii inferioris) are superficial to FAMM flap dissection and are not discussed in detail.

Nerves

The buccinator muscle receives motor innervation from the deep buccal branch of the facial nerve (VII), with minor contributions from branches of the zygomatic and mandibular divisions. The buccal branch of the facial nerve courses beneath the zygomaticus and levator labii superioris and supplies the buccinator by diving medially to reach the posterior surface of the muscle at the level of the masseter.

The long buccal branch (buccal nerve or buccinator nerve) of the anterior division of the mandibular nerve (V_3) emerges from the lateral pterygoid superficial to the internal maxillary artery just before the latter reemerges from between the two heads of the lateral pterygoid. The nerve passes obliquely in an inferior and anterior direction crossing over the medial pterygoid. In so doing, it runs parallel and posterior to the buccal branch of the internal maxillary artery. The long buccal branch finally reaches the buccinator at its posterior and superior corner, pierces the muscle, and supplies sensory innervation to the buccal mucosa and the skin of the cheek near the angle of the mouth (Fig. 13-2).[24]

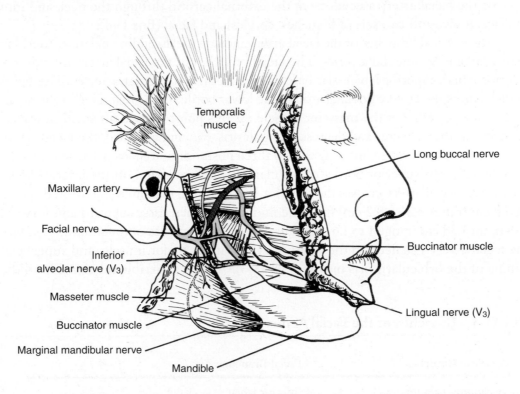

Fig. 13-2   Relationship of the motor and sensory branches to the buccinator muscle. The long buccal nerve from the anterior division of the mandibular nerve (V_3) enters the buccinator at its posterior and superior border. It lies deep to the maxillary artery as it exits the lateral pterygoid muscle. The posterior division of V_3 gives off the inferior alveolar nerve into the mandible and the lingual nerve along the lingual surface of the mandible. The facial nerve (VII) gives off the marginal mandibular branch superficial to the masseter, which is reflected away from the mandible. The deep buccal branch of the buccal nerve from the facial nerve enters the posterior border of the buccinator caudal to the long buccal nerve. (Modified from Carstens MH, Stofman GM, Hurwitz DJ, et al. The buccinator myomucosal island pedicle flap: anatomic study and case report. Plast Reconstr Surg 88:39, 1991.)

Arteries

The buccinator is supplied by two large vascular pedicles: the buccal artery (internal maxillary) and facial artery. The buccal pedicle passes under the lateral pterygoid and runs forward and downward to penetrate and perfuse the posterior half of the buccinator. The internal maxillary artery also sends minor contributions from the lesser palatine and posterosuperior alveolar branches. The facial artery branches into the muscle just as it crosses the mandible. The buccinator also receives minor vascular contributions from perforators of the infraorbital artery. Musculomucosal flaps based on the buccinator muscle have a Mathes/Nahai type III classification. This rich blood supply forms the basis for the buccinator musculomucosal flaps described by Bozola et al[20] (buccal artery) and Carstens et al[24] (facial artery). The buccinator and its blood supply also form the foundation of the FAMM flap.[23]

As the facial artery ascends from the external carotid through the neck and into the face, it gives off two sets of branches: cervical and facial (Box 13-1).

The cervical branches of the facial artery include the ascending palatine, tonsillar, glandular, and submental arteries. The facial branches of the facial artery include the inferior labial, superior labial, alar base, lateral nasal, and angular arteries. The facial branch enters the face by hooking around the lower border of the mandible in the notch at the anterior edge of the masseter muscle. At this point it gives off small muscular branches to the masseter and depressor anguli oris. Moving cephalad, the facial artery follows a tortuous course, infusing two to three posterior and inferior branches to the buccinator at the superior border of the mandible before giving off the inferior labial artery. The facial artery crosses the superior border of the mandible at a mean distance of 6.5 cm (range 5.3 to 8.2 cm) from the midline and then passes upward and forward to a point 1.38 cm (range 1 to 1.6 cm) lateral to the commissure of the mouth.[25-27] Here the facial artery lies deep to the risorius, zygomaticus major muscle, and superficial lamina of the orbicularis oris muscle (Fig. 13-3).[23] It has a variable relationship to the

Box 13-1   Branches of the Facial Artery

Cervical Branches	Facial Branches
Ascending palatine	Inferior labial
Tonsillar	Superior labial
Glandular	Lateral nasal
Submental	Alar base
	Angular

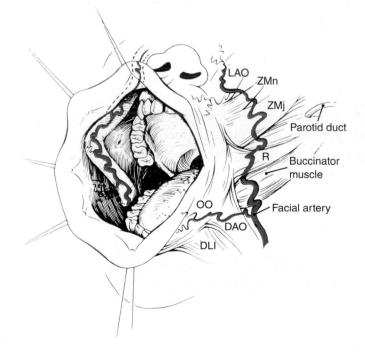

Fig. 13-3   The course of the facial artery and its relationship to the parotid duct and facial muscles. (*DAO*, Depressor anguli oris; *DLI*, depressor labii inferioris; *LAO*, levator anguli oris; *OO*, orbicularis oris; *R*, risorius; *ZMj*, zygomaticus major; *ZMn*, zygomaticus minor.) (Modified from Pribaz JJ, Stephens W, Crespo L, et al. A new intraoral flap: facial artery musculomucosal [FAMM] flap. Plast Reconstr Surg 90:421, 1992.)

levator labii superioris alaeque nasi muscle. At this point the facial artery gives off multiple perforators to the cheek and the superior labial artery, and then continues as the angular artery before reaching the medial canthus.

In the face, the named branches of the facial artery anastomose with their corresponding branches from the contralateral side, and also with branches of the internal maxillary, infraorbital, and ophthalmic arteries (Fig. 13-4).[25] The facial artery is symmetrical in only two thirds of dissections, and it may terminate prematurely or follow a circuitous route.[27] For example, in 50 facial artery cadaveric dissections, Niranjan[27] found that the facial artery terminated as an angular artery in 68%, a lateral nasal vessel in 26%, a superior labial vessel in 4%, and as an alar base vessel in 2% of cadavers. The author also identified an aberrant, long circuitous course in 10%. Knowledge of the anatomic variations of the facial artery is useful in planning a FAMM flap. Variations in the facial artery course or termination necessitate preoperative arterial mapping with Doppler ultrasound and digital palpation.

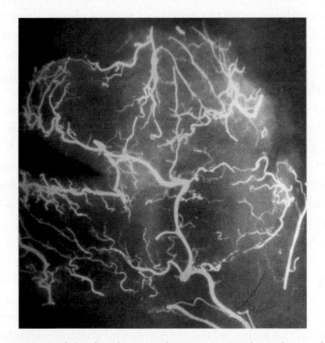

Fig. 13-4   This angiogram of the facial artery shows its major branches and their anastomoses with branches of the internal maxillary and infraorbital arteries. Facial artery connections with the ophthalmic artery are not shown. (Reprinted from British Journal of Oral and Maxillofacial Surgery, Volume 37, Dupoirieux L, Plane L, Gard C, et al, Anatomical basis and results of the facial artery musculomucosal flap for oral reconstruction, pages 25-28, copyright 1999, with permission from Elsevier.)

Veins

The FAMM flap has excellent venous outflow and rarely becomes congested. This may, in part, result from three overlapping pathways of buccinator drainage: the pterygoid plexus, the facial vein, and the maxillary vein. Recent evidence, however, may suggest that in addition to these primary pathways, there is a small but significant submucosal network of venae comitantes that contribute to flap drainage.[25]

The pterygoid plexus forms a large delta of veins situated between the temporalis and lateral pterygoids, and partly between the medial and lateral pterygoids. It receives tributaries from veins draining branches of the internal maxillary artery, including the sphenopalatine, middle meningeal, deep temporal, pterygoid, masseteric, buccinator, alveolar, and some palatine veins. This plexus communicates freely with the anterior facial vein and branches of the ophthalmic vein through the inferior orbital fissure.

The facial vein begins at the root of the nose and is a direct continuation of the angular vein. It is lateral and posterior to the facial artery and follows a less tortuous course. The vein runs obliquely downward and backward beneath the zygomaticus and levator labii superioris, descends along the anterior border, and then runs on the superficial surface of the masseter. Here the facial vein receives the deep facial vein, which drains the anterior tributaries of the pterygoid venous plexus along with the superior and inferior labial, buccinator, and masseteric veins. The vein then crosses over the body of the mandible and passes obliquely backward, beneath the platysma and cervical fascia, superficial to the submaxillary gland, digastric, and stylohyoid. It unites with the retromandibular vein to form the common facial vein, which crosses the external carotid artery and enters the internal jugular vein at a variable point below the hyoid bone. Interestingly, the facial artery and vein do not commonly travel together in the cheek.[27] At the superior border of the mandible, the facial vein is 0.4 cm (range 0 to 1.2 cm) posterior to the artery. At the level of the commissure, the vein is 1.1 cm (range 0.4 to 2 cm) posterior to the artery. At a point where the artery crosses a line drawn from the ala nasi to the superior border of the pinna, the facial vein is 1.5 cm (range 0.3 to 2.3 cm) posterior to the artery.

The maxillary vein is formed as the posterior tributaries of the pterygoid plexus join together at the level of the mandibular ramus. After leaving the infratemporal fossa, the maxillary vein passes backward between the sphenomandibular ligament and the neck of the mandible. It joins the superficial temporal to form the retromandibular vein within the parotid gland, superficial to the external carotid artery but beneath the facial nerve, between the ramus of the mandible and the sternocleidomastoid muscle.

Dupoirieux et al[25] studied the gross and microscopic anatomy of the FAMM flap by mapping the facial artery with red latex dye. Their histologic analysis indicated that an extensive submucosal venous plexus exists in the FAMM flap pedicle (Fig. 13-5). In the absence of a named vein in the flap, this rich submucosal plexus may provide the venous outflow that allows free mobility of the flap without venous congestion. However, this point remains to be proved.

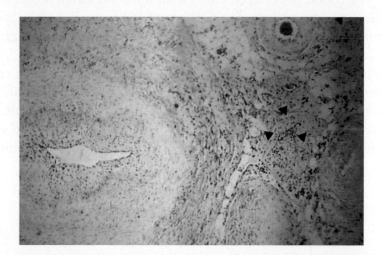

Fig. 13-5 This histologic section of a FAMM pedicle shows microscopic veins *(arrows)* surrounding the artery (hematoxylin and eosin stain, original magnification 50×). In the absence of a named vein in the FAMM pedicle, these small submucosal venae comitantes may provide adequate drainage. (Reprinted from British Journal of Oral and Maxillofacial Surgery, Volume 37, Dupoirieux L, Plane L, Gard C, et al, Anatomical basis and results of the facial artery musculomucosal flap for oral reconstruction, pages 25-28, copyright 1999, with permission from Elsevier.)

Parotid Duct

Stensen's duct (parotid duct) arises from the anterior border of the parotid gland and parallels the zygomatic arch 1.5 cm (approximately 1 fingerbreadth) inferior to the inferior margin of the arch. It runs superficial to the masseter muscle and then turns medially 90 degrees to pierce the buccinator muscle at the level of the second maxillary molar, where it opens into the oral cavity. Using surface landmarks, Stensen's duct lies midway between the zygomatic arch and the corner of the mouth along a line between the upper lip philtrum and tragus. The buccal branch of CN VII runs with the parotid duct. The duct measures 4 to 6 cm in length and 5 mm in diameter. An accessory parotid gland and duct are noted in 20% of people.[28] The accessory gland is typically found overlying the masseter, and the accessory duct usually lies cranial to Stensen's duct.

SURGICAL TECHNIQUE

In preparation for flap harvesting, the defect is mapped and measured. Silk (2-0) retraction stitches are placed along the ipsilateral upper/lower lips and commissure. The FAMM flap can be designed superiorly (retrograde flow) or inferiorly (antegrade flow)

(Fig. 13-6).[23] The course of the facial artery is outlined intraorally with Doppler ultrasound. The flap is centered over the facial artery in a boomerang or oblique design, extending from the retromolar trigone to the level of the ipsilateral gingival labial sulcus at the level of the alar margin. The width of the flap averages 1.5 to 2 cm and is well anterior to Stensen's duct. (The flap can be wider, but this often causes buccal mucosal tethering.) In early work on axial cheek island flaps, Sasaki et al[29] cannulated and transplanted the duct when the flap design included its orifice. This, however, is never necessary with the FAMM flap, because the flap is always situated well anterior to Stensen's duct, and the flap design is tailored according to reconstructive need.

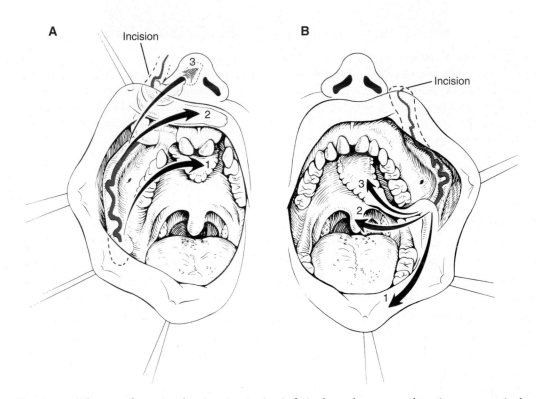

Fig. 13-6   The arc of rotation has its pivot point inferiorly at the retromolar trigone, superiorly at the gingival labial sulcus, or anywhere in between depending on the reconstructive need *(arrows).* **A,** The superiorly based FAMM flap may be used to reconstruct defects of the anterior hard palate, alveolus, maxillary antrum, nasal floor/septum, upper lip (sulcus and vermilion), and orbit. **B,** The inferiorly based FAMM flap may be used to reconstruct defects of the posterior hard and soft palate, tonsillar fossa, alveolus, floor of mouth, cheek, and lower lip (sulcus and vermilion). (Modified from Pribaz JJ, Stephens W, Crespo L, et al. A new intraoral flap: facial artery musculomucosal [FAMM] flap. Plast Reconstr Surg 90:421, 1992.)

Dissection begins at the distal end of the flap, with an incision through the mucosa and buccinator. The facial artery is identified, ligated, and divided. The rest of the flap is scored, and dissection proceeds just deep to the facial vessels, taking only a small hemicuff of the deep layer of the overlying buccinator muscle and orbicularis muscle near the oral commissure. The flap is usually 8 to 10 mm thick. It is crucial to raise the facial artery with the flap so that the entire flap remains axial; however, the facial vein is never taken with the flap. This axial supply allows the development of long, narrow flaps with length/width ratios as high as 5:1. Lengths of 8 to 9 cm can be developed and based either superiorly or inferiorly with a mucosal pedicle base, as long as a reasonable (judgment call) soft tissue base is maintained to ensure adequate venous drainage. Surprisingly, the flaps rarely appear congested despite the conspicuous absence of a named vein. We believe that the extensive submucosal venous plexus adapts to provide adequate drainage to the pterygoid, buccal, or facial veins (see Fig. 13-5). Moreover, the hearty vascularity of this flap enables it to be folded or doubled back on itself to provide both oral and nasal resurfacing of a palate.

The arc of rotation has its pivot point inferiorly at the retromolar trigone, superiorly at the gingivobuccal sulcus, or anywhere in between depending on the flap design. The FAMM flap can be rotated 180 degrees and transposed across the retromolar area, passed over the mandibular/maxillary alveolus through edentulous spaces, or tunneled through the gingivobuccal sulci to reach the nasal or maxillary antrum. We have rarely created an alveolar trough, but commonly have used a bite block to protect the pedicle. The arc of rotation allows superiorly based FAMM flaps to reach the anterior hard palate, alveolus, maxillary antrum, nasal floor/septum, upper lip (sulcus and vermilion), and orbit. Inferiorly based FAMM flaps may be used to reconstruct defects of posterior hard and soft palate, tonsillar fossa, alveolus, floor of mouth, cheek, and lower lip (sulcus and vermilion). Because the facial artery runs a tortuous course, an additional 4 to 5 cm of pedicle length could be obtained under mild tension to unfurl the serpentine coils of the vessel. We, however, resist this temptation and uniformly inset FAMM flaps without tension.

Unlike buccinator musculomucosal flap donor sites, which may require skin grafting or healing by secondary intention, the narrow pedicle FAMM donor site is closed in two layers. We approximate the buccinator muscle and mucosa, taking care to avoid Stensen's duct.

Box 13-2   Advantages of the FAMM Flap

Axial flow	Long length/width ratio
	Reliable
	Good bulk, can be folded or doubled over
Versatile	Superior or inferiorly based
	Long arc of rotation
	Transposition flap
	Island or multiple island flaps
	Completed in one stage
Like tissue	Good color, texture, and moisture match for oronasal lining
	No hair
	No external scar

MODIFICATIONS

The FAMM flap is versatile and has many advantages compared with skin grafts, other local flaps, or free tissue transfers (Box 13-2). It has a long length/width ratio, provides similar tissue, avoids hair-bearing skin, and contains mucus secretory glands. There are many different uses for the FAMM flap. We describe some specific technical modifications for common applications.

Oronasal Fistula

To date, the most common indication for a FAMM flap is a wide palatal cleft that has failed a conventional attempt at closure. In most cases, we use local turndown flaps for nasal lining, then insert cancellous iliac bone grafts and cover it with a FAMM flap. In palatal reconstruction, the FAMM flap can be based either superiorly or inferiorly.[23] If there is a gap in the alveolar ridge, we prefer to use a superiorly based flap. Fig. 13-7 presents a young adult with an oronasal fistula after an attempted bilateral cleft lip/palate repair. The patient underwent a one-stage closure with a superiorly based flap that was passed through a gap in the alveolar ridge. In patients with intact dentition, we use a superiorly based FAMM flap and a two-stage approach. We pass the FAMM flap behind the last maxillary molar and then insert a bite block for 10 days. At a second stage, the bite block is removed and the FAMM flap is divided and inset. The superiorly based FAMM flap can also be performed in one stage for patients with intact dentition by simultaneously raising a retromolar turnover flap to line the nasal side of the oronasal fistula and then pedicling the FAMM flap into the trough created by raising the turnover flap.

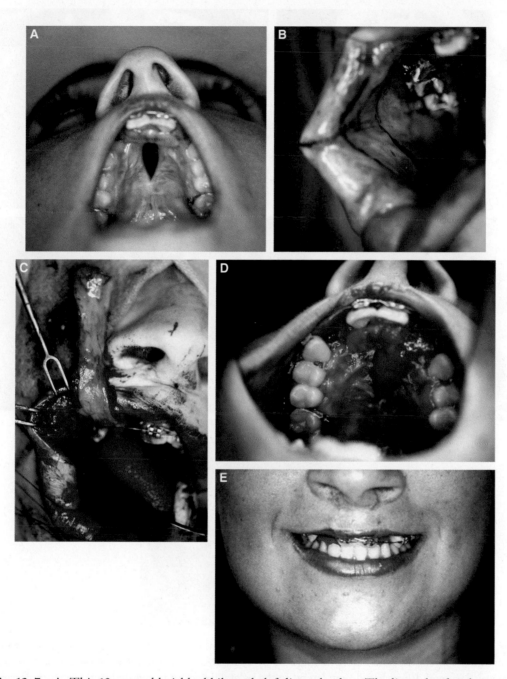

Fig. 13-7   A, This 12-year-old girl had bilateral cleft lip and palate. The lip and soft palate were closed in infancy, leaving a residual cleft of hard palate and bilateral alveolus. **B,** A right superiorly based FAMM flap was designed. **C,** A one-stage closure was performed using local turndown flaps for nasal lining, cancellous bone graft, and a superiorly based flap passed through a gap in the alveolar ridge. **D,** Appearance of the flap 4 weeks after palate closure. **E,** The patient has a normal smile without nerve weakness.

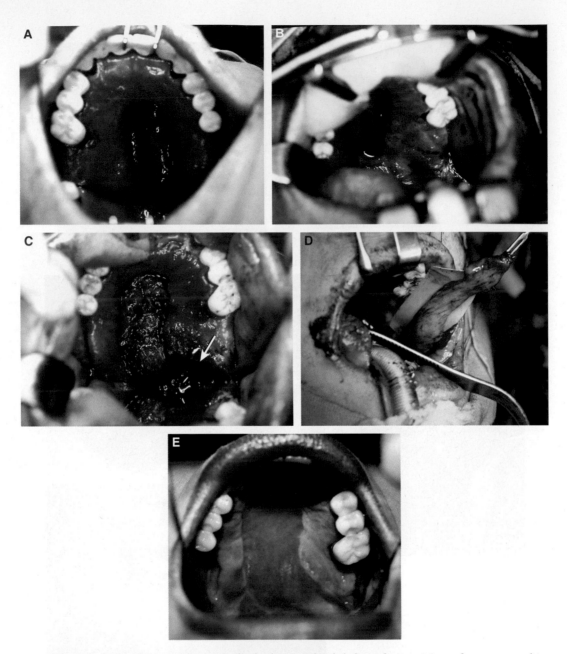

Fig. 13-8 A, This 61-year-old woman had a large palatal defect after excision of a recurrent histiocytoma. The hard palate defect measured 2 by 3 cm. **B,** A medially based mucoperiosteal palatal
flap was designed. It was based 1 cm lateral to the palatal defect and extended to the retromolar area
at the base of an inferiorly based FAMM flap. **C,** The palatal flap was turned over for nasal lining.
The newly created trough *(arrow)* in the retromolar area created space for the FAMM flap. **D,** The
inferiorly based FAMM flap was elevated. **E,** Three months after the FAMM flap was inset the palatal
defect is well healed. (From Matros E, Swanson EW, Pribaz JJ. A modification of the facial artery
musculomucosal flap for palatal reconstruction in patients with intact dentition. Plast Reconstr Surg
125:645, 2010.)

More recently, we have treated oronasal fistulas with an inferiorly based FAMM flap (Fig. 13-8).[30] Typically, nasal lining is created by elevating a medially based mucoperiosteal flap. (The lateral extent of the mucoperiosteal flap extends laterally to the base of the FAMM flap.) The mucoperiosteal flap is elevated, turned over, and inset into the palatal defect creating nasal lining. The donor site defect of the mucoperiosteal flap creates a trough to allow space for the interiorly based FAMM flap (see Fig. 13-8, C). Once pedicled and inset, the flap provides oral mucosal lining for the palatal defect.

Although we have used superiorly based and inferiorly based FAMM flaps to treat oronasal fistulas of the hard palate, others have cleverly used FAMM flaps to reconstruct soft palate defects. Dolderer et al[31] described an extended trilaminar FAMM flap that included a portion of a redundant paralyzed ptotic lower lip in a 75-year-old oral squamous cell cancer survivor. The patient had a substantial reduction in velopharyngeal insufficiency and resolution of his oral incompetence. Although it is unlikely that these exact circumstances would often coexist to permit this same opportunity, the authors demonstrated the versatility of the FAMM flap.

Lip and Vermilion Reconstruction

Numerous techniques for lip and vermilion reconstruction have been described. Schulten[32] (1894) described the double-pedicle flap of the upper lip for repairing a missing prolabium segment in the lower lip. Lexer[33] (1909) described a tongue flap. Other types of local advancement flaps were described by Friedlander,[34] Spira and Stal,[35] and Kolhe and Leonard.[36] For superficial resurfacing of the vermilion, a cross-lip mucosal flap was described by Mazzola and Lupo,[37] and then again by Standoli.[38] This flap borrows labial mucosa from the inner surface of one lip to resurface the vermilion of the other lip. Sakai et al[39] and then Iwahira et al[40] described an interesting technique that incorporated bilateral island vermilion flaps or sliding-door flaps. Kawamoto[41] and Lew et al[42] described unipedicle and bipedicle cross-lip vermilion flaps. Ahuja[43] described mucosal free grafts. He used labia minora grafts for vermilion reconstruction. Rayner and Arscott[44] introduced the buccinator musculomucosal flap in 1987. In their report, a sensate musculomucosal random flap from the buccal mucosa was used to resurface the vermilion. Bozola et al[20] modified this flap slightly. They described an axial buccinator musculomucosal flap based on the buccal artery. Carstens et al[24] described a buccinator musculomucosal flap based on the facial artery. More recently, Ono et al[45] described a buccal musculomucosal flap that was also based on the facial artery.

The FAMM flap is ideal for reconstructing the inner, moist lip mucosa, because it consists of similar tissue with the same color, texture, and moisture as the native lip (Fig. 13-9).[46] When used for vermilion reconstruction, some drying of the mucosa will occur, but otherwise a good color match can be obtained. Also the flap bulk helps to restore lip fullness in cases of total lip loss. When used for lip reconstruction, the FAMM flap has the advantage of being completed in one stage compared with tongue flaps and cross-lip flaps, which require a second stage for division and inset of the flap. This can be particularly useful in patients who cannot be expected to follow postoperative instructions.[47] Compared with other buccal flaps, the oblique orientation of the FAMM flap is more amenable for transposition in lip reconstruction. Although very large buccal musculomucosal flaps of the entire cheek can be safely raised because of the rich blood supply of the region, we have attempted to minimize donor site morbidity by raising long, thin FAMM flaps. A single FAMM flap can, for example, be used to reconstruct as much as three quarters of the lower lip vermilion.[47] Axial FAMM flaps are thin and robust (providing adequate bulk to the lip) and allow the donor defect to be easily closed. The oblique orientation of the flap allows resuturing of the muscular layer in a favorable direction for minimal interference with facial expression.

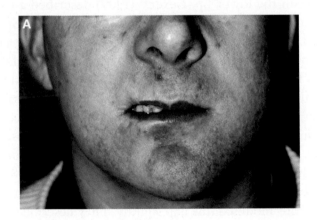

Fig. 13-9   A, This 33-year-old man had craniofacial microsomia and a deficiency of the vermilion portion of the right upper lip that created a "snarling" appearance.

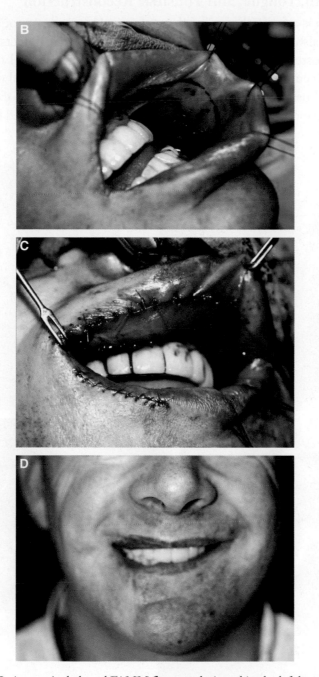

Fig. 13-9, cont'd B, A superiorly based FAMM flap was designed in the left buccal mucosa. **C,** The FAMM flap was transposed into the upper lip. **D,** The patient demonstrates a satisfactory functional outcome. (**A** to **C** from Pribaz JJ, Meara JG, Wright S, et al. Lip and vermilion reconstruction with the facial artery musculomucosal flap. Plast Reconstr Surg 105:864, 2000.)

Floor of Mouth, Tongue, and Tonsillar Reconstruction

The FAMM flap is a facile choice for floor of mouth, tongue, or tonsillar fossa reconstruction. It can also be used to cover partial mandibulectomy defects and as an adjunct for mandibular osteoradionecrosis.[48] The inferiorly based FAMM flap can be passed through a trough cut in the alveolar ridge or around the most distal mandibular molar. Older, alcohol-consuming, cigarette-smoking patients with floor of mouth or tongue cancer often have poor dentition, and the FAMM flap can be passed between decaying teeth (Fig. 13-10).

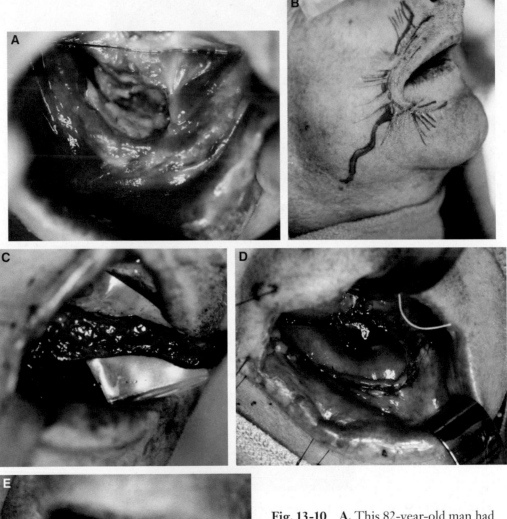

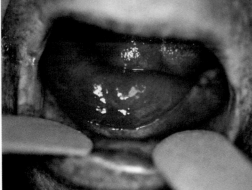

Fig. 13-10   **A,** This 82-year-old man had radionecrosis of the floor of the mouth after treatment for squamous cell carcinoma. **B,** Surface markings show the course of the facial artery and its relationship to perioral musculature. **C,** A right inferiorly based FAMM flap was developed. **D,** The flap was inset and folded back on itself. **E,** The reconstruction is stable 6 months postoperatively.

The conventional FAMM flap can be as long as 8 to 9 cm; however, we have increased flap length by splitting the distal end of the flap and extending the harvest into the upper and lower lips (Fig. 13-11). Once elevated, the arms of the Y-shaped flap are sewn together to create an extended I-shaped flap. We have routinely obtained an additional 4 to 5 cm using the Y-I design.

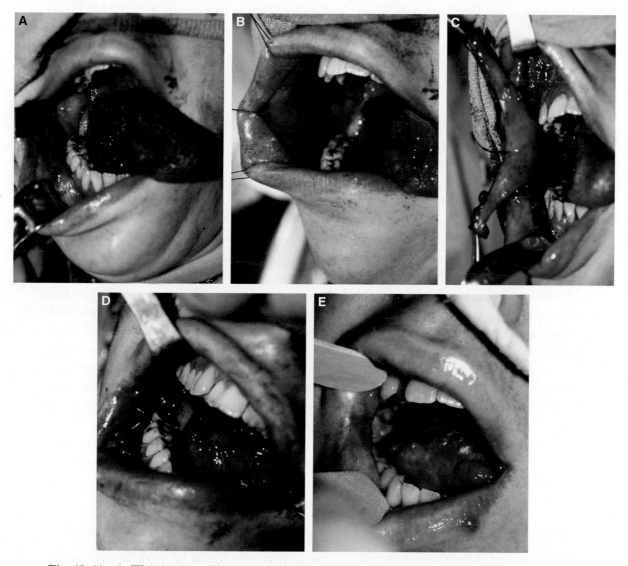

Fig. 13-11 A, This 48-year-old patient had a large tongue defect after excision of a squamous cell carcinoma. **B,** An inferiorly based Y-shaped FAMM flap was designed with extensions into the upper and lower lip. **C,** Once elevated, the arms of the Y-shaped flap were sewn together to create an extended I-shaped flap. **D,** The I-shaped flap was inset. **E,** Three weeks after inset the FAMM flap is well healed.

The FAMM flap is an ideal choice for intraoral reconstruction because of the ease of harvest, proximity to the defects, similar mucosal lining, absence of external scar, and low complication rate. Moreover, the FAMM flap does not require any modification in planning the neck dissection during the ablative portion of the operation other than to preserve the facial artery. If, however, the facial artery is ligated during the ablative operation, it may still be possible to perform a FAMM flap. The facial arteries anastomose through the inferior labial arteries as well as a horizontal mental artery; therefore, if the facial artery is ligated, an inferiorly based (antegrade flow) FAMM flap may still be harvested ipsilaterally based on flow from the contralateral inferior labial artery.[49] Prudent surgical judgment is essential. In the oral cavity, the FAMM flap offers supple ground on which a dental prosthesis can be abutted, and an elastic cushion against prosthetic loading.[50]

Nasal Lining for Septal or Total Nasal Reconstruction

Acquired septal perforations or total nasal loss can present challenging reconstructive problems. A variety of flaps and grafts are necessary to provide coverage, lining, and support; here we focus on restoring the nasal lining. Kazanjian and Roopenian[51] lined the nose with folded forehead flaps or nasolabial flaps. Other surgeons used temporoparietal or radial forearm fascial free flaps.[52,53] In 1998 Duffy et al[54] described the septal mucosal reconstruction of a patient with Wegener's saddle-nose deformity using bilateral FAMM flaps and costal cartilage for support. The authors approached the nasal antra through bilateral lateral rhinotomy incisions. The atrophic, chronically inflamed, friable, ulcerated mucosa was debrided, and intranasal scarring was released. When the nasal dorsum was exposed, the authors found that most of the cartilaginous septum and upper and lower lateral cartilages were absent. Bilateral superiorly based FAMM flaps were raised and tunneled through bilateral upper gingivobuccal incisions and into the nasal passages. After placing the costal cartilage grafts for dorsal and columellar support, the FAMM flaps were inset without tension and redundant. In this setting, the bulkiness of the flaps was expected to cause postoperative nasal airway obstruction, so intranasal debulking was performed 3 weeks after inset.

The FAMM flap works well for nasal lining, because it provides highly vascular coverage for cartilage or bone grafts and thereby reduces postoperative infection. In addition, the FAMM flap provides tissue very similar to nasal mucosa and, theoretically, should moisten the nasal passageway and humidify inspired air.

Orbital Reconstruction

Our anatomic dissections demonstrate that a superiorly based FAMM flap will reach the orbital area. Theoretically, a pedicle flap could be used to reconstruct eyelid lining; however, we are not aware of any clinical reports of a FAMM flap used for this purpose.

PITFALLS

Elevation and inset of a FAMM flap are straightforward, but three pitfalls must be avoided. First, the flap must be axially supplied by the facial artery along its entire length. We ensure an axially based flap by first elevating the distal edge of the FAMM flap, then identifying the facial artery, and finally ligating it. As the dissection proceeds proximally, we tailor our flap design to follow the serpiginous course of the facial artery. Because the FAMM flap may primarily drain through the submucosal venous plexus, the flap cannot be designed as an island flap. Second, the extraordinary vascularity of the FAMM flap will support a length/width ratio of 5:1; however, we must caution against creating a flap more than 2.5 to 3 cm wide to avoid cheek tethering. In the early 1990s, we experimented with wide (3 cm or more) FAMM flaps, but occasionally had to perform a z-plasty to release a cheek contracture. Last, the facial artery runs a tortuous course; therefore an additional 4 to 5 cm of pedicle length may be obtained under mild tension to unfurl the serpentine coils of the vessel. We, however, suggest resisting this temptation and insetting the FAMM flap without tension.

References

1. McDowell F. Ancient ear lobe and rhinoplastic operation in India (from the Sushruta Samhita c 600 BC. Translated from the Sanskrit and published by KKL Bhishagratna, Calcutta, 1907). Plast Reconstr Surg 43:515, 1969.
2. Almast SC. History and evolution of the Indian method of rhinoplasty. In Transactions of the Fourth International Congress of Plastic and Reconstructive Surgery, Rome and Amsterdam, Oct 1967, Excerpta Medica Foundation.
3. Sinha RN. The story of plastic surgery. Patna Med J 7:173, 1950.
4. Thiersch C. Vershluss eines loches im harten gaumen durch die weichtheile der wange. Arch Heilk 9:159, 1868.
5. Rosenthal W. Verschluss traumatischer gaumendefekte durch weichteile des gesichts. Zentralbl Chir 43:596, 1916.
6. Esser JF. Deckung von gaumenderfekten mittels gestielter naso-labial hautlappen. Dtsch Z Chir 57:280, 1918.
7. Schuchardt K. Plastiche Operatione im Mund-und Kiefer-Bereicht. Berlin: Urban & Schwarzenberg, 1959.
8. Barron JN, Emmett AJ. Subcutaneous pedicle flaps. Br J Plast Surg 18:51, 1965.
9. Trevaskis AE, Rempel J, Okunski W, et al. Sliding subcutaneous-pedicle flaps to close a circular defect. Plast Reconstr Surg 46:155, 1970.
10. Strahan RW, Sorosky R, Williams D. Vascular pedicled island flaps: use in head and neck reconstructive surgery. Arch Otolaryngol 92:588, 1970.
11. Lejour M. One-stage reconstruction of nasal skin defect with local flaps. Chir Plast 1:254, 1972.
12. Georgiade NG, Mladick RA, Thorne FL. The nasolabial tunnel flap. Plast Reconstr Surg 43:463, 1969.
13. Elliot RA Jr. Use of nasolabial skin flap to cover intraoral defects. Plast Reconstr Surg 58:201, 1976.
14. Rose EH. One-stage arterialized nasolabial island flap for floor of mouth reconstruction. Ann Plast Surg 6:71, 1981.
15. Filiberti AT. Plastic closure of a septal perforation. Ann Chir Otorhinolaryngol 96:1, 1965.
16. Tipton JB. Closure of large septal perforations with a labial-buccal flap. Plast Reconstr Surg 46:514, 1970.

17. Jackson IT. Closure of secondary palatal fistulae with intra-oral tissue and bone grafting. Br J Plast Surg 25:93, 1972.

18. Kaplan EN. Soft palate repair by levator muscle reconstruction and a buccal mucosal flap. Plast Reconstr Surg 56:129, 1975.

19. Maeda K, Ojimi H, Utsugi R, et al. A T-shaped musculomucosal buccal flap method for cleft palate surgery. Plast Reconstr Surg 79:888, 1987.

20. Bozola AR, Gasques JA, Carriquiry CE, et al. The buccinator musculomucosal flap: anatomic study and clinical application. Plast Reconstr Surg 84:250, 1989.

21. Rayner CR. Oral mucosal flaps in midfacial reconstruction. Br J Plast Surg 37:43, 1984.

22. Carstens MH, Stofman GM, Sotereanos GC, et al. A new approach for repair of oro-antral-nasal fistulae. The anteriorly based buccinator myomucosal island flap. J Craniomaxillofac Surg 19:64, 1991.

23. Pribaz JJ, Stephens W, Crespo L, et al. A new intraoral flap: facial artery musculomucosal (FAMM) flap. Plast Reconstr Surg 90:421, 1992.

    This article is the index description of the FAMM flap. The authors described the anatomy, technical aspects, and clinical applications of superiorly and inferiorly based FAMM flaps.

24. Carstens MH, Stofman GM, Hurwitz DJ, et al. The buccinator myomucosal island pedicle flap: anatomic study and case report. Plast Reconstr Surg 88:39, 1991.

25. Dupoirieux L, Plane L, Gard C, et al. Anatomical basis and results of the facial artery musculomucosal flap for oral reconstruction. Br J Oral Maxillofac Surg 37:25, 1999.

    The gross and histologic analysis of the FAMM flap described in this article provided evidence that the rich submucosal plexus may supply the venous outflow that allows free mobility of the flap without venous congestion.

26. Zhao Z, Li S, Yan Y, et al. New buccinator myomucosal island flap: anatomic study and clinical application. Plast Reconstr Surg 104:55, 1999.

27. Niranjan NS. An anatomical study of the facial artery. Ann Plast Surg 21:14, 1988.

    This anatomic study of the vascular pattern of the FAMM flap provided a detailed description of the variations of the course of the facial artery and its relationship to the FAMM pedicle.

28. Frommer J. The human accessory parotid gland: its incidence, nature, and significance. Oral Surg Oral Med Oral Pathol 43:671, 1977.

29. Sasaki TM, Baker HW, McConnell DB, et al. Cheek island flap for the replacement of critical limited defects of the upper aerodigestive tract. Am J Surg 152:435, 1985.

30. Matros E, Swanson EW, Pribaz JJ. A modification of the facial artery musculomucosal flap for palatal reconstruction in patients with intact dentition. Plast Reconstr Surg 125:645, 2010.

31. Dolderer JH, Hussey AJ, Morrison WA. Extension of the facial artery musculomucosal flap to reconstruct a defect of the soft palate. Scan J Plast Reconstr Surg Hand Surg 45:208, 2011.

32. Schulten MV. En methodatt erstta en defekt af ena lappen medelst en bryggformad lamba fran den anra. Fin Lakaresallsk Handl 35:859, 1894.

33. Lexer E. Wangenplastik. Dtsch Z Chir 100:206, 1909.

34. Friedlander AH. Modified lip stripping with reconstruction of a new vermilion border. N Y State Dent J 42:27, 1976.

35. Spira M, Stal S. V-Y advancement of a subcutaneous pedicle in vermilion lip reconstruction. Plast Reconstr Surg 72:562, 1983.

36. Kolhe PS, Leonard AG. Reconstruction of the vermilion after "lip-shave". Br J Plast Surg 41:68, 1988.

37. Mazzola RF, Lupo G. Evolving concepts in lip reconstruction. Clin Plast Surg 11:583, 1984.

38. Standoli L. Cross lip flap in vermilion reconstruction. Ann Plast Surg 32:214, 1994.

39. Sakai S, Soeda S, Terayama I. Bilateral island vermilion flaps for vermilion border reconstruction. Ann Plast Surg 20:459, 1988.

40. Iwahira Y, Yataka M, Maruyama Y. The sliding door flap for repair of vermilion defects. Ann Plast Surg 41:300, 1998.

41. Kawamoto HK Jr. Correction of major defects of the vermilion with a cross-lip vermilion flap. Plast Reconstr Surg 64:315, 1979.
42. Lew D, Clark R, Jimenez F, et al. The bipedicled lip flap for reconstruction of the vermilion border in the patient with a severe perioral burn. Oral Surg Oral Med Oral Pathol 63:526, 1987.
43. Ahuja RB. Vermilion reconstruction with labia minora graft. Plast Reconstr Surg 92:1418, 1993.
44. Rayner CR, Arscott GD. A new method of resurfacing the lip. Br J Plast Surg 40:454, 1987.
45. Ono I, Gunji H, Tateshita T, et al. Reconstruction of defects of the entire vermilion with a buccal musculomucosal flap following resection of malignant tumors of the lower lip. Plast Reconstr Surg 100:422, 1997.
46. Pribaz JJ, Meara JG, Wright S, et al. Lip and vermilion reconstruction with the facial artery musculomucosal flap. Plast Reconstr Surg 105:864, 2000.
    This article described a novel approach to lip reconstruction using a FAMM flap.
47. Baj A. FAMM Flap reconstruction of the inferior lip vermilion: surgery during early infancy. J Plast Reconstr Aesthet Surg 61:425, 2008.
48. Ayad T. Reconstruction of floor of mouth defects by the facial artery musculo-mucosal flap following cancer ablation. Head Neck 30:437, 2008.
49. Park C. New perioral flaps: anatomic study and clinical applications. Plast Reconstr Surg 101:268, 1994.
50. Hatoko M. Use of facial artery musculomucosal flap for closure of soft tissue defects of the mandibular vestibule. Int J Oral Maxillofac Surg 31:210, 2002.
51. Kazanjian VH, Roopenian A. Median forehead flaps in the repair of defects of the nose and surrounding areas. Trans Am Acad Ophthalmol Otolaryngol 60:557, 1956.
52. Upton J, Ferraro N, Healy G, et al. The use of prefabricated fascial flaps for lining of the oral and nasal cavities. Plast Reconstr Surg 94:573, 1994.
53. Winslow CP, Cook TA, Burke A, et al. Total nasal reconstruction: utility of the free radial forearm fascial flap. Arch Facial Plast Surg 5:159, 2003.
54. Duffy FJ Jr, Rossi RM, Pribaz JJ. Reconstruction of Wegener's nasal deformity using bilateral facial artery musculomucosal flaps. Plast Reconstr Surg 101:1330, 1998.

14

Submental Artery Perforator Flap

Jeong Tae Kim

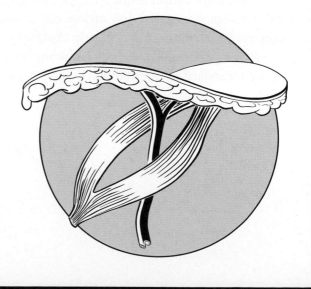

The ideal flap for reconstructing facial defects should be thin, reliable, and a good color and texture match. Various random-pattern flaps, such as the supraclavicular flap or platysma musculocutaneous flap, provide a good color match for the face. However, their use has been limited by poor flap mobility, an unacceptable donor scar, unreliability, and a paucity of tissue. The result can be disappointing because of partial flap loss. Tissue expansion methods supply sufficient coverage with pliable skin but require staged operations that increase the cost of treatment. Although free flap transfers offer the advantage of repairing complex facial defects in one stage, their color and texture show a definite demarcation compared with the facial skin. Unlike these flaps, the submental artery perforator (SMAP) flap is a reliable flap for reconstructing facial defects. It has many advantages over other regional or distant flaps, such as the forehead, deltopectoral, and pectoralis flaps, which produce poor aesthetic results or considerable donor site morbidity. These latter flaps should be reserved as a second option.

Resurfacing is one of the main applications of perforator flaps.[1] The submental area is an optimal donor site for facial resurfacing. Since the first report of the submental island flap by Martin et al,[2] the flap has been used as an island and free flap to cover facial defects. The submental flap can be regarded as a perforator flap based on a consistent perforator. This vessel is consistently located at either the medial or lateral border of the anterior belly of the digastric muscle. As with perforators elsewhere in the body, the location is not always symmetrical in the neck.[3] Harvest of the submental flap without the underlying mylohyoid or digastric muscles was described before the concept of perforators was clearly explained.[4] The submental flap can successfully be elevated as a perforator flap by excluding the anterior belly of the digastric muscle and using a standard submental flap design or a reverse-pattern submental flap.[3-6]

ANATOMY

The submental area is supplied by the submental and facial arteries. Above the inferior mandibular border, the facial artery runs under the marginal mandibular branch of the facial nerve and orbicularis oris muscle (Fig. 14-1). This vessel runs a tortuous course accompanied by its venae comitantes and anastomoses with the dorsal nasal artery at its termination. The venae comitantes of the facial artery are small in diameter. Unlike the artery, the facial vein runs a relatively straight course just under the facial nerve branches and zygomaticus muscles, several to 10 mm apart from the facial artery. The vessel communicates with the posterior facial vein to form the common facial vein, draining into the internal jugular vein. The facial vein measures 2.2 to 3.2 mm in diameter, and the common facial vein is 2.4 to 3.5 mm.[5] This vein is big enough to allow sufficient venous drainage and receives tributaries from the transverse facial vein, inferior orbital vein, and veins from the facial muscles, buccal fat pad, and eyelids. The venae comitantes of the facial artery have valves against reverse flow. Therefore additional venous drainage afforded by the facial vein is required when a reverse submental perforator flap is performed.

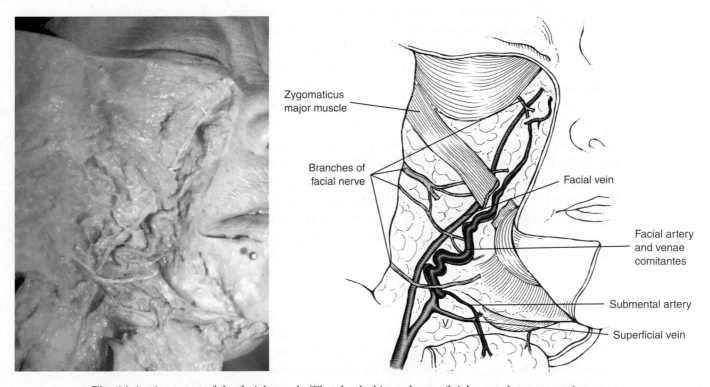

Fig. 14-1 Anatomy of the facial vessels. The cheek skin and superficial musculoaponeurotic system are elevated on a fresh cadaver. Deep to the branches of the facial nerve and zygomaticus major muscle, the facial vein runs a straight course with many tributaries lateral to the highly tortuous facial artery and its venae comitantes. Two perforators at both borders of the anterior belly of the digastric muscle supply the submental territory. A superficial vein runs a different course from the submental artery and its venae comitantes.

The submental artery runs a tortuous and constant course along the inferior mandibular border, until it reaches the lateral border of the anterior belly of the digastric muscle (Fig. 14-2). The diameter of this artery is 1 to 1.5 mm and averages 2 mm at its origin.[6] Variations in the origin of the submental artery have been reported. These include an independent origin from the carotid artery (1 of 56 dissections) or a more proximal origin from the facial artery.[2] The submental artery is the largest of the cervical branches at a distance of 5 to 6.5 cm away from its origin from the facial artery.[2,7] At this level it runs on the mylohyoid muscle just inferior to the body of the mandible, and deep to the anterior belly of the digastric muscle. At the mandibular symphysis, the terminal branch of the submental artery connects with the contralateral terminal branch and curves upward around the mandibular border, dividing into a superficial and a deep branch in the lower lip. The deep branch runs between the muscle of the lower lip and the bone, where it anastomoses with the sublingual branch of the lingual artery and with the mylohyoid branch of the inferior alveolar artery.[4]

The submental artery is accompanied by small venae comitantes. The venous system drains into the facial vein, common facial vein, and external jugular vein.[8] The submental vein is separate from the submental artery and its venae comitantes (see Fig. 14-2). This vein runs a relatively straight course superior and superficial to the submandibular gland, draining into the common facial vein. The submental vein runs adjacent to but not with the submental artery and its venae comitantes. The submental artery and vein meet at the lateral border of the anterior belly of the digastric muscle and run together from this point to supply a reliable perforator to the overlying skin.

Even though the tiny venae comitantes cannot always overcome the resistance of the valve in the proximal draining veins, they are reliable in the submental perforator flap. However, the venae comitantes in the reverse pattern are too tiny to sufficiently accommodate the venous return. Therefore the additional venous drainage afforded by the submental vein is required for successful reconstruction, and this vein should be included in the reverse submental perforator flap. Although some surgeons have suggested a separate venous anastomosis to a suitable vein close to the recipient site as a strategy to overcome the consistent valve of the venae comitantes,[9,10] inclusion of a separate superficial submental vein solves this problem.[3] Even though dissection of the submental vein can be complicated, it obviates the need to perform a microscopic venous anastomosis.

There is a consistent perforator located at the lateral border of the anterior belly of the digastric muscle. Medial to the lateral border of this belly, the submental vessels run close to the inferior mandibular border and give rise to minor branches to the periosteum, lower lip, anterior belly of the digastric muscle, neighboring muscles, and a medial perforator located at the medial border of the belly. The perforator flap can be elevated based on either one or both of these perforators, which are generally reliable.

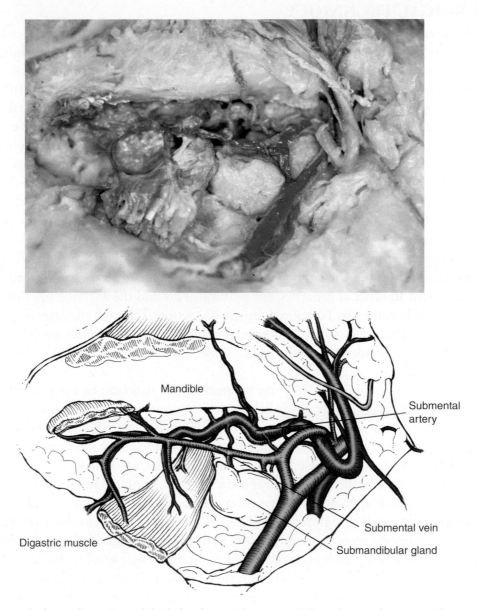

Fig. 14-2 Cadaver dissection of the left submental territory. The submental artery with its tiny venae comitantes runs a tortuous course along the inferior mandibular border. The submental vein is located superficial to the submandibular gland and meets the submental pedicle at the lateral border of the anterior belly of the digastric muscle.

SURGICAL TECHNIQUE

The patient is placed in the supine position with the neck extended. The upper limit of the flap is marked 1 to 4 cm below the inferior mandibular border from the midline to both mandibular angles to hide the scar as much as possible. The lower limit is defined just above the cervicomental angle to achieve a maximum width consistent with direct closure. Depending on the defect, the length of the skin paddle can be designed to both facial arteries and extended to both angles of the mandible. Beyond this point, the vascular supply is unreliable and the final scar is conspicuous.[8] The width of the flap depends on the patient's age and skin redundancy, which is estimated with a pinch test and can be used to determine if primary closure is possible. The spindle-shaped flap is outlined symmetrically in a horizontal fashion to maintain the natural submental contour after primary closure of the donor defect. After an incision through the platysma muscle is made, dissection continues in the subplatysmal plane.

There are three approaches to the submandibular perforator flap: lateral, inferior, and superior. Initially, the lateral approach is the easiest way to become familiar with the anatomy. In other approaches, the perforator around the anterior belly of the digastric muscle can easily be injured during dissection. Through the lateral approach, the submental artery is isolated from the proximal facial artery, and pedicle dissection proceeds along the tortuous course of this vessel until the anterior belly of the digastric muscle is reached.

In the inferior approach,[2,7-9,11] the submandibular gland can be a good landmark to use to find the pedicle. After the pedicle is located, dissection proceeds with traction on the gland,[11] because several twigs are given off to the gland, lymph nodes, and surrounding muscles that require ligation. Care must be taken to avoid injuring the marginal mandibular nerve and venae comitantes. This approach facilitates dissection of the submental vein and is the most useful approach for dissecting the reverse perforator flap.

The superior approach[4,6,10,12] has several advantages. Dissection of both facial and submental arteries is straightforward. There is less risk of injury to the marginal mandibular nerve, easy separation of the pedicle from the submandibular gland, and easy access to submental lymph nodes should intraoperative biopsy be required in patients with cancer. With the complete identification of the marginal mandibular nerve, the facial vessels are easily identified and dissection proceeds to the origin of the submental artery. The superior approach is also convenient for dissecting the reverse-pattern flap. After downward traction is applied to the submandibular gland, small twigs supplying the gland are ligated or cauterized, and the submental pedicles are then easily exposed. The submental pedicle is located deeply, close to the bone, between the submandibular gland and mylohyoid muscle; therefore careful dissection along the mandibular border is required to avoid separating the skin paddle from the pedicle and to ensure identification of the pedicle during dissection. Dissection continues to the lateral perforator and anterior belly of the digastric muscle. The flap is elevated based on the perforator. If the lateral perforator is not available or is absent, the anterior belly of the digastric muscle should be split open to approach the medial perforator. In some cases, the muscle belly can be included for a musculocutaneous flap, particularly if a bulky reconstruction is required. After identification of one or both perforators from the submental artery, the flap is elevated based on the perforator with or without the digastric muscle. The flap is transposed to the recipient site through an incision or a subcutaneous tunnel without tension, and extreme care must be taken to avoid twisting or kinking the perforator pedicle. Drainage of the donor site is necessary for a few days postoperatively.

Because of the symmetrical design of the SMAP flap, the side contralateral to the pedicle may be elevated in advance to facilitate identification of the medial perforator. This maneuver can also be useful as a preliminary exercise in perforator pedicle dissection.[13] Usually a unilateral perforator is enough to perfuse the contralateral side across the midline in symmetrically designed flaps.[6] However, excessive flap thinning can cause partial flap loss. In such cases supercharging the contralateral pedicle should be considered.

Elevation of the musculocutaneous flap, which includes the anterior belly of the digastric muscle, can be carried out more easily than elevation of the perforator flap. The musculocutaneous pattern is considered for bulky reconstruction, or if bolstering the flap's blood supply is desired. In some patients, harvesting the anterior belly of the digastric muscle enhances postoperative neck contour, because an aesthetic criterion of a youthful neck is a curving cervicomental angle of 105 to 120 degrees.[14] Therefore fullness of the submental area can be corrected by splitting the anterior belly of the digastric muscle in obese and elderly patients.[15]

Small venae comitantes are easily injured during dissection, leading to problems with venous drainage or venous-related partial flap loss.[4,8,10] Temporary congestion is sometimes initially observed in the perforator flap. Therefore it is often better to include some surrounding tissue with the pedicle instead of completely skeletonizing the perforator pedicle. This is particularly true if bulk and arc of rotation are not an issue.

Pedicle length can be increased by several methods.[10] Dividing the facial vessels distal to the origin of the submental artery provides an additional 1 to 2 cm of pedicle length. A longer pedicle can be obtained by dividing the straight facial vein and anastomosing it to a suitable vein at the recipient site. The reverse pattern is also an effective method for further pedicle advancement.[3,10] For this pattern, it is better to include the superficial submental vein and ligate the proximal facial artery to the branching point of the submental artery. Dissection along the distal facial artery is carried out underneath the marginal mandibular nerve to move the pivotal point cranially from the nerve. The distal facial vein runs more lateral to the artery and has sufficient connections to the neighboring veins, compared with the venae comitantes. Therefore this vein can accommodate reverse venous flow against the valves.

With the neck slightly flexed, the donor site can generally be closed primarily without tension for defects up to 7 to 8 cm. If necessary, the caudal neck skin can be mobilized to facilitate closure. Closure is not a problem in older patients who generally have sufficient neck skin laxity to allow closure of large defects.[16] A width of at least 5 cm can be obtained in younger patients, and a width of 6 to 8 cm in elderly patients.[2,8]

In my experience, closure of defects up to 7 cm wide is fairly easy, and is successfully done without difficulty in younger patients[2-4] (Fig. 14-3). Superior undermining is contraindicated to prevent injuries of the marginal mandibular nerve and lower lip eversion. In some obese patients, closure is performed under tension, and neck contour can be improved after closure. Natural cervicomental contour can be obtained by several fixations of the lower flap to the periosteum of the hyoid bone. The scar is well hidden in the submental area even in patients requiring skin grafts to achieve complete closure of the donor defect.

Surface Landmarks

The origin of the submental artery is 5.5 cm (4 to 7 cm) anterior to the angle of the mandible and 7 mm (3 to 15 mm) from the mandibular border. The surface marking of its termination is a point 8 mm (2 to 12 mm) behind the mandibular border and 6 mm (4 to 8 mm) lateral to the midline.[10] In injection studies and clinical applications,[2,6,12] the vascular territory of the flap includes the submandibular area, part of the chin, and part of the lower lip. The flap's vascular territory measures from 4 by 5 cm to 7 by 15 cm. In another cadaver injection study,[6] the submental artery supplied the ipsilateral upper neck and a variable area across the midline as large as 10 by 16 cm. The maximum dimension (clinical) of this area was reported to be 7 by 15 cm. According to that injection study,[6] the pedicle showed good perfusion on the contralateral side and, in my experience, the possible dimensions can reliably be extended to the contralateral angle of the mandible across the midline.

The main submental perforator was reported to be approximately 5.5 cm lateral and 3 cm inferior to the lateral commissure.[7] However, the reliable perforators are found at both borders of the anterior belly of the digastric muscle, even though they are not always symmetrical. These perforators are useful in situations requiring a long pedicle.

Vascular Anatomy

There have been several studies of the submental area perforators. According to the cadaveric studies of Whetzel and Mathes,[17] the submental skin territory is supplied predominantly by one perforator that characteristically gives off three or four branches to supply the separate subcutaneous islands of dermis. Another study reported that cutaneous perforators range from one to four in number, with one perforator piercing the platysma and dividing into many branches in the subdermal plane.[2] According to this study, this perforator originates 3 to 15 mm from the mandibular border (average 7 mm) and 4 to 7 cm from the mandibular angle (average 5.5 cm). In my own studies, I have examined the location and number of submental perforators in 24 submental areas in four barium-injected fresh cadavers and eight clinical dissections.

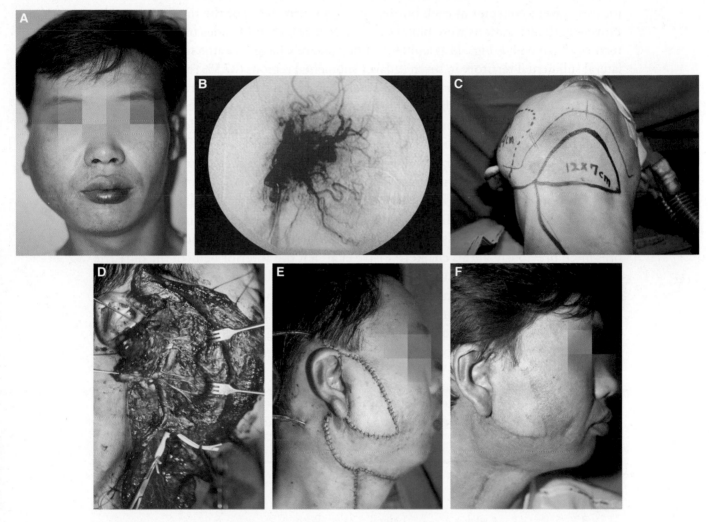

Fig. 14-3 **A,** A 27-year-old patient presented with an arteriovenous malformation of the right cheek. **B,** A preoperative angiogram showed the vascular malformation in the right parotid gland. **C,** A 12 by 7 cm submental perforator flap was designed in a symmetrical spindle shape. **D,** The defect was exposed after radical excision of the lesion, including the parotid gland and skin. **E,** Postoperative view after resurfacing with the flap, which had a sufficient arc of rotation. **F,** The postoperative course was uneventful. The flap provided a good color match and a well-contoured submental curve.

We found one or two reliable perforators always present on each side, and their locations were constant at each border of the anterior belly of the digastric muscle. However, their locations were not always symmetrical on both sides of the submental territory (Table 14-1, Figs. 14-4 and 14-5). Only one reliable perforator supplied the unilateral submental territory in seven cadaver submental regions (87.5%) and nine clinical dissections (56.3%). Furthermore, these perforators were distributed asymmetrically in all cadaveric and clinical dissections (62.5%). The perforator was located only at the medial border of the anterior belly of the digastric muscle in seven sides, at the lateral border in nine sides, and at both borders in eight sides (see Fig. 14-5). These anatomic data based on the perforator concept prove the reliability of the perforator flap, even when the anterior belly of the digastric muscle is excluded.

Harvesting the anterior belly of the digastric muscle is controversial. Some surgeons suggest that the anterior belly should be included[6,11,12]; others maintain that its inclusion is not necessary.[2-10] This controversy can be clarified based on the anatomic data presented previously in this chapter.[3] Pistre et al[8] left the anterior belly of the digastric muscle intact in their initial trial and progressively included it because it improved venous drainage. Venous congestion is not caused by exclusion of the anterior belly of the digastric muscle, but by insufficient venous drainage through the venae comitantes. When the venae comitantes are collapsed or spastic during pedicle dissection, inclusion of the submental vein is recommended.

Table 14-1   Number of Reliable Submental Perforators and Their Location Relative to the Anterior Belly of the Digastric Muscle

Case Number	Type	Right	Left
1	Cadaver	Lateral	Medial
2	Cadaver	Lateral	Medial
3	Cadaver	Lateral	Both
4	Cadaver	Lateral	Medial
5	Clinical	Both	Both
6	Clinical	Medial	Medial
7	Clinical	Both	Lateral
8	Clinical	Lateral	Medial
9	Clinical	Lateral	Both
10	Clinical	Lateral	Both
11	Clinical	Both	Both
12	Clinical	Medial	Lateral

From Kim JT, Kim SK, Koshima I, et al. An anatomic study and clinical applications of the reversed submental perforator-based island flap. Plast Reconstr Surg 109:2204-2210, 2002.
Both, Present on each side of the anterior belly of the digastric muscle; *Lateral,* lateral to the digastric muscle; *Medial,* medial to the digastric muscle.

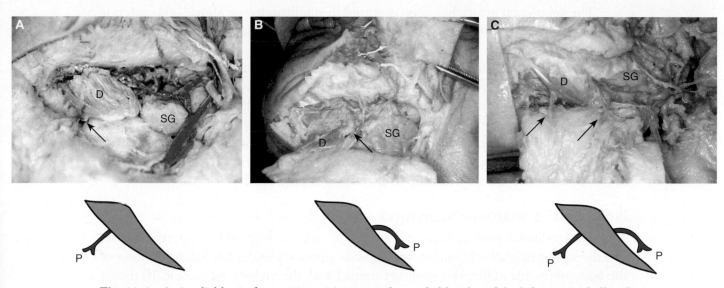

Fig. 14-4 **A,** A reliable perforator *(arrow)* is seen at the medial border of the left anterior belly of the digastric muscle. **B,** A reliable perforator *(arrow)* at the lateral border of the left anterior belly of the digastric muscle. **C,** Two reliable perforators *(arrows)*, one at each border of the left anterior belly of the digastric muscle. (*D*, Digastric muscle; *P,* perforator; *SG,* submandibular gland.)

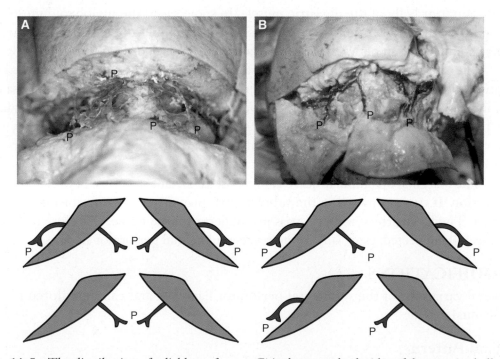

Fig. 14-5 The distribution of reliable perforator *(P)* is shown on both sides of the anterior belly of the digastric muscle. **A,** Symmetrical locations of the reliable perforators. **B,** Asymmetrical locations.

The submental artery has been reported to run deep to[6] or above[12] the anterior belly of the digastric muscle. According to an anatomic study by Faltaous and Yetman,[6] the submental artery is deep to the anterior belly of the digastric muscle in 70% of cases, and it runs superficial to the belly in the other 30%. They reported that several perforators supply the overlying skin through the platysma muscle, and that two major perforators come off proximal and distal to the digastric muscle. These anatomic finding are in agreement with my anatomic study. Even though minor perforators come directly through the anterior belly of the digastric muscle, they are too tiny to isolate. Nevertheless, one or both of the reliable perforators at each border of the anterior belly of the digastric muscle are available to adequately supply the flap.

Neighboring Anatomic Structures

The submandibular gland is located between the anterior belly of the digastric muscle and the stylomandibular ligament, and extends superiorly under the inferior border of the body of the mandible. It is in direct contact with the mylohyoid muscle, its motor nerve, and the submental vessels. When the submental artery and its venae comitantes pass superiorly and medially over the gland, they are embedded in a tortuous groove on its surface and give several small branches to the gland. Branches to the submandibular gland and lymph nodes can be a good landmark for identifying the neighboring submental vessels.

The mylohyoid muscle forms the floor of the dissection during elevation of the submental perforator flap. This flat triangular muscle is situated immediately superior to the anterior belly of the digastric muscle. In some cases, the mylohyoid muscle is joined with the anterior belly of the digastric muscle. The submental artery and its venae comitantes run between the muscle and mandibular border.

The digastric muscle consists of two fleshy bellies; only the anterior belly is relevant to the anatomy of this flap. The anterior belly arises from the digastric fossa on the inner side of the inferior mandibular border close to the symphysis, and inserts into the hyoid bone. The muscle is supplied by small twigs from the submental artery, and the reliable perforators branch from the submental artery and vein at the anterior and posterior borders of this belly.

The marginal mandibular nerve is the most important structure in the submental dissection. It curves upward in the subplatysmal plane near the inferior mandibular border. The facial artery and vein pass just underneath the nerve; therefore it should be carefully dissected, especially in the reverse submental perforator flap.

MODIFICATIONS

Several variations of the submental perforator flap exist and can be tailored to the individual patient.

Island Pattern

The island pattern of the submental perforator flap has a wide arc of rotation and can reach the whole homolateral face, including the temple, cheek, and periauricular area (see Fig. 14-3). Apart from the temple, the flap does not reach the forehead or any part of the oral cavity.[2] Intraoral reconstruction with the perforator island flap provides an alternative if the surgeon wants to avoid a free flap. The flap is particularly amenable to reconstruction of the oral commissure and intraoral reconstruction.[16] An island or bipedicle pattern[8] can be raised for the upper lip and nasal lining, or for reconstructing any bearded area of an adult man; however, a hair-bearing flap may not be appropriate for nasal or intraoral resurfacing (Fig. 14-6). For forehead reconstruction, the Y-V procedure facilitates lengthening of the vein.[18] Because the facial vein is taut compared with the tortuous facial artery, the Y-V procedure allows mobilization of the flap by up to 5 cm.[8] The submental flap is also extremely useful as a local pedicle flap as opposed to a regional flap. This is illustrated in Figs. 14-7 and 14-8.

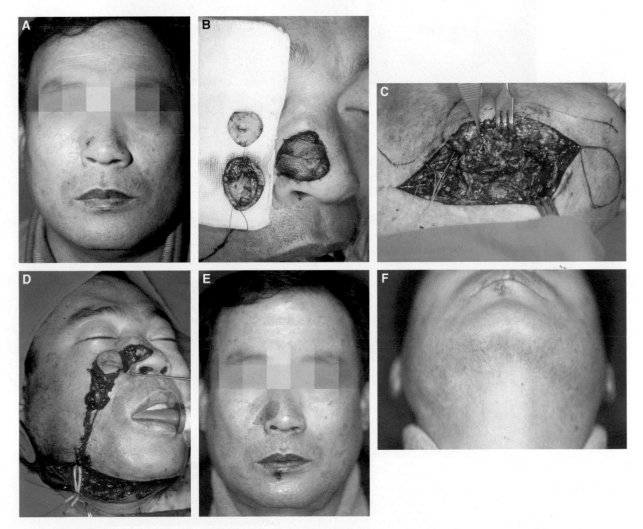

Fig. 14-6 **A,** A 49-year-old patient presented with a recurrent basal cell carcinoma of the right lateral side of the nose. **B,** A large defect involving the ala resulted after Mohs micrographic surgery for complete removal of the lesion. **C,** The superior approach was performed, and the submental pedicle was identified with traction on the submandibular gland. **D,** The pedicle was elongated further with a reverse pattern. The flap was passed under the marginal mandibular nerve to reach the defect. **E,** Reconstruction provided good contour of the nose, but the hair-bearing skin of the flap was evident. **F,** The donor scar was well hidden after primary closure.

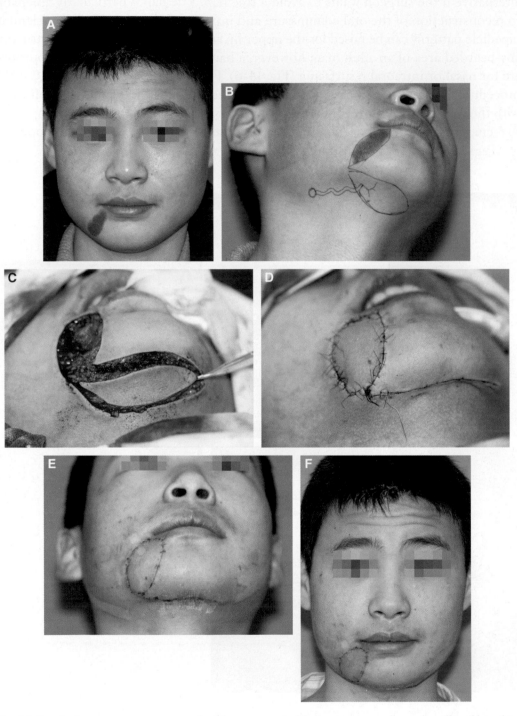

Fig. 14-7   A, A young man presented with a congenital hairy nevus on the right side of his chin. **B,** The defect was planned, and a pedicle submental flap was designed. **C,** The defect was created, and the flap was prepared as an island flap. **D,** The flap was rotated into the defect as a propeller flap, and the donor defect was closed. **E** and **F,** The patient is shown in the early postoperative period. (Case courtesy Daping Yang, MD.)

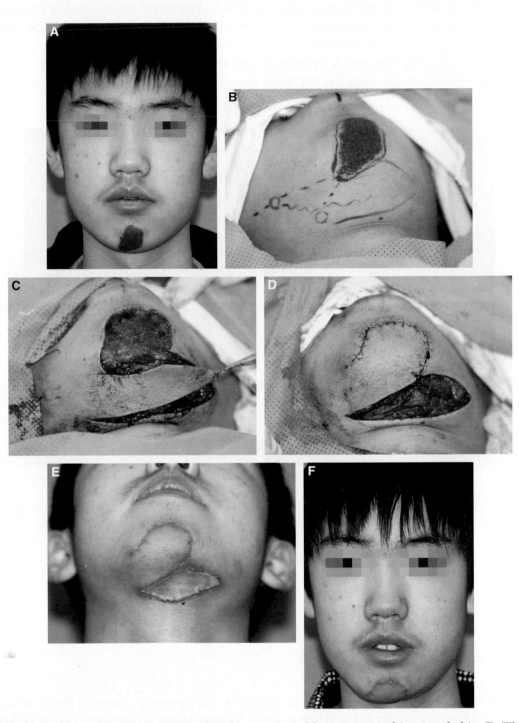

Fig. 14-8 **A,** A young man presented with a congenital hairy nevus in his central chin. **B,** The excision was marked and a submental flap planned. **C,** The defect was created and the flap prepared. **D,** The flap was not islanded but was rotated into the defect. **E,** The donor defect was skin grafted. **F,** The patient is shown postoperatively. (Case courtesy Daping Yang, MD.)

The perforator island flap can also be used as a turnover flap for lining pharyngocutaneous or esophagocutaneous fistulas, or other such defects. In this case, the flap has the advantage of being less bulky than other regional flaps (Fig. 14-9). The extended submental island lip flap, which includes the full-thickness of the central lower lip (mucosomusculocutaneous flap), has also been reported for fistula repair.[19]

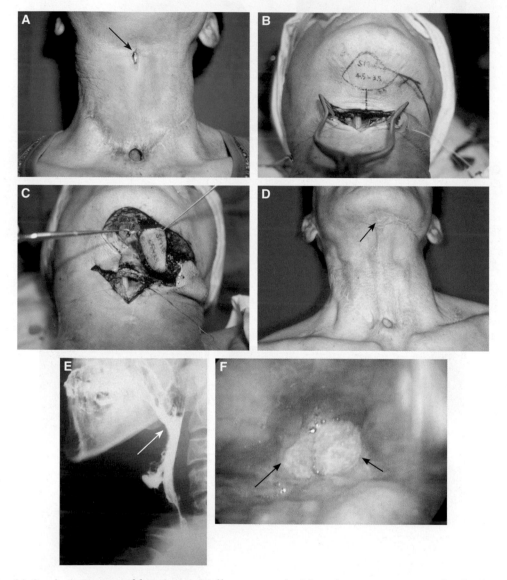

Fig. 14-9 **A,** A 52-year-old patient initially presented with a pharyngocutaneous fistula *(arrow)* after total laryngectomy for laryngeal cancer. There was no evidence of recurrence, but the patient had serious dysphagia because of food leakage. **B,** After debridement, there was a 3 by 4 cm defect of the hypopharynx. A 3.5 by 4.5 cm submental perforator island flap was designed. **C,** The flap was turned over to patch the defect and create an inner lining, and a split-thickness skin graft was used to cover the outer surface after closure of the donor defect. **D,** The fistula was completely repaired *(arrow)*. **E,** Barium studies performed after the operation show a patent lumen with no leakage *(arrow)*. **F,** The inner-lining skin of the patched flap *(arrows)* is intact on esophagoscopy.

Free Pattern

The submental perforator flap can also be reliably used as a free flap. It is particularly elegant in forehead or periorbital reconstruction.

Reverse Island Pattern

The arc of rotation of the flap can be lengthened by using reverse flow based on the distal facial vessels.[2,4,10] Using this variant, the flap can reach the nose, upper lip, moustache, and midface regions (Fig. 14-10). Martin et al[2] described the possibility of dissecting the distally based flap. They employed the reverse pattern as a distally based flap, and

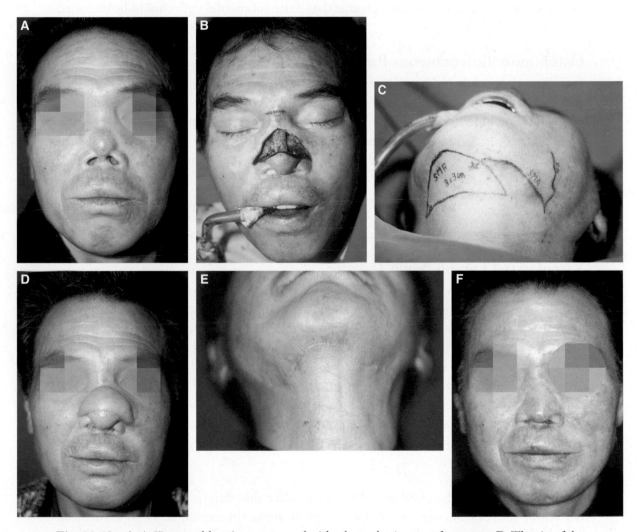

Fig. 14-10 A, A 57-year-old patient presented with a hypoplastic nose after noma. **B,** The tip of the nose was reconstructed by hinging the retruded distal nose, and reconstructing the nasal dorsum with a cantilever calvarial bone graft. **C** and **D,** An 8 by 3 cm submental perforator flap was designed as a reverse-pattern flap and passed through the tunnel to reach the defect. **E,** The donor scar was well concealed without obliteration of the cervicomental angle. **F,** The nose was adequately reconstructed with an additional debulking procedure. The color match was excellent.

proposed that the marginal mandibular branch of the facial nerve restricts the pivot point of the pedicle. Another report states that the postoperative course of the reverse pattern flap is hazardous because of the high risk of facial nerve injury during the dissection.[8] Nevertheless, the pedicle can be safely passed underneath the marginal mandibular nerve. Using this maneuver, a more cranial pivot point can be obtained with no restriction or compression of the pedicle. This modification allows the flap to reach the midface, including the nose.[3] Accordingly, the term *reverse flap* is more appropriate than distally based flap, because the flow in the pedicle becomes reversed after flap elevation.

The reverse submental perforator flap is susceptible to venous congestion.[4] A bluish tinge can initially be observed but gradually subsides in the postoperative period. Based on our knowledge of the anatomic data,[3] the submental vein should be included to increase reliability.

Osteo(musculo)cutaneous Pattern

Including the mylohyoid muscle or anterior belly of the digastric muscle allows a bulky flap to be planned and increases flap reliability. A 10 by 2 cm segment of mandibular rim can be included as an osteocutaneous flap to reconstruct the malar or zygomatic bone defects.[2,4,8] A successful composite flap must incorporate a cuff of the mylohyoid muscle; the outlines of the mandible are not altered by using the inner cortex of bone.[2,8]

Fascioplatysmal Flap

Soft tissue defects can be filled with the fascioplatysmal flap, which includes the platysma muscle and adipose tissue after deepithelialization of the skin paddle.

Vascularized Lymph Node Transfer

Submandibular or cervical lymph nodes can be included in the submental flap to create a draining flap for lymphedema. After flap inset, lymph nodes and draining lymphatic channels in the flap function to drain lymphatic fluids surrounding the submental flap directly to the recipient vein through the pedicle vein. Cervical lymphatic groups are more functional than submandibular groups. The submandibular gland and tortuous facial vessels winding near the gland should be dissected carefully to maintain lymphatic channels in the flap between the skin and deep lymph nodes. The submental flap with vascularized lymph nodes is less bulky than the inguinal flap with vascularized lymph nodes (Fig. 14-11).

Others

Tissue expansion can be employed to obtain a wider thin flap or to facilitate closure of the donor site. Special care is necessary in positioning the expander. With expansion, venous drainage is redistributed from the top of the expanded skin to the periphery; therefore overexpansion can jeopardize flap survival if redirection of venous flow fails. Following expansion, half of the expanded skin is used for the flap, and the other half is used to reduce tension of the donor site closure.

A prefabricated superficial temporal fascia flap has been combined with a submental perforator flap to line and cover the cheek in patients with noma defects.[11] This

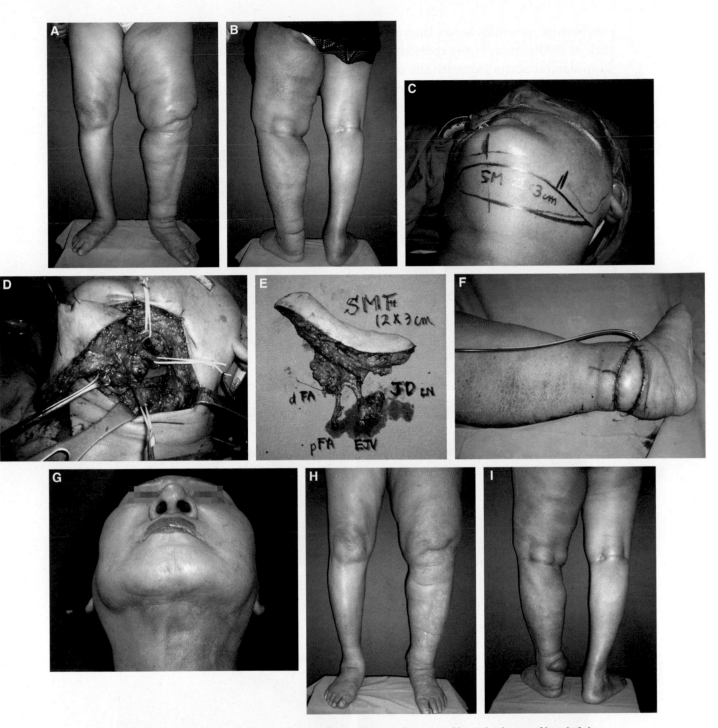

Fig. 14-11 **A** and **B,** A 73-year-old woman had a 20-year history of lymphedema of her left lower extremity. **C,** A 12 by 3 cm submental flap was designed. **D,** The flap was dissected, with careful preservation of jugulodigastric lymph nodes and their draining channels. **E,** The flap was harvested. **F,** The flap was inset in the left ankle, functioning as a new lymphatic draining site to the underlying recipient vein. **G-I,** The patient is shown 10 months postoperatively. The circumference measured at midthigh and midcalf is reduced significantly. She is more comfortable walking and stepping up and down. (*dFA,* Distal facial artery; *EJV,* external jugular vein; *JDLN,* jugulodigastric lymph nodes; *pFA,* proximal facial artery; *SMF,* submental flap.)

combination provides better thickness and color match than other conventional flaps such as deltopectoral or pectoralis major flaps. The entire flap can be used with only an ipsilateral perforator with the contralateral skin paddle. Because the contralateral side of the flap is reliable, even based on an ipsilateral perforator, the contralateral skin paddle can be used for inner lining in nasal reconstruction (Fig. 14-12).

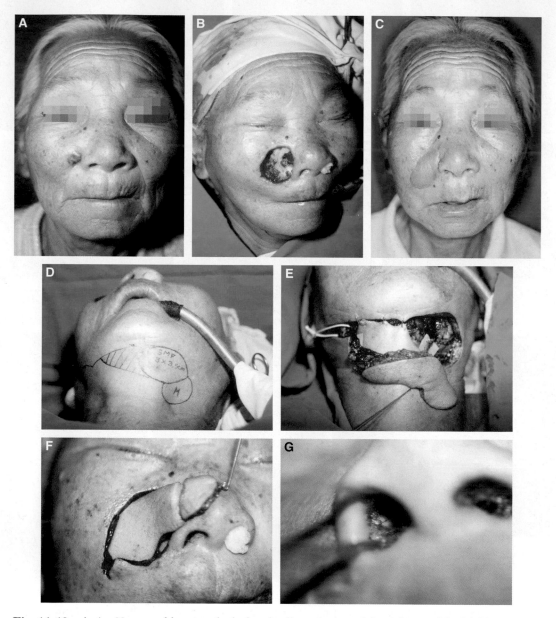

Fig. 14-12   **A,** An 83-year-old patient had a basal cell carcinoma of the right nasolabial fold. **B,** Mohs micrographic surgery revealed that the defect extended to the bone and through the nasal cavity. For this reason, flap coverage was required. **C,** Good resurfacing was achieved with a reverse submental perforator island flap. **D,** A submental perforator flap with a 7 by 3 cm skin paddle was designed with a distal island component for inner lining. **E,** A contralateral submental vein was combined for supercharging to the flap to relieve possible congestion. **F,** The reverse flap reached the defect, and the distal island paddle provided inner lining of the nostril. **G,** The reconstructed inner lining was well maintained after the operation.

PITFALLS

In patients with head and neck skin cancer, the submental lymph nodes may be involved and included in the flap, potentially spreading the malignant cells after flap transfer.[8] However, metastatic submental or submandibular nodes can be located before flap elevation. Furthermore, the nodes can be prophylactically cleared when the flap is harvested.

The SMAP flap usually provides thin and pliable skin, but its thickness varies depending on the patient's age and degree of obesity. An osteocutaneous or musculocutaneous flap is planned for filling defects or for dimensional reconstructions. The flap can be surprisingly bulky if adipose tissue is thick.

The marginal mandibular nerve can be injured, and extreme care is necessary during this part of the dissection.[8] This complication has been reported to be as high as 16%[10]; however, it can be avoided by identifying the nerve through the superior approach. Pistre et al[8] showed that dissecting the nerve was not necessary by staying close to the posterior aspect of the platysma muscle from the angle of mandible to the midline. Careful dissection of the nerve is indispensable to improve the arc of rotation and prevent pedicle kinking in the reverse flap.

It is difficult to separate the submandibular gland from facial vessels, especially in vascularized lymph node transfers. The gland should be fixed after flap harvest to prevent gland ptosis.

For nasal reconstruction, the SMAP flap has several disadvantages compared with the forehead flap. These include hair-bearing skin, thickness of the musculocutaneous flap, and difficulty in shaping the flap.[20] Partial or complete flap loss is less likely to occur as our knowledge of anatomy improves. This flap can safely be used in patients who have received radiation in a therapeutic dose, although there is a risk of difficulty with donor site closure.[21]

CONCLUSION

The SMAP flap has proved to be an excellent regional flap in reconstructing facial and neck defects. Its advantages include a wide arc of rotation, excellent color and texture match, and a well-hidden donor site. The flap is reliable and relatively easy to elevate. It is a good choice for facial resurfacing, because it matches the color and texture of facial skin. The flap is reliable, having a constant vascular pedicle, and it is as versatile as an island, reverse island, or free flap. Its mobile arc of rotation reaches the temporal, midface, and lower face regions. The oral cavity can also be reconstructed using the SMAP flap. In this application, the flap can have a pedicle length of up to 8 cm.[13] A longer pedicle is available with a reverse-pattern flap. A donor site up to 8 cm in width can be closed primarily with no obliteration of the cervicomental angle, particularly in elderly patients with ample skin laxity.[3] The donor scar is concealed within the submental area and is more acceptable than the scar of the supraclavicular flap. The SMAP flap can also be a useful alternative to a radial forearm free flap, because free tissue transfer is avoided. The flap provides one more option in the area of facial resurfacing or intraoral reconstruction.

References

1. Kim JT, Koo BS, Kim SK. The thin latissimus dorsi perforator-based free flap for resurfacing. Plast Reconstr Surg 107:374-382, 2001.

2. Martin D, Pascal JF, Baudet J, et al. The submental island flap: a new donor site. Anatomy and clinical applications as a free or pedicled flap. Plast Reconstr Surg 92:867-873, 1993.
    The authors described a new island flap based on the submental artery and used for reconstructing facial defects. They discussed its advantages, including an extended territory.

3. Kim JT, Kim SK, Koshima I, et al. An anatomical study and clinical applications of the reversed submental perforator-based island flap. Plast Reconstr Surg 109:2204-2210, 2002.
    This article described a reverse submental flap based on the perforator concept. Cadaver studies were used to verify the location of these perforators. The reverse pattern has proved useful for midface resurfacing and nose reconstruction.

4. Yilmaz M, Menderes A, Barutcu A. Submental artery island flap for reconstruction of the lower and mid face. Ann Plast Surg 39:30-35, 1997.
    The various components of the submental island flap, with muscle or bone, were discussed. Complications and drawbacks were described and compared with other papers.

5. Wang JG, Chen WL, Ye HS, et al. Reverse facial artery-submental artery deepithelialised submental island flap to reconstruct maxillary defects following cancer ablation. J Craniomaxillofac Surg 39:499-502, 2011.
    The authors assessed the reliability of this flap and concluded that it is safe, quick, and simple to elevate.

6. Faltaous AA, Yetman RJ. The submental artery flap: an anatomic study. Plast Reconstr Surg 97:56-60, 1996.
    The authors reviewed their anatomic studies of the submental artery and vein, including the location of these vessels relative to the anterior belly of the digastric muscle. Anterior belly should be included in the flap for reliability.

7. Pistre V, Pelissier P, Martin D, et al. The submental flap: its uses as a pedicled or free flap for facial reconstruction. Clin Plast Surg 28:303-309, 2001.
    This article summarized anatomy, surgical technique, and clinical results using the submental flap for facial reconstruction. The advantages and disadvantages were compared with the long-term clinical experience.

8. Pistre V, Pelissier P, Martin D, et al. Ten years of experience with the submental flap. Plast Reconstr Surg 108:1576-1581, 2001.
    The authors discussed their clinical experience with the submental flap in 31 cases over the past 10 years, including the composite flap. Complications were described, and technical advancement in flap harvesting was introduced.

9. Kitazawa T, Harashina T, Taira H, et al. Bipedicled submental island flap for upper lip reconstruction. Ann Plast Surg 42:83-86, 1999.

10. Sterne GD, Januszkiewicz JS, Hall PN, et al. The submental island flap. Br J Plast Surg 49:85-89, 1996.

11. Barthelemy I, Martin D, Sannajust JP, et al. Prefabricated superficial temporal fascia flap combined with a submental flap in noma surgery. Plast Reconstr Surg 109:936-940, 2002.
    This article presented the various clinical applications of the submental flap, with operative techniques. Several methods of obtaining a long, reliable pedicle by additional dissection were described.

12. Curran AJ, Neligan P, Gullane PJ. Submental artery island flap. Laryngoscope 107:1545-1549, 1997.

13. Vural E, Suen JY. The submental island flap in head and neck reconstruction. Head Neck 22:572-578, 2000.

14. Ellenbogen R, Karlin JV. Visual criteria for success in restoring the youthful neck. Plast Reconstr Surg 66:826-837, 1980.

15. Connell BF, Shamoun JM. The significance of digastric muscle contouring for rejuvenation of the submental area of the face. Plast Reconstr Surg 99:1586-1590, 1997.

16. Daya M, Mahomva O, Madaree A. Multistaged reconstruction of the oral commissures and upper and lower lip with an island submental flap and nasolabial flap. Plast Reconstr Surg 108:968-971, 2001.

17. Whetzel TP, Mathes SJ. Arterial anatomy of the face: an analysis of vascular territories and perforating cutaneous vessels. Plast Reconstr Surg 89:591-603, 1992.
    This article showed the vascular territory of the submental area according to latex injection results. The angiosome of the submental area is known to be supplied predominantly by one perforator that gives several branches for separate islands of dermis.

18. Martin D, Legaillard P, Bakhach J, et al. Reverse flow YV pedicle extension: a method of doubling the arc of rotation of a flap under certain conditions. Ann Chir Plast Esthet 39:403-414, 1994.

19. Janssen DA, Thimsen DA. The extended submental island lip flap: an alternative for esophageal repair. Plast Reconstr Surg 102:835-838, 1998.

20. Pribaz JJ, Fine NA, Orgill DP. Discussion of Faltaous AA, Yetman RJ. The submental artery flap: an anatomic study. Plast Reconstr Surg 97:56-60; discussion 61-62, 1996.

21. Wu Y, Tang P, Qi Y, et al. Submental island flap for head and neck reconstruction: a review of 20 cases. Asian J Surg 21:247-252, 1998.

[illegible faded reference text]

Upper Extremity

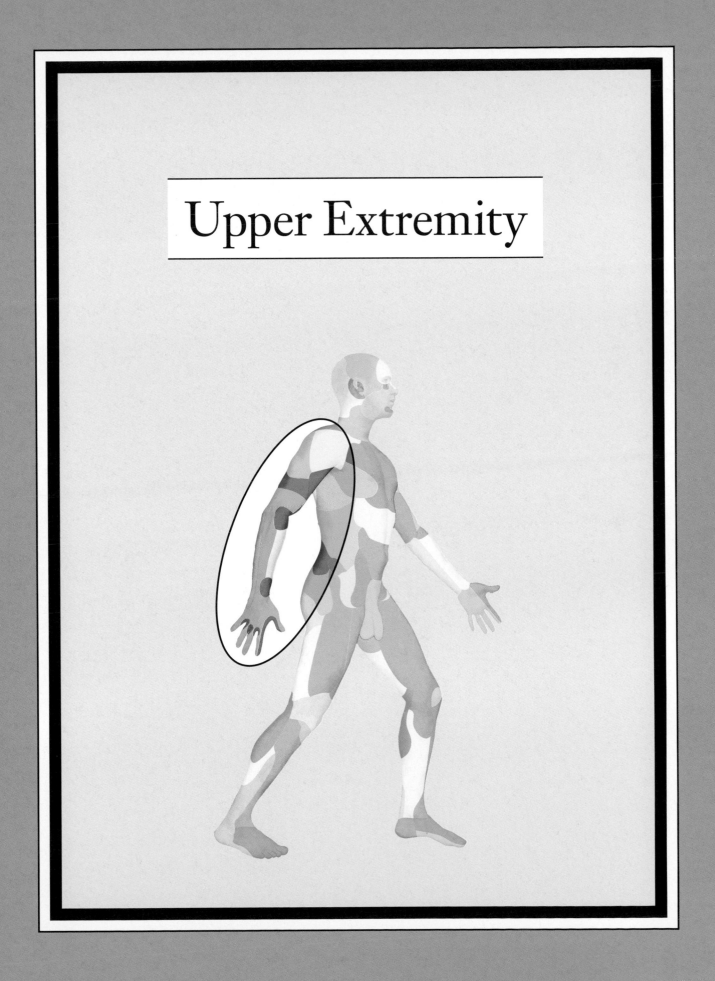

15

Vascular Supply of the Integument of the Upper Extremity

Binu Prathap Thomas
Christopher R. Geddes
Maolin Tang
Steven F. Morris

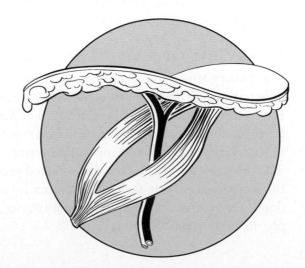

The upper extremity is commonly involved in severe soft tissue injuries requiring coverage by a regional pedicle flap or microvascular free tissue transfer. Knowledge of the cutaneous vascular supply is important for flap design. Because it is often preferable to harvest skin flaps from the injured limb, reconstructive surgeons benefit from a detailed understanding of the flap vascular anatomy of upper extremity flaps. The work of pioneers in the study of vascular anatomy of the integument has greatly advanced our understanding of this anatomy.[1-6]

This chapter describes the vascular supply to the integument of the upper extremity. Information presented is based on data obtained in our series of dissection studies. Fresh human cadavers were injected using a modification of the lead oxide–gelatin injection technique originally performed by Salmon,[3,4] and later modified by Rees and Taylor.[7] The anatomic technique is described in detail in Chapter 4. Techniques used to interpret and record data included digital photography, Microsoft Excel spreadsheets (Microsoft Corporation, Redmond, WA), Adobe Photoshop (version 7.0; Adobe, San Jose, CA) to convert the angiograms from individual radiographs to collage form and to shade territories in color, and Scion Image for Windows (Scion Corporation, Frederick, MD) to calculate the area of the vascular territories.

This chapter includes a synopsis of the main vascular architecture of the upper extremity, an overview of the cutaneous vascularity, and a description of anatomic regions and the principal vascular territories. Potential flaps based on perforator vessels are also described with the description of various source vessels in this chapter.

OVERVIEW OF VASCULAR ANATOMY

The axillary artery and its terminal branches provide the principal arterial supply to the upper arm. The brachial artery begins at the lower border of the teres major muscle as the continuation of the axillary artery. The vessel runs down the medial aspect of the arm and divides into the radial and ulnar arteries in the cubital fossa. The radial and ulnar arteries and the anterior and posterior interosseous arteries supply the forearm. The palmar aspect of the hand is supplied predominantly by the ulnar artery through the superficial palmar arch. The dorsum is supplied by the radial artery through the dorsal metacarpal arteries. The digital arteries arising from the arches in the hand supply the fingers and thumb (Fig. 15-1).

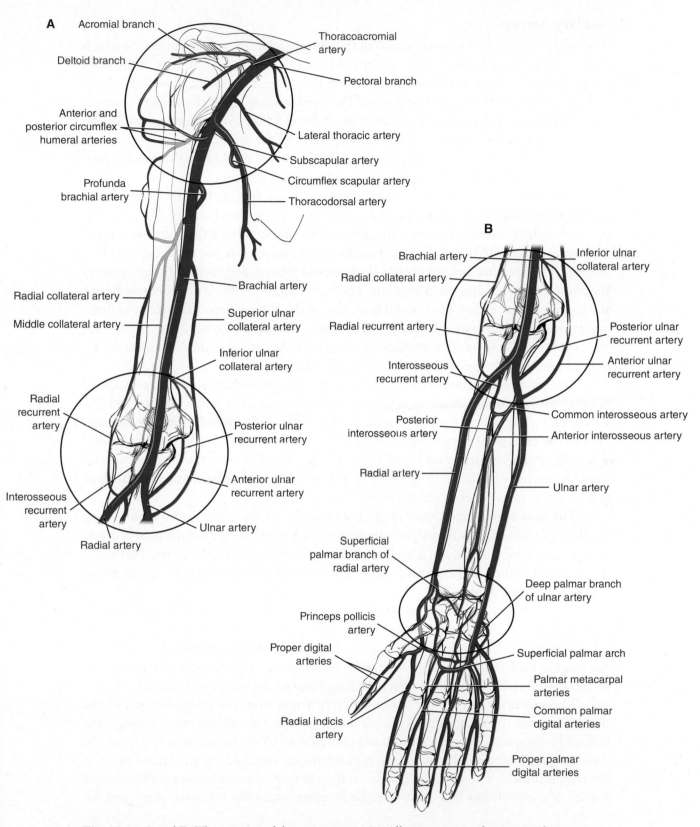

Fig. 15-1   A and **B,** The arteries of the upper extremity. All cutaneous perforators in the upper extremity can be traced to one of the named source vessels that make up the various vascular territories.

Axillary Artery

The axillary artery is the continuation of the third part of the subclavian artery, which begins at the lateral border of the first rib and extends to the lower border of the teres major muscle.[8] The artery is crossed by the pectoralis minor muscle, which divides it into proximal, posterior, and distal parts. The surface anatomy of the axillary artery is marked with the patient's arm abducted by drawing a line from the midpoint of the clavicle to the palpable pulsation on the lateral wall of the axilla.

The branch from the first part of the axillary artery is the superior thoracic artery. It is not involved in the cutaneous supply of the upper extremity.

The thoracoacromial artery arises from the second part of the axillary artery and divides into pectoral, acromial, clavicular, and deltoid branches (see Fig. 15-1, *A*). The pectoral branch descends between the pectoral muscles, supplying them and the breast, and anastomoses with the intercostal branches of the internal thoracic and lateral thoracic arteries. The acromial branch crosses the coracoid process deep to the deltoid, pierces the muscle, and reaches the acromion. The vessel anastomoses with the branches of the suprascapular artery, the deltoid branches of the thoracoacromial artery, and the posterior circumflex humeral artery. The acromial branch also contributes to the skin over the shoulder through musculocutaneous branches at the superior border of the deltoid muscle near the acromioclavicular joint (Fig. 15-2).

The clavicular branch of the thoracoacromial artery lies between the clavipectoral fascia and the pectoralis major muscle and supplies the sternoclavicular joint and subclavius muscle. The deltoid branch crosses the pectoralis minor muscle with the cephalic vein in the deltopectoral groove to supply the deltoid and pectoralis major muscles. This artery gives a cutaneous branch that supplies the skin over the anterior deltoid muscle near the middle of this groove. Manchot[1] referred to this cutaneous branch as the "anterior subcutaneous deltoid artery."

The subscapular artery arises from the third part of the axillary artery, runs along the distal border of the subscapularis muscle, and anastomoses with the lateral thoracic artery, intercostal arteries, and deep branch of the transverse cervical arteries. This vessel is the largest branch of the axillary artery. The perforators from the subscapular artery are described in Chapter 29.

The anterior circumflex humeral artery also arises from the third part of the axillary artery at the distal border of the subscapularis muscle. The vessel runs horizontally behind the coracobrachialis muscle and the short head of the biceps muscle, anterior to the surgical neck of the humerus. The artery anastomoses with the posterior circumflex humeral artery after traversing under the long head of the biceps and deltoid muscles.

The posterior circumflex humeral artery arises from the axillary artery at the distal border of the subscapularis muscle and runs with the axillary nerve through the quadrangular space. The artery winds around the neck of the humerus and supplies the shoulder joint, deltoid, teres major and minor muscles, and the long and lateral heads of the triceps muscle. The vessel gives a descending branch to anastomose with the deltoid branch of the profunda brachial artery, the anterior circumflex humeral artery, and the acromial branches of the suprascapular and thoracoacromial arteries (see Fig. 15-2). The posterior circumflex humeral artery primarily supplies the deltoid muscle and the skin over the posterior shoulder area. A number of variations are possible for this vessel.[6] A large cutaneous branch is given off from the posterior circumflex humeral artery that has been consistently found in our dissections. Manchot[1] referred to this branch as the "posterior subcutaneous deltoid artery."

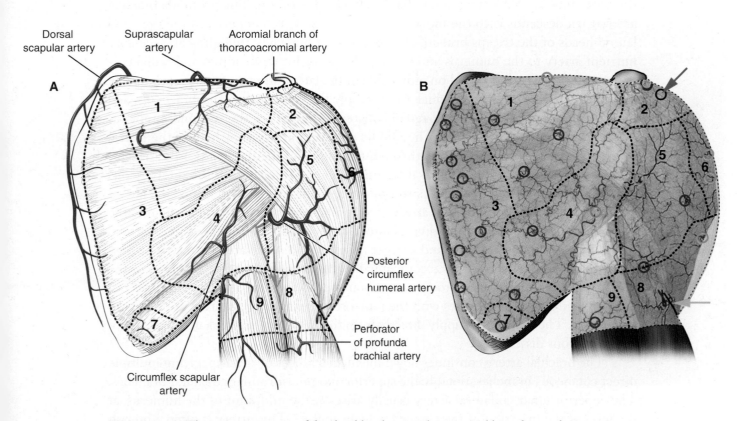

Fig. 15-2   A, The posterior aspect of the shoulder showing the principal branches to the integument. **B,** An angiogram of the integument of the posterior aspect of the right shoulder from a human cadaver injected with lead oxide and gelatin. *Red circles* identify musculocutaneous perforators and *blue circles* show septocutaneous perforators. Anatomic territories of the cutaneous blood supply are numbered. The *green arrow* points to the wire marking the posterior insertion of the deltoid muscle, and the *blue arrow* points to the wire marking the top of the humerus. (*1,* Suprascapular artery; *2,* acromial branch of the thoracoacromial artery; *3,* dorsal scapular artery or superficial transverse cervical artery; *4,* circumflex scapular artery; *5,* posterior circumflex humeral artery; *6,* anterior circumflex humeral artery; *7,* lateral branches of the intercostal arteries; *8,* profunda brachial artery; *9,* direct cutaneous branch of the axillary artery.)

Brachial Artery

The brachial artery and its branches primarily supply the arm. The artery begins at the lower border of the teres major muscle as a continuation of the axillary artery and terminates as the radial and ulnar arteries at the elbow, just inferior to the lacertus fibrosus (Fig. 15-3; see Fig. 15-1, *A*).

The profunda brachial artery branches off immediately from the beginning of the brachial artery at the proximal arm, from the posteromedial aspect. It gives off the ascending deltoid branch immediately after its formation. The profunda brachial artery then descends with the radial nerve in the spiral groove between the long and lateral heads of the triceps brachii. Here it gives off branches, including an accessory nutrient artery to the humerus and the middle (posterior descending) and radial collateral arteries, which proceed on either side of the lateral intermuscular septum. The muscular arteries from the brachial artery supply the coracobrachialis, brachialis, and biceps muscles. The middle and radial collateral arteries are the terminal branches of the profunda brachial artery. The middle collateral artery runs behind the lateral intermuscular septum and passes through the long and medial head of the triceps. It then passes behind the humeral diaphysis and anastomoses with the interosseous recurrent artery, arising from the posterior interosseous artery posterior to the lateral epicondyle.[6] The radial collateral artery accompanies the radial nerve. Proximal to the lateral intermuscular septum, it divides into a smaller anterior radial collateral artery, which follows the radial nerve, and a larger posterior radial collateral artery. The posterior radial collateral artery is accompanied by the posterior cutaneous nerve of the arm. It gives off numerous septocutaneous branches to the skin of the lateral aspect of the arm, and then anastomoses with the radial recurrent artery anterior to the lateral epicondyle. The cutaneous supply directly from the profunda brachial artery was quite variable in our dissections.

The brachial artery continues down the medial aspect of the arm, giving multiple direct cutaneous branches, notably the superior and inferior ulnar collateral branches. The superior ulnar collateral artery usually arises at the midpoint of the humerus, at the level of the insertion of the coracobrachialis muscle. This artery is often a branch of the profunda brachial artery and accompanies the ulnar nerve behind the medial epicondyle. The superior ulnar collateral artery anastomoses with the posterior ulnar recurrent artery. The inferior ulnar collateral (supratrochlear) artery begins 5 cm proximal to the elbow and passes between the median nerve and the brachialis muscle, giving an anterior descending branch that anastomoses with the anterior ulnar recurrent artery. The inferior ulnar collateral artery then pierces the medial intermuscular septum and anastomoses with a branch from the middle collateral branch of the profunda brachial artery.

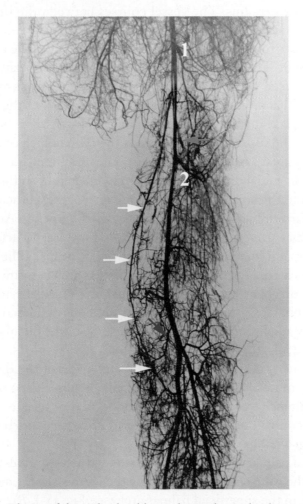

Fig. 15-3 This arterial cast of the right shoulder and arm shows the direct cutaneous branches of the axillary artery *(1)* and the profunda brachial artery *(2)*. The superior ulnar collateral artery anastomoses *(yellow arrows)* with the inferior ulnar collateral artery *(blue arrow)* and ulnar recurrent artery. The *green arrow* points to the direct cutaneous branch of the proximal brachial artery.

Radial Artery

The radial artery is the direct continuation of the brachial artery, beginning at the level of the neck of the radius. The vessel courses between the brachioradialis and flexor carpi radialis muscles, to the radial styloid process in the forearm. At the wrist, the radial artery passes to the dorsal aspect of the carpus under the tendons of the first extensor compartment. The artery crosses the scaphoid and trapezium in the anatomic snuffbox to pass between the heads of the first dorsal interosseous muscle to reach the palmar aspect of the hand. In the hand, the radial artery crosses the palm at first deep to the oblique head, and then between the oblique and transverse heads of the adductor pollicis muscle. The vessel anastomoses with the deep branch of the ulnar artery to complete the deep palmar arch (see Fig. 15-1, *A*). The main branches of the radial artery in the forearm are the radial recurrent artery given off laterally in the antecubital fossa, muscular branches to the adjacent muscles along its length, septocutaneous branches supplying the forearm integument, and palmar carpal branches. At the dorsal aspect of the wrist, the radial artery gives off the first dorsal metacarpal artery and the dorsal carpal arch. In the palm, the main branches are the princeps pollicis and the radialis indicis arteries, which are given off as the deep palmar arch is formed.

The radial recurrent artery, the largest branch of the radial artery in the forearm, arises in the antecubital fossa, passes between the divisions of the radial nerve to ascend deep to the brachioradialis muscle, and anastomoses with the radial collateral artery at the elbow (see Fig. 15-1, *A*).

The palmar carpal branch of the radial artery arises at the distal border of the pronator quadratus muscle. The artery passes medially, anterior to the distal radius, to anastomose with a branch from the ulnar artery to form the cruciate palmar carpal arch. This arch receives contributions from the anterior interosseous artery and a recurrent branch from the deep palmar arch.

The superficial palmar branch arises as the radial artery curves around the carpus and descends into the palm through or over the thenar muscles to anastomose with the ulnar artery and form the superficial palmar arch (see Fig. 15-1, *B*).

Ulnar Artery

The ulnar artery, which is the larger of the two terminal branches of the brachial artery, begins in the antecubital fossa and traverses the medial aspect of the forearm, lateral to the flexor carpi ulnaris muscle up to the wrist. The ulnar artery lies in a deeper plane than the radial artery and passes through Guyon's canal to enter the palm. The proximal branches of the ulnar artery are the anterior and posterior ulnar recurrent arteries (given off medially from the parent artery) and the common interosseous artery (given off laterally), which divides into the anterior and posterior interosseous arteries in the antecubital fossa (see Fig. 15-1, *B*). The anterior ulnar recurrent artery is also referred to as the *epitrochlear artery*.[3] In the forearm, the ulnar artery provides muscular branches to the adjacent muscles—flexor carpi ulnaris, flexor digitorum profundus, and pronator quadratus—and skin of the forearm over the medial aspect. In the proximal forearm, the ulnar artery gives rise to several musculocutaneous perforators that pass through the flexor muscles. In the distal forearm, the ulnar artery gives rise to a series of small septocutaneous perforators that supply the volar forearm skin and skin of the forearm over the medial aspect. The terminal branches of the ulnar artery in the wrist and hand are the palmar carpal branch, the dorsal carpal branch, and the deep palmar branches.

Anterior Interosseous Artery

The anterior interosseous artery arises from the common interosseous artery, almost immediately after it originates from the ulnar artery. The vessel courses on the anterior aspect of the interosseous membrane along with the anterior interosseous nerve lying between the flexor digitorum profundus and flexor pollicis longus muscles. The anterior interosseous artery supplies these muscles and then passes posterior to the pronator quadratus muscle. The anterior and posterior interosseous arteries lie on either side of the interosseous membrane. There are approximately three to five communications between these two vessels. The anterior interosseous artery gives a dorsal perforating branch that traverses the interosseous membrane at the proximal margin of the pronator quadratus muscle and terminates as a cutaneous branch supplying the integument on the dorsum of the wrist.

Posterior Interosseous Artery

The posterior interosseous artery is a branch of the common interosseous artery that emerges behind the interosseous membrane at the distal border of the supinator muscle. It is accompanied by the posterior interosseous nerve before the nerve forms terminal branches to supply the extensor muscles. The artery lies in the septum between the fifth and sixth extensor compartments, which contain the extensor digiti minimi and extensor carpi ulnaris muscles, respectively. The posterior interosseous artery gives the interosseous recurrent branch proximally, which proceeds superiorly to form part of an anastomosis around the elbow joint.

Deep Palmar Arch

The deep palmar arch is classically formed by the anastomoses of the terminal radial artery with the deep palmar branch of the ulnar artery at the level of the metacarpal bases. Many variations are noted in the formation of the deep palmar arch. This arch has been classified as two groups, depending on whether the contributing arteries anastomose completely or incompletely. The deep palmar arch is classified as *group I* if the arch is complete, with anastomoses of the two arteries. Coleman and Anson[9] reported this pattern in 97% of specimens. Group I is further subdivided into the following four types, defined by the vessels that form the arch:

- Type A: The arch is formed by the radial artery and the superior ramus of the deep branch of the ulnar artery.
- Type B: The arch is formed by the radial artery and inferior ramus of the deep branch of the ulnar artery.
- Type C: The arch is formed by the ramus of the deep branch of the ulnar artery and the radial artery.
- Type D: The arch is formed by the superior ramus of the deep branch of the ulnar artery and an enlarged superior perforating artery of the second intermetacarpal space.

The deep palmar arch is classified as *group II* if the arch is incomplete and the contributing arteries do not anastomose. Coleman and Anson[9] reported this pattern in 3% of dissections. Group II is subdivided into the following two types:

- Type A: The inferior deep branch of the ulnar artery joins the perforating branch of the second intermetacarpal space.
- Type B: The radial artery anastomoses with the perforating artery of the second intermetacarpal space, and the deep branch of the ulnar artery joins the perforating branch of the third intermetacarpal space.

The branches of the deep palmar arch are the palmar metacarpal, perforating, and recurrent branches. The palmar metacarpal arteries are extremely variable in size and range from three to six in number.[9] The princeps pollicis and radialis indicis arteries to the thumb and index finger, respectively, may arise from a common trunk as the first palmar metacarpal artery, or separately as the first and second palmar metacarpal arteries. The remaining palmar metacarpal arteries run in the second to fourth intermetacarpal spaces and join the common digital arteries, which are the terminal branches of the superficial palmar arch.

Perforating branches of the deep palmar arch pass through the second to fourth intermetacarpal spaces to anastomose with the dorsal metacarpal arteries, or may even form the dorsal metacarpal arteries. These branches provide the basis for the dorsal metacarpal artery flap (Chapter 20). Recurrent branches ascend proximally from the deep palmar arch to contribute to the palmar carpal arch, and to supply individual carpal bones.

Superficial Palmar Arch

The superficial palmar arch is formed by the ulnar artery in the palm, lateral to the pisiform, and curves laterally in line with the distal border of the fully extended thumb. Many variations in the formation have been described.[9] The superficial palmar arch has been classified as two groups, depending on whether the arch is complete or incomplete. The arch is classified as *group 1* if the arch is complete. This group is further subdivided into the following five types, according to the vessels that anastomose to form the arch:

- Type A: The arch is formed by the ulnar artery and the superficial branch of the radial artery. This pattern is the classical description of the superficial palmar arch.
- Type B: The arch is formed entirely from the ulnar artery and is the most common type seen (37% of specimens).
- Type C: The arch is formed by the ulnar artery and enlarged median artery.
- Type D: The arch is formed by the ulnar artery, the superficial branch of the radial artery, and the median arteries.
- Type E: The arch is formed by the ulnar artery and a branch of the deep arch.

The superficial palmar arch is classified as *group II* if the arch is incomplete, or if the ulnar artery does not supply the thumb and index finger.

The branches from the arch, the three common palmar digital arteries, join with the corresponding palmar metacarpal arteries from the deep palmar arch and divide into two proper palmar digital arteries. These arteries run along the contiguous sides of all four fingers. Coleman and Anson[9] have described even branching patterns of the superficial palmar artery.

Dorsal Carpal Arch

The dorsal carpal arch provides vascularity to the dorsum of the hand and is formed by the radial, ulnar, or interosseous artery branches. Six types of arches are described[9]:

- Type 1: The arch is formed by the anastomoses of the dorsal carpal branch of the radial artery, the posterior interosseous artery, and the anterior interosseous artery.
- Type 2: The arch is formed by the dorsal carpal branches of the radial, ulnar, and interosseous arteries.
- Type 3: The arch is formed solely by the dorsal carpal branch of the radial artery.
- Type 4: The arch is formed by the dorsal carpal branches of the radial and ulnar arteries.
- Type 5: The arch is formed by the dorsal carpal branches of the ulnar and interosseous arteries.
- Type 6: The dorsal arch is absent.

PERFORATOR GROUPS WITH SOURCE VESSELS

In our dissections, we identified 15 cutaneous vascular territories in the upper arm. Each territory was supplied by a named source artery that provided a variable number of cutaneous perforators (Fig. 15-4). The precise location and number of perforators in each territory were quite variable.[1] Despite this variability among individual perforators, the cutaneous areas or vascular territories supplied by the source vessels were relatively

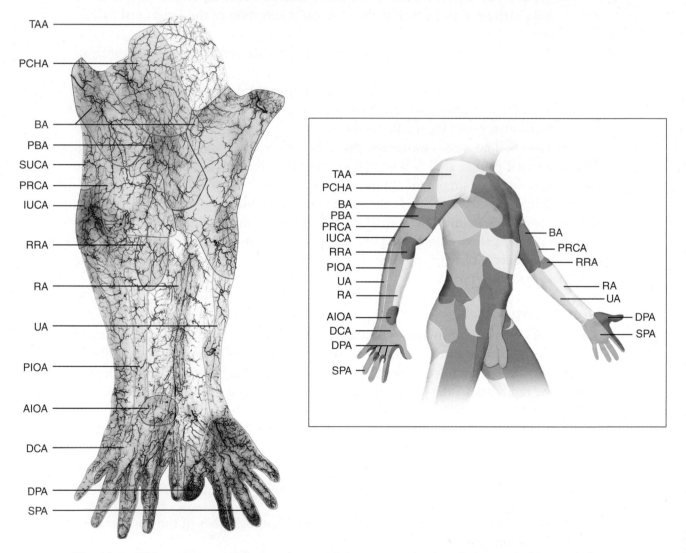

Fig. 15-4   This angiogram of the integument of the upper extremity of a human cadaver was obtained using the lead oxide and gelatin injection technique. The vascular territories of the upper limb are shown in different colors. Each color corresponds to a different source artery. To prepare this angiogram, a medial incision was made along a line from the axilla over the medial epicondyle, and along the ulnar aspect of the forearm and hand. (Vascular territories are listed in Table 15-1.)

uniform. Table 15-1 presents observations from our dissections, including the average area of the integument supplied by each perforator and the ratio of the area supplied by the musculocutaneous perforators and septocutaneous perforators. The integument of the upper extremity constitutes approximately 10% of the total surface area of the body. An average of 48 ± 19 perforators (at least 0.5 mm diameter) in 15 vascular territories supplied the integument of the upper extremity (see Fig. 15-4). Septocutaneous arteries predominated in the shoulder, elbow, distal forearm, and hand regions. Musculocutaneous perforators were more numerous in the upper arm and proximal forearm. The average perforator in the upper extremity was approximately 0.7 ± 0.2 mm in diameter and supplied an average of 35 cm².

Table 15-1 Cutaneous Vascular Territories of the Upper Extremity

Code	Vascular Territory	Number (≥0.5 mm)	Superficial Length (mm)	Diameter (mm)	Total Area (cm²)	Area/ Perforator (cm²)	Area of Region (%)	Ratio (MC/SC)
Shoulder and Arm								
TAA	Thoracoacromial artery	3 (± 1)	37 (± 18)	0.8 (± 0.2)	109 (± 48)	36 (± 25)	6 (± 3)	9:1
PCHA	Posterior circumflex humeral artery	3 (± 2)	49 (± 16)	1.0 (± 0.2)	113 (± 54)	43 (± 20)	6 (± 3)	9:1
SUCA	Superior ulnar collateral artery	2 (± 1)	56 (± 34)	0.9 (± 0.2)	94 (± 29)	39 (± 21)	5 (± 2)	1:9
PBA	Profunda brachial artery	4 (± 2)	28 (± 12)	0.7 (± 0.2)	131 (± 30)	31 (± 20)	7 (± 2)	7:3
BA	Brachial artery	6 (± 4)	30 (± 14)	0.7 (± 0.4)	162 (± 42)	27 (± 19)	9 (± 2)	1:1
PRCA	Posterior radial collateral artery	2 (± 1)	49 (± 15)	1.0 (± 0.2)	64 (± 31)	32 (± 35)	3 (± 2)	3:2
Forearm								
IUCA	Inferior ulnar collateral artery	2 (± 1)	35 (± 12)	0.8 (± 0.2)	63 (± 20)	31 (± 13)	3 (± 1)	3:7
RRA	Radial recurrent artery	2 (± 1)	37 (± 18)	0.7 (± 0.3)	55 (± 27)	32 (± 8)	2 (± 1)	4:1
RA	Radial artery	5 (± 5)	32 (± 25)	0.6 (± 0.2)	180 (± 68)	35 (± 48)	10 (± 4)	7:3
UA	Ulnar artery	7 (± 2)	27 (± 14)	0.6 (± 0.2)	186 (± 58)	26 (± 7)	10 (± 3)	3:2
PIOA	Posterior interosseous artery	5 (± 2)	21 (± 11)	0.5 (± 0.1)	116 (± 43)	22 (± 15)	6 (± 2)	9:1
AIOA	Anterior interosseous artery	3 (± 1)	21 (± 10)	0.5 (± 0.1)	27 (± 12)	9 (± 6)	1 (± 1)	4:1
Hand								
DCA	Dorsal carpal arch	1*	32	0.5	116	117	6	0:1
DPA	Deep palmar arch	1*	36	1.5	85	85	5	0:1
SPA	Superficial palmar arch	1*	65	1.8	171	171	9	0:1

*Territories DCA, DPA, and SPA were analyzed as a single perforator.
MC, Musculocutaneous; *SC*, septocutaneous.

Anatomic Subregions

The upper extremity integument has been divided into the following three subregions based on arbitrary boundaries to facilitate description: shoulder and arm, forearm, and hand (see Table 15-1).

The shoulder and arm subregion is bounded by the anterior (deltopectoral groove), superior, and posterior margins of the deltoid muscle to the elbow flexion crease. The forearm subregion extends from the elbow flexion crease to the wrist. The hand subregion includes the wrist and hand.

Shoulder and Arm

The principal source vessels of the vascular territories of the shoulder and arm subregion are the thoracoacromial and posterior circumflex humeral arteries (Fig. 15-5). The upper arm is supplied by the brachial artery medially and the profunda brachial artery laterally. Perforators emerge mainly along the medial and lateral intermuscular septum (Figs. 15-6 and 15-7).

The medial aspect of the arm may be divided into two regions: one anterior and one posterior to the brachial artery (see Fig. 15-6). The anterior area is supplied by direct branches from the brachial artery. The posterior area is supplied by two large branches from the brachial artery: the posterior brachial cutaneous artery superiorly and the superior ulnar collateral artery inferiorly. The lateral aspect of the arm is supplied through direct branches of the profunda brachial artery and the posterior radial collateral artery and middle collateral branches.

Thoracoacromial Artery Territory

The major perforators to the skin over the anterior shoulder arise from the deltoid branch of the thoracoacromial artery, which descends in the deltopectoral groove (see Figs. 15-1, *A*, and 15-6). Near the middle of the deltopectoral groove, the deltoid branch of the thoracoacromial artery turns superficially to supply the skin. A prominent cutaneous perforator from this artery supplying the skin has been called the *anterior subcutaneous deltoid artery*.[1,2,10,11] The diameter of the main perforator was 0.8 ± 0.2 mm in our dissections. There were 3 ± 1 perforators given from the thoracoacromial artery to supply skin over the anterior aspect of the deltoid. In 75% of specimens, these branches were musculocutaneous, emerging through the marginal fibers of the deltoid muscle. The average superficial pedicle length was 37 ± 18 mm, and the diameter of the thoracoacromial artery at its origin was 2.5 ± 0.5 mm. The total area of the territory was 109 ± 48 cm^2, and the musculocutaneous/septocutaneous perforator ratio was 9:1. The cutaneous branches anastomosed with those from the posterior aspect, usually near the middle of the shoulder region. The thoracoacromial artery, with the deltoid branch and the cutaneous area it supplies, can be used as a potential perforator flap with reliable vascularity and consistent anatomy.

Posterior Circumflex Humeral Artery Territory

The posterior circumflex humeral artery arises from the axillary artery and traverses the quadrangular space to reach the subdeltoid area (see Figs. 15-2 and 15-5). A large perforator called the *posterior subcutaneous deltoid artery* has been reported and described

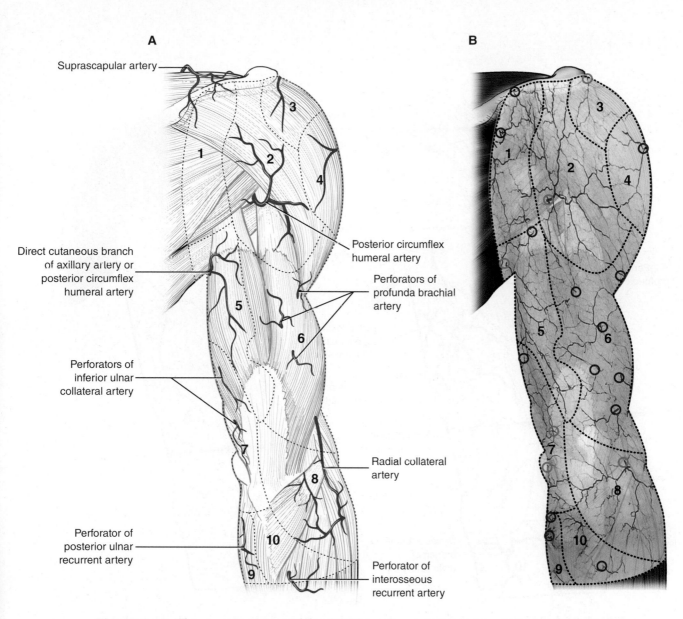

Fig. 15-5 A, The posterior aspect of the shoulder and arm showing the principal branches to the integument. **B,** This angiogram of the integument of the posterior aspect of the right shoulder and arm is from a human cadaver injected with lead oxide and gelatin. *Red circles* identify musculocutaneous perforators; *blue circles* show septocutaneous perforators. Anatomic territories of the cutaneous blood supply are numbered as follows: *1,* Suprascapular artery; *2,* posterior circumflex humeral artery; *3,* deltoid branch of the thoracoacromial artery; *4,* anterior circumflex humeral artery; *5,* direct cutaneous branch of the axillary artery; *6,* profunda brachial artery; *7,* inferior ulnar collateral artery; *8,* radial collateral artery; *9,* posterior ulnar recurrent artery; *10,* interosseous recurrent artery.

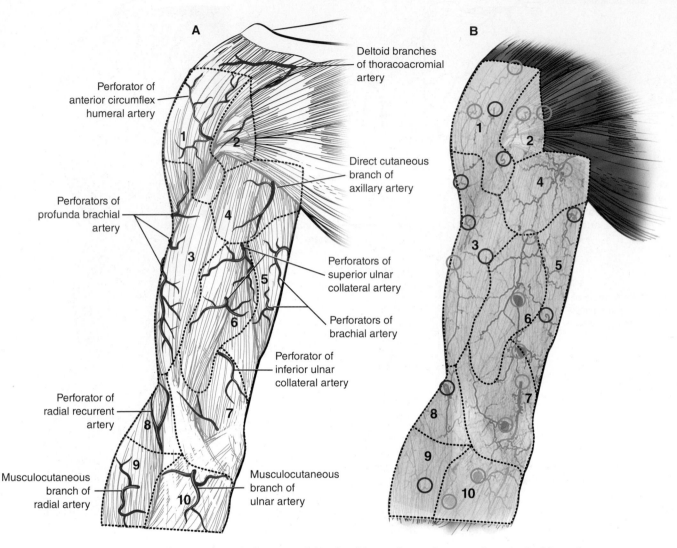

Fig. 15-6 A, The anteromedial aspect of the shoulder and arm showing the principal branches to the integument. **B,** An angiogram of the integument of the anteromedial aspect of the right shoulder and arm from a human cadaver injected with lead oxide and gelatin. Anatomic territories of cutaneous blood supply are numbered as follows: *1,* Anterior circumflex humeral artery; *2,* deltoid branches of the thoracoacromial arteries; *3,* profunda brachial artery; *4,* direct cutaneous branch of the axillary artery; *5,* brachial artery; *6,* superior ulnar collateral artery; *7,* inferior ulnar collateral artery; *8,* radial recurrent artery; *9,* musculocutaneous branch of the radial artery; *10,* musculocutaneous branch of the ulnar artery.

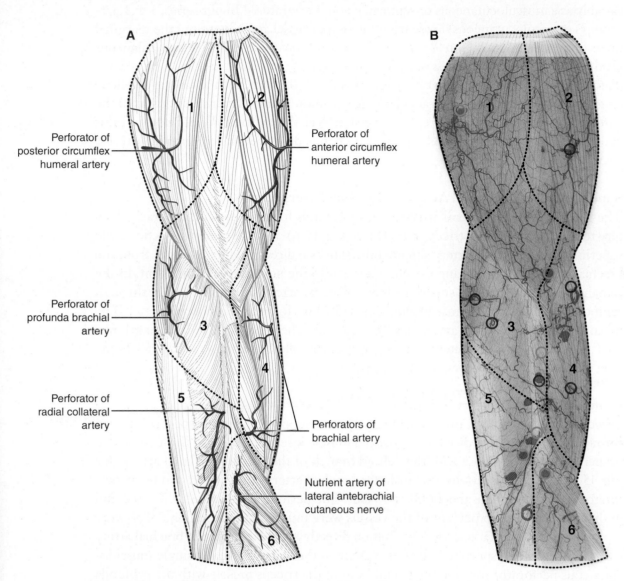

A

Perforator of
posterior circumflex
humeral artery

Perforator of
anterior circumflex
humeral artery

Perforator of
profunda brachial
artery

Perforator of
radial collateral
artery

Perforators of
brachial artery

Nutrient artery of
lateral antebrachial
cutaneous nerve

B

Fig. 15-7 A, The lateral aspect of the shoulder and arm showing the principal branches to the integument. **B,** An angiogram of the integument of the lateral aspect of the right shoulder and arm from a human cadaver injected with lead oxide and gelatin. *Red circles* identify musculocutaneous perforators; *blue circles* represent septocutaneous perforators. Anatomic territories of cutaneous blood supply are numbered as follows: *1,* Posterior circumflex humeral artery; *2,* anterior circumflex humeral artery; *3,* profunda brachial artery; *4,* brachial artery; *5,* radial collateral artery; *6,* inferior ulnar collateral artery.

variably as a musculocutaneous or septocutaneous perforator.[1,2] In our series, 3 ± 2 perforators (musculocutaneous) arose from the source vessel and penetrated the marginal fibers of the deltoid muscle in 91% of the dissections (musculocutaneous/septocutaneous ratio was 9:1). The average area of the vascular territory was 113 ± 54 cm². The average diameter of the source vessel at its origin was 2.5 ± 0.3 mm, with an average pedicle length of 6 to 8 cm to the quadrangular space. Salmon reported contributions from the anterior circumflex humeral artery to the skin over the deltoid. We did not find this contribution in our dissections. The deltoid flap is described based on the posterior circumflex humeral artery.[12,13]

Superior Ulnar Collateral Artery or Brachial Artery Territory

The superior ulnar collateral artery territory extends from the axis of the brachial artery to the midline of the triceps muscle (see Fig. 15-6). In 30% of our dissections, the superior ulnar collateral artery supplied the skin as a direct cutaneous vessel from the brachial artery, accompanying the ulnar nerve into the posterior compartment. In the remaining dissections, the superior ulnar collateral artery supplied the skin through septocutaneous (95%) or musculocutaneous (5%) perforators, numbering 2 ± 1. The mean area supplied by the artery was 94 ± 29 cm². The superficial pedicle length was 56 ± 34 mm, and the diameter of the superior ulnar collateral artery was 0.9 ± 0.2 mm. The medial arm flap is based on this vessel.[14-16]

Profunda Brachial Artery Territory

Direct branches from the profunda brachial artery supply the lateral aspect of the arm through direct branches distal to the deltoid muscle insertion, and also through medial branches that anastomose with the deltoid branch of the throacoacromial artery (see Fig. 15-7). In our dissections, the profunda brachial artery contributed two to six perforators with an average area of 131 ± 30 cm². The perforators averaged 0.7 ± 0.2 mm in diameter. Sixty-two percent of the vessels were musculocutaneous, and 38% were septocutaneous. The cutaneous contribution directly from the profunda brachial artery was variable. In one specimen, the only supply to the skin was from a single musculocutaneous perforator through the lateral head of the triceps muscle with the profunda brachial artery traversing the spiral groove. In another dissection, the posterior brachial cutaneous artery originated from the profunda brachial artery. The major branch from the profunda brachial artery, the posterior radial collateral artery, is considered as a separate territory because of its important contribution to the lateral aspect of the arm.

Brachial Artery Territory

The brachial artery sends perforators to the skin on either side of the biceps muscle and to skin over the insertion of the deltoid muscle (see Figs. 15-3 and 15-6). In our series, the number of perforators supplying this territory ranged from 2 to 10 (average 6 ± 4). Perforators coursed between the biceps and brachialis muscles to supply the skin over the lateral bicipital groove, from the deltoid muscle insertion as far down as the elbow flexion crease near the insertion of the biceps tendon. The musculocutaneous/septocutaneous perforator ratio was 1:1 in this territory. The average area supplied by the brachial artery was 162 $\pm$ 42 cm^2. The mean diameter of the perforators was 0.7 $\pm$ 0.4 mm. The superficial length of the perforator vessel was 30 $\pm$ 14 mm.

A consistent, large cutaneous branch from the brachial artery with a mean diameter of 1.5 mm and a pedicle length of 6.2 cm has been observed. This branch, the posterior brachial cutaneous artery, supplies the posterior brachial arm flap[17,18] (see Fig. 15-3).

Posterior Radial Collateral Artery Territory

There is confusion in the literature regarding the terminology and anatomy of the branches from the profunda brachial artery. According to Cormack and Lamberty,[6,19] there are two terminal branches from the profunda brachial artery. The middle and the radial collateral arteries are the terminal branches of the profunda brachial artery. The middle collateral artery runs posterior to the lateral intermuscular septum, passes through the long and medial head of the triceps and behind the humeral diaphysis, and anastomoses with the interosseous recurrent artery arising from the posterior interosseous artery, posterior to the lateral epicondyle.[6] The radial collateral artery accompanies the radial nerve. Proximal to the lateral intermuscular septum, it divides into a smaller anterior radial collateral artery, which follows the radial nerve, and a larger posterior radial collateral artery. The posterior radial collateral artery is accompanied by the posterior cutaneous nerve of the arm and gives off numerous septocutaneous branches to the skin of the lateral and distal half of the arm through septocutaneous perforators. There were 2 $\pm$ 1 perforators in our dissections. The average area of skin supplied was 64 $\pm$ 31 cm^2. The posterior radial collateral artery had a diameter of 1.6 $\pm$ 0.2 mm, and averaged 5.8 cm in length, beginning at its origin from the profunda brachial artery. The superficial pedicle length was 49 $\pm$ 15 mm. The musculocutaneous/septocutaneous perforator ratio was 3:2.

The posterior radial collateral artery has been extensively used with the skin area it supplies as the lateral arm flap, especially for upper extremity reconstruction[20-24] (see Chapter 16). This vessel can be used as an osteocutaneous flap, because branches from the posterior radial collateral artery also supply the lateral aspect of the lower half of the humerus. The radial recurrent artery anastomoses with the posterior radial collateral artery and can be included in the flap harvest.

Taylor and Palmer[5] have included the posterior radial collateral artery territory with the profunda brachial artery angiosomes. In this book, the artery has been labeled as a separate territory because of the consistency of the area supplied (unlike the profunda brachial artery territory) and because of its importance as the pedicle for the lateral arm flap.

The Forearm

Three main vessels supply most of the forearm. These vessels are the radial, ulnar, and posterior interosseous arteries, with minor contribution from the anterior interosseous artery. At the elbow, perforators originating from the extensive anastomoses around the elbow from the collateral and recurrent branches of the brachial, radial, and ulnar arteries supply the skin. The anterior interosseous artery contributes to the supply of the dorsal radial aspect of the distal forearm through a dorsal perforating cutaneous branch (see Fig. 15-1, *B*).

Inferior Ulnar Collateral and Ulnar Recurrent Artery Territories

The inferior ulnar collateral and ulnar recurrent arteries are considered together because of the variability and inverse relationship shown by these source vessels in supplying the medial aspect of the elbow (see Figs. 15-1, *A*, and 15-3). The anterior ulnar recurrent artery is also referred to as the *epitrochlear artery*.[3] In our series, an average of 2 ± 1 perforators were found in this territory. The mean vessel diameter was 0.8 ± 0.2 mm, with a superficial length of 35 ± 12 mm. The average area supplied by each perforator was 63 ± 20 cm². The musculocutaneous/septocutaneous perforator ratio was 3:7. Flaps raised on either pedicle can be useful for soft tissue coverage in the elbow region.

Radial Recurrent and Interosseous Recurrent Artery Territories

The radial recurrent and interosseous recurrent artery territories are considered together because of the variability and inverse relationship shown by these source vessels in supplying the lateral aspect of the elbow. In our dissections, there was an average of 2 ± 1 perforators from these source vessels. The average perforator diameter was 0.7 ± 0.3 mm. The musculocutaneous/septocutaneous perforator ratio was 4:1. The perforators supplied an area of 55 ± 27 cm² and had an average superficial pedicle length of 37 ± 18 mm.

The radial recurrent artery is otherwise referred to as the *epicondylar artery*.[3] These recurrent vessels anastomose with the posterior radial collateral artery over the lateral epicondyle. This anastomosis has been used in harvesting a reverse lateral arm flap for local coverage around the elbow.[25,26]

Radial Artery Territory

In our dissections, septocutaneous and musculocutaneous perforators from the radial artery supplied the lateral half of the forearm. These vessels ranged in number from 4 to 7 (mean 5). The perforators were generally musculocutaneous in the proximal forearm and septocutaneous in the distal forearm. The average vessel diameter was 0.6 ± 0.2 mm, and the average area supplied was 80 ± 68 cm². The superficial length of the perforator averaged 32 ± 25 mm. The musculocutaneous/septocutaneous perforator ratio was 7:3 (Fig. 15-8).

The radial artery provides many options for flap harvest.[27] Its numerous septocutaneous perforators allow harvest of proximally and distally based flaps (see Chapter 19). It is one of the most versatile flaps based pedicled and free skin, fascia, and osteocutaneous flaps. Perforator flaps have been based on branches of the radial artery to preserve the vessel. Two consistent perforators from the radial artery (one proximal and one distal) that have been used for this purpose are noted in our angiograms. The proximal perforator is the inferior cubital artery[28-31]; the distal perforator is a septocutaneous perforator located just proximal to the wrist.[27,30,32] The inferior cubital artery can arise from the radial or the radial recurrent arteries, and is located between the deep branch of the cephalic vein and the medial cubital vein. This artery is the most proximal perforator from the radial artery. A flap size of approximately 4 by 17 cm has been reported.[6,29,33]

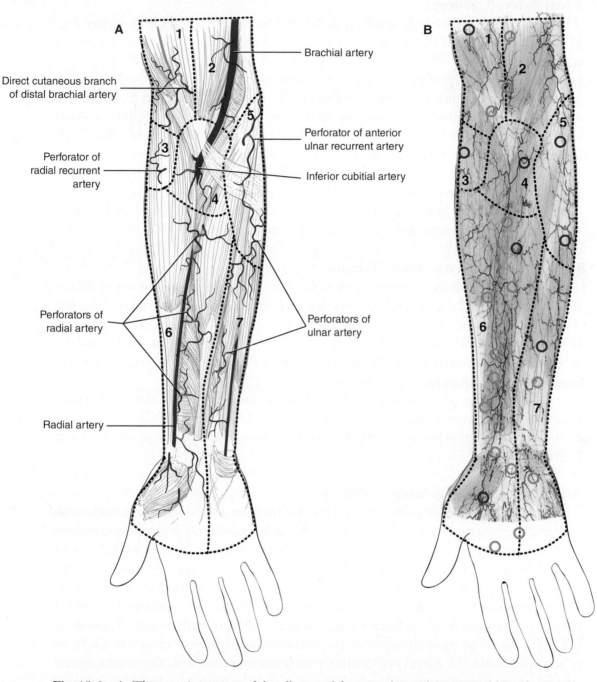

Fig. 15-8 A, The anterior aspect of the elbow and forearm shows the principal branches to the integument. **B,** The corresponding angiogram of the skin of the volar forearm showing cutaneous perforators. *Red circles* demonstrate musculocutaneous perforators, and *blue circles* show septocutaneous perforators. Anatomic territories of cutaneous blood supply are numbered as follows: *1,* Posterior radial collateral artery; *2,* brachial artery; *3,* radial recurrent artery; *4,* inferior cubital artery; *5,* anterior ulnar recurrent artery; *6,* radial artery; *7,* ulnar artery.

Ulnar Artery Territory

The ulnar artery consistently supplied the medial forearm in our dissections (see Fig. 15-8). There were four to nine perforators from the ulnar artery, supplying an area of approximately 190 cm². Most of the perforators were musculocutaneous (69%) and penetrated the flexor carpi ulnaris muscle. The mean superficial perforator pedicle length was 27 ± 14 mm. In one dissection, the ulnar artery originated directly from the axillary artery and proceeded subcutaneously along the arm and forearm. This path is reported in approximately 10% of dissections and has been used as a fasciocutaneous flap.[34] Although the ulnar artery is not as commonly used in flap surgery as the radial artery, it provides a reliable flap that can be used as a pedicle or free flap.[35-37] In particular, the dorsal branch of the ulnar artery has been used in a pedicle flap for local coverage.[38] A consistent perforator supplying skin over the dorsum of the hand has been described as the *ulnar parametacarpal flap* and can be harvested as a perforator flap.[39,40]

Posterior Interosseous Artery Territory

The posterior interosseous artery supplied the skin of the dorsal forearm in our dissections through 5 ± 2 discrete perforators that were approximately 0.5 mm in diameter. These vessels provided an average skin area of 116 ± 43 cm². The superficial length of the perforator pedicle was 21 ± 11 mm. The close relation between the branches of the posterior interosseous nerve is of importance during flap harvest. The musculocutaneous/septocutaneous perforator ratio was 9:1 (Fig. 15-9).

The posterior interosseous artery flap has been used for upper extremity reconstruction as a cutaneous and osteocutaneous flap[30,41-43] (see Chapter 14). The difficulties encountered with this flap have included venous congestion, thus prompting its use as a free flap.

Anterior Interosseous Artery Territory

The anterior interosseous artery supplied the skin over the distal dorsal forearm through its dorsal perforating branch, which is given off near its entry into the pronator quadratus muscle. An average total area of 27 ± 12 cm was supplied. The number of perforators ranged from 2 to 4 (mean 3 ± 1). The dorsal perforating branch pierces the interosseous membrane and emerges between the muscles of the first extensor compartment and the extensor digitorum communis tendons, approximately 4 cm proximal to Lister's tubercle. The superficial perforator length was 21 ± 10 mm with a mean diameter of 0.5 ± 0.1 mm. The musculocutaneous/septocutaneous perforator ratio was 4:1. In six of our specimens, the dorsal perforating branch anastomosed with the intercompartmental supraretinacular artery,[1,2] which has provided the source for vascularized bone grafts for scaphoid nonunions.[44] The dorsal perforating branch then gave off three to four branches to supply the skin over the distal third of the dorsum of the forearm. This dorsal perforator of the anterior interosseous artery has been used primarily as a pedicle "posterior interosseous flap and also as a free flap."[45]

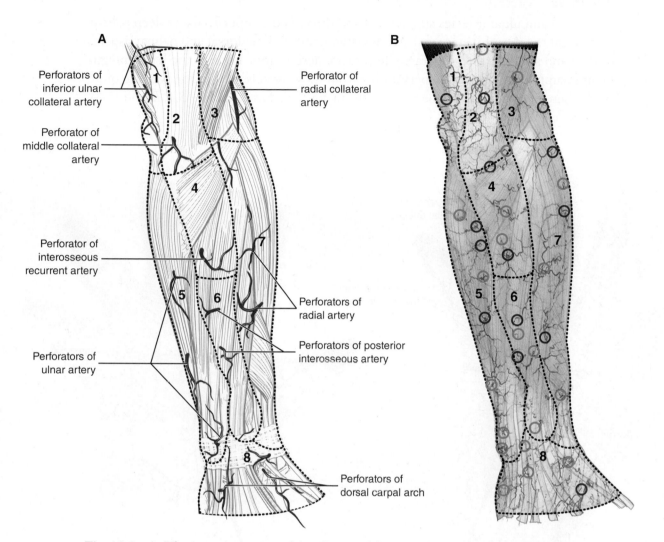

Fig. 15-9 **A,** The posterior aspect of the elbow and forearm shows the principal branches to the integument. **B,** An angiogram of the integument of the posterior aspect of the right elbow and forearm from a human cadaver injected with lead oxide and gelatin. *Red circles* identify musculocutaneous perforators; *blue circles* show territories of cutaneous blood supply and are numbered as follows: *1,* Inferior ulnar collateral artery; *2,* middle collateral artery; *3,* radial collateral artery; *4,* interosseous recurrent artery; *5,* ulnar artery; *6,* posterior interosseous artery; *7,* radial artery; *8,* dorsal carpal arch.

The Hand

The radial and ulnar arteries supply the hand through the superficial and deep palmar arches and the dorsal metacarpal arteries (Fig. 15-10).[46] The dorsal and palmar aspects of the hand are described separately for ease of description. Though the hand integument is supplied profusely by perforators from these vessels, the perforators are quite small; therefore we will describe them by the major branches (see Figs. 15-1, *B*, and 15-4).

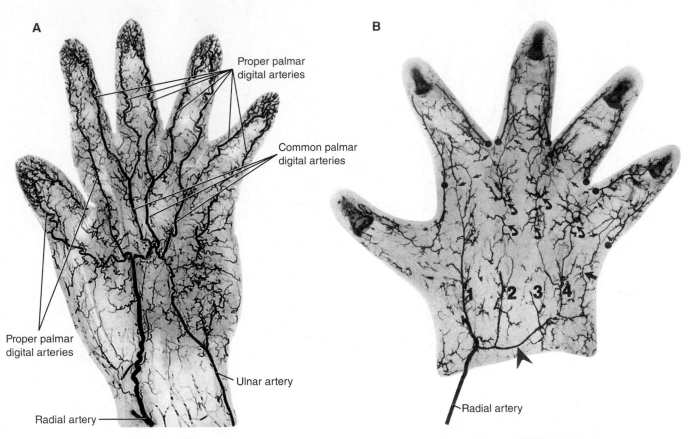

Fig. 15-10   A, This angiogram of human hand volar skin was obtained using the lead oxide and gelatin arterial injection technique. It shows the radial and ulnar arteries, superficial palmar arch, common palmar digital arteries, radial and ulnar proper digital arteries to each digit, and anastomotic pathways between each of the main arteries. Note the dense concentration of small vessels at the fingertips. **B,** This angiogram of human hand dorsal skin was obtained using the lead oxide and gelatin arterial injection technique. The radial artery provides the main arterial supply to the dorsal skin. The dorsal carpal arch *(large arrow)* and the dorsal metacarpal arteries *(1 through 4)* are shown. Note the perforating branches to the dorsum from the palmar digital arteries *(curved arrows)*, which supply for dorsal metacarpal artery flap. The volar digital skin has been incised in the midline of each digit to show the vascular anastomoses between the palmar digital arteries *(black circles)* and the dorsal skin *(small arrows)*. (From Yang D, Morris SF. Reversed dorsal digital and metacarpal island flaps supplied by the dorsal cutaneous branches of the palmar digital artery. Ann Plast Surg 46:444-449, 2001.)

Superficial Palmar Arch Territory

The palm and fingers are usually supplied by the superficial and deep palmar arches. The superficial palmar arch supplies the skin over the palm and the ulnar three fingers, the ulnar half of the index finger, and the skin over the dorsum of the fingers through the dorsal branches of the digital arteries. Small branches from the superficial palmar arch pierce the palmar aponeurosis to supply the skin in the palmar triangle. A perforator-based flap from the radial aspect of the midpalm, and based on perforators from the terminal branch of the superficial palmar arch and the princeps pollicis artery, was described for coverage of thumb defects,[47,48] and for palmar coverage in surgery for Dupuytren's disease.[49]

Deep Palmar Arch Territory

The deep palmar arch supplies the thumb and the index finger over the palmar aspect by the princeps pollicis and radialis indicis arteries, and the dorsal aspect of the hand through the perforating branches. The perforating branches arose through the second, third, and fourth intermetacarpal spaces in our dissections to supply the dorsal skin of the hand through a direct cutaneous branch. This branch also communicates with the dorsal metacarpal artery of the corresponding area, or may be solely supplied by the dorsal metacarpal artery if the perforating branch is absent. An ingenious cutaneous flap has been described based on the direct cutaneous branch supplying the dorsum of the hand.[50]

Dorsal Metacarpal and Dorsal Carpal Arch Territory

The vascular anatomy of the dorsal metacarpal and dorsal carpal arch area has been well analyzed and described.[9,46,51] The dorsum of the hand and fingers is supplied by three major groups of arteries. The dorsal metacarpal arteries supply the proximal two thirds of the hand. The dorsal perforating branches of the deep palmar arch supply the distal third of the hand and proximal dorsal fingers. The dorsal cutaneous branches of the palmar digital arteries and the dorsal digital branches of the dorsal metacarpal arteries supply the dorsal aspect of the fingers.[46,51]

The dorsal metacarpal arteries supply the proximal aspect of the dorsal skin of the hand[46,51] (see Fig. 15-10). These arteries arise from the radial artery and the dorsal carpal arch. Our studies demonstrated that the first dorsal metacarpal artery arises directly from the radial artery and travels along the radial aspect of the second metacarpal bone. The second, third, and fourth dorsal metacarpal arteries arise from the dorsal carpal arch and run distally along the third, fourth, and fifth metacarpal bone, respectively. These arteries lie deep to the extensor tendons and supply the skin by minute branches given at intervals from the parent vessel. At the neck of the metacarpal, the dorsal perforating branches from the deep palmar arch supply the dorsal skin of the hand. These anastomose with the dorsal metacarpal arteries at the distal metacarpal level.

The dorsal perforating branches of the deep palmar arch supply the distal third of the dorsum of hand. These branches reach the skin through one to two perforators in the second, third, and fourth intermetacarpal spaces at the level of the metacarpal neck. They anastomose with branches from the dorsal metacarpal arteries proximally, the dorsal cutaneous branches of the palmar digital arteries distally, and with adjacent perforating branches laterally. The vascular anatomy of dorsal digital and dorsal meta-carpal flaps has been extensively studied.[46,51,52]

Flaps based on the dorsal metacarpal arteries have been used extensively to re-construct defects of the hand, especially the thumb,[46,53-55] and index finger.[56] Various flap modifications have been described.[57-61] The dorsum of the digits has two cutane-ous vascular sources: the dorsal digital branches of the dorsal metacarpal arteries and the dorsal cutaneous branches of the palmar digital arteries. The anastomoses between branches of these two vessels are seen in the proximal phalanx area. The palmar digital arteries supply the dorsal skin beyond the distal third of the proximal phalanx. In the small finger, the dorsal carpal branch of the ulnar artery anastomoses with the ulnar dorsal branches of the palmar digital arteries. Koshima and colleagues[62] have recently described flaps based on the perforators from the digital artery.

VARIABILITY IN VASCULAR ANATOMY

It is well known that there is considerable variation in vascular anatomy. In the course of the dissections that were the basis of this and the other anatomic chapters in this book, we observed considerable variation in both the main source vessels supplying perforators to the skin and in the perforators themselves. Without large sample sizes, it is difficult to predict the frequency of vascular variability. Surgeons must consider the possibility of vascular variability when planning surgical procedures in the upper limb. It is important to use all of the available information, including physical examination, Doppler studies, and possibly arteriograms, before surgery to determine if any variability in the vasculature exists and whether there has been any change to the vasculature as a result of tumors or trauma. Tountas and Bergman[63] have compiled an excellent review of the topic of vascular variability in the upper limb.

References

1. Manchot C, ed. Die Hautarterien des Menschlichen Körpers. Leipzig: FCW Vogel, 1889.
2. Morain WD, Ristic J, eds. The Cutaneous Arteries of the Human Body [translation]. New York: Springer-Verlag, 1983.
3. Salmon M, ed. Arteries of the Skin. London: Churchill Livingstone, 1988.
4. Salmon M, ed. Arteries of the Muscles of the Extremities and the Trunk. St Louis: Quality Medical Publishing, 1994.
5. Taylor GI, Palmer JH. The vascular territories (angiosomes) of the body: experimental study and clinical applications. Br J Plast Surg 40:113-141, 1987.
6. Cormack GC, Lamberty BG, eds. The Arterial Anatomy of Skin Flaps. London: Churchill Livingstone, 1986.
7. Rees MJ, Taylor GI. A simplified lead oxide cadaver injection technique. Plast Reconstr Surg 77:141-145, 1986.
8. Warwick W, ed. Gray's Anatomy. London: Churchill Livingstone, 1989.
9. Coleman SS, Anson BJ. Arterial patterns in the hand based upon a study of 650 specimens. Surg Gynecol Obstet 113:409-424, 1961.
   This paper presented the results of an extensive study of the vasculature of 650 hands. The arches of the hand were examined in great detail and the variations reported. Classifications of the various patterns were well tabulated and illustrated.

10. Nakajima K, Ide Y, Abe S, et al. Anatomical study of the pectoral branch of thoracoacromial artery. Bull Tokyo Dent Coll 38:207-215, 1997.

11. Geddes CR, Tang ML, Yang D, et al. An assessment of the anatomical basis of the thoracoacromial artery perforator flap. Can J Plast Surg 11:23-27, 2003.

12. Russell RC, Guy RJ, Zook EG, et al. Extremity reconstruction using the free deltoid flap. Plast Reconstr Surg 76:586-595, 1985.

13. Volpe CM, Peterson S, Doerr RJ, et al. Forequarter amputation with fasciocutaneous deltoid flap reconstruction for malignant tumors of the upper extremity. Ann Surg Oncol 4:298-302, 1997.

14. Hentz VR, Pearl RM, Kaplan EN. Use of the medial upper arm skin as an arterialised flap. Hand 12:241-247, 1980.

15. Gao XS, Mao ZR, Yang ZN, et al. Medial upper arm skin flap: vascular anatomy and clinical applications. Ann Plast Surg 15:348-351, 1985.

16. Breidenbach WC, Adamson W, Terzis JK. Medial arm flap revisited. Ann Plast Surg 18:156-163, 1987.

17. Matlaub HS, Ye Z, Yousif NJ, et al. The medial arm flap. Ann Plast Surg 29:517-522, 1992.

18. Masquelet AC, Rinaldi S. Anatomical basis of the posterior brachial skin flap. Anat Clin 7:155-160, 1985.

19. Cormack GC, Lamberty BG. Fasciocutaneous vessels in the upper arm: application to the design of new fasciocutaneous flaps. Plast Reconstr Surg 74:244-250, 1984.

    The authors described principles of the blood supply to the upper arm and explained the role of fasciocutaneous perforators emerging along the medial and lateral intermuscular septa. They reported the available length and diameter of the middle collateral artery, from which perforators arise on the lateral side, and described a flap based on this vessel.

20. Katsaros J, Schusterman M, Hanel DP, et al. The lateral upper arm flap: anatomy and clinical applications. Ann Plast Surg 12:489-500, 1984.

    In this pioneer article, the authors described the anatomy and clinical applications of the lateral arm on the posterolateral aspect of the distal upper arm. They evaluated the area supplied by the posterior radial collateral artery, a direct continuation of the profunda brachii.

21. Scheker LR, Kleinert HE, Hanel DP. Lateral arm composite tissue transfer to ipsilateral hand defects (Part 1). J Hand Surg Am 12:665-672, 1987.

22. Scheker LR, Lister GD, Wolff TW. The lateral arm free flap in releasing severe contracture of the first web space. J Hand Surg Br 13:146-150, 1988.

23. Waterhouse N, Healy C. The versatility of the lateral arm flap. Br J Plast Surg 43:398-402, 1990.

24. Teoh LC, Khoo DB, Lim BH. Osteocutaneous lateral arm flap in hand reconstruction. Ann Acad Med Singapore 24(Suppl 4):15-20, 1995.

25. Lai CS, Lin SD, Chou CK, et al. The reverse lateral arm flap, based on the interosseous recurrent artery for cubital fossa burns. Br J Plast Surg 47:341-345, 1994.

26. Lai CS, Tsai CC, Liao KB, et al. The reverse lateral arm adipofascial flap for elbow coverage. Ann Plast Surg 39:196-200, 1997.

27. Yang D, Morris SF, Geddes CR, et al. Reversed forearm flap supplied by septocutaneous perforator of the radial artery: anatomical basis and clinical applications. Plast Reconstr Surg 112:1012-1016, 2003.

28. Lamberty BG, Cormack GC. The forearm angiotomes. Br J Plast Surg 35:420-429, 1982.

29. Lamberty BG, Cormack GC. The antecubital fascio-cutaneous flap. Br J Plast Surg 36:428-433, 1983.

30. El-Khatib H, Zeidan M. Island adipofascial flap based on distal perforators of the radial artery: an anatomic and clinical investigation. Plast Reconstr Surg 100:1762-1766, 1997.

31. El-Khatib HA. Island fasciocutaneous flap based on the proximal perforators of the radial artery for resurfacing of burned cubital fossa. Plast Reconstr Surg 100:919-925, 1997.

32. Koshima I, Moriguchi T, Etoh H, et al. The radial artery perforator-based adipofascial flap for dorsal hand coverage. Ann Plast Surg 35:474-479, 1995.

33. Ho AM, Chang J. Radial artery perforator flap. J Hand Surg Am 35:308-311, 2010.

34. Devansh. Superficial ulnar artery flap. Plast Reconstr Surg 97:420-426, 1996.

35. Lovie MJ, Duncan GM, Glasson DW. The ulnar artery forearm free flap. Br J Plast Surg 37:486-492, 1984.

36. Koshima I, Lamberty BG, Cormack GC. The forearm angiotomes. Br J Plast Surg 35:420-429, 1982.

37. Guimberteau J, Goin JL, Panconi B, et al. The reverse ulnar artery forearm island flap in hand surgery: 54 cases. Plast Reconstr Surg 81:925-932, 1988.

38. Becker C, Gilbert A. [The ulnar flap] Handchir Mikrochir Plast Chir 20:180-183, 1988.

39. Bakhach J, Saint Cast Y, Gazarian A, et al. [Ulnar parametacarpal flap. Anatomical study and clinical application] Ann Chir Plast Esthet 40:136-147, 1995.

40. Bakhach J, Martin D, Baudet J. [Ulnar parametacarpal flap. Experience with 10 clinical cases] Ann Chir Plast Esthet 41:269-276, 1996.

41. Penteado CV, Masquelet AC, Chevrel JP. The anatomic basis of the fascio-cutaneous flap of the posterior interosseous artery. Surg Radiol Anat 8:209-215, 1986.

42. Angrigiani C, Grilli D, Dominikow D, et al. Posterior interosseous reverse forearm flap: experience with 80 consecutive cases. Plast Reconstr Surg 92:285-293, 1993.

43. Shibata M, Iwabuchi Y, Kubota S, et al. Comparison of free and reversed pedicled posterior interosseous cutaneous flaps. Plast Reconstr Surg 99:791-802, 1997.

44. Sheetz KK, Bishop AT, Berger RA. The arterial blood supply of the distal radius and its potential use in vascularized pedicled bone grafts. J Hand Surg Am 20:902-914, 1995.

45. Shibata M, Ogishyo N. Free flaps based on the anterior interosseous artery. Plast Reconstr Surg 97:746-755, 1996.

46. Yang D, Morris SF. Reversed dorsal digital and metacarpal island flaps supplied by the dorsal cutaneous branches of the palmar digital artery. Ann Plast Surg 46:444-449, 2001.

47. Kim KS, Kim ES, Hwang JH, et al. Thumb reconstruction using the radial midpalmar (perforator-based) island flap (distal thenar perforator-based island flap). Plast Reconstr Surg 125:601-608, 2010.

48. Seyhan T. Reverse thenar perforator flap for volar hand reconstruction. J Plast Reconstr Aesthet Surg 62:1309-1316, 2009.

49. Pelissier P, Gardet H, Sawaya E, et al. Anatomical study of the palmar intermetacarpal perforator flap. J Hand Surg Eur Vol 34:224-226, 2009.

50. Quaba AA, Davison PM. The distally-based dorsal hand flap. Br J Plast Surg 43:28-39, 1990.

51. Yang D, Morris SF. Vascular basis of dorsal digital and metacarpal skin flaps. J Hand Surg Am 26:142-146, 2001.

   The vascular anatomy of dorsal digital skin flaps and the vascular anastomoses between the dorsal cutaneous branch of the palmar digital artery and the dorsal digital branches of the dorsal metacarpal artery at the level of the proximal phalanx were studied. There were two sources of the arterial supply to the dorsum of the digit: (1) the dorsal digital branches of the dorsal metacarpal artery and (2) the dorsal cutaneous branches of the palmar digital artery.

52. Dautel G, Borrelly J, Merle M, et al. Dorsal vascular network of the first web space. Anatomical bases of the kite flap. Surg Radiol Anat 11:109-113, 1989.

53. Foucher G, Braun JB. A new island flap transfer from the dorsum of the index to the thumb. Plast Reconstr Surg 63:344-349, 1979.

54. Earley MJ, Milner RH. Dorsal metacarpal flaps. Br J Plast Surg 40:333-341, 1987.

   The history of dorsal metacarpal flaps and their anatomic basis were described. The origin, course, branches, and termination of the dorsal metacarpal arteries were illustrated. The second dorsal metacarpal flap was performed in two patients, and possible difficulties were discussed.

55. Earley MJ. The second dorsal metacarpal artery neurovascular island flap. J Hand Surg Br 14:434-440, 1989.

56. Battiston B, Artiaco S, Antonini A, et al. Dorsal metacarpal artery perforator-based propeller flap for complex defect of the dorsal aspect in the index finger. J Hand Surg Eur Vol 34:807-809, 2009.

57. Yousif NJ, Ye Z, Sanger JR, et al. The versatile metacarpal and reverse metacarpal artery flaps in hand surgery. Ann Plast Surg 29:523-531, 1992.

58. El-Khatib HA. Clinical experiences with the extended first dorsal metacarpal artery island flap for thumb reconstruction. J Hand Surg Am 23:647-652, 1998.

59. Karacalar A, Ozcan M. U-I flap. Plast Reconstr Surg 102:741-747, 1998.

60. Katsaros J, Tan F, Zoltie N. The use of the lateral arm flap in upper limb surgery. J Hand Surg Am 16:598-604, 1991.

61. Chen SL, Chou TD, Chen SG, et al. The boomerang flap in managing injuries of the dorsum of the distal phalanx. Plast Reconstr Surg 106:834-839, 2000.

    A quantitative data summary table for the cutaneous vascular territories of the upper extremity was presented. All values are averages, plus or minus the standard deviation for the number, diameter, length, and areas calculated from the authors' series. The area of each vascular territory and the area supplied by each perforator were calculated from digital angiograms of the region.

62. Koshima I, Urushibara K, Fukuda N, et al. Digital artery perforator flaps for finger tip reconstructions. Plast Reconstr Surg 118:1579-1584, 2006.

63. Tountas CP, Bergman RA, eds. Anatomic Variations of the Upper Extremity. London: Churchill Livingstone, 1993.

16

Lateral Arm Perforator Flap

Michel Saint-Cyr
Luis R. Scheker

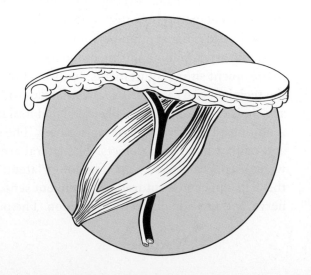

The lateral arm flap has assumed a major role in reconstructive surgery since it was first described by Song et al[1] in 1982 for the treatment of a burn scar contracture of the face and neck. Because of its superior design versatility, reliable anatomy, and ease of elevation, indications for this flap continue to grow. These indications have been well described by Schusterman et al,[2] Katsaros et al,[3] Rivet et al,[4] and Scheker et al[5] for reconstruction of the extremities and the head and neck.

The reconstructive ideal involves replacing traumatized or deficient structures with tissues of identical characteristics in a manner that minimizes donor site morbidity. The lateral arm perforator flap balances these requirements well by providing thin, potentially sensate skin with a good color match, comparable texture, and pliability for reconstructing the extremities and head and neck region. Donor site morbidity is limited to the ipsilateral upper extremity. Unlike the comparable radial forearm flap, the lateral arm perforator flap does not sacrifice a major artery of the hand. The flap can be raised with the patient in the supine position, which allows a more efficient two-team approach. Depending on the patient's body habitus, the donor site can be closed primarily in most cases if flap width is 6 cm or less.[6]

Modifications of the lateral arm flap have developed as the popularity of the flap has increased. Details of these modifications have been well described by Katsaros et al.[7] This flap has been used as an adipofascial flap covered with a split-thickness skin graft when thin, dorsal hand coverage is required.[8-10] It also allows good tendon gliding without excess subcutaneous bulk that results with the standard fasciocutaneous lateral arm flap. The intermuscular septum perforators originating from the dominant posterior radial collateral artery allow splitting of the flap into different segments that can be tailored to the recipient site's requirements. Insetting both portions of the split flap side by side at the recipient site can increase the total flap width and allow direct closure of the donor site. This variation is especially useful in dorsal hand coverage following avulsion injuries requiring a large area of skin replacement. The split flap can also cover combined dorsal and palmar hand skin defects. The lateral arm flap can provide protective sensation when used as a sensate flap. The lower lateral cutaneous nerve of the arm innervates this flap and can be sutured to a recipient sensory nerve, such as branches of the radial nerve, and provide protective sensation. The posterior cutaneous nerve of the forearm can also be harvested with the flap and used as a vascularized nerve graft of up to 10 cm in length; however, this procedure causes anesthesia in the proximolateral portion of the forearm. The osteofasciocutaneous variation of the lateral arm flap is ideally suited for reconstructing small bony defects such as those that occur with the metacarpals or metatarsals.[11,12] A segment of 1 to 1.5 cm by 10 to 15 cm of humerus can be harvested with the flap based on muscle and periosteal branches emanating from the posterior radial collateral artery. A composite flap using a segment of triceps tendon measuring 2 by 10 cm can also be useful for reconstructing tendon defects when minimal excursion is required (for example, Achilles tendon defects).[13] Another modification of the lateral arm flap is the extended lateral arm flap (lateral forearm flap).[14-19] Compared with the lateral arm flap, this variation has the advantages of a longer pedicle and thinner skin, and it does not cause residual anesthesia in the forearm. The lateral arm flap and its extended lateral arm flap variation are also well suited for reconstructing noncircumferential hypopharyngeal defects and contour deformity defects in the head and neck region, as shown by Ninkovic et al[20] and Marques Faria et al.[21]

ANATOMY

The extended lateral arm flap encompasses the skin and underlying soft tissue of the distal half of the lateral arm and the proximal third of the dorsolateral forearm. The longitudinal axis of the flap is centered over a line running from the deltoid muscle insertion to the lateral epicondyle of the humerus with the patient's elbow extended (Fig. 16-1). This line corresponds to the lateral intermuscular septum of the arm where the dominant pedicle of the flap—the posterior radial collateral artery—and its two venae comitantes are found.

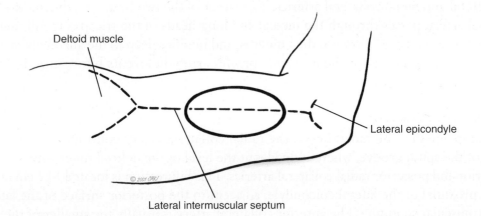

Fig. 16-1 The longitudinal axis of the flap is centered over a line running from the deltoid insertion to the lateral epicondyle of the humerus. (From Christine M. Kleinert Institute for Hand and Mircosurgery, Inc., Louisville, Kentucky.)

Lateral Intermuscular Septum

The arm is enclosed in a strong sheath of deep fascia known as the *brachial fascia*. This fascia is continuous with the pectoral and axillary fascia superiorly and attaches to the epicondyles of the humerus and the olecranon of the ulna inferiorly. The medial and lateral intermuscular septa extend from the brachial fascia and separate the arm into anterior and posterior fascial compartments. After extending from the brachial fascia, the lateral and medial intermuscular septa attach to the lateral and medial supracondylar ridge of the humerus, respectively. The anterior flexor compartment contains the biceps brachii, coracobrachialis, and brachialis muscles, the proximal portion of the brachioradialis muscle, and the accompanying nerves and vessels. The posterior compartment forms the extensor compartment and contains the triceps brachii muscle. The lateral arm flap is based on the lateral intermuscular septum, which contains the posterior radial collateral artery and the posterior cutaneous nerve of the forearm. The lateral intermuscular septum is bordered by the muscle bellies of the brachialis and brachioradialis muscles anteriorly, and the triceps brachii muscle posteriorly.

Vascular Anatomy
Profunda Brachii Artery

The profunda brachii artery provides the main vascular supply to the lateral arm flap and represents the first and largest branch of the brachial artery. This artery has the most superior origin of all branches of the brachial artery, arising from the proximal segment of the brachial artery below the insertion of the latissimus dorsi muscle. It gives rise to several muscular branches on the medial aspect of the arm. After accompanying the radial nerve in the spiral groove, the profunda brachii artery emerges between the medial and lateral heads of the triceps brachii muscle, where it supplies all three heads of this muscle and the humerus. The artery then divides into two branches: the middle collateral and radial collateral arteries. The larger of the two branches, the middle collateral artery, passes through the medial and long heads of the triceps brachii muscle, follows the posterior border of the humerus, and ramifies deep to the anconeus muscle. The average diameter of the profunda brachii artery before its bifurcation is 2 mm (range 1.2 to 3.5 mm).[4]

Radial Collateral Artery

Accompanied by the radial nerve, the radial collateral artery continues to the distal end of the spiral groove, where it divides at the level of the deltoid tuberosity into the anterior and posterior radial collateral arteries. This bifurcation is located 10.2 cm (average) proximal to the lateral epicondyle, adjacent to the posterior surface of the lateral intermuscular septum.[12] The anterior collateral artery is usually the smaller of the two terminal branches. This vessel passes through the lateral intermuscular septum with the radial nerve and courses distally between the brachialis and brachioradialis muscles, where it enters the flexor compartment of the arm immediately distal to the bifurcation of the radial collateral artery (Fig. 16-2). The posterior radial collateral artery is the main artery of the lateral arm flap and enters the lateral intermuscular septum at a level close to the distal insertion of the deltoid muscle. At this point, the artery is found within the lateral intermuscular septum, between the brachialis and brachioradialis muscles anteriorly and the triceps brachii muscle posteriorly (Fig. 16-3). It remains

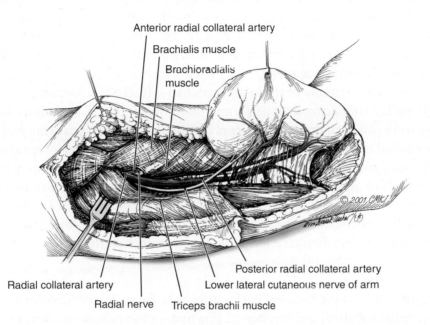

Fig. 16-2 The radial collateral artery divides into two terminal branches: the anterior and posterior radial collateral arteries. (From Christine M. Kleinert Institute for Hand and Mircosurgery, Inc., Louisville, Kentucky.)

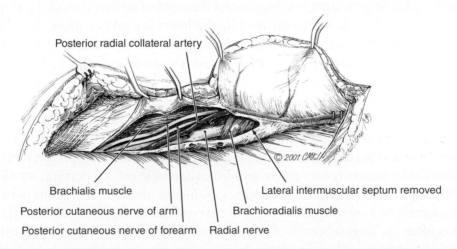

Fig. 16-3 The posterior radial collateral artery courses within the lateral intermuscular septum between the brachialis and brachioradialis muscles medially and the triceps brachii muscle laterally. (From Christine M. Kleinert Institute for Hand and Mircosurgery, Inc., Louisville, Kentucky.)

within the lateral intermuscular septum, intimately attached to the lateral border of the humerus, where it gives off periosteal and muscular branches. Along its course within the lateral intermuscular septum, the posterior radial collateral artery gives rise to four or five septocutaneous perforators 1 to 15 cm proximal to the lateral epicondyle. These perforators pass to the deep fascia and subsequently supply the skin. The most proximal branch is found very close to the posterior cutaneous nerve of the forearm, and the largest branch is located 10 cm (average) proximal to the lateral epicondyle.[8,9] The posterior radial collateral artery courses distally, posterior to the lateral epicondyle of the humerus. The vessel anastomoses with the interosseous recurrent artery and contributes to the collateral circulation of structures around the elbow, including the skin, elbow joint, and aponeurosis.

The vascular anatomy of the lateral arm flap is basically constant, with few variations. Of the 125 lateral arm flaps performed at our institution, variations in the vascular anatomy were found in only two patients (1.6%). Both of these patients had a double posterior radial collateral artery running parallel within the lateral intermuscular septum. The superficial branch perfused the proximal portion of the flap, whereas the deeper branch occupied the usual position of the posterior radial collateral artery and perfused the distal portion of the flap near the lateral epicondyle. Flap perfusion was established by anastomosing the superficial branch end to side to the deep branch, and anastomosing the deep branch end to side to the recipient artery.

Perforator Vessels

An average of 4.5 septocutaneous perforators arise from the profunda brachii artery–posterior radial collateral artery system.[10] The first septocutaneous branch is found close to the bifurcation of the radial collateral artery, 10.7 cm (average) proximal to the lateral epicondyle of the humerus.[12] A second septocutaneous branch to the lateral arm flap originates from the posterior radial collateral artery, 7.8 cm (average) from the lateral epicondyle. This branch often has the greatest diameter of all branches of the posterior radial collateral artery. It is accompanied by the lower lateral cutaneous nerve of the arm and the posterior cutaneous nerve of the forearm as they enter the subcutaneous tissue. A mean of 3.8 muscle perforators pass from the posterior radial collateral artery posteriorly to the triceps brachii muscle; a mean of 2.4 perforators pass anteriorly to supply the biceps muscle.[10] These perforators are distributed 2 to 10 cm proximal to the lateral epicondyle. Fascial perforators originate from the posterior radial collateral artery within the intermuscular septum and course superficially toward the fascia, where they follow anterior and posterior directions. An average of 2.3 true fascial perforators can be found directed posteriorly over the triceps brachii muscle and 1.8 perforators directed anteriorly over the brachioradialis muscle. A dominant proximal cutaneous perforator can consistently be located approximately 10 cm cephalad to the lateral epicondyle. This branch is often the largest branch of the posterior radial collateral artery. These fascial perforators terminate either directly in fascia or give rise to cutaneous branches, thus offering the possibility of separate fascial and cutaneous perfusion.

Venous Anatomy

Venous drainage of the lateral arm flap is provided by superficial and deep venous systems connected by communicating veins. Superficial veins of the lateral arm drain through the cephalic vein, which is located in the superficial fascia along the anterolateral surface of the biceps muscle. The deeper system consists of one or two venae comitantes that accompany the posterior radial collateral artery. Both systems can provide adequate venous drainage to the flap, but the largest of the two venae comitantes is preferred because of its proximity to the artery during anastomosis. When using the deeper system, the cephalic vein can be used as an interpositional conduit to revascularize structures distal to the flap.

Neural Anatomy

Radial Nerve

The radial nerve passes through the spiral groove of the humerus and gives rise to two important nerves: the lower lateral cutaneous nerve of the arm and the posterior cutaneous nerve of the forearm. The radial nerve then pierces the lateral intermuscular septum, runs anterior to it, and leaves the arm by coursing between the brachialis and brachioradialis muscles.

Lower Lateral Cutaneous Nerve of the Arm

The lower lateral cutaneous nerve of the arm is the sensory nerve to the lateral arm flap and originates from the radial nerve in the spiral groove. The nerve pierces the lateral intermuscular septum, passes anterior to it, and ramifies in the lateral skin of the distal half of the arm (Fig. 16-4). It provides sensory innervation to the skin from the distal lateral arm down to the olecranon region.

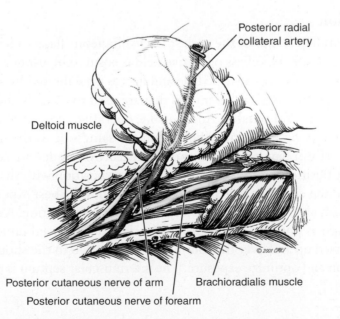

Fig. 16-4 The lower lateral cutaneous nerve of the arm (posterior cutaneous nerve of the arm) runs with the posterior radial collateral artery and innervates the flap. (From Christine M. Kleinert Institute for Hand and Mircosurgery, Inc., Louisville, Kentucky.)

Posterior Cutaneous Nerve of the Forearm

The posterior cutaneous nerve of the forearm supplies sensory innervation to the skin of the proximal posterolateral aspect of the forearm. This nerve originates from the radial nerve in the spiral groove, usually 1 to 5 cm below the origin of the lower lateral cutaneous nerve of the arm. The nerve closely follows the posterior radial collateral artery. It pierces the lateral intermuscular septum and then runs anterior to it, passing through the lateral head of the triceps brachii muscle to reach the subcutaneous level. Although this nerve is closely associated with the flap and its pedicle, it does not provide sensation to the flap. However, it can be used as a vascularized nerve graft of up to 10 cm to bridge nerve defects in the recipient hand or the facial nerve. If an extended lateral arm flap is used, then the posterior cutaneous nerve of the forearm should be included with the flap and sutured to a recipient sensory nerve to provide protective sensation.

SURGICAL TECHNIQUE
Surface Landmarks

The cutaneous area supported by the lateral arm flap is located along a line drawn from the insertion of the deltoid muscle to the lateral humeral epicondyle (see Fig. 16-1). This line is the central axis of the flap and represents the lateral intermuscular septum in which the posterior radial collateral artery courses. Maximal flap dimensions vary from 8 by 10 cm to 15 by 14 cm.[3] A safe zone where the flap can be harvested is represented by a rectangular area proximal to the lateral epicondyle that is 12 cm in length and one third the circumference of the arm in width.[4] The lateral arm flap can also be extended up to 12 cm distal to the lateral epicondyle when an extended lateral arm flap is required. Harvesting the flap as distally as possible and caudal to the lateral epicondyle yields a thinner extended lateral arm flap (lateral forearm flap) with a significantly longer pedicle.

Flap Elevation

The lateral arm flap is one of the easiest fasciocutaneous flaps to harvest for the following reasons: a safe, bloodless operative field is ensured by using a tourniquet; optimal visualization of the vascular pedicle and nerves is facilitated by shoulder and arm mobilization; and the surgical landmarks that are used to identify the vascular pedicle are easily identified and reliable. Additionally, operative morbidity can be limited to the same extremity by harvesting the flap on the same side as the defect. Whenever possible, we perform flap harvesting and reconstruction under an axillary block. Surgery begins by positioning the patient in the supine position with the arm abducted to 90 degrees and the elbow flexed. This position provides the best exposure, and the arm and shoulder can always be mobilized later for better visualization. A sterile tourniquet is placed as high as possible on the arm. A stockinette is placed under the tourniquet and then reversed up and over the tourniquet and sutured to the shoulder to minimize distal migration and optimize exposure. The intermuscular septum is outlined by drawing a line from the deltoid insertion to the lateral epicondyle. This line can be extended into the forearm if an extended lateral arm flap is used. A template design is tailored to the defect and centered over the line corresponding to the lateral intermuscular septum to maximize pedicle length (Fig. 16-5, *A* through *D*). Dissection begins with a perpendicular skin incision along the posterior and distal border of the flap. This incision is carried down until the deep brachial fascia is visualized. The incision proceeds through the deep fascia and includes an extra 2 cm cuff of fascia from the original skin flap design. The additional fascia can be used to increase flap bulk or to provide additional coverage. Dissection proceeds in a subfascial plane from a posterior-distal to anterior-superior direction until the lateral intermuscular septum is encountered. Flap

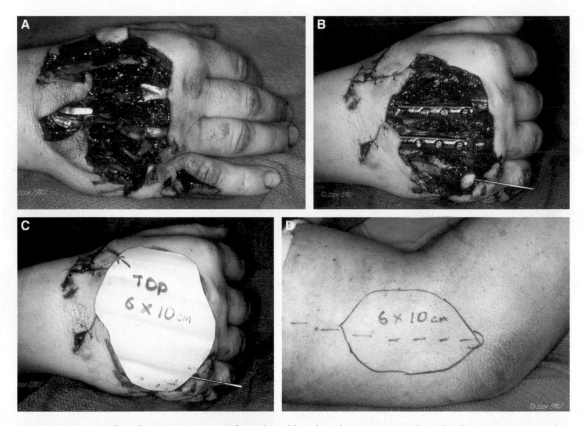

Fig. 16-5 A, Flap elevation sequence for a dorsal hand avulsion injury with multiple open metacarpal fractures and extensor tendon and dorsal skin loss. **B,** The wound is debrided, and open reduction and internal fixation of metacarpal fractures are performed. **C,** A template of the skin deficit is designed with proper orientation of the vascular pedicle. **D,** A line is drawn from the deltoid insertion to the lateral epicondyle that corresponded to the lateral intermuscular septum. The predesigned template of the deficit is centered and marked over the main axis of the flap along the intermuscular septum.

elevation starts posteriorly, because the plane of dissection is more easily identified and developed over the triceps brachii muscle and tendon (Fig. 16-5, *E* through *G*). There are no triceps brachii fiber origins attached to either the posterior aspect of the lateral intermuscular septum or the deep fascia. As a result, posterior flap elevation is relatively quick and easy, but careful coagulation of all small vessels is crucial to avoid donor site hematoma and flap bleeding when circulation is restored. Small perforator vessels can be seen within the fascia and followed to the posterior radial collateral artery. As dissection proceeds from a posterior to anterior direction, the pedicle can be seen within the lateral intermuscular septum (Fig. 16-5, *H*). Dissection progresses proximally to expose the pedicle along its entire length from the lateral epicondyle to the deltoid insertion. When the pedicle is completely visualized from its posterior aspect, anterior dissection of the flap begins (Fig. 16-5, *I*). The skin is incised along the anterior border

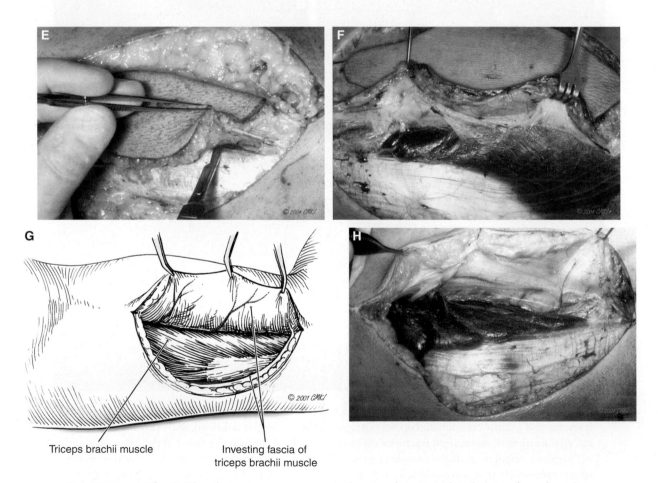

Triceps brachii muscle   Investing fascia of
                                triceps brachii muscle

Fig. 16-5, cont'd   E, Flap dissection starts posteriorly, over the triceps brachii muscle and tendon. **F** and **G,** An easy plane of dissection is carried out between the triceps brachii muscle epimysium and the lateral arm flap deep fascia. **H,** The pedicle is visualized along its entire course within the lateral intermuscular septum after posterior flap dissection.

of the flap with an extra 2 cm of deep fascia included. Flap elevation progresses from an anterior to posterior direction toward the lateral intermuscular septum using sharp dissection to divide fibers of the brachioradialis muscle from the lateral intermuscular septum. When the vascular pedicle is seen in its entirety from the anterior aspect, the septum can be safely separated from the lateral border of the humerus (Fig. 16-5, *J*). This separation proceeds from distal to proximal and becomes easier, because the distance between the humerus and the pedicle increases proximally. The pedicle is transected just distal to the bifurcation of the radial collateral artery into its posterior and anterior branches. Pedicle length can also be extended by ligating the anterior radial collateral artery. Dissection continues into the spiral groove until the pedicle length is adequate. A proximal longitudinal skin incision can also be made to facilitate proximal pedicle exposure. The tailored skin flap is inset into the defect (Fig. 16-5, *K* and *L*).

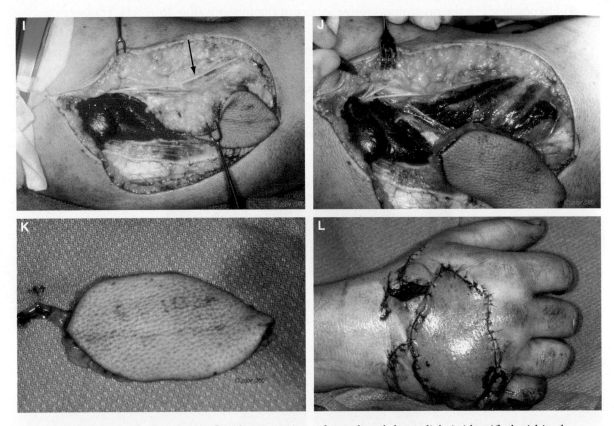

Fig. 16-5, cont'd   I, Anterior flap dissection is performed, and the pedicle is identified within the lateral intermuscular septum. The posterior cutaneous nerve of the forearm *(arrow)* is preserved (seen here entering the flap). **J,** The pedicle is separated from its humeral attachment within the lateral intermuscular septum. **K,** The lateral arm flap is harvested. **L,** The flap is inset into the dorsal hand wound after extensor tendon reconstruction. Tendon grafts are passed through the subcutaneous layer of the flap.

Three important nerves are identified during flap elevation: the radial nerve, the lower lateral cutaneous nerve of the arm, and the posterior cutaneous nerve of the forearm. Proximally, the radial nerve must be protected. This nerve lies anterior to the posterior radial collateral artery before coursing between the brachialis and brachioradialis muscles. To avoid postoperative neuropraxia, the radial nerve must be carefully retracted. The lower lateral cutaneous nerve of the arm, which originates from the radial nerve proximally within the spiral groove, innervates the flap and must be included if a sensate tissue transfer is planned. The posterior cutaneous nerve of the forearm also originates from the radial nerve, approximately 1 to 5 cm distal to the origin of the lower lateral cutaneous nerve of the arm within the spiral groove. This nerve pierces the lateral intermuscular septum, passes anterior to it, and runs closely with the posterior radial collateral artery before piercing the lateral head of the triceps brachii muscle and reaching the skin. This nerve can also be harvested as a vascularized nerve graft up to 10 cm in length. Whenever possible, this nerve is preserved to prevent anesthesia or painful hypesthesia in the proximoposterior aspect of the forearm (Fig. 16-5, *M*). Transection of the nerve can be required in up to 50% of patients during pedicle dissection. If the posterior cutaneous nerve of the arm is transected, it should be repaired to minimize the risks of anesthesia or painful hypesthesia in the proximolateral forearm region.

Final range of motion can be maximized with aggressive postoperative hand therapy (Fig. 16-5, *N* and *O*). Any flap revision or debulking can be performed safely 6 months after surgery.

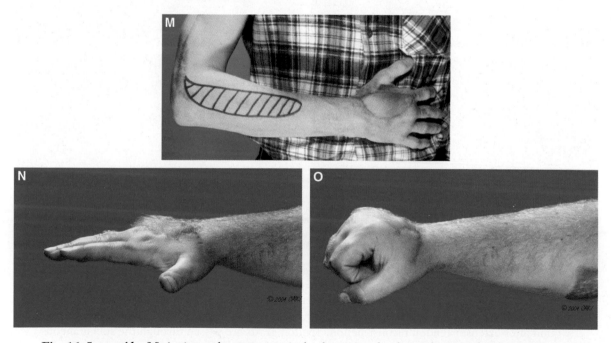

Fig. 16-5, cont'd   M, At 6 months postoperatively, the patient has hypesthesia in the proximolateral aspect of the forearm resulting from transection of the posterior cutaneous nerve of the forearm. **N** and **O,** Final range of motion 6 months postoperatively. (From Christine M. Kleinert Institute for Hand and Mircosurgery, Inc., Louisville, Kentucky.)

MODIFICATIONS
Adipofascial Flap

The lateral arm flap can be used as an adipofascial or fascial free flap when very thin pliable coverage is required such as dorsal hand coverage with reconstruction of extensor tendon gliding surfaces (Fig. 16-6). This flap is also useful in ear and nose reconstruction where preserving the underlying cartilage is important. Harvesting the flap is similar to the standard fasciocutaneous flap elevation technique except that skin and some of the subcutaneous tissues are not included with the flap. A variable amount of fat can be harvested with the fascia, depending on the recipient site requirements. With the patient placed in the supine position, a curvilinear or straight line is drawn from the deltoid muscle insertion to the lateral epicondyle. This line corresponds to the lateral intermuscular septum and central axis of the flap. A curvilinear or longitudinal incision is made along this line. The flap is harvested as an adipofascial flap that contains up to seven fascial branches originating from the posterior radial collateral artery within the lateral intermuscular septum, with the largest one found approximately 10 cm proximal to the lateral epicondyle.[10,12] Micropaque injection studies have shown that fascial perfusion by the posterior radial collateral artery extends posteriorly over the triceps brachii muscle and anteriorly to the septum between the biceps and the brachialis muscles.

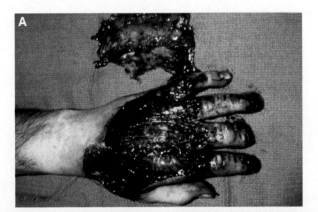

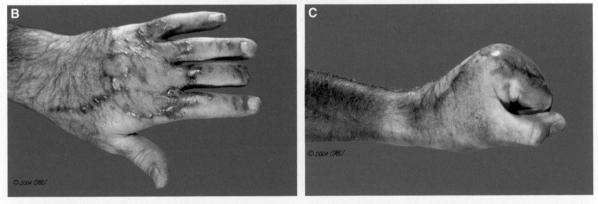

Fig. 16-6 **A,** Left hand dorsal skin avulsion injury with harvested adipofascial lateral arm free flap before inset and anastomosis. **B** and **C,** Six months postoperatively, the adipofascial flap and split-thickness skin graft are well healed and final range of motion is good. (From Christine M. Kleinert Institute for Hand and Mircosurgery, Inc., Louisville, Kentucky.)

Adipofascial flaps of up to 9 by 12 cm have been safely elevated. When using a split- or full-thickness skin graft, we prefer to graft the deep surface of the flap. This side contains fewer transected small vessels and decreases the chance of hematoma formation. Once elevated, the fascial flap can be split into separate segments, each containing a fascial branch and used for reconstructing separate defects. A composite flap can also be used when fascia is combined with triceps tendon, triceps brachii or brachialis muscle, a segment of humerus, nerve, or a segment of skin.

Osteocutaneous Flap

Periosteal branches of the posterior radial collateral artery allow the posterolateral aspect of the humerus to be harvested as a vascularized bone graft (Fig. 16-7). At least one or two direct branches of the posterior radial collateral artery to the humerus can be found 2 to 7 cm proximal to the lateral epicondyle.[11] Bone should be harvested at this level, and because of this direct blood supply to the humerus, harvesting a surrounding

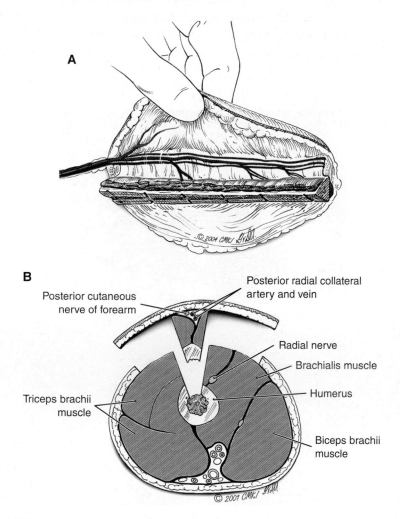

Fig. 16-7 A, Osteocutaneous lateral arm flap. **B,** Cross-sectional view. (From Christine M. Kleinert Institute for Hand and Mircosurgery, Inc., Louisville, Kentucky.)

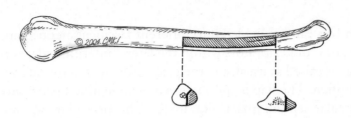

Fig. 16-8 Osteotomy cuts through the lateral humerus. (From Christine M. Kleinert Institute for Hand and Mircosurgery, Inc., Louisville, Kentucky.)

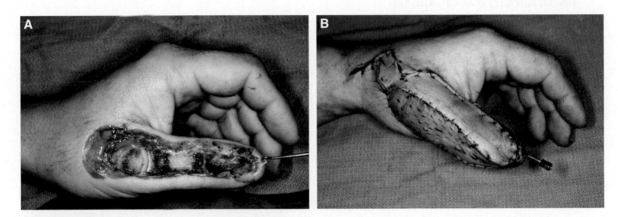

Fig. 16-9 **A,** Avulsion injury involving the dorsal aspect of the left thumb, distal and proximal phalanges, and distal metacarpal. **B,** An osteocutaneous lateral arm free flap is used to resurface the dorsal thumb defect and provide a vascularized bone segment for stable fusion of the interphalangeal and metacarpophalangeal joints of the thumb.

muscle cuff is not necessary. A segment measuring 10 to 15 cm by 1 to 1.5 cm can be used. Special attention must be given to the orientation of the osteotomy cuts. To minimize the risks of a stress fracture, the osteotomy cuts should be oriented obliquely instead of perpendicular to the long axis of the humerus (Fig. 16-8). Small to medium-sized bony defects of the phalanges, metacarpals, and metatarsals are especially amenable to reconstruction with this flap (Fig. 16-9).

Neurosensory Flap

The neurosensory flap is raised in a fashion similar to the fasciocutaneous flap. The lower lateral cutaneous nerve of the arm provides sensation to the lateral arm flap. This nerve can be included during dissection and sutured to a recipient sensory cutaneous nerve, such as a branch of the radial sensory nerve, and will provide protective but not discriminating sensation. A segment of up to 10 cm of the posterior cutaneous nerve of the forearm can also be included with the flap and used as a vascularized nerve graft. However, harvesting this nerve results in an area of anesthesia in the proximal lateral aspect of the forearm.

Split Flap

The lateral arm flap can be divided into different fasciocutaneous flaps based on the number and location of perforators within the lateral intermuscular septum. The fasciocutaneous flap is raised as usual, and the perforators within the lateral intermuscular septum are identified. The flap is split between two identified perforators, leaving the lateral intermuscular septum intact (Fig. 16-10). This procedure allows each segment of the flap to be oriented in a different direction, with direct donor site closure (for example, side by side to increase the effective width of the flap [Fig. 16-11] or as two separate skin paddles for coverage of through-and-through defects [Fig. 16-12]). The flap segments produced from this modification can be a combination of skin, bone, fascia, muscle, tendon, and fat.

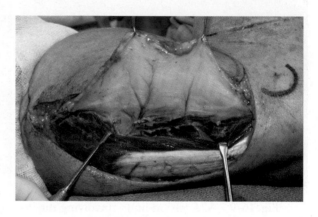

Fig. 16-10   The lateral arm free flap is elevated over the triceps muscle, and the posterior radial collateral artery is identified within the septum between the triceps brachii and brachioradialis muscles. Note the distinct cutaneous perforators originating from the pedicle, which allow the flap to be split into two distinct skin paddles.

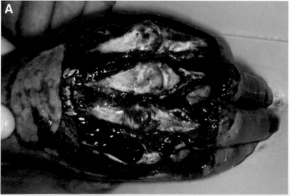

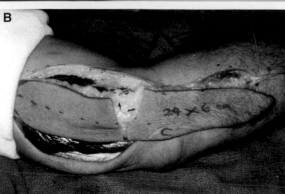

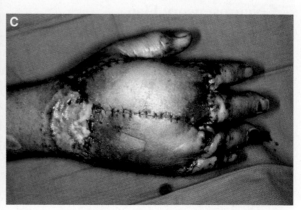

Fig. 16-11   **A,** This large dorsal hand avulsion injury is shown after debridement and before flap coverage. **B,** A split lateral arm free flap is based on separate perforators, allowing both skin paddles to be placed side by side for greater width coverage. **C,** Two-week postoperative result.

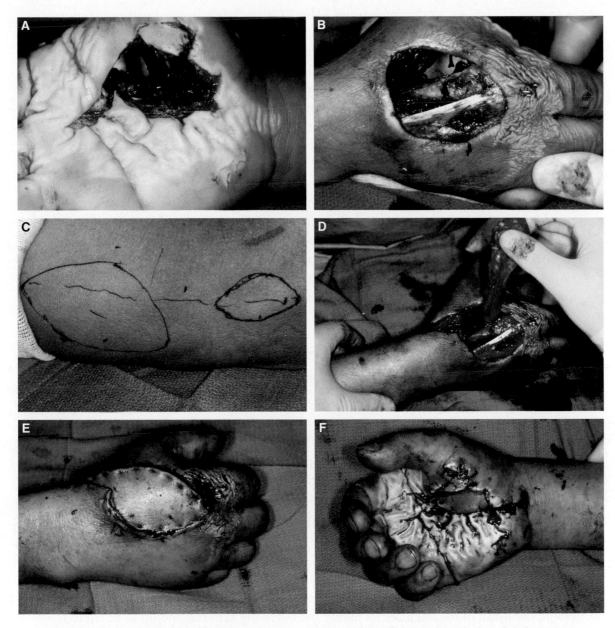

Fig. 16-12 **A** and **B,** Volar and dorsal views of a through-and-through right hand defect. **C,** A split skin paddle lateral arm free flap is designed. **D,** A deepithelialized segment of the flap is passed through the defect. **E** and **F,** The inset flap is shown.

Vascularized Triceps Tendon Flap

A segment of triceps tendon measuring 10 by 2 cm can safely be used without compromising function of the triceps brachii muscle. Segments of triceps tendon up to 10 by 5 cm have been reported without complications.[13] When including a segment of the triceps brachii muscle, a thin wedge of the muscle's lateral head is also harvested to preserve the posterior musculocutaneous perforators to the tendon graft. Extension of the skin paddle distal to the lateral epicondyle in the form of an extended lateral arm flap (lateral forearm flap) also provides thinner skin coverage over tendon reconstruction in the extremities (for example, Achilles tendon or ankle coverage).

Musculofascial Flap

A portion of the lateral head of the triceps brachii muscle can be included with the flap to add necessary bulk for contour defects and to fill dead space.[22] Vascularized muscle has the potential advantages of reducing the bacterial count and enhancing resistance to infection in contaminated wounds. Segmental muscle branches from the posterior radial collateral artery, which are found along the length of the muscle, are left intact and harvested with the flap to ensure adequate perfusion to the muscle.

Flow-Through Flap

A subcutaneous vein such as the cephalic vein can be harvested with the flap and used as a flow-through conduit for revascularization of structures distal to the flap. The posterior radial collateral artery can also be used to revascularize structures distal to the flap, such as the thumb.

Extended Lateral Arm Flap (Lateral Forearm Flap)

In the elbow region, the posterior radial collateral artery follows a progressively more superficial course before emptying into the epicondylar and olecranon plexus and supplying terminal branches that perfuse the skin of the lateral forearm flap. Multiple vascular anastomoses are located between the posterior radial collateral artery and the interosseous recurrent artery, superficial to the deep fascia in the lateral elbow region. These anastomoses create a rich plexus and offer variability in flap design. Controversy exists as to whether or not the posterior radial collateral artery continues as a true axial vessel past the lateral epicondyle.[19] When extending the classic lateral arm flap past the elbow, inclusion of the deep fascial plexus and overlying skin can add up to 12 cm to the flap.[15] Posterolateral forearm skin can be harvested separately without lateral arm skin. This modification offers the advantages of thinner skin, less anesthesia in the forearm, and a longer pedicle. The posterior cutaneous nerve of the forearm can be included to provide protective sensation to the flap. The combined lateral arm–lateral forearm flap offers a unique variability in subcutaneous thickness, which can be useful in head and neck reconstruction.

Pedicle Length Extension

An additional 6 to 8 cm of pedicle length can be obtained by splitting the triceps brachii muscle between the lateral and long heads to expose the entire length of the profunda brachii artery in the spiral groove.[23] A tunnel is developed under the lateral head of the

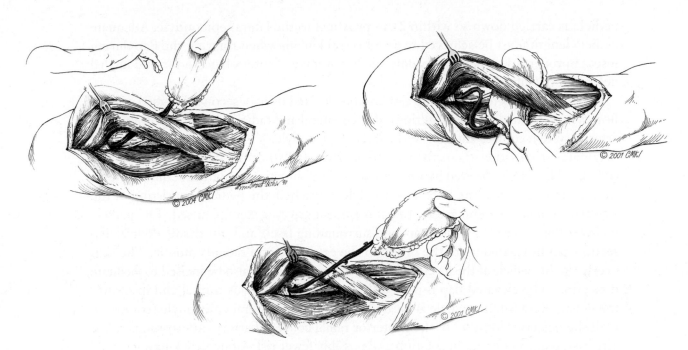

Fig. 16-13   Pedicle length is extended by passing the skin paddle under the triceps brachii muscle. (From Christine M. Kleinert Institute for Hand and Mircosurgery, Inc., Louisville, Kentucky.)

triceps brachii muscle, through which the flap or its pedicle is passed (Fig. 16-13). The origin of the profunda brachii artery from the brachial artery can usually be reached through this tunnel.

Reverse Lateral Arm Flap

Reconstructing periolecranon soft tissue defects can be a formidable challenge in patients with trauma, infection, or decubitus ulcers. The lateral arm flap is ideal for covering elbow defects by providing skin with similar texture, color, and thickness. The reverse lateral arm flap is a distally based flap that uses reversed arterial flow from one of two recurrent arterial systems that anastomose with the posterior radial collateral artery to ensure flap survival. These systems include the interosseous recurrent artery and the radial recurrent artery. Culbertson and Mutimer[24] have described the "flow-through" posterior radial collateral artery–interosseous recurrent artery system. Near the elbow, the posterior radial collateral artery passes posterior to the lateral epicondyle and anastomoses with a branch of the ulnar artery—the interosseous recurrent artery—and a branch of the posterior interosseous artery. Injection studies by Katsaros et al[3] have demonstrated that skin paddles measuring more than 8 by 10 cm can be harvested on this posterior radial collateral artery–interosseous recurrent artery reverse vascular supply. Flap elevation is similar to the standard flap elevation technique. The distal pedicle must not be skeletonized to prevent damage to the arterial inflow and venous drainage of the flap. The pedicle is dissected with a strip of surrounding fascia and subcutaneous fat measuring 2.5 to 3 cm in width. The flap is delivered to the defect site either through a generous subcutaneous tunnel or through an incised skin bridge. Dissection of the pedicle is carried down to within 2 cm proximal to the lateral epicondyle. Adequate pedicle length must be achieved to avoid vessel kinking when rotating the flap during inset. A properly designed skin paddle allows coverage of anterior, posterior, and medial defects of the elbow.

The reverse lateral arm flap can also be elevated using a second reversed arterial flow system formed by the posterior radial collateral and radial recurrent arteries. This arterial system courses anterior to the lateral epicondyle.[25] The radial recurrent artery originates from either the proximal radial artery (64%) or the distal brachial artery (18%).[26] The flap is elevated in a proximal to distal direction using the standard elevation technique. When the lateral epicondyle is reached, the pedicle consisting of the posterior radial collateral artery–radial recurrent artery system is raised. The pedicle includes the underlying periosteum and surrounding fascia and soft tissue. Pedicle dissection can be carried up to the origin of the extensor carpi radialis muscle. The skin overlying the pedicle at the level of the lateral epicondyle can also be incised to facilitate dissection. The elevated flap is passed through a subcutaneous tunnel and inset into the defect. Because the pedicle is located anterior to the lateral epicondyle (compared with the posterior location of the posterior radial collateral artery–interosseous radial artery system), a safer arc of rotation and possibly fewer risks of pedicle kinking can be achieved. Türegün et al[27] have presented further refinements for this flap, including measuring the skin paddle dimensions with the elbow in full flexion, marking the flap as close to the lateral epicondyle as possible. This method of measurement allows flap coverage over a complete range of motion, with skin of comparable thickness and color. The patient wears an extension splint for 1 week postoperatively to minimize the risk of pedicle kinking and to maximize blood flow. For coverage of trauma-related defects of the elbow, preoperative angiography helps ensure the patency of either the interosseous recurrent artery or the radial recurrent artery.

The reverse lateral arm perforator flap can also be used as an adipofascial flap instead of a fasciocutaneous flap, and it is based on the posterior radial collateral artery–interosseous radial artery system.[28] Flap elevation is similar to that of the reverse fasciocutaneous flap; however, skin is not elevated. With this modification a larger flap can be raised without concerns about primary donor site closure. Minimal closure tension creates a scar that does not tend to widen, and flap debulking can be tailored to the requirements of the recipient site.

Lateral Arm Advancement Flap

Soft tissue defects surrounding the elbow can also be reconstructed using a proximally based lateral arm flap designed as a V-Y flap, rotation-advancement flap, or island flap.[29] This flap is harvested using a standard technique, and proper elevation and mobilization of the posterior radial collateral artery is crucial for adequate distal advancement of the flap.

Skin Expansion

Pretransfer tissue expansion increases flap dimensions, facilitating direct closure of the donor site. Primary donor site closure is possible with flaps having dimensions of up to 11 by 18 cm.[30]

PITFALLS

Disadvantages of the lateral arm flap include the presence of hair in some individuals. In these patients, the flap is harvested more distally, in the nonglabrous portion of the arm and proximal forearm. Excess subcutaneous fat can be problematic and is also avoided by using a more distally based flap. Whenever possible, sacrifice of the posterior cutaneous nerve of the forearm should be avoided. We commonly reanastomose this nerve if it is transected during pedicle dissection. A lateral forearm flap prevents this problem, because the skin paddle is innervated by the posterior cutaneous nerve of the forearm. The radial nerve is closely related to the vascular pedicle, and care must be taken not to damage it as it courses through the spiral groove. Undue tension applied during primary closure can also yield an unsightly, widened scar. This problem is compounded if a skin graft is used for donor site closure. Proper skin paddle design, including a split flap or even an alternate flap, can alleviate or prevent this problem.

CONCLUSION

The lateral arm flap is a reliable tool for reconstructive surgeons. Its anatomy is predictable, making flap harvest relatively simple and straightforward. Pedicle diameter is adequate for microsurgery, and its length can be increased by designing the skin paddle more distally in the arm or proximal forearm. This modification also provides a flap with thinner, less glabrous skin, and is advantageous when resurfacing defects in areas that require minimal subcutaneous fat, such as the ankle, dorsum of the hand, hypopharynx, and contour deformities of the head and neck region. The lateral arm flap does not require sacrificing a major artery of the hand and lends itself well to numerous modifications, because it has multiple fasciocutaneous perforators and branches to muscle, tendon, and bone. This anatomy allows the design of composite flaps that can be tailored to meet the requirements of complex defects. In upper extremity reconstruction, the flap can be raised ipsilateral to the defect, thus limiting all morbidity to the same region. Protective sensation can be provided as well as revascularization of structures distal to the flap. Primary donor site closure can usually be accomplished if flap width is limited to 6 cm, depending on the patient's body habitus.

References

1. Song R, Song Y, Yu Y, et al. The upper arm free flap. Clin Plast Surg 9:27-35, 1982.
2. Schusterman M, Acland RD, Banis JC, et al. The lateral arm flap: an experimental and clinical study. In Williams HB, ed. Transactions of the Eighth International Congress of Plastic and Reconstructive Surgery. Montreal, Canada, June 1983.
3. Katsaros J, Schusterman M, Beppu M, et al. The lateral upper arm flap: anatomy and clinical applications. Ann Plast Surg 12:489-500, 1984.

    The authors described the vascular anatomy of the lateral arm flap in 32 cadaveric dissections along with details of the flap's anatomy, innervation, and vascular branches to the humerus. A series of 23 patients was also presented with the following flap components: standard fasciocutaneous flap (n = 16), triceps tendon flap (n = 1), innervated flap (n = 1), fascial flap (n = 3), and vascularized humerus osseous flap (n = 1). A single flap failure was reported. The authors advocated the use of this flap in upper extremity and head and neck reconstruction.

4. Rivet D, Buffet M, Martin D, et al. The lateral arm flap: an anatomic study. J Reconstr Microsurg 3:121-132, 1987.

5. Scheker LR, Kleinert HE, Hanel DP. Lateral arm composite tissue transfer to ipsilateral hand defects. J Hand Surg 12(5 Pt 1):665-672, 1987.

> *This was a clinical study of 29 patients who underwent hand reconstruction with an ipsilateral lateral arm flap. Thirteen emergency free flaps and 16 elective free flaps were performed with an overall success rate of 96.5%. Indications for surgery included degloving of the dorsum of the hand, first web space contracture release following electrical burns, extravasation injury, chronic ulceration following thermal injury, unstable skin grafts, and exposed hardware. Composite flaps consisting of skin, fat, and fascia were used in 25 cases, and a flow-through flap to revascularize nonviable digits was used in two cases. The anatomy of the lateral arm flap was described in detail as well as important landmarks and harvesting techniques. This flap is advocated for ipsilateral composite reconstruction of the upper extremity without sacrifice of a major artery of the hand.*

6. Scheker LR, Lister GD, Wolff TW. The lateral arm free flap in releasing severe contracture of the first web space. J Hand Surg 1:146-150, 1988.

> *This article described the usefulness of the innervated lateral arm flap in reconstructing severely contracted first web spaces in a series of nine patients. Indications for surgery included first web space contracture following trauma, electrical burn injury, and laceration of the median and ulnar nerves. A temporary internal splint using a bent Kirschner wire in a "W" shape was used to maintain the first web space dimensions during flap healing. Flap survival was 100% and all procedures resulted in an angle of palmar abduction of at least 40 degrees between the first and second metacarpals.*

7. Katsaros J, Tan E, Zoltie N, et al. Further experience with the lateral arm flap. Plast Reconstr Surg 87:902-910, 1991.

> *The authors described in detail their 7-year experience using the lateral arm free flap and its various modifications in 150 patients. The overall free flap survival rate was 97.3%. Complications included transient nerve palsies (n = 4) and a posterior nerve palsy (n = 1); all of the patients recovered. This article illustrated the versatility of the lateral arm flap through its numerous modifications, which included the split flap (n = 18), osteocutaneous flap (n = 11), vascularized triceps tendon flap (n = 6), neurosensory flap (n = 5), and adipofascial flap (n = 5).*

8. Yousif NJ, Warren R, Matloub HS, et al. The lateral arm fascial free flap: its anatomy and use in reconstruction. Plast Reconstr Surg 86:1138-1145, 1990.

> *The vascular, microscopic, gross, and radiographic anatomy of the lateral arm fascial flap was studied in 20 fresh cadavers after blue latex injection of the brachial artery. The posterior radial collateral artery vascularized the flap and provided at least four fascial branches that were located from 1 to 15 cm proximal to the lateral epicondyle. Dimensions of up to 12 by 9 cm can be harvested with good axial perfusion. The authors also described a series of seven patients who underwent reconstruction of the upper extremity (n = 5) and head and neck region (n = 2) with the lateral arm fascial flap. They stressed the value of this flap in preserving fine underlying cartilaginous anatomy in ear and nose reconstruction, and in providing thin coverage with a gliding surface in upper extremity reconstruction.*

9. Ulusal BG, Lin YT, Ulusal AE, et al. Free lateral arm flap for 1-stage reconstruction of soft tissue and composite defects of the hand: a retrospective analysis of 118 cases. Ann Plast Surg 58:173-178, 2007.

10. Summers AN, Sanger JR, Matloub HS. Lateral arm fascial flap: microarterial anatomy and potential clinical applications. J Reconstr Microsurg 16:279-286, 2000.

11. Haas F, Rappl T, Koch H, et al. Free osteocutaneous lateral arm flap: anatomy and clinical applications. Microsurgery 23:87-95, 2003.

12. Hennerbichler A, Etzer C, Gruber S, et al. Lateral arm flap: analysis of its anatomy and modification using a vascularized fragment of the distal humerus. Clin Anat 16:204-214, 2003.

13. Smit JM, Darcy CM, Audolfsson T, et al. Multilayer reconstructions for defects overlying the Achilles tendon with the lateral-arm flap: long-term follow-up of 16 cases. Microsurgery. 2012 Mar 31. [Epub ahead of print]

14. Depner C, Erba P, Rieger UM, et al. Donor-site morbidity of the sensate extended lateral arm flap. J Reconstr Microsurg 28:133-138, 2012.

15. Brandt KE, Khouri RK. The lateral arm/proximal forearm flap. Plast Reconstr Surg 92:1137-1143, 1993.

   The authors described the vascular anatomy of the lateral arm/proximal forearm flap in 10 cadaveric dissections following blue latex injection and in 14 clinical cases using 15 flaps. Indications for surgery included reconstruction of the upper extremity (n = 7), lower extremity (n = 5), and penis (n = 3). The average flap dimensions were 24 by 10 cm and ranged from 35 by 12 cm to 14 by 5 cm. The flaps extended past the lateral epicondyle for an average of 9.3 cm (range 6 to 12 cm). The posterior collateral artery was found to terminate in a rich vascular plexus composed of the olecranon anastomosis and branches of the radial recurrent artery. Inclusion of this plexus during flap elevation allows the possibility of extending the lateral arm flap up to 12 cm past the lateral epicondyle, or of using the proximal forearm skin only as a separate flap with a longer pedicle. Advantages of this modification over the standard lateral arm flap include thinner sensate skin and a longer pedicle length.

16. Shibata M, Hatano Y, Iwabuchi Y, et al. Combined dorsal forearm and lateral arm flap. Plast Reconstr Surg 96:1423-1429, 1995.

17. Fogdestam I, Tarnow P, Kalaaji A. Extended free lateral arm flap with preservation of the posterior cutaneous nerve of the forearm. Scand J Plast Reconstr Hand Surg 30:49-55, 1996.

18. Lanzetta M, Bernier M, Chollet A, et al. The lateral forearm flap: an anatomic study. Plast Reconstr Surg 99:460-464, 1997.

   Twelve fresh cadaver arms were dissected and injected with either methylene blue or latex. The posterior radial collateral artery was cannulated close to the lateral epicondyle and injected with methylene blue to determine the distal cutaneous flare, which averaged 15 cm (range 13 to 18 cm) distal to the lateral epicondyle. Latex injections were also performed in five arms and radiographed. The posterior radial collateral artery was shown to constantly divide proximal to the lateral epicondyle into an anterior and posterior division. The anterior division is the nutrient artery of the flap and extends along the lateral surface of the forearm, centered on the brachioradialis, 11 cm (average) before arborizing into a rich vascular plexus. Thirteen clinical cases were described in which the lateral forearm flap was used. This flap provides a longer pedicle length, thinner skin, and fewer sensory deficits at the donor site.

19. Tan BK, Lim BH. The lateral forearm flap as a modification of the lateral arm flap: vascular anatomy and clinical implications. Plast Reconstr Surg 105:2400-2404, 2000.

20. Ninkovic M, Harpf C, Schwabegger AH, et al. The lateral arm flap. Clin Plast Surg 28:367-374, 2001.

21. Marques Faria JC, Rodrigues ML, Scopel GP, et al. The versatility of the free lateral arm flap in head and neck soft tissue reconstruction: clinical experience of 210 cases. J Plast Reconstr Aesthet Surg 61:172-179, 2008.

22. Gordon DJ, Small JO. The addition of muscle to the lateral arm and radial forearm flaps for wound coverage. Plast Reconstr Surg 89:563-566, 1992.

23. Moffett TR, Madison SA, Derr JW, et al. An extended approach for the vascular pedicle of the lateral arm free flap. Plast Reconstr Surg 89:259-267, 1992.

24. Culbertson JH, Mutimer K. The reverse lateral upper arm flap for elbow coverage. Ann Plast Surg 18:62-68, 1987.

25. Coessens B, Vico P, De Mey A. Clinical experience with the reverse lateral arm flap in soft-tissue coverage of the elbow. Plast Reconstr Surg 92:1133-1136, 1993.

   Clinical experience with the reverse lateral arm flap for coverage of medium-sized defects of the posterior elbow in five patients was reviewed. The authors performed lead oxide injections and subsequent radiographic examination to map the vascular supply of the reverse lateral arm flap. The distal end of the posterior collateral artery anastomosed constantly in the epicondylar region with two recurrent arteries: the interosseous recurrent artery and the recurrent radial artery. Either of these arteries can be used as the vascular supply to the flap, but the authors prefer to use the recurrent radial artery, which lies anterior to the lateral epicondyle, because it offers a gentler arc of rotation with less risk of pedicle kinking.

26. Revol MP, Lantieri L, Loy S, et al. Vascular anatomy of the forearm muscles: a study of 50 dissections. Plast Reconstr Surg 88:1026-1033, 1991.

27. Türegün M, Nisanci M, Duman H, et al. Versatility of the reverse lateral arm flap in the treatment of post-burn antecubital contractures. Burns 31:212-216, 2005.

28. Lai CS, Tsai CC, Liao KB, et al. The reverse lateral arm adipofascial flap for elbow coverage. Ann Plast Surg 39:196-200, 1997.

29. Lazarou SA, Kaplan IB. The lateral arm flap for elbow coverage. Plast Reconstr Surg 91:1349-1354, 1993.

30. Shenaq SM. Pretransfer expansion of a sensate lateral arm free flap. Ann Plast Surg 19:558-562, 1987.

17

Posterior Interosseous
Artery Perforator Flap

Minoru Shibata

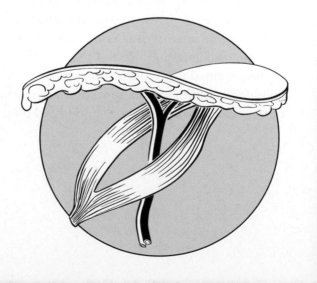

When selecting reconstructive procedures for the hand, an acceptable final appearance and good function must be considered. The introduction of the posterior interosseous artery flap by Zancolli and Angrigiani[1] and Penteado et al[2] therefore captured the attention of many surgeons who reconstruct the upper extremity. Skin flaps elevated on perforators from the posterior interosseous artery provide thin skin with an excellent color and quality match for covering soft tissue of the hand, especially on its dorsal aspect. Functional reconstruction of the hand often requires tedious, complicated procedures. Simultaneous soft tissue coverage is occasionally needed. In these circumstances, the reverse pedicle posterior interosseous artery perforator (PIOAP) flap is an extremely useful tool. Despite several potential pitfalls, this flap can be useful for reconstructing defects of the upper extremity.

ANATOMY

The PIOAP flap is a septocutaneous flap supplied by the posterior interosseous artery. This artery courses distally on the septum between extensor digiti minimi and extensor carpi ulnaris muscles and gives off interstitial arteries that run perpendicular to the skin on the dorsoulnar aspect of the forearm.[2-5] The number of these perforating vessels is variable; however, there are usually three branches,[3,4] one with a large diameter and two with intermediate diameters. After piercing the fascia, the interstitial arteries immediately form a suprafascial vascular network that produces a second plexiform network in the subcutaneous tissue plane. Care must be exercised because all of these perforating vessels are located in the middle third of the forearm, and no reliable perforators are found in the proximal third of the forearm. If a distally based pedicle flap is designed in the proximal third of the forearm to extend distal to the MP joint level, some of the adipofascia of the middle third of the forearm needs to be attached to the flap as part of the pedicle to capture the suprafascial plexus fed by its perforators (Fig. 17-1).

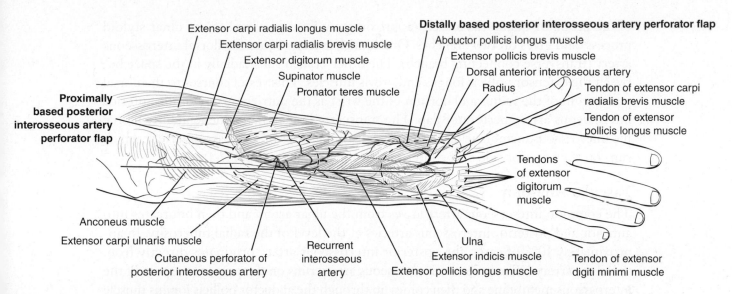

Fig. 17-1 Vascular anatomy of the posterior interosseous artery perforator (PIOAP) flap.

The PIOAP flap is used as an island flap. It is characterized by the vascular pedicle running along on the septum between the extensor digit minimi and extensor carpi ulnaris muscles. A loop is created that anastomoses with the dorsal branch of the anterior interosseous artery and with the dorsal carpal arterial arch, allowing the flap to be used as a reverse pedicle island flap. The arc of rotation is defined by the sum of the length of the flap, the length of the posterior interosseous artery in the septum, and the length to the pivot point around the distal radioulnar joint. The fasciocutaneous perforators (interstitial arteries) delivered from the posterior interosseous artery form the suprafascial vascular network. This network takes on the character of a vascular axis and extends proximally or distally, allowing elongation of the island flap.

SURGICAL TECHNIQUE
Surface Landmarks

The PIOAP flap is designed on a line between the lateral humeral epicondyle and the distal radioulnar joint. The posterior interosseous artery arises from the common interosseous artery and runs posterior to the supinator muscle, entering at the junction of the middle and proximal thirds of the line. The middle-sized perforator branch to the posterior forearm skin is usually located in the middle third of the forearm. The flap has to be designed to involve these skin perforators in the middle third of the forearm. It can be extended proximally or distally on the same fascia in the dorsal aspect of the forearm.

The distally based posterior interosseous artery pedicle flap is based on the dorsal branches of the anterior interosseous artery. The vascular anastomosis between anterior and posterior interosseous arteries is a very consistent finding that was confirmed in 97.1% to 100% of cadaveric limbs.[2-7] The dorsal branch of the anterior interosseous artery pierces the interosseous membrane in the distal forearm at the proximal edge of the pronator quadratus muscle (approximately 5 cm proximal to the ulnar styloid process) and gives off two branches. One branch travels to join the dorsal interosseous artery (transverse connecting branch). The other branch runs radially in the space between the extensor pollicis longus and brevis muscles. This vessel courses to the dorsal periosteum of the radius and dorsum of the wrist as the nutrient artery of the anterior interosseous artery perforator flap. The transverse branch may independently pierce the interosseous membrane distal to the trunk of the anterior interosseous artery, which runs on the anterior side of the interosseous membrane (see Fig. 17-1).

Vascular Anatomy

The common interosseous artery arises from the ulnar artery and then bifurcates into anterior and posterior interosseous arteries at the level of the radial tuberosity. In approximately 10% of cases, the posterior interosseous artery originates directly from the ulnar artery.[2] The posterior interosseous artery runs on the posterior aspect of the interosseous membrane and then comes up through the abductor pollicis longus muscle belly at the junction of the proximal and middle third of the forearm. The vessel gives off the ascending recurrent branch proximally and descends along the posterior septum. The artery travels between the extensor digiti minimi and extensor carpi ulnaris muscles from the junction of the middle and proximal thirds of the forearm to the distal radioulnar joint. Doppler ultrasound may be helpful to detect the course of the posterior interosseous artery running on the posterior septum. More precise confirmation of the course of the artery may be possible with CT angiography.[8] The posterior interosseous vessels travel with the posterior interosseous nerve, giving off several fascial perforators at the wrist level. The proximal cutaneous perforator usually has a larger diameter. The fasciocutaneous perforators run in a tortuous fashion and form a suprafascial vascular network after piercing the fascia. The terminal arteries to the skin form a second plexus within the plane of subcutaneous tissue.

The posterior interosseous artery travels distally to the proximal edge of the extensor retinaculum. This site is the most distal pivot point of a reverse pedicle PIOAP flap. The artery communicates with the dorsal branch of the anterior interosseous artery around the proximal wrist joint and courses beneath the extensor retinaculum. The posterior interosseous artery continues distally and anastomoses to the dorsal carpal arch. This anastomosis allows the PIOAP flap to be employed as a distally based flap with the pivot point placed at the proximal border of the distal radioulnar joint (see Fig. 17-1).

Neighboring Flaps and Anatomic Structures
Anterior Interosseous Artery Perforator Flap

The anterior interosseous artery perforator flap is a cutaneous flap based on the posterior branch of the anterior interosseous artery, and is also known as the anterior interosseous flap.[9,10] This branch supplies the distal third of the dorsal aspect of the forearm, which is nearly the same territory included in the PIOAP flap, with the additional region of the entire wrist area.

The anterior interosseous artery originates from the common interosseous artery and travels distally with the anterior interosseous nerve on the anterior side of the interosseous membrane. This artery gives off a dorsal branch that penetrates the interosseous membrane at the proximal edge of the pronator quadratus muscle, approximately

5 cm proximal to the radial styloid process. This branch continues distally with the terminal branch of the posterior interosseous nerve and gives off two branches. One branch courses radially between the extensor pollicis longus and brevis muscles, and enters the deep fascia to supply the dorsal distal third of the forearm and entire dorsal wrist.[3,10] One branch descends along the ulna to the wrist joint, creating an arch with the posterior interosseous artery.

Dorsoulnar Flap Based on Distal Branches of the Ulnar Artery (Becker's Flap)

The dorsoulnar branch of the ulnar artery arises 2 to 5 cm proximal to the pisiform bone. This branch supplies the skin through the space dorsal to the flexor carpi ulnaris muscle and palmar to the extensor carpi ulnaris muscle. The branch bifurcates into a short descending (distal) branch and relatively long ascending (proximal) branch. The skin flap based on this ascending branch can be designed on the space between the palmaris longus and extensor digitorum communis muscles, up to 20 cm proximally.[11] See Chapter 18 for additional information.

Lateral Arm Flap

The lateral arm flap is nourished by the septal artery, which originates from the posterior descending branch of the profunda brachii artery. The septal artery runs distally on the septum between the brachialis and triceps brachii muscles. The vessel continues to run between the brachioradialis and brachialis muscles in the distal portion of the arm, and anastomoses with the posterior recurrent radial artery in the lateral elbow region. The anatomy of this flap is very consistent and can be elevated either as a free or a pedicle flap. Pedicle flaps can be used to cover the shoulder or elbow as a proximally or distally based flap, respectively. The flap can be extended to the proximal third of the forearm to obtain a thinner flap. See Chapter 16 for additional information.

APPLICATIONS
Coverage of Large Defects in the Forearm and Hand
Extended Posterior Interosseous Artery Perforator–Lateral Arm Flap

The lateral arm flap can be designed to include the dorsoulnar aspect of the proximal third of the forearm to obtain thinner skin.[12] The proximal forearm area can also be included in the PIOAP flap. The PIOAP and lateral arm flaps can be combined in a Siamese-type flap.[13] In a similar fashion, Harii[14] designed the microvascular musculocutaneous flap by combining groin and latissimus dorsi flaps to reconstruct large defects in the upper or lower extremities. The extended PIOAP–lateral arm flap can be rotated proximally or distally by keeping one of the vascular pedicles intact and anastomosing the other vascular pedicle to the vessels in the recipient area. It should be possible to mobilize distantly by dividing both source pedicles and anastomosing these vessels in the recipient bed. However, dissection of this larger flap takes more time and requires more difficult and tedious preparation for two pairs of vascular pedicles appropriate for anastomosis. Extending the flap over to the defect with either pedicle as the pivot point requires only a single vascular pedicle preparation and anastomosis. This maneuver ensures survival of the pedicled side of the flap if the vascular anastomosis fails. This procedure would be especially useful as the salvage procedure for severe traumatic cases.

Distally Based Posterior Interosseous Artery Flap

The distal anastomosis of the anterior and posterior interosseous arteries is the most important anatomic structure for the survival of the reverse pedicle PIOAP flap. This anastomosis is a very reliable anatomic finding. Careful dissection around the wrist joint (approximately 2 cm proximal to the ulnar head) is required to preserve this transverse arterial connection.

If the caliber of the posterior interosseous artery becomes minute in the middle or distal third of the dorsal forearm, two options exist. First, the dissection is stopped and the donor site is closed if the dissection has not been completed. Alternatively, the reverse pedicle flap can be converted to a free flap by anastomosing the proximal end of the PIOAP flap, where vessel caliber is large enough to successfully perform vascular anastomosis. These decisions can be made after dissecting the posterior interosseous artery.

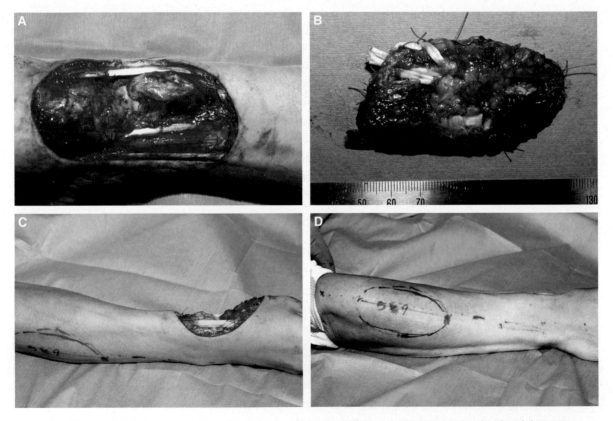

Fig. 17-2 This 51-year-old man developed a malignant fibrous histiocytoma in the distal forearm and wrist area. **A** and **B,** The tumor was resected widely to include the radial artery and radial sensory nerve, and tendons of the abductor pollicis longus, flexor carpi radialis, and extensor pollicis brevis muscles. **C** and **D,** A reverse pedicle PIOAP flap was designed to cover the soft tissue defect.

Other methods can be used to provide arterial inflow and venous outflow through fascial extension of adjacent cutaneous flaps. Therefore a deepithelialized adipofascial extension of either the anterior interosseous artery perforator flap or the dorsoulnar flap based on distal branches of the ulnar artery should augment flap vascularity (Figs. 17-2 through 17-4).

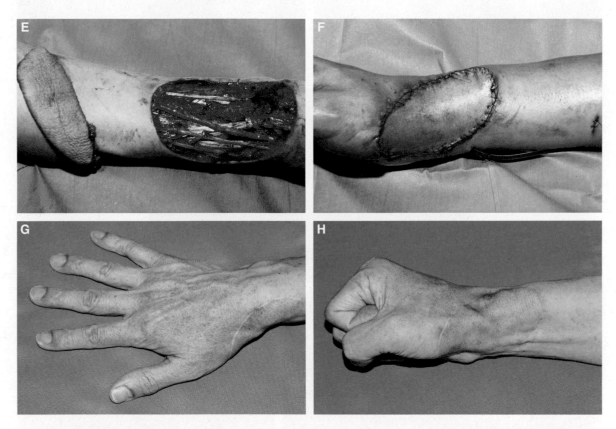

Fig. 17-2, cont'd E, The radial artery was reconstructed with a vein graft. The tendon defects of the abductor pollicis longus, flexor carpi radialis, and extensor pollicis brevis muscles were reconstructed using a palmaris longus graft. The flap was raised. **F,** The flap was inset in the defect. **G** and **H,** Two years and 10 months after surgery, the patient has radial sensory nerve function. The vein graft to the radial artery is patent, and the skin color and contour match are excellent.

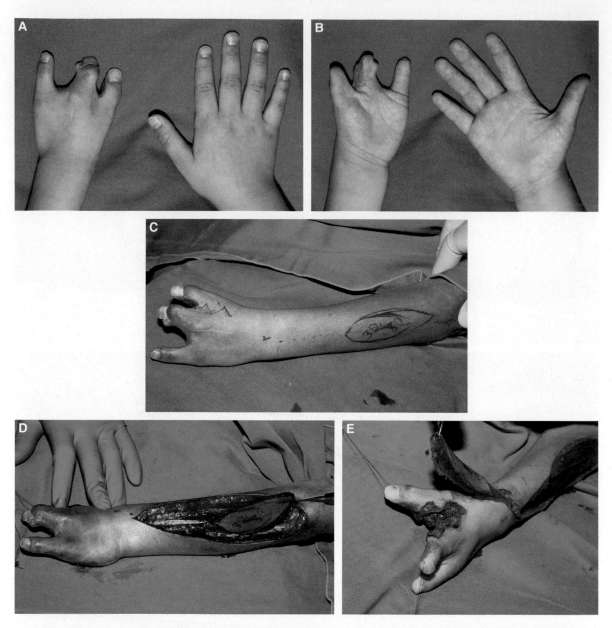

Fig. 17-3   A and **B,** This boy, 3 years and 4 months old, presented with brachysyndactyly of the left thumb. He had undergone previous surgery for closure of the left interdigital space and separation of the syndactyly of the two radial digits. **C,** The surgical plan was to widen the first interdigital space and remove the second metacarpal bone. A pedicle PIOAP flap was planned for coverage of the soft tissue defect created by the widened first web space. **D** and **E,** The flap was elevated and transposed into the first web space soft tissue defect. The donor site was closed primarily.

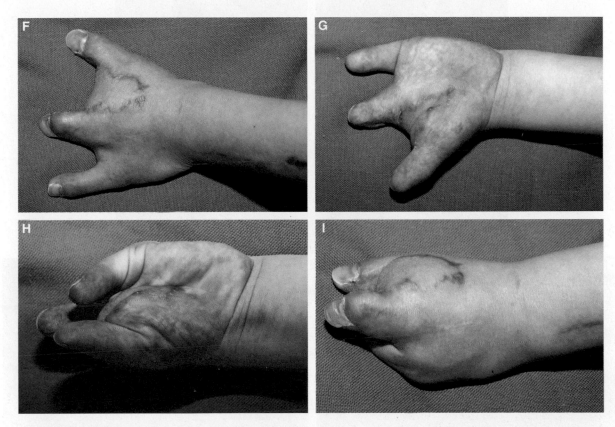

Fig. 17-3, cont'd   F-I, The patient is shown 5 months postoperatively. The flap has healed well with good color match and an acceptable donor site scar.

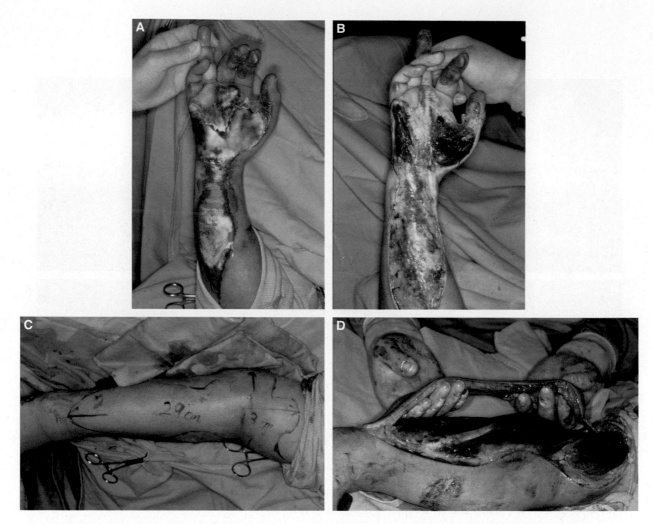

Fig. 17-4   **A,** This 39-year-old man was injured with a hot press. **B,** The wound was extensive after debridement of the full-thickness eschar. **C,** A large combined posterior interosseous flap and lateral arm flap was designed measuring 29 by 13 cm. **D,** The flap was elevated with the anterior interosseous artery intact distally and a posterior radial collateral artery intact proximally.

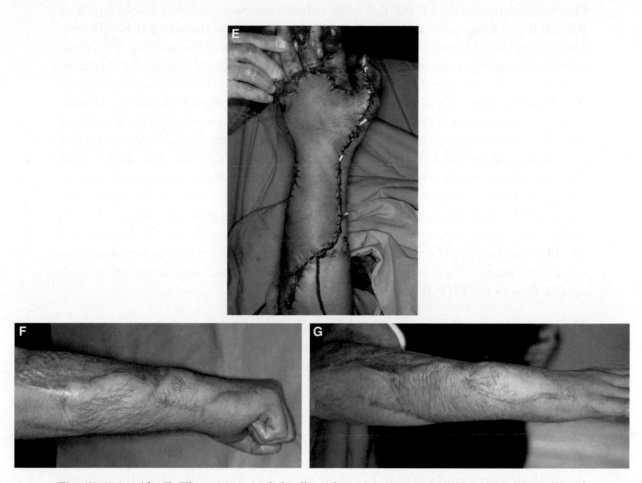

Fig. 17-4, cont'd   E, The posterior radial collateral artery was anastomosed to the common digital artery of the fourth web space. The dorsal branch of the anterior interosseous artery was maintained and provided excellent vascularity to the flap. **F** and **G,** Healing was complete and without complications. Functional and cosmetic results were excellent.

MODIFICATIONS
Anterior Interosseous Artery Fascial Flap

One modification of the PIOAP flap is the anterior interosseous artery fascial flap. The PIOAP flap is designed as usual; however, dissection distal to the skin flap is different. Distal radial dorsal forearm adipofascia is included at the base of the skin flap. This distal adipofascia extension provides additional vascularity from a distal to proximal direction. The cutaneous perforator from the dorsal branch of the anterior interosseous artery is visualized through a fascial incision over the ulnar third of distal radius bone. If more distal vascular pedicle is required, the interosseous membrane overlying the anterior interosseous artery piercing site is divided distally, and then the underlying anterior interosseous artery trunk is divided proximal to the branching site. The dorsal radial wrist adipofascia, which is supplied by the terminal branch of the anterior interosseous artery, can be elevated with the pedicle at the distal radioulnar joint as the pivot point. More simply, pedicle dissection is stopped after confirming that the posterior branch of the anterior interosseous artery extends into the elevating pedicle. In this case, the proximal border has to be shifted proximally to compensate for a more proximally located pivot point. This procedure provides significant vascular augmentation through reverse flow to the PIOAP flap.

Dorsoulnar Flap Based on Distal Branches of the Ulnar Artery

In this modification of the PIOAP flap, the dorsoulnar forearm fascia is included in the flap as the distal fascial extension to integrate the nonreverse arterial inflow and venous returning system of the dorsoulnar flap based on distal branches of the ulnar artery.[11]

Dissection distal to the flap on the ulnar side is different from dissection of the standard PIOAP flap. The fascia over the flexor carpi ulnaris muscle is exposed and incised longitudinally at the radial border of the muscle. This fascia is elevated in the dorsoulnar direction to locate the ascending branch of the dorsal ulnar artery. The dorsal ulnar artery emerges from the ulnar artery 2 to 5 cm proximal to the pisiform bone. The distal radioulnar joint is the pivot point of the PIOAP flap and is located 2.5 cm proximal to the pisiform bone. For this reason, this modified PIOAP flap with fascial extension of the dorsoulnar forearm flap is rotated with the original pivot point for the PIOAP flap. This procedure is easier to perform than the modification for the anterior interosseous artery fascial flap.

PITFALLS
Anatomic Variation

The posterior interosseous artery may become very small as it travels distally in approximately 6% of the cases.[4] In these patients, flap harvest may have to be terminated or converted to the free flap.[15] In approximately 8% of the cases, the origin of the skin perforator is located quite distally. This problem can be solved by using the perforator supplying the distal adipofascia. Nerves crossing the arterial system may be managed with a neurotomy and immediate repair to regain near-normal muscle power.

Venous Congestion

Venous congestion is often observed. A serious problem can be avoided by elevating the cutaneous vein with the flap pedicle.

Subcutaneous Passage of the Flap and Pedicle Tension

Tethered fibers in the subcutaneous tunnel must be eliminated to avoid compression of the vascular pedicle, which can undergo postoperative swelling in the tunnel. Tension on the pedicle and external compression must be avoided.

Primary Donor Site Closure With Excess Tension

Primary closure of the donor site is crucial to minimize donor site morbidity. However, if too much tension is created by the closure, a condition similar to compartment syndrome may occur. If too much tension is suspected after primary closure, sutures should be removed. The wound should be closed loosely and early secondary closure considered.

Flap necrosis of various degrees requires additional use of another flap in up to 14% of patients.[15] Despite the limitations of the PIOAP flap, many papers conclude that this flap is one of the most useful tools for coverage of the dorsal hand or thumb.[6,7,16] Limitations of this flap may be minimized by applying modifications described in this chapter.

References

1. Zancolli EA, Angrigiani C. Posterior interosseous island forearm flap. J Hand Surg 13:130-135, 1988.
   > *These authors were among the first to develop the posterior interosseous flap. This paper presented an anatomic study of the posterior interosseous artery flap involving 20 cadavers and 25 clinical cases.*
2. Penteado CV, Masquelet AC, Chevrel JP. The anatomic basis of the fasciocutaneous flap of the posterior interosseous artery. Surg Radiol Anat 8:209-215, 1986.
   > *The authors presented one of the earliest studies of the anatomy of the posterior interosseous artery flap. Seventy cadavers and 12 clinical cases were reviewed.*
3. Bayon P, Pho RW. Anatomical basis of dorsal forearm flap. J Hand Surg 13:435-439, 1988.
   > *This paper reported on the anatomic basis of the posterior interosseous arterial flap using 35 upper limbs and supplies useful information for clinical elevation of the flap.*
4. Büchler U, Frey HP. Retrograde posterior interosseous flap. J Hand Surg 16:283-292, 1991.
   > *The authors conducted a retrospective clinical study of 36 distally based posterior interosseous flap procedures and analyzed anatomic variations, causes of hypoperfusion, and flap survival rates.*
5. Costa H, Soutar DS. The distally based island posterior interosseous flap. Br J Plast Surg 41:221-227, 1988.
6. Angrigiani C, Grilli D, Dominikow D, et al. Posterior interosseous reverse forearm flap: experience with 80 consecutive cases. Plast Reconstr Surg 92:285-293, 1993.
7. Costa H, Comba S, Martins A, et al. Further experience with the posterior interosseous flap. Br J Plast Surg 44:449-455, 1991.
8. Rozen WM, Hong MK, Ashton MW, et al. Imaging the posterior interosseous artery with computed tomographic angiography. Ann Plast Surg 65:300-301, 2010.
9. Martin D, Rivet D, Boileau R, et al. The posterior radial epiphysis free flap: a new donor site. Br J Plast Surg 42:499-506, 1989.
   > *This was the first paper to report on skin and osteocutaneous flaps based on the posterior branch of the anterior interosseous artery flap.*

10. Shibata M, Ogishyo N. Free flaps based on the anterior interosseous artery. Plast Reconstr Surg 97:746-755, 1996.

These authors reported on free vascularized nerve and skin flaps based on the anterior interosseous artery, including the first clinical case of a free cutaneous flap based on the posterior branch of the anterior interosseous artery.

11. Becker C, Gilbert A. The ulnar flap. Handchir Mikrochir Plast Chir 20:180-183, 1988.

12. Kuek LB, Chuan TL. The extended lateral arm flap: a new modification. J Reconstr Microsurg 7:167-173, 1991.

13. Shibata M, Hatano Y, Iwabuchi Y, et al. Combined dorsal forearm and lateral arm flap. Plast Reconstr Surg 96:1423-1429, 1995.

14. Harii K. Muscle and musculocutaneous flap. In Microvascular Tissue Transfer. Tokyo: Igaku-Shoin, 1983.

15. Shibata M, Iwabuchi Y, Kubota S, et al. Comparison of free and reversed pedicled posterior interosseous cutaneous flaps. Plast Reconstr Surg 99:791-802, 1997.

The authors compared free and pedicle posterior interosseous artery flaps for coverage of the hand and distal forearm. Three pedicle flaps with reverse flow were used as the combined flap with a lateral arm flap to cover larger defects.

16. Vogelin E, Langer M, Büchler U. How reliable is the posterior interosseous artery island flap? A review of 88 patients. Handchir Mikrochir Plast Chir 34:190-194, 2002.

The authors retrospectively studied 88 cases of reverse pedicle posterior interosseous flaps and concluded that this flap is ideal for reconstruction of the thumb web and dorsal hand.

18

Ulnar Artery Perforator Flap

Daping Yang
Ammar S. Al Dhamin
Steven F. Morris

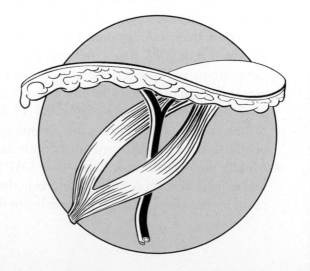

Lovie et al[1] originally described the ulnar forearm flap as a free flap in 1984. This flap mirrors the versatility of the radial forearm flap in that a skin island can be raised either as a free flap or as a reverse-flow island flap. The ulnar forearm flap is based on the septocutaneous perforators of the ulnar artery. The ulnar forearm flap is a good option for hand reconstruction, because it provides thin and pliable skin, a large consistent pedicle, and the possibility of combination with muscle (flexor carpi ulnaris), tendon (palmaris longus), sensory nerve, and bone (ulna). Compared with the radial forearm flap, the ulnar forearm flap offers several advantages such as ease of donor site closure, cosmetic acceptability, and hairlessness.[2,3] Both the radial forearm flap and ulnar forearm flap have characteristics that make them suitable options for reconstructing defects in the upper extremity and head and neck regions. However, both of these forearm island flaps require sacrificing one of the major arteries to the hand, which could jeopardize hand vascularity. The true ulnar artery perforator (UAP) flap includes skin from the ulnar forearm or hand based on an ulnar artery perforator, with preservation of the ulnar artery. The flap can be harvested from the proximal, middle, or distal forearm.

CLASSIFICATION OF FLAPS

- **Proximal ulnar perforator flaps**   El-Khatib et al[4] have described a proximal ulnar adipofascial perforator flap based on proximal perforators of the ulnar artery to correct contracture of elbow burn scars. The vascular supply of the flap is the fasciocutaneous perforators originating from either the proximal ulnar artery or the anterior ulnar recurrent artery. Maruyama et al[5] reported on an ulnar recurrent artery fasciocutaneous flap in 1987, based on the posterior ulnar recurrent artery. They described the anatomy of the anterior and posterior recurrent ulnar arteries and used this flap successfully in nine cases for elbow reconstruction. Mateev et al[6] used the posterior ulnar recurrent artery perforator flap (PURAP) in 22 cases for elbow and forearm reconstruction, highlighting the advantages of this donor site, which include thin, pliable skin with a well-concealed donor site.

- **Middle ulnar perforator flaps**   The UAP flap from the middle third of the forearm can be used to cover soft tissue defects in the forearm such as the donor defect of the radial forearm flap. Donor site morbidity of the radial forearm flap is well documented, with partial loss of split-thickness grafts occurring in 16% to 35% of cases.[7-11] Several techniques have been described that facilitate primary closure of small to medium-sized donor defects. Elliot et al[12] used the ulnar artery–based V-Y transposition flap to close small radial forearm donor defects primarily. Yii and Niranjan[13] successfully used a forearm fascial flap with a split-thickness skin graft to reconstruct distal forearm and hand defects (mostly free radial forearm flap donor defects) that were not suitable for closure with ulnar-based skin flaps. This flap was based on the ulnar artery and/or the anterior interosseous artery. The large fascial flap was supplied by a single perforator of the ulnar artery. No additional scar was incurred, because the fascial flap was harvested through the incision used for harvesting the radial forearm flap.

To facilitate closure of the radial donor defect, Hsieh et al[14] developed a bilobed flap based on a fasciocutaneous perforator of the ulnar artery. The bilobed flap is designed along the ulnar artery, adjacent to the radial forearm flap donor site. The pivot point of the flap is located approximately 8 cm proximal to the pisiform bone. There are one or two perforators from the ulnar artery near the pivot point. The bilobed flap includes a large lobe and a small lobe. The large lobe is used for repairing the radial forearm donor defect and the small lobe for closing the large lobe defect.

- **Distal ulnar perforator flaps** In the distal third of the forearm, an island flap based on a single dorsal perforator of the ulnar artery has been used. Becker and Gilbert[15,16] (1988 and 1990) described a flap from the ulnar border of the distal dorsal forearm based on the dorsal branch of the ulnar artery. This flap can be rotated 180 degrees to reconstruct defects on the dorsum of the hand without disrupting the ulnar artery.[17] However, the vascular pedicle is short, limiting flap mobility. To obtain a greater arc of rotation, Karacalar and Özcan[18] designed the flap more proximally, based on the ascending branch of the dorsal branch of the ulnar artery in a subcutaneous pedicle flap. A longer vascular pedicle was obtained to repair skin defects around the wrist.

In 1998, Bertelli and Pagliei[19] developed a reverse perforator flap distally based on the dorsal branches of the ulnar artery and nerve. The flap is raised on the distal half of the forearm and ulnar aspect of the hand, and its rotation point is located dorsally near the metacarpophalangeal joints. Blood supply to the flap is maintained by the anastomosis of the dorsal branch of the ulnar artery with the dorsal intermetacarpal arteries and with the digital arteries in the fourth web space. Karacalar and Özcan[20,21] reported a similar reverse perforator flap with the rotation point more proximal, near the insertion of the extensor carpi ulnaris muscle. Blood supply to this flap is maintained by the anastomosis between the descending branch of the dorsal branch of the ulnar artery and the dorsal carpal arch around the wrist. This flap is based on the descending branch, and reverse flow is ensured by the dorsal carpal arch through the descending branch. The distally based ulnar perforator flap has become a popular and widely used choice for hand reconstruction, and several large series have highlighted the flap's advantages and reliability.[21-26]

ANATOMY

The territory of the ulnar artery abuts that of the radial artery on the anterior midline of the forearm. The ulnar artery territory passes around the ulnar border of the forearm, extending onto the dorsal surface to the subcutaneous border of the ulna (Fig. 18-1). The boundary between ulnar and radial territories varies; however, it generally overlies the palmaris longus muscle. In some cases, there are relatively fewer ulnar artery perforators, and the ulnar territory is partly taken over by radial or posterior interosseous perforators.[27-29]

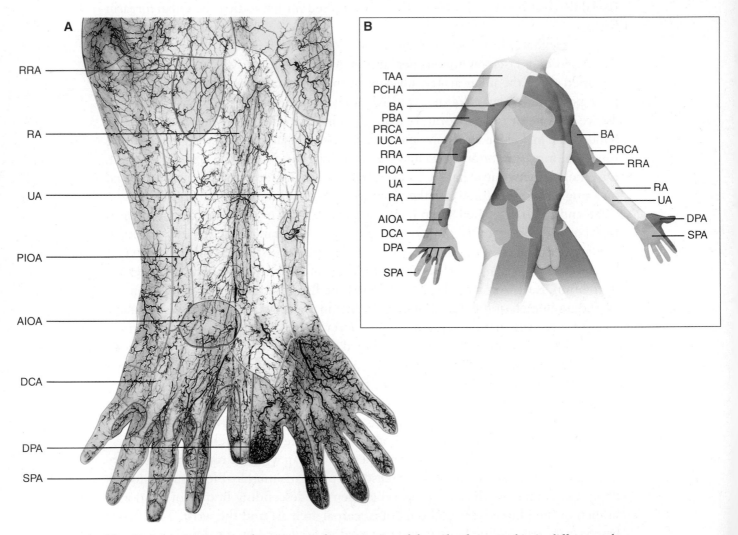

Fig. 18-1   A, Angiogram showing vascular territories of the volar forearm skin in different colors. **B,** The vascular territories of the upper limb. (*AIOA,* Anterior interosseous artery; *BA,* brachial artery; *DCA,* dorsal carpal arch; *DPA,* deep palmar arch; *IUCA,* inferior ulnar collateral artery; *PBA,* profunda brachial artery; *PCHA,* posterior circumflex humeral artery; *PIOA,* posterior interosseous artery; *PRCA,* posterior radial collateral artery; *RA,* radial artery; *RRA,* radial recurrent artery; *SPA,* superficial palmar arch; *TAA,* thoracoacromial artery; *UA,* ulnar artery.)

Our anatomic and angiographic studies demonstrate the distribution of the perforators of the ulnar artery, which supply the volar forearm and wrist[28] (Figs. 18-2 through 18-4; see Fig. 18-1). These perforators tend to become smaller from proximal to distal in the forearm, as the ulnar artery diminishes in caliber. Most of the perforators longitudinally anastomose with each other along the course of the main artery. These perforators form a deep fascial plexus and are arranged longitudinally along the main arterial axis. There are reduced-caliber choke anastomoses oriented transversely between the perforators of the radial, ulnar, and posterior interosseous arteries. These anastomoses form a plexus of longitudinally and horizontally oriented perforators. This information is useful clinically, especially when a Doppler probe is used to design customized flaps.

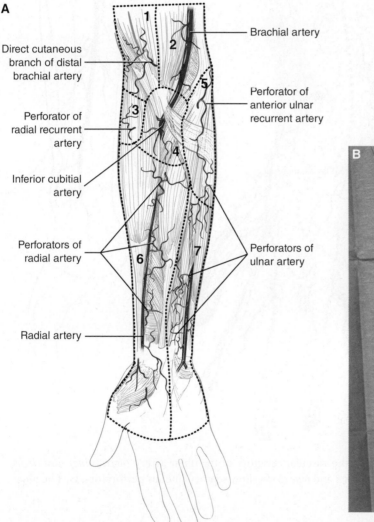
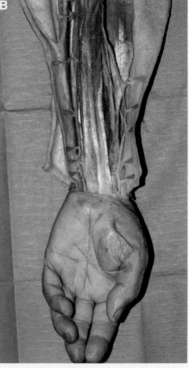

Fig. 18-2 A, The vascular architecture of the volar forearm. **B,** Cadaver dissection of perforators of the ulnar and radial arteries. Note the series of small, fairly short perforators *(blue arrows)* arising from both the radial and ulnar arteries. Ulnar artery perforators arise between flexor carpi ulnaris and palmaris muscle tendons in the distal forearm. Radial artery perforators arise between the flexor carpi radialis and brachioradialis muscle tendons in the distal forearm.

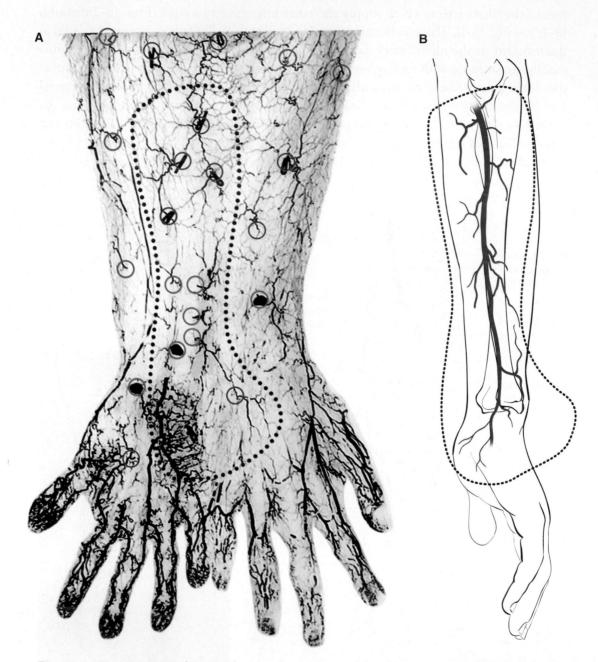

Fig. 18-3   **A,** Angiogram showing the vascular territory of the ulnar artery *(dotted line). Red circles* indicate musculocutaneous perforators, and *blue circles* show septocutaneous perforators. **B,** The ulnar artery and its perforators.

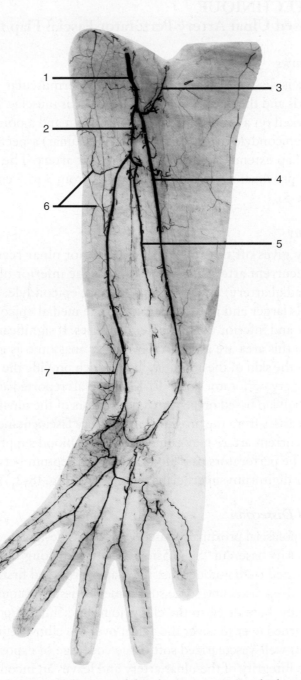

Fig. 18-4 Angiogram showing perforators of the ulnar artery. (*1*, Brachial artery; *2*, ulnar artery; *3*, radial recurrent artery; *4*, radial artery; *5*, anterior interosseous artery; *6*, proximal perforators from the ulnar artery; *7*, dorsal branch of the ulnar artery.)

SURGICAL TECHNIQUE
Proximally Based Ulnar Artery Perforator Fascial Flap for Elbow Scar Contracture
Surface Landmarks

The ulnar artery is dissected as it runs along the intermuscular septum between the flexor carpi ulnaris and the flexor digitorum superficialis muscles. The longitudinal axis of the flap is marked on a line connecting the pisiform and a point 2 cm lateral to the medial humeral epicondyle on the anteromedial (or ulnar) aspect of the forearm. The axial line of the flap extends distally along the ulnar artery. The surface landmark of the origin of the proximal ulnar perforators varies from 3 to 5 cm distal to the elbow joint line (Fig. 18-5).

Vascular Anatomy

The ulnar artery gives off the anterior and posterior ulnar recurrent arteries. The anterior ulnar recurrent artery anastomoses with the inferior ulnar collateral artery (branch of the radial artery) anterior to the medial epicondyle. The posterior ulnar collateral artery is larger and passes posterior to the medial epicondyle to anastomose with the superior and inferior ulnar collateral arteries. If significant branches from the brachial artery to this area are absent, this vascular anastomosis gives off a number of small branches to the skin of the anterior elbow, which provide the vascular basis for the ulnar recurrent artery perforator flap.[27] El-Khatib et al[4] reported an anatomic study of a pedicle adipofascial flap based on proximal perforators of the ulnar artery. The vascular supply of the flap arises from the proximal ulnar artery fasciocutaneous perforators. The anterior ulnar recurrent artery may contribute to the blood supply of the flap through its perforators. The perforators pass along the fascial septum between the flexor carpi ulnaris and flexor digitorum superficialis muscles (see Fig. 18-2, A).

Flap Design and Dissection

The fascial or adipofascial proximally based UAP flap is designed to incorporate at least two perforators at its base. An "S" incision is centered along the longitudinal axis of the flap and deepened to the subdermis. The flap is dissected first at the distal end and includes both the deep fascia and some subcutaneous tissue if required. The pivot point of the flap is usually 4 cm distal to the elbow joint line. The adipofascial/fascial flap is then rotated or turned over to cover the defect over the elbow region, and skin grafted. This flap provides well-vascularized soft tissue coverage of exposed elbow structures, yet maintains the integrity of the ulnar artery and leaves an inconspicuous donor site.

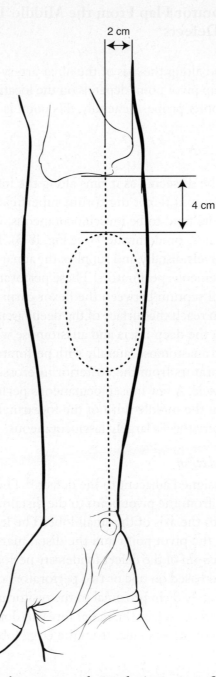

2 cm

4 cm

Fig. 18-5 The proximally based ulnar artery perforator fasciocutaneous flap design. The *long dotted line* represents the longitudinal axis of the flap and extends from the pisiform bone to a point 2 cm lateral to the medial humeral epicondyle.

Ulnar Artery Perforator Flap From the Middle Third of the Forearm for Radial Donor Defects

Surface Landmarks

A skin island is marked along the axis of the ulnar artery on the middle or distal third of the forearm. The flap pivot point depends on the location of perforators that may be identified using a Doppler probe. Generally, this point is approximately 8 cm proximal to the pisiform bone.

Vascular Anatomy

The ulnar artery can be dissected as it runs along the intermuscular septum between the flexor carpi ulnaris and flexor digitorum superficialis muscles. In the proximal forearm, the perforators tend to be musculocutaneous, whereas in the distal forearm septocutaneous perforators predominate[28] (see Fig. 18-3). The ulnar artery, accompanied by the ulnar nerve, travels distally and supplies the ulnar territory with a series of five to six smaller septocutaneous perforators. These perforators pass anterior to the ulnar nerve along the fascial septum between the flexor carpi ulnaris and flexor digitorum superficialis muscles to reach the surface of the deep fascia. The perforators tend to fan out predominantly on the deep fascia and anastomose with each other longitudinally. These perforators also anastomose laterally with perforators from the radial artery, and posteriorly with perforators from the posterior interosseous artery on the superficial surface of the deep fascia. A few musculocutaneous perforators may pierce the flexor carpi ulnaris muscle in the middle third of the forearm; however, the blood supply to the skin of the ulnar territory is largely fasciocutaneous.

Flap Design and Dissection

The bilobed flap is designed adjacent to the defect.[14] The axis of the large lobe is perpendicular to the line from the pivot point to the distalmost margin of the defect, and is also perpendicular to the axis of the small lobe. The length of both flaps is equal to the distance between the pivot point and the distal margin of the defect. The flap is dissected first at the margin of the defect to identify perforators of the ulnar artery. The bilobed flap is elevated based on one or two perforators of the ulnar artery around the pivot point (approximately 8 cm proximal to the pisiform bone). The large lobe of the flap is rotated 90 degrees to repair the radial forearm donor defect, and the small lobe is rotated to cover the resultant defect from the large lobe.

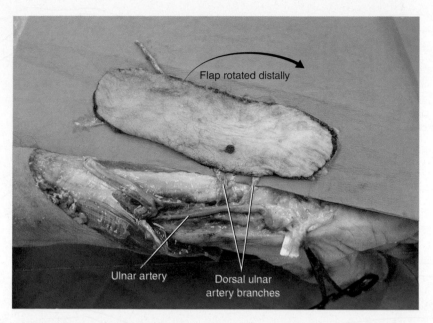

Flap rotated distally

Ulnar artery

Dorsal ulnar
artery branches

Fig. 18-6 The distally based dorsal UAP flap design. The flap can be based on a consistent dorsal perforator of the ulnar artery and be used for hand reconstruction, particularly along the ulnar border, dorsum, and palm of the hand.

Distally Based Dorsal Ulnar Artery Perforator Flap for Hand Reconstruction

Surface Landmarks

In the distal third of the forearm, the ulnar artery gives off its dorsal branch 2 to 7 cm proximal to the pisiform bone. The distally based dorsal UAP flap is outlined on the dorsal ulnar aspect of the distal forearm. The potential area of the flap is 6 by 16 cm, with the length extending from the distal third of the forearm to the distal third of the dorsal surface of the hand[19] (Fig. 18-6). The flap can be used for reconstructing the palm, dorsum, or ulnar border of the hand.[21-26]

Vascular Anatomy

The diameter of the dorsal branch of the ulnar artery is 0.9 to 1.8 mm at its origin from the ulnar artery (see Fig. 18-4). The dorsal branch of the ulnar artery runs obliquely from the palmar to the dorsal surface, passing deep to the flexor carpi ulnaris muscle and superficial to the ulnar nerve. It then gives off a fasciocutaneous branch that divides into an ascending branch and a descending branch. The ascending branch runs along the ulnar border of the forearm and anastomoses proximally with a cutaneous perforator from the ulnar artery on the superficial surface of the deep fascia. The descending

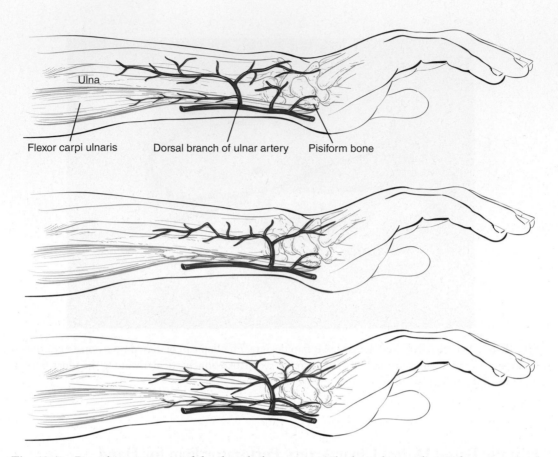

Fig. 18-7   Branching patterns of the dorsal ulnar artery. The branches to the pisiform, proximal forearm, and distal forearm can arise from the ulnar artery as a single trunk (72%), in two branches (24%), or as three separate branches (4%). (Modified from Becker C, Gilbert A. The dorsal ulnar artery flap. In Gilbert A, Masquelet AC, Hentz VR, eds. Pedicle Flaps of the Upper Extremity. London: Martin Dunitz, 1990.)

branch passes between the ulnar head and the pisiform bone, accompanied by the dorsal branch of the ulnar nerve, and anastomoses with the dorsal carpal arch (dorsal carpal vascular network). The descending branch also anastomoses with cutaneous perforators at the dorsum of the hand.[20] Becker and Gilbert[16] described a number of variations in the branching pattern of the dorsal ulnar artery; it was absent in only 1 of 100 forearms studied (Fig. 18-7).

Flap Dissection
The base of the flap is located dorsally, close to the ulnar head. The dorsal branch of the ulnar artery is dissected in the wrist, and it is ligated close to its origin. The fasciocutaneous flap is then dissected in a proximal to distal direction. The deep fascia should be included in the flap, and the distally based pedicle is elevated with the subcutaneous tissue to preserve the anastomosis. Venous drainage is maintained by the intact veins in the subcutaneous pedicle of the flap.

CASE EXAMPLES

This 55-year-old man's left hand was crushed in an industrial ice machine and was managed elsewhere with dressings for several weeks (Fig. 18-8). The wound was full thickness, with ulnar nerve and artery damage. The nerve was intact, but a 3 cm length of the artery was thrombosed.

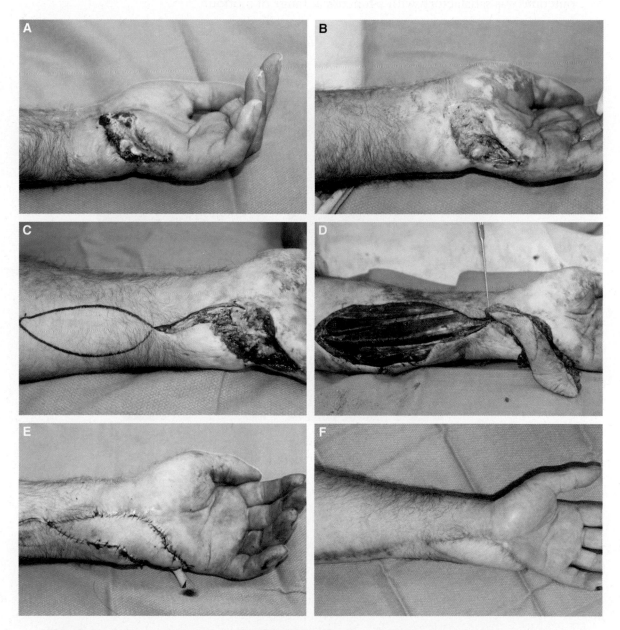

Fig. 18-8   A, The patient presented with a full-thickness wound extending to the carpus, with associated ulnar nerve and artery injuries. **B,** The nonviable debris in the wound was debrided, and the ulnar nerve and artery were dissected and examined. The ulnar nerve was intact although injured. The ulnar artery was thrombosed over a span of 3 cm. **C,** An ulnar perforator flap was designed on the most distal intact perforator of the ulnar artery. **D** and **E,** The ulnar perforator flap was inset. **F,** The patient is shown 6 months postoperatively with slow recovery of ulnar sensation.

This 29-year-old man presented with an electrical burn injury to his right hand (Fig. 18-9). He was seen at our hospital 7 days after the injury and had with tissue necrosis on the dorsum of the hand. The wound was debrided, and a reverse pedicle dorsal UAP flap was elevated, supplied by the dorsal carpal arch through the dorsal branch of the ulnar artery. The flap was transferred to the dorsum of the hand through a subcutaneous tunnel. It survived completely. The patient required physiotherapy. The ultimate outcome was satisfactory, with a functional range of motion.

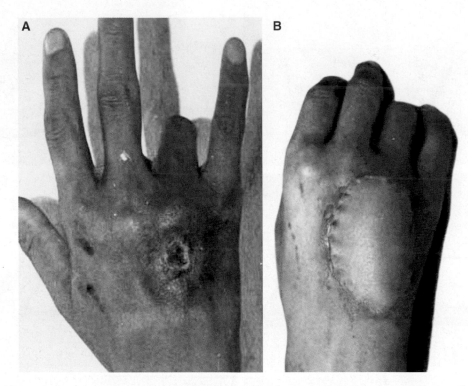

Fig. 18-9 A, Preoperative view of a lesion in the dorsal aspect of the hand caused by an electrical burn. **B,** The skin defect was covered with a reverse dorsal UAP flap based on the dorsal branch of the ulnar artery.

MODIFICATIONS

The ulnar artery forearm flap is quite similar to that of the radial forearm flap, and in many ways has similar versatility. The flap may include muscle (flexor carpi ulnaris), tendon (palmaris longus), nerve, and bone (ulna), similar to the radial forearm flap.

Ulnar Forearm Adipofascial Perforator Flap for Distal Forearm and Hand Defects

The forearm adipofascial flap consists of subcutaneous fat and fascia of the forearm. Yii and Niranjan[13] successfully used the fascial flap with a split-thickness skin graft to reconstruct distal forearm and hand defects (mostly free radial forearm flap donor defects), based on the ulnar artery and/or anterior interosseous artery. A fascial flap may be supplied by a single perforator of the ulnar artery. This flap is easy to raise and leaves no donor site defect.

Free Ulnar Fasciocutaneous Perforator Flap With a Segment of the Ulnar Artery

Free perforator flaps based on a single forearm perforator would require supramicrosurgical skills. For practical reasons, it is advisable to include a segment of the ulnar artery. The flap is elevated as a septocutaneous perforator flap with a very short segment (1 to 1.5 cm) of the ulnar artery included in the inverted-T–shaped arterial pedicle. Both ends of the ulnar artery segment could be anastomosed in the recipient site for a through-flow type of reconstruction. The ends of the donor ulnar artery are anastomosed to restore continuity of the vessel.[30] The diameter of the dorsal branches of the ulnar artery and nerve is suitable for anastomosis. Therefore this flap could be used as a sensate free flap.

Ulnar Forearm Osteocutaneous Perforator Flap

The dorsal branch of the ulnar artery gives off branches to the periosteum of the ulna. Anastomosis between the anterior interosseous artery and the dorsal branch of the ulnar artery is consistently found along the insertion of the pronator quadratus muscle on the ulna. Several periosteal branches are identified from this vascular arcade. Bertelli and Pagliei[19] reported that a distally based osteocutaneous perforator flap could be designed with the periosteal supply to the ulna (Fig. 18-10).

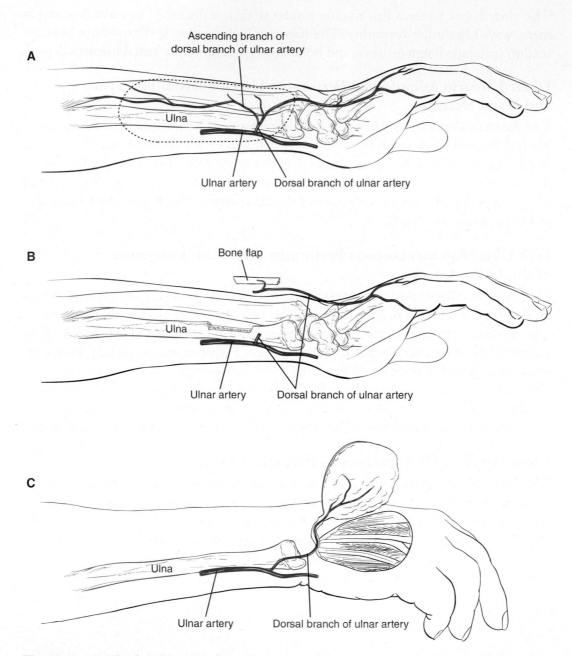

Fig. 18-10 **A,** The dorsal branch of the ulnar artery splits into ascending and descending branches, which can both be used to design flaps. The distally based dorsal UAP flap is outlined with a *dotted line.* **B,** A vascularized segment of ulna can be distally based on the anastomosis with dorsal metacarpal arteries. **C,** The dorsal branch of the ulnar artery can be used to design proximally based skin flaps from the dorsum of the hand.

PITFALLS
Anatomic Variability

Important considerations in harvesting a UAP flap are the variable location and size of the artery's perforators. A Doppler examination alone is often inadequate for predicting the location and size of the perforators because of interference from the radial and ulnar arteries. Preoperative CT angiography may be helpful but is expensive and time consuming, and may not be appropriate in a trauma situation. The surgical plan needs to be determined once the exact perforator size and position are known; therefore the flap harvest requires a flexible plan. Simic et al[31] found an anomalous superficial ulnar artery during anatomic dissection. It originated from the brachial artery, approximately 6 cm distal to the profunda brachial artery. Becker and Gilbert[16] reported the absence of the dorsal branch of the ulnar artery in 1% of dissections (1 of 100). Bertelli and Pagliei[19] found that the dorsal branch of the ulnar artery arises from the anterior interosseous artery in 7.7% of dissections (2 of 26). Therefore, if partial necrosis or blisters occur on the distally based dorsal UAP flap, it may be caused by poor vascular anastomoses between the dorsal branch of the ulnar artery and the dorsal carpal arch around the wrist, and not from the flap design beyond the vascular territory. If insufficient vascularity is noted in the elevated dorsoulnar flap after the tourniquet is released, we suggest that the elevated flap be converted from a reverse pedicle flap to a free flap. This conversion is achieved by anastomosing the proximal stump of the dorsal branch of the ulnar artery, which is attached to the flap.

Venous Congestion

A large superficial vein should be included with the pedicle of the flap to augment venous return rather than providing venous drainage only through the tiny reversed concomitant veins associated with the arterial perforator. Despite this effort, traction or pressure on the pedicle may result in venous congestion. The flap should be carefully examined before leaving the operating room to make certain that venous outflow is not compromised.

References

1. Lovie MJ, Duncan GM, Glasson DW. The ulnar artery forearm free flap. Br J Plast Surg 37:486-492, 1984.
2. Koshima I, Iino T, Fukuda H, et al. The free ulnar forearm flap. Ann Plast Surg 18:24-29, 1987.
3. Christie DR, Duncan GM, Glasson DW. The ulnar artery free flap: the first 7 years. Plast Reconstr Surg 93:547-551, 1994.
4. El-Khatib H, Mahboub T, Ali T. Use of an adipofascial flap based on the proximal perforator of the ulnar artery to correct contracture of elbow burn scars: an anatomic and clinical approach. Plast Reconstr Surg 109:130-136, 2002.
   A pedicle adipofascial flap based on the most proximal two to four perforators of the ulnar artery was used to repair elbow defects after release of a burn scar contracture. An anatomic dissection was performed to determine the location and dimensions of the flap.

5. Maruyama Y, Onishi K, Iwahira Y. The ulnar recurrent fasciocutaneous island flap: reverse medial arm flap. Plast Reconstr Surg 79:381-387, 1987.

6. Mateev MA, Trunov L, Hyakusoku H, et al. Analysis of 22 posterior ulnar recurrent artery perforator flaps: a type of proximal ulnar perforator flap. Eplasty 10:E2, 2010.

7. Timmons MJ, Missotten FE, Poole MD, et al. Complications of radial forearm flap donor sites. Br J Plast Surg 39:176-178, 1986.

8. Boorman JG, Brown JA, Sykes PJ. Morbidity in the forearm flap donor arm. Br J Plast Surg 40:207-212, 1987.

9. Bardsley AF, Soutar DS, Elliot D, et al. Reducing morbidity in the radial forearm flap donor site. Plast Reconstr Surg 86:287-292, 1990.

10. Swanson E, Boyd JB, Manktelow RT. The radial forearm flap: reconstructive applications and donor-site defects in 35 consecutive patients. Plast Reconstr Surg 85:258-266, 1990.

11. Richardson D, Fisher SE, Vaughan ED, et al. Radial forearm flap donor-site complications and morbidity: a prospective study. Plast Reconstr Surg 99:109-115, 1997.

12. Elliot D, Bardsley AF, Batchelor AG, et al. Direct closure of the radial forearm flap donor defect. Br J Plast Surg 41:358-360, 1988.

13. Yii NW, Niranjan NS. Fascial flaps based on perforators for reconstruction of the defects in the distal forearm. Br J Plast Surg 52:534-540, 1999.

    Twenty fascial flaps were used to reconstruct defects in the distal forearm, wrist, and hand in 18 patients over a 2-year period. In 16 patients the flaps were based on a single fascial feeding vessel or "perforator" arising from the anterior interosseous artery and/or ulnar artery when the radial artery had been used as the donor vessel in free flap reconstruction elsewhere in the body. No flaps were lost.

14. Hsieh CH, Kuo YR, Yao SF, et al. Primary closure of radial forearm flap donor defects with a bilobed flap based on the fasciocutaneous perforator of the ulnar artery. Plast Reconstr Surg 113:1355-1360, 2004.

    A bilobed flap based on the fasciocutaneous perforator of the ulnar artery was designed to repair the radial forearm flap donor defect. The large lobe of the flap was used for repairing the donor defect, and the small lobe covered the resultant defect from the large lobe. This flap is suitable for closing medium-sized defect.

15. Becker C, Gilbert A. The ulnar flap: description and application. Eur J Plast Surg 11:79-82, 1988.

16. Becker C, Gilbert A. The dorsal ulnar artery flap. In Gilbert A, Masquelet AC, Hentz VR, eds. Pedicle Flaps of the Upper Extremity. London: Martin Dunitz, 1990.

17. Holevich-Madjarova B, Paneva-Holevich E, Topkarov V. Island flap supplied by the dorsal branch of the ulnar artery. Plast Reconstr Surg 87:562-566, 1991.

18. Karacalar A, Özcan M. Use of a subcutaneous pedicle ulnar flap to cover skin defects around the wrist. J Hand Surg Am 23:551-555, 1998.

19. Bertelli JA, Pagliei A. The neurocutaneous flap based on the dorsal branches of the ulnar artery and nerve: a new flap for extensive reconstruction of the hand. Plast Reconstr Surg 101:1537-1543, 1998.

    Using information from their anatomic study, the authors developed a neurocutaneous flap distally based on the dorsal branch of the ulnar artery and nerve. The flap was raised on the hand and distal forearm, with its rotation point located dorsally near the metacarpophalangeal joint. The flap was used clinically to repair skin defects on the hand.

20. Karacalar A, Özcan M. The distally based ulnar artery forearm flap supplied by the dorsal carpal arch. Ann Plast Surg 41:304-306, 1988.

21. Karacalar A, Özcan M. Preliminary report: the distally pedicled dorsoulnar forearm flap for hand reconstruction. Br J Plast Surg 52:453-457, 1999.

    The authors modified the standard dorsoulnar flap based on the dorsal branch of the ulnar artery to a distally based dorsoulnar flap based on the vascular anastomoses between the dorsal branch of the ulnar artery and the dorsal carpal arch. This modification provided a longer pedicle and increased the arc of rotation.

22. Ignatiadis IA, Giannoulis FS, Mavrogenis AF, et al. Ulnar and radial artery based perforator adipofascial flaps. EEXOT 59:101-108, 2008.

23. Liu DX, Wang H, Li XD, et al. Three kinds of forearm flaps for hand skin defects: experience with 65 cases. Arch Orthop Trauma Surg 131:675-680, 2011.

24. Ignatiadis IA, Mavrogenis AF, Avram AM, et al. Treatment of complex hand trauma using the distal ulnar and radial artery perforator-based flaps. Injury 39(Suppl 3):S116-S124, 2008.

25. Sauerbier M, Unglaub F. Perforator flaps in the upper extremity. Clin Plast Surg 37:667-676, 2010.

26. Page R, Chang J. Reconstruction of hand soft-tissue defects: alternatives to the radial forearm fasciocutaneous flap. J Hand Surg Am 31:847-856, 2006.

27. Cormack GC, Lamberty BG. The Arterial Anatomy of Skin Flaps, 2nd ed. Edinburgh: Churchill Livingstone, 1994.

28. Kanellakos GW, Yang D, Morris SF. Cutaneous vasculature of the forearm. Ann Plast Surg 50:387-392, 2003.

29. Inoue Y, Taylor GI. The angiosomes of the forearm: anatomic study and clinical implication. Plast Reconstr Surg 98:195-210, 1996.

30. Arnstein PM, Lewis JS. Free ulnar artery forearm flap: a modification. Br J Plast Surg 55:356-357, 2002.

31. Simic P, Borovecki F, Jalsovec D, et al. The superficial ulnar artery originating from the left brachial artery. Ital J Anat Embryol 109:13-18, 2004.

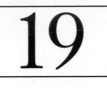

Radial Artery
Perforator Flap

Daping Yang
Jenny Fei Yang
Steven F. Morris

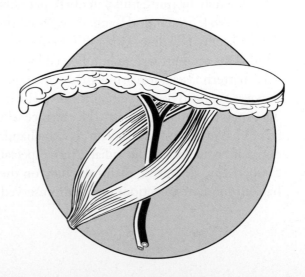

The radial forearm flap was originally described as a free flap by Yang et al[1] in 1981 and was popularized in the English-language literature by Song et al[2] in 1982. Also in 1982, Lu et al[3] described the use of a distally based, axial-pattern, radial forearm fasciocutaneous flap based on the radial artery and vena comitans for reconstruction of soft tissue defects of the hand. The radial forearm free flap and distally based pedicle flap rapidly became popular for head and neck and extremity reconstruction because of its advantages, including reliable vascularity, thin pliable skin, hairlessness, possible sensibility, and ease of dissection. Since then, several other investigators have reported on the versatility of the reverse radial forearm flap for upper extremity reconstruction.[4,5] Biemer and Stock[6] and Foucher et al[7] described successful cases of thumb reconstruction by inclusion of a segment of radius as an osteocutaneous flap, and inclusion of vascularized tendon and nerve.

The advantages of using the radial forearm flap for hand reconstruction are numerous. However, two major disadvantages for the donor site are the sacrifice of the radial artery, which may possibly jeopardize hand vascularity, and poor donor site scarring. The donor site, particularly if a skin graft is required, is often obvious, and there may be associated tendon exposure with skin graft loss. Vascular complications of radial forearm flap or radial artery harvest have been reported, including digital or hand ischemia, vascular insufficiency, hypothenar hammer syndrome, and digital cold intolerance.[8] The flap may be quite bulky in obese patients.

In 1984, Soutar and Tanner[5] reported the first successful case of a fascial forearm flap and split-thickness skin graft for coverage of exposed tendons on the dorsum of the hand. This account was soon followed by several series describing the use of a reverse axial-pattern fascial forearm flap for coverage of the hand. The major advantage of this flap was reduced donor site morbidity, which was attributed to harvesting fascia alone. The major disadvantage was the sacrifice of the radial artery, with permanent loss of its contribution to the circulation of the hand. There are definite vascular changes that occur after the loss of the radial artery, especially in cold climates. Timmons[9] performed a superb and definitive anatomic study on the radial forearm flap using ink, latex, and barium sulphate injections on 56 unpreserved cadaveric forearms.

To overcome these drawbacks, the radial artery perforator (RAP) flap with preservation of the radial artery was developed in the 1990s. Zhang[10] reported on 10 cases using a reverse forearm pedicle fasciocutaneous flap with preservation of the radial artery for hand reconstruction. To understand the vascular basis of this flap, Chang[11] performed an anatomic study in 1990 to show that the pivot point of the pedicle was located 1.5 cm proximal to the radial styloid process. In 1992, Goffin et al[12] also performed an anatomic study of the perforators of the distal radial artery. A flap based on the distal perforators of the radial artery was raised on the dorsolateral aspect of the distal third of the forearm in seven clinical cases. Bertelli and Khoury[13] and Bertelli and Kaleli[14] introduced the concept of a neurocutaneous flap whose arterial vascularization is provided by the vascular plexus around and inside the cutaneous nerve. They reported on reverse neurocutaneous island flaps for reconstructions in the distal third of the forearm. The flap is distally based on a pedicle that includes the lateral antebrachial cutaneous nerve and cephalic vein. The vascular supply of the flap is the paraneural vascular plexus, which is formed by perforators from the radial artery. In 1994, Weinzweig et al[15] reported their anatomic study and clinical experiences with the distally based radial forearm fasciosubcutaneous flap, supplied by radial artery perforators situated 5 to 8 cm proximal to the radial styloid process.

The RAP flap is generally based on a single perforator, either proximally or distally. The proximally based radial forearm fasciocutaneous flap, based on the inferior cubital artery, may be used as a local perforator flap or as a microvascular free flap. The inferior cubital artery is the largest perforator arising from the radial artery. Because of its wide arc of rotation, this perforator flap may be useful for covering exposed elbow joints or prostheses, and is capable of reaching the olecranon region.[16]

The distally based radial forearm fasciocutaneous flap is vascularized by the perforators of the distal radial artery. The skin flap is along the axis of the radial artery; the pivot point of its adipofascial pedicle (usually 3 cm in width) is approximately 2 to 4 cm above the radial styloid process. The venous outflow of the flap is provided by the cephalic vein, with accompanying veins of the radial artery left behind. This flap not only preserves the radial artery but also provides a more acceptable donor site. It is easy to raise and transfer, and does not require microsurgical techniques. This flap could potentially be used as an innervated flap without requiring microsurgical technique, with the inclusion of the lateral cutaneous nerve of the forearm. The flap is a very useful and reliable alternative for reconstructing soft tissue defects of the hand. The advantage of this flap is its constant and reliable blood supply with preservation of the main radial artery.[15,17-19] Distally based composite flaps from the radial forearm including other tissues, such as the periosteum, tendon, and nerve, have been introduced.[20-22] The RAP flap has become a reliable and well-accepted successor to the radial forearm flap, with significant advantages.[23-31]

ANATOMY

Forearm skin is thin, pliable, and generally an excellent donor site for reconstruction of the hand, upper extremity, and head and neck regions. It is principally supplied by the radial and ulnar arteries and their branches. The pattern of blood supply to the forearm skin is analogous to that of the lower leg skin. Although there are a few musculocutaneous perforators in the proximal forearm, most of the blood supply comes from fasciocutaneous perforators arising from the radial, ulnar, anterior interosseous, and posterior interosseous arteries (Fig. 19-1). These arteries reach the surface by passing along the intermuscular fascial septa. A significant plexus is formed by branches of these perforators at the level of the deep fascia.[9]

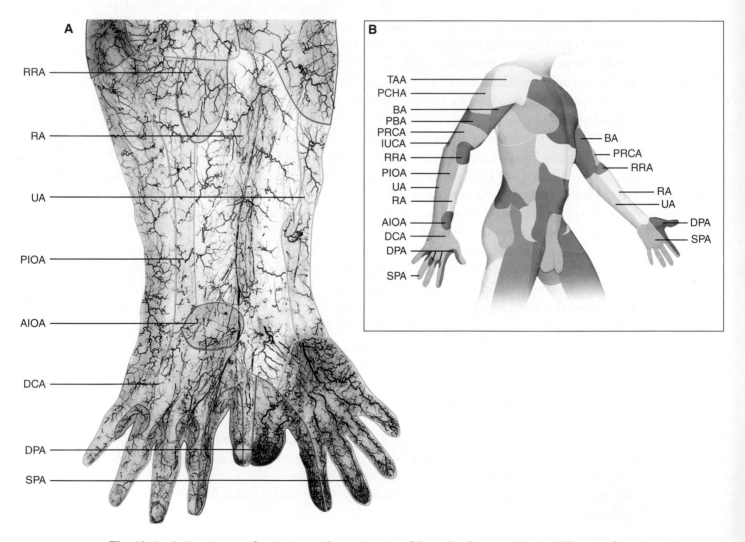

Fig. 19-1   A, Angiogram showing vascular territories of the volar forearm skin in different colors. **B,** Vascular territories of the upper limb. (*AIOA,* Anterior interosseous artery; *BA,* brachial artery; *DCA,* dorsal carpal arch; *DPA,* deep palmar arch; *IUCA,* inferior ulnar collateral artery; *PBA,* profunda brachial artery; *PCHA,* posterior circumflex humeral artery; *PIOA,* posterior interosseous artery; *PRCA,* posterior radial collateral artery; *RA,* radial artery; *RRA,* radial recurrent artery; *SPA,* superficial palmar arch; *TAA,* thoracoacromial artery; *UA,* ulnar artery.)

The radial artery supplies the major part of the volar forearm between the elbow and wrist (Fig. 19-2). The anatomic territory of the radial artery comprises the lateral (radial) half of the volar surface of the forearm, as well as the lateral (radial) border and lateral (radial) portion of the posterior surface. The boundary between the radial and ulnar territories varies but generally overlies the palmaris longus muscle.

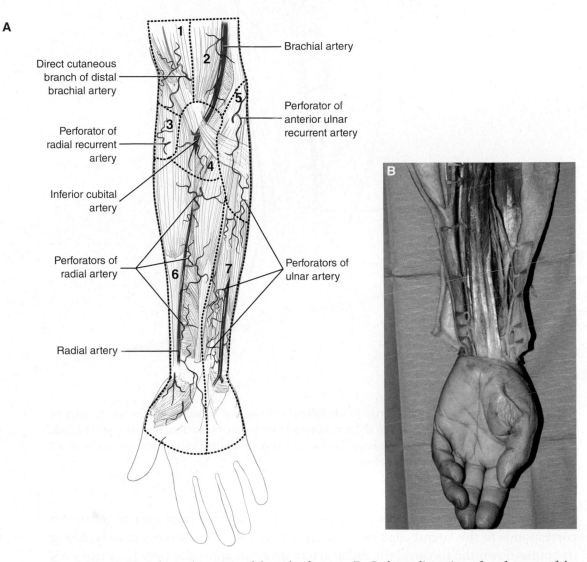

A, Direct cutaneous branch of distal brachial artery

Brachial artery

Perforator of radial recurrent artery

Perforator of anterior ulnar recurrent artery

Inferior cubital artery

Perforators of radial artery

Perforators of ulnar artery

Radial artery

Fig. 19-2 A, Vascular architecture of the volar forearm. **B,** Cadaver dissection of perforators of the radial and ulnar arteries. Note the series of small, fairly short perforators *(blue arrows)* arising from both the radial and ulnar arteries. Radial artery perforators arise between the flexor carpi radialis and brachioradialis muscle tendons in the distal forearm. Ulnar artery perforators arise between flexor carpi ulnaris and palmaris muscle tendons in the distal forearm.

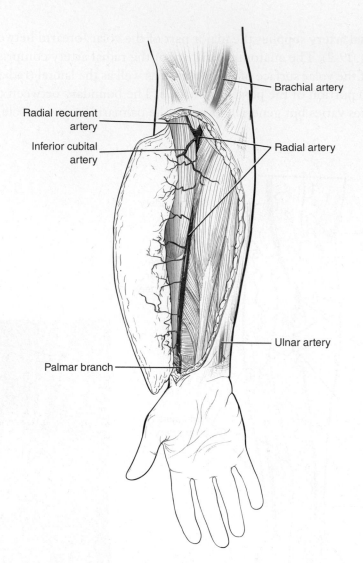

Brachial artery

Radial recurrent
artery

Inferior cubital
artery

Radial artery

Ulnar artery

Palmar branch

Fig. 19-3   The radial artery gives rise to the following branches: radial recurrent artery, inferior cubital artery, a series of perforators in the forearm, and the terminal branches, palmar carpal branch, and superficial palmar branch. Cutaneous, fasciocutaneous, or adipocutaneous flaps can be based on any suitably situated and sized perforator or branch.

The lateral boundary between the radial and posterior interosseous territories corresponds to the lateral edge of the extensor digitorum communis muscle. Along its course down the forearm, the radial artery gives off approximately 12 perforators to the skin along the fascial septum[19] (Fig. 19-3). These perforators arise between the brachioradialis and pronator teres muscles in the proximal third of the forearm, and between the brachioradialis and flexor carpi radialis muscles in the distal two thirds of the forearm. Distally, one or two of these perforators may be between the tendons of the flexor carpi radialis and flexor digitorum superficialis muscles. These forearm perforators within the fascial plexus are oriented predominantly along the longitudinal axis in the proximal two thirds of the forearm; they are oriented more transversely in the distal third[32,33] (Fig. 19-4).

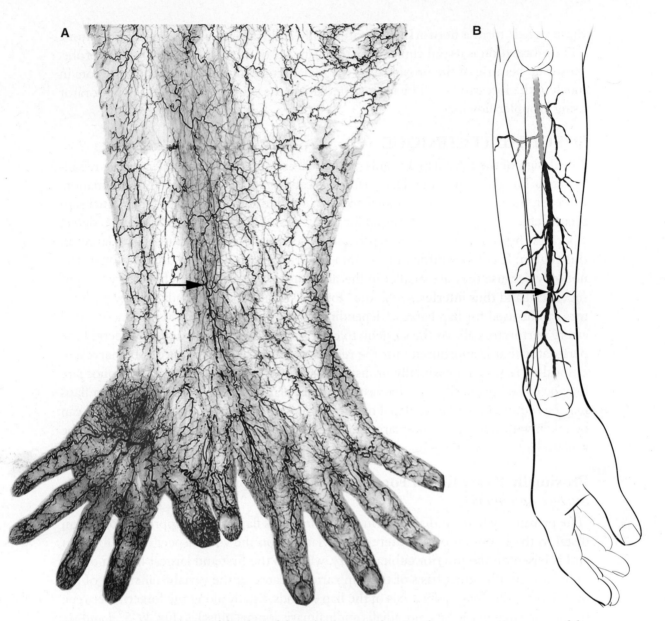

Fig. 19-4 A, Arteriogram of the skin of the volar forearm showing the accompanying artery of the superficial branch of the radial nerve *(arrow).* **B,** Most of the cutaneous branches of the radial artery longitudinally anastomose with each other *(arrow)* along the course of the main artery.

Our anatomic and angiographic studies have demonstrated the distribution of radial artery perforators (see Figs. 19-1 and 19-2). These perforators tend to become smaller in diameter toward the distal end of the forearm, as the radial artery diminishes in caliber.[9,32] Most of the radial artery perforators anastomose longitudinally with each other along the course of the main artery and form a deep fascial plexus oriented along the main arterial axis. This favors the design of longitudinally oriented perforator flaps. In addition, transversely oriented, reduced-caliber choke anastomoses are located between the perforators of the radial, ulnar, and posterior interosseous arteries. Together these vessels form a network of longitudinally and transversely oriented perforators. This information is useful clinically in the planning of skin flaps with a Doppler probe. However, because of the proximity of the radial artery to the individual perforators in much of the forearm, it is difficult to differentiate the source vessel from the perforator using Doppler flowmetry.

SURGICAL TECHNIQUE

The design of the RAP flap depends on the size and location of the defect being reconstructed. The radial artery and its perforators can be identified by Doppler examination; however, the proximity of the radial artery makes it difficult to identify individual septocutaneous perforators in the distal forearm. Surgeons are much more likely to detect a perforator preoperatively in the proximal forearm because these vessels are larger in this region. It is more difficult to find radial artery perforators in the distal forearm, not only because they are smaller in this area but also because the radial artery is more superficial and thus interferes with the Doppler signal. Any of the radial artery perforators can be used for flap harvest, depending on the surgical plan. The variety of radial artery perforators allows the surgeon to customize the reconstruction by selecting the perforator that is appropriate for the reconstructive plan. The flaps can be harvested as local or regional, proximally or distally based flaps or as free flaps. The donor site may be closed primarily after harvesting a small flap, or a skin graft or local skin flaps may be required for a larger flap. For a free RAP flap harvest, a cuff of radial artery can be taken with the vessels to enlarge the pedicle diameter, and the radial artery can be repaired after harvest.

Proximally Based Radial Forearm Fasciocutaneous Flap

Surface Landmarks

The proximally based radial forearm fasciocutaneous flap base lies approximately 4 cm distal to the midpoint of the interepicondylar line on the volar aspect of the forearm and is based on the inferior cubital artery, which is the first and largest branch of the radial artery. The exact basis of the flap varies because of the variable anatomy of the perforators. The longitudinal axis of the flap extends distally along the forearm between the lateral edge of the brachioradialis and palmaris longus muscles (Fig. 19-5, *A* and *B*).

Vascular Anatomy

The inferior cubital artery (mean diameter 1.1 mm)[33] is the largest perforator arising proximally from the radial artery in the antecubital fossa. It reaches the skin by passing superficially in the fascia between the brachioradialis and pronator teres muscles or through either muscle. Cormack and Lamberty[16,34,35] found that the perforator arose from the radial recurrent artery rather than the radial artery itself in 16 of 37 dissected cadaver arms. Magden et al[36] described numerous variations in the origin of the inferior cubital artery (Fig. 19-5, *C*). The surface landmark of the origin of the inferior cubital perforator varies from 2 to 5 cm (average 4 cm) distal to the midpoint of the interepicondylar line on the anterior aspect of the forearm (see Fig. 19-5).

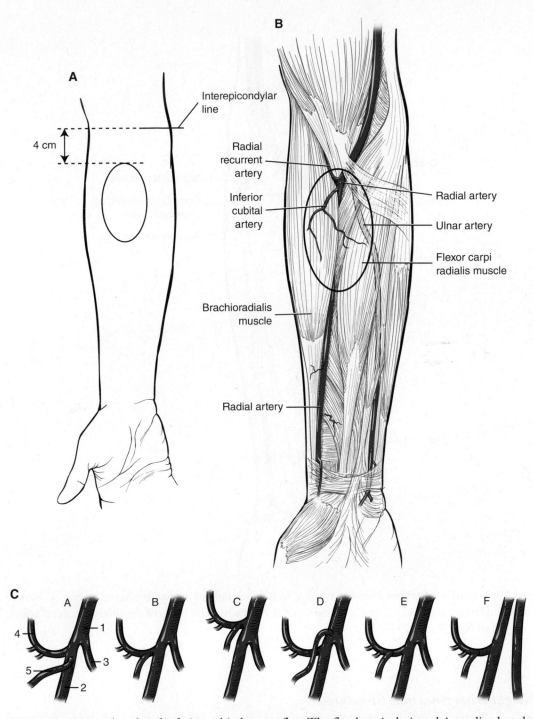

Fig. 19-5   A, Landmarks of inferior cubital artery flap. The flap base is designed 4 cm distal to the midpoint of the interepicondylar line on the volar aspect of the forearm. **B,** The proximally based radial forearm fasciocutaneous flap design based on the cubital artery branch. The flap axis can be designed distally along the forearm. **C,** Patterns of origin of the inferior cubital artery. *(A)* The inferior cubital artery *(5)* arises from the radial artery *(2)* in 62%; *(B)* from the radial recurrent artery *(4)* in 2.5%; *(C)* from the radial recurrent artery, which originates from the brachial artery *(1)*, in 7.5%; *(D)* from the brachial artery in 2.5%; and *(E)* from the radial artery, which has an aberrant proximal origin, in 2.5% of cadaver dissections.

Continued

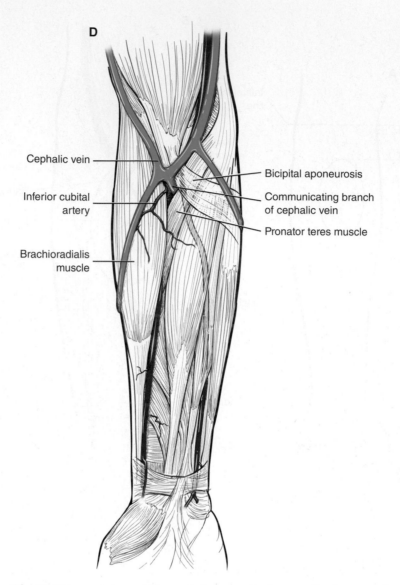

Fig. 19-5, cont'd   D, Vein anatomy relative to inferior cubital artery flap harvest after. (**C** and **D** modified from Magden O, Icke C, Arman C, et al. An anatomical study of the inferior cubital artery. Eur J Plast Surg 20:24, 1997.)

Neighboring Anatomic Structures

The cephalic vein gives off a cubital branch and a deep branch that communicates with the venae comitantes of the radial artery. In the fork of this inverted V, the inferior cubital perforator reaches the skin (Fig. 19-5, *D*). From this point, the inferior cubital perforator tends to run distally along the line of the cephalic vein, directly toward the radial styloid process. Venous drainage of the forearm flap is mainly through the superficial venous system. The area of skin lying along the line of the cephalic vein is supplied by the lateral cutaneous nerve of the arm.

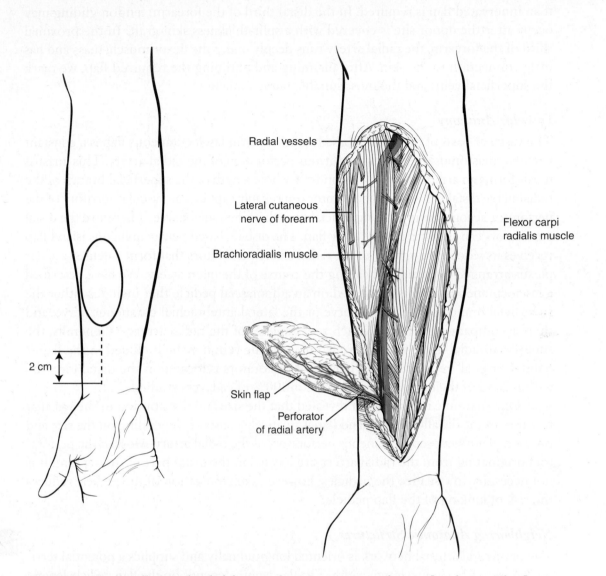

Fig. 19-6 The distally based radial forearm fasciocutaneous perforator flap design. The flap is marked along the axis of the radial artery at the proximal border of the forearm. The pivot point of the pedicle is about 2 cm above the radial styloid process.

Distally Based Radial Forearm Fasciocutaneous Flap
Surface Landmarks

The distally based radial forearm fasciocutaneous flap design includes a skin island marked along the axis of the radial artery, in the proximal border of the forearm. The pivot point of the pedicle is approximately 3 to 4 cm proximal to the radial styloid process (Fig. 19-6). The ideal place for flap elevation is the middle third of the forearm; however, flaps may be raised wherever an adequately sized perforator is suitably positioned for the planned reconstruction. This is also the best place to incorporate a part of the radius if an innervated flap is required. In the distal third of the forearm, tendon gliding may occur after the donor site is covered with a split-thickness skin graft. In the proximal third of the forearm, the radial artery runs deeply under the flexor muscle mass and has little connection to the skin. After planning and outlining the required flap, we mark the superficial veins and the most suitable nerve branches.

Vascular Anatomy

The vascular basis of the distally based radial forearm fasciocutaneous flap is a constant vascular anastomosis between the various perforators of the radial artery. This anastomosis forms an arterial network around the whole length of the superficial branch of the radial nerve distally. The distal perforator can reliably capture the vascular territory of the perforator accompanying the superficial branch of the radial nerve. Therefore the distal perforators can supply a reverse-flow flap. The distally based neurocutaneous island flap receives its vascular supply from the radial artery perforators that form a dense vascular plexus arranged longitudinally along the course of the main artery. We have described a fasciocutaneous flap distally based on an adipofascial pedicle that includes either the superficial branch of the radial nerve or the lateral antebrachial cutaneous nerve, and their accompanying arteries, which are branches of the radial artery.[19] Generally, the superficial radial nerve is preserved. The cephalic vein may be included in the flap.[28] Saint-Cyr et al[8] reported that a cluster of perforators is located in the distal forearm, within 2 cm of the radial styloid process in 100% of cadavers studied.

Our anatomic investigation revealed that the size and distribution of the vascular territory of the distally based island flap is relatively constant, depending on the size and position of adjacent septocutaneous perforators of the radial artery. Most of the perforators originating from the radial artery are located in the distal part of the septum. It is not necessary to visualize the pedicles; however, skeletonization of the pedicle reduces the risk of kinking of the flap pedicle.

Neighboring Anatomic Structures

The perineural arterial network is oriented longitudinally and supplies a potential territory of up to 5 cm in maximum width. The flap length depends on the flap pedicle length. The longer the pedicle, the smaller the required skin island flap. The upper margin of the flap is located at a level 10 cm distal to the elbow. For hand reconstruction, the base of the flap can be located on a suitable perforator from 2 to 8 cm proximal to the radial styloid process, depending on the required pedicle length. The flap pivot point is generally located about 2 cm from the radial styloid process and should be centered over one or more of the radial perforators. The deep fascia can be included in the flap as needed, but is not essential for flap vascularity.

CASE EXAMPLES

An injury to this 21-year-old boy's hand resulted in soft tissue defects on the dorsum of the hand and first web, and contracture of the first web space. A 10 by 4 cm radial forearm perforator flap without radial artery was designed in the distal two thirds of the forearm. The distal perforator pedicle was located 2 cm proximal to the radial styloid process. The flap was used to cover the defect on the dorsal side of the hand and first web. It was possible to close the donor area directly, and the flap healed well, without complications (Fig. 19-7).

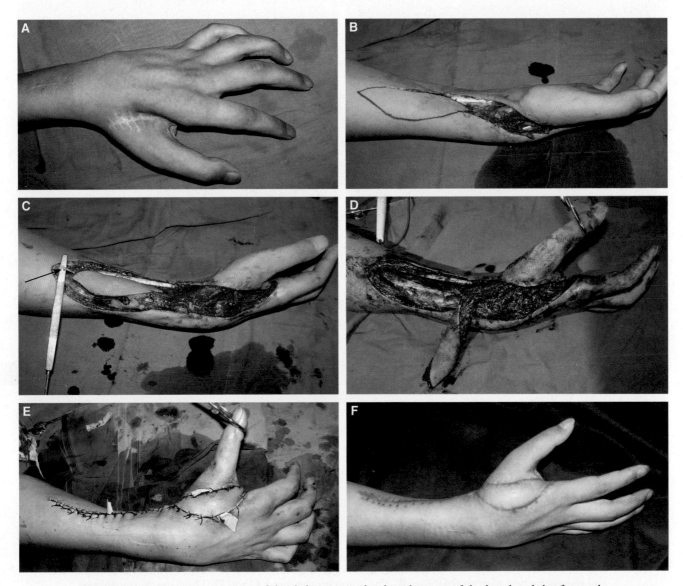

Fig. 19-7   A, Preoperative view of the deformity in the dorsal aspect of the hand and the first web, and first web space contracture. **B,** A RAP flap was designed based on the radial artery perforator *(arrow)*. **C,** The flap was dissected, and the lateral cutaneous nerve of the forearm *(arrow)* was identified. **D,** Flap elevation. The distal perforator pedicle was located 2 cm proximal to the radial styloid process. **E,** The soft tissue deformity was covered with the perforator flap, and the donor site was closed directly. **F,** Late follow-up result. The flap survived completely.

This 61-year-old patient was referred from another hospital after an incomplete resection of a Merkel cell carcinoma. The previous pathology report showed involvement of the deep margin of resection. Therefore a complete resection of the area with wider, deep and lateral margins was undertaken. After resection, an RAP flap was designed adjacent to the wound to reconstruct the defect. The donor site was grafted with split-thickness skin. Both the flap and skin graft healed uneventfully (Fig. 19-8).

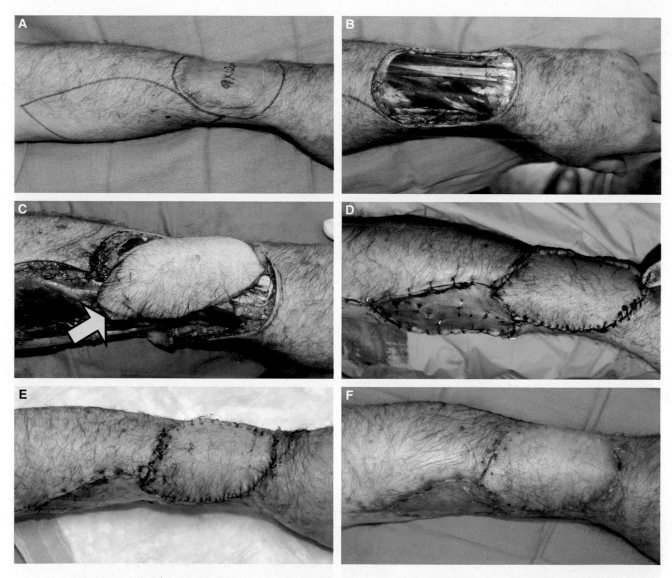

Fig. 19-8   A, Planning included reexcision of Merkel cell carcinoma from the dorsum of the left wrist and reconstruction with an RAP flap. **B,** The lesion was resected. **C** and **D,** The flap was transferred and inset. **E,** Initial healing. **F,** One month postoperatively, the flap and skin graft are completely healed.

This 25-year-old woman was involved in an industrial accident that resulted in an injury to the dorsal aspect of her right hand and wrist and the distal third of her forearm, with tendon and skin loss (Fig. 19-9). Her extensor pollicis longus and extensor indicis tendons were repaired. The soft tissue defect was covered with a reverse radial forearm island flap based on a radial artery perforator, which accompanies the superficial branch of the radial nerve. The flap size was 12 by 8 cm. The donor site wound was resurfaced with a split-thickness graft. The flap survived completely, but flap bulkiness was evident. The flap was debulked 6 months later and extensor tendon grafting was performed on the third finger so that the patient could achieve normal extension.

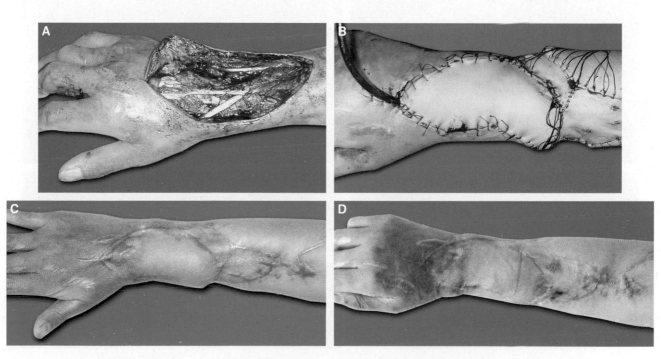

Fig. 19-9 A, Preoperative view of a soft tissue defect on the dorsal aspect of the hand and the distal third of the forearm, with tendon and skin loss. **B,** The skin defect was covered with a reverse radial forearm island flap based on a radial artery perforator. The donor site was covered with a split-thickness graft. **C,** The flap survived completely, but flap bulkiness was evident. **D,** The flap was debulked 6 months postoperatively.

This 20-year-old farmer presented with injuries to the extensor tendon and soft tissue of the dorsal hand and wrist (Fig. 19-10). Bone was exposed. The injuries were caused by an accident involving farming machinery. The skin defect was covered with a reverse radial forearm island flap based on the perforator of the radial artery. The flap size was 13 by 8 cm. The donor site wound was covered with a split-thickness graft. The flap survived completely.

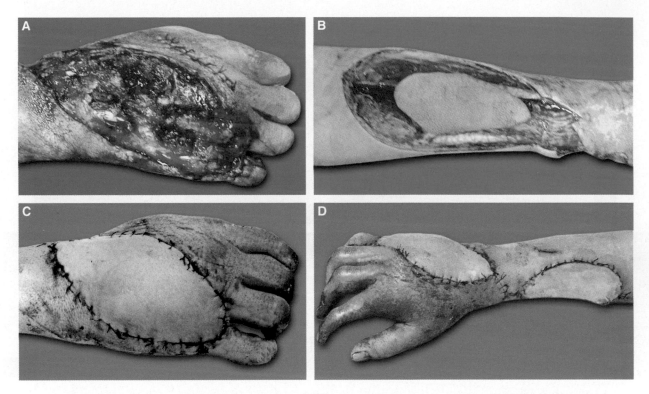

Fig. 19-10 **A,** Dorsal hand and wrist wound following a farming injury. **B,** An RAP flap was performed to reconstruct the soft tissue loss. **C** and **D,** The flap and skin graft survived completely.

This 22-year-old man presented after a crush injury to his left hand (Fig. 19-11). When the patient was seen at our hospital 10 days after the injury, the ulnar aspect of the hand and little finger were necrotic. We amputated the little finger and excised the necrotic soft tissue. The exposed bone was covered with a free RAP flap with a 1.5 cm segment of the radial artery. The venous outflow of the flap was provided by the cephalic vein. The donor radial artery was repaired primarily. Both ends of the radial artery were anastomosed with the ulnar artery in the recipient site to create a through-flow situation. The flap size was 14 by 10 cm. The donor site wound was resurfaced with split-thickness graft. The flap survived completely.

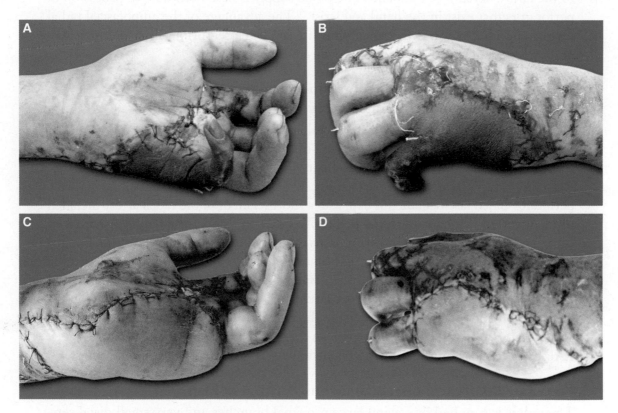

Fig. 19-11 A and **B,** Anterior and posterior views of a crush injury of the left hand with resulting necrosis of the little finger and ulnar part of the hand. **C** and **D,** The little finger was amputated and the necrotic tissue resected. The skin defect and exposed bone were covered with a free radial forearm perforator flap with a 1.5 cm segment of the radial artery. The flap survived completely.

MODIFICATIONS

The radial forearm is a very versatile donor site, because many kinds of proximally or distally based flaps can be raised by including perforators anywhere along the radial artery axis. RAP flaps can also be designed to include periosteum (of the radius), tendon (palmaris longus), nerve (lateral cutaneous nerve of the forearm or superficial radial nerve), bone (radius), or any combination of these for different applications.

Radial Artery Fascial or Adipofascial Perforator Flap

Distally based radial artery perforator hand and forearm fascial or adipofascial flaps consist of the fascia and subcutaneous fat and fascia of the forearm respectively.[20,24] These flaps are easy to elevate and can cover surfaces ranging from an individual finger to the entire dorsum of the hand. The blood supply is based on the rich profusion of perforators that exist in the hand and wrist.[20] The advantage of the adipofascial radial forearm perforator flap is that the donor site can be closed primarily, avoiding a skin graft, which results in a superior donor site aesthetic outcome.[24]

Free Radial Forearm Fasciocutaneous Perforator Flap With a Segment of the Radial Artery

Free flaps based exclusively on distal radial artery fasciocutaneous perforators would require supramicrosurgical skills because of the small vessel diameter. For practical reasons, it is advisable to include a segment of the radial artery into such a flap design to facilitate vascular anastomoses (see Fig. 19-11). The flap is elevated as a distal row perforator-based fasciocutaneous flap, with a short segment of the radial artery included in the inverted-T–shaped arterial pedicle. Venous outflow of the flap is provided by the cephalic vein, with accompanying veins of the radial artery left behind. The donor radial artery is repaired primarily. Anastomosis of both ends of the radial artery in the recipient site creates a through-flow situation, which may create physiologic flow in the radial artery perforator and reduce circulatory complications in the flap. Considering the possible sequelae of sacrificing the radial artery, this technique is obviously advantageous, especially in patients with an abnormal preoperative Allen test. This free RAP flap with anastomoses of large-diameter vessels is very easy to raise and transfer.[19]

Free Radial Forearm Osteocutaneous Perforator Flap

The radius is supplied by several large proximal branches and very small distal septoperiosteal branches of the radial artery. The middle of the bone receives a nutrient artery from the anterior interosseous artery. The distal portion of the bone receives one or two small septoperiosteal branches from the anterior interosseous artery. The radius also receives blood from the posterior interosseous artery through attached muscles.

The free radial forearm osteocutaneous perforator flap has been successfully transferred for one-stage reconstruction of total nasal loss. This thin flap consists of vascularized radius and superficial adipose tissue without deep fascia. The flap is nourished by a single perforator of the radial artery and a cutaneous vein. The advantages of this flap over a radical forearm flap are minimal donor site morbidity and simpler dissection of the radial artery.[20,26]

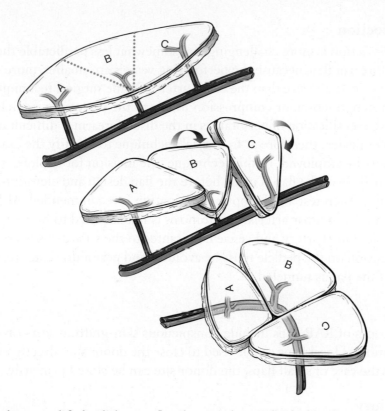

Fig. 19-12 A shape-modified radial artery flap showing three individual perforator flaps harvested from the radial artery. These can be combined to reconstruct a differently shaped defect. Harvesting three individual flaps allows primary donor site closure. (Modified from Mateev MA, Ogawa R, Trunov L, et al. Shape-modified radial artery perforator flap method: analysis of 112 cases. Plast Reconstr Surg 123:1533, 2009.)

Shape-Modified Radial Artery Perforator Flap Method

Mateev et al[27] have described a radial artery skin flap technique in 112 cases to reduce donor site morbidity, relying on an understanding of the pattern of perforators of the radial artery. In this surgical technique, the authors designed a series of individual flaps based on individual radial artery perforators, which were combined to reconstruct the deformity, allowing primary closure of the donor site rather than using a skin graft (Fig. 19-12).[27] The advantages of the techniques, including the versatility of multiple skin paddles and fewer donor site problems related to skin grafting, are somewhat tempered by the need to sacrifice the radial artery. However, for hand reconstruction where there may be multiple soft tissue defects, this technique could be particularly applicable.

PITFALLS
Possible Complications

The possible complications of an RAP flap include partial or complete flap necrosis, radial nerve injury resulting in hypoesthesia or dysesthesia of the forearm and hand, and hypertrophic or unattractive forearm scarring from incisions or skin grafting the donor site.

Flap Dissection

RAP flap dissection is more challenging and somewhat less predictable than dissection of a radial forearm flap, because the perforating vessels are smaller, more delicate, and variable in position and size than the radial artery. Gentle surgical technique is required to avoid stretch, traction, or compression injury to the perforator pedicle of the flap. Preoperative identification of perforators in the distal forearm is difficult using a hand-held Doppler device; therefore a "free style" technique to identify the exact perforator location must be employed. In this technique, the incision for exploring the planned perforator pedicle of the flap is made before the flap design and elevation. Performing a preoperative Allen test and Doppler examination is recommended. Although a patent palmar radial to ulnar arterial anastomosis is not required to harvest an RAP flap, patency of the radial artery and venae comitantes to the wrist level is essential to flap survival. Tension on the pedicle must be avoided, and perforator compression must be alleviated if the flap is tunneled.

Scarring

The drawbacks of RAP flaps include conspicuous skin-grafting scars on the forearm. A combination of local flaps can be used to close the donor site directly to avoid a skin graft, or in the case of small flaps, the donor site can be closed primarily.

Nerve Injury

Postoperative hypoesthesia or paresthesia in the radial nerve distribution can occur after RAP flap harvest. If the superficial branch of the radial nerve is sacrificed, the sensibility of the radial side of the hand is lost and painful neuromata may result. There is a plexus of arteries surrounding the radial nerve that provides enriched vascular supply in the axis of the nerve. However, sacrifice of the radial nerve results in significant morbidity and should be avoided. The lateral cutaneous nerve of the forearm can be included in the flap, and the morbidity that results from its harvest is usually well accepted.

Venous Congestion

Some surgeons advocate ligating the cephalic vein at the distal end of the flap to prevent venous congestion. Others preserve the cephalic vein in the flap. We have not observed any problems preserving the cephalic vein in our 26 cases.[17] Matei et al[26] reported superficial flap epidermolysis in 12% of a series of 63 forearm perforator flaps, which may suggest that venous insufficiency is a potential problem with the small vein size in perforator flaps.

References

1. Yang G, Chen B, Gao Y, et al. The forearm free skin flap transplantation. Natl Med J China 61:139, 1981.
   This article was the first published account of the radial forearm flap.
2. Song R, Gao Y, Song Y, et al. The forearm flap. Clin Plast Surg 9:21, 1982.
3. Lu KH, Zhong DC, Chen B, et al. [The forearm radial arterial turnover flap and its clinical applications] Zhonghua Wai Ke Za Zhi 20:695, 1982.
4. Reis D, Moss AL. One-stage repair with vascularised tendon grafts in a dorsal hand injury using the "Chinese" forearm flap. Br J Surg 36:473, 1983.

5. Soutar DS, Tanner NS. The radial forearm flap in the management of soft tissue injuries of the hand. Br J Plast Surg 37:18, 1984.

6. Biemer E, Stock W. Total thumb reconstruction: a one-stage reconstruction using an osteo-cutaneous forearm flap. Br J Plast Surg 36:52, 1983.

7. Foucher G, van Genechten F, Merle N, et al. A compound radial artery forearm flap in hand surgery: an original modification of the Chinese forearm flap. Br J Plast Surg 37:139, 1984.

8. Saint-Cyr M, Mujadzic M, Wong C, et al. The radial artery pedicle perforator flap: vascular analysis and clinical implications. Plast Reconstr Surg 125:1469, 2010.

9. Timmons MJ. The vascular basis of the radial forearm flap. Plast Reconstr Surg 77:80, 1986.

   In this definitive anatomic study of the radial forearm flap, the author dissected 56 cadavers using various techniques including ink, latex, and barium sulphate injections.

10. Zhang YT. [The use of reversed forearm pedicled fascio-cutaneous flap in treatment of hand trauma and deformity (report of 10 cases)] Chin J Plast Surg 4:41, 1988.

11. Chang SM. The distally based radial forearm fascia flap. Plast Reconstr Surg 85:150, 1990.

12. Goffin D, Brunelli F, Galbiatti A, et al. A new flap based on the distal branches of the radial artery. Ann Chir Main Memb Super 11:217, 1992.

13. Bertelli JA, Khoury Z. Neurocutaneous axial island flaps in the forearm: anatomical, experimental and preliminary results. Br J Plast Reconstr Surg 46:489, 1993.

14. Bertelli JA, Kaleli T. Retrograde flow neurocutaneous island flaps in the forearm: anatomic basis and clinical results. Plast Reconstr Surg 95:851, 1995.

15. Weinzweig N, Chen L, Chen ZW. The distally based radial forearm fasciosubcutaneous flap with preservation of the radial artery: an anatomic and clinical approach. Plast Reconstr Surg 94:675, 1994.

    The authors investigated the contribution of the distal radial artery and its superficial and deep branches to the fasciosubcutaneous plexus of the forearm by dissecting 17 fresh cadaver forearms. They used a distally based radial forearm fasciosubcutaneous flap with preservation of the radial artery for repairing soft tissue defects of the hand.

16. Cormack GC, Lamberty BG, eds. The Arterial Anatomy of Skin Flaps, 2nd ed. Edinburgh: Churchill Livingstone, 1994.

17. Koshima I, Moriguchi T, Etoh II, et al. The radial artery perforator-based adipofascial flap for dorsal hand coverage. Ann Plast Surg 35:474, 1995.

    This flap is classified as one of the distally based septocutaneous flaps, which are supplied by the dorsal superficial branch of the radial artery.

18. Jeng SF, Wei FC. The distally based forearm island flap in hand reconstruction. Plast Reconstr Surg 102:400, 1998.

    The authors performed the distally based forearm island flap in 12 patients with soft tissue defects of the hand. The skin flap is supplied by the perforators of the distal radial artery, and the pivot point of its subcutaneous pedicle is approximately 2 to 4 cm above the radial styloid process.

19. Yang D, Morris SF, Tang M, et al. Reversed forearm island flap supplied by the septocutaneous perforator of the radial artery: anatomical basis and clinical applications. Plast Reconstr Surg 112:1012, 2003.

    The authors studied cutaneous perforators of the radial artery adjacent to the superficial branch of the radial nerve and the lateral antebrachial cutaneous nerve in 10 fresh cadavers using a lead oxide mixture to create an overall map of the cutaneous vasculature and source vessels. The accompanying arteries were located along the lateral antebrachial cutaneous nerve and the superficial branch of the radial nerve. Vascular communication among these cutaneous vessels was evaluated to determine the cutaneous vascular territory of the radial forearm flap. They described clinical experience using the reversed forearm island flap for hand reconstruction in five patients.

20. Medalie DA. Perforator-based forearm and hand adipofascial flaps for the coverage of difficult dorsal hand wounds. Ann Plast Surg 48:477, 2002.

    The distally based hand and forearm adipofascial flaps consist of the subcutaneous fat and fascia of the hand and/or forearm, and their blood supply is based on the rich profusion of perforators in the hand and wrist.

21. Safak T, Akyurek M. Free transfer of the radial forearm flap with preservation of the radial artery. Ann Plast Surg 45:97, 2000.

22. Koshima I, Tsutsui T, Nanba Y, et al. Free radial forearm osteocutaneous perforator flap for reconstruction of total nasal defects. J Reconstr Microsurg 18:585, 2002.

    A case in which a radial forearm osteocutaneous perforator flap was transferred for one-stage reconstruction of total nasal loss. This flap consists of vascularized radial bone and superficial adipose tissue and is nourished by a single perforator of the radial artery.

23. Ozkan O, Akyurek M, Csokunfirat K, et al. The free radial artery septal perforator vessel-based flap. Plast Reconstr Surg 115:2062, 2005.

24. Page R, Chang J. Reconstruction of hand soft-tissue defects: alternatives to the radial forearm fasciocutaneous flap. Am J Hand Surg 31:847, 2006.

25. Ignatiadis IA, Mavrogenis AF, Avram AM, et al. Treatment of complex hand trauma using the distal ulnar and radial artery perforator-based flaps. Injury 39(Suppl 3):S116, 2008.

26. Matei I, Georgescu A, Chiroiu B, et al. Harvesting of forearm perforator flaps based on intraoperative vascular exploration: clinical experiences and literature review. Microsurgery 28:321, 2008.

27. Mateev MA, Ogawa R, Trunov L, et al. Shape-modified radial artery perforator flap method: analysis of 112 cases. Plast Reconstr Surg 123:1533, 2009.

28. Sauerbier M, Unglaub F. Perforator flaps in the upper extremity. Clin Plast Surg 37:667, 2010.

29. Ho AM, Chang J. Radial artery perforator flap. Am J Hand Surg 35:308, 2010.

30. Gao W, Yan H, Li Z, et al. The free dorsoradial forearm perforator flap. Anatomical study and clinical application in finger reconstruction. Ann Plast Surg 66:53, 2011.

31. Liu DX, Wang H, Li XD, et al. Three kinds of forearm flaps for hand skin defects: experience of 65 cases. Arch Orthop Trauma Surg 131:675, 2011.

32. Kanellakos GW, Yang D, Morris SF. Cutaneous vasculature of the forearm. Ann Plast Surg 50:387, 2003.

33. Inoue Y, Taylor GI. The angiosomes of the forearm: anatomic study and clinical implication. Plast Reconstr Surg 98:195, 1996.

34. Lamberty BG, Cormack GC. The forearm angiotomes. Br J Plast Surg 35:420, 1982.

35. Lamberty BG, Cormack GC. The antecubital fasciocutaneous flap. Br J Plast Surg 36:428, 1983.

36. Magden O, Icke C, Arman C, et al. An anatomical study of the inferior cubital artery. Eur J Plast Surg 20:24, 1997.

20

Hand Flaps

Michel Saint-Cyr
Amit Gupta

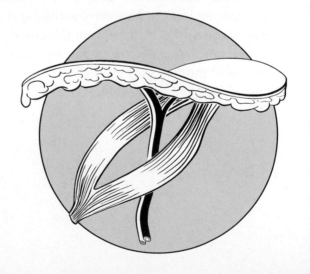

Innovations in skin flap design have led to a gradual evolution in the use and utility of skin flaps in hand surgery. This evolution is driven by our goals of optimizing tissue replacement, minimizing donor site expenditure, and maintaining function. Improved knowledge of the hand's vascular anatomy is the main reason for the variety of flap designs that exist today. Early flap designs were principally based on a random blood supply and were used as transposition, rotation, or advancement flaps. Although these flaps are still indicated today, they offer limited advancement and occasionally require a two-stage procedure, which can impede early mobilization.[1-3]

An *island flap* can be defined as a flap that is sustained by an identifiable vascular pedicle and attached to its donor site by that pedicle alone. The development of the neurovascular island flap by Littler[4,5] in 1956 was an important step forward in that surgeons could now transfer a skin island based on a specific neurovascular pedicle. Many island flaps were subsequently developed, including the first dorsal metacarpal artery (FDMA) flap (kite flap), described by Foucher and Braun[6] in 1979. Flaps could now be transposed, rotated, or advanced into a defect based on a predictable blood supply. Other anatomic studies improved our knowledge of the hand's dorsal blood supply and further demonstrated the versatility of island flaps.[7-10] It was recognized that abundant and expendable dorsal skin could be transferred to reconstruct myriad defects, based on either antegrade or retrograde flow from the dorsal metacarpal arteries (DMAs).[11-12] Refinements in island flap design also brought about a better appreciation of the vascular communications between the volar and dorsal vascular networks of the hand and digits. Standard DMA flaps from the dorsum of the hand were eventually harvested as perforator flaps based on cutaneous perforators from the metacarpal arteries. Early examples of this flap were the second through fourth metacarpal artery perforator flaps first described by Quaba and Davison.[13] Key advantages of these flaps include one-stage reconstruction, straightforward elevation, and low donor site morbidity. These perforator flaps are based on cutaneous perforators found just distal to the juncturae tendinae, at the level of the metacarpal neck in the second to fourth intermetacarpal spaces. Vascular connections between the DMA and proper palmar digital (PPD) arteries, through the dorsal digital branches, also allowed extended versions of these flaps.[14] These flaps could now be pivoted past the metacarpal neck, at the proximal phalanx level, to reach the distal phalanx based on retrograde flow from the dorsal digital branches. The clinical results were confirmed by Yang and Morris' vascular anatomic studies[15] of dorsal digital and metacarpal skin flaps. Flow through dorsal digital branches formed the basis for various homodigital and heterodigital antegrade and retrograde flaps, all of which have significantly increased our reconstructive options in the past 10 years.[16-19]

Axial vessels such as the dorsal metacarpal, palmar metacarpal, and digital arteries give off numerous cutaneous perforators and communicating branches along their course. All of these cutaneous perforators originating from either the digital or metacarpal arteries can give rise to potential perforator flaps in the hand. Sound knowledge of vascular anatomy allows surgeons more freedom to select optimal flaps for their patients. New perforator-based flap designs will undoubtedly be developed as our knowledge of the hand's vascular anatomy expands.

DORSAL METACARPAL ARTERY FLAPS

The dorsal aspect of the hand represents an invaluable and expendable donor site for reconstructing a variety of defects. Thorough knowledge of the vascular anatomy of the dorsal skin of the hand and the digits has led to many innovative flap designs for this area, and is an important prerequisite for their safe application. The blood supply to the dorsal skin of the hand and digits is provided by (1) the DMAs, which vascularize the proximal portion of the hand, and (2) the dorsal perforating metacarpal arterial branches from the deep palmar arch, which supply the distal hand and proximal phalanx.[15] These two major arterial systems form the basis for direct and reverse DMA flaps.

First Dorsal Metacarpal Artery Flap

The FDMA flap (kite flap), described by Foucher and Braun,[6] provides two major applications in hand reconstruction: (1) dorsal hand wound coverage and (2) thumb reconstruction.

Anatomy

In Foucher's anatomic study[6] of 30 injected cadaveric hands, the FDMA originated from the radial artery in 28 specimens and from the dorsalis superficialis antebrachialis artery in 2 (Fig. 20-1). From there, it courses distal to the extensor pollicis longus tendon, and proximal to the radial artery's entry between both heads of the first dorsal interosseous muscle. The FDMA travels parallel to the dorsal surface of the second metacarpal, and superficial to the first dorsal interosseous muscle fascia, with some fibers occasionally

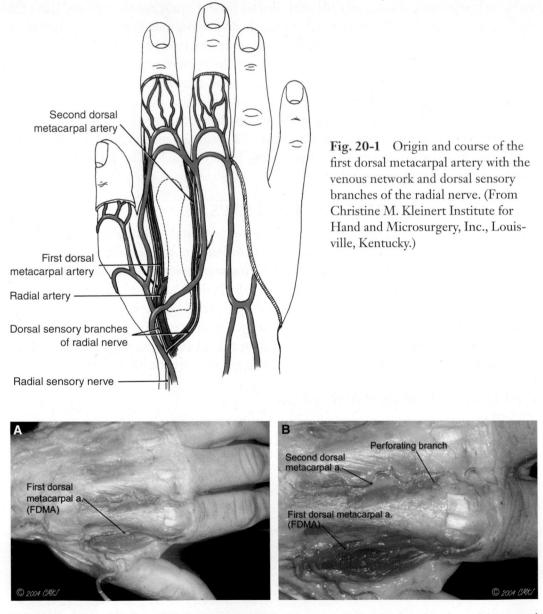

Second dorsal
metacarpal artery

First dorsal
metacarpal artery

Radial artery

Dorsal sensory branches
of radial nerve

Radial sensory nerve

Fig. 20-1   Origin and course of the first dorsal metacarpal artery with the venous network and dorsal sensory branches of the radial nerve. (From Christine M. Kleinert Institute for Hand and Microsurgery, Inc., Louisville, Kentucky.)

A

First dorsal
metacarpal a.
(FDMA)

© 2004 CMKI

B

Perforating branch

Second dorsal
metacarpal a.

First dorsal metacarpal a.
(FDMA)

© 2004 CMKI

Fig. 20-2   The path of the FDMA. **A,** The FDMA courses parallel to the dorsal surface of the second metacarpal, and superficial to the first dorsal interosseous muscle fascia. Fibers occasionally cover the vessel. **B,** It continues distally and anastomoses at the level of the metacarpal neck with dorsal perforating branches from the palmar metacarpal arteries of the deep palmar arch. (From Christine M. Kleinert Institute for Hand and Microsurgery, Inc., Louisville, Kentucky.)

covering the vessel (Fig. 20-2, *A*). The FDMA then continues distally and anastomoses at the level of the metacarpal neck with dorsal perforating branches from the palmar metacarpal arteries of the deep palmar arch (Fig. 20-2, *B*). These perforator branches form the basis of the reverse-flow FDMA island flap. They anastomose with three different arterial systems: (1) distally with the dorsal branches of the PPD arteries, (2) proximally with branches of the DMA, and (3) laterally with adjacent DMA perforating branches. Angiographic studies by Yang and Morris[15] confirmed the presence of vascular connections between the dorsal digital branches of the second through fourth DMA arteries and the dorsal branches of the PPD arteries. These connections make it possible to harvest an extended reverse DMA flap based on retrograde flow from the dorsal branches of the PPD artery.

Surgical Technique

Surface Landmarks

The FDMA flap is designed over the dorsum of the index finger's proximal phalanx along the midradial and midulnar lines of the finger (Fig. 20-3). Distal and proximal limits include the proximal interphalangeal (PIP) joint and metacarpophalangeal (MCP) joint, respectively; however, an extended flap can also be harvested by including skin from the dorsum of the middle phalanx. Inclusion of the dorsal skin of the MCP joint can make dissection of the pedicle safer, because the layer of subcutaneous tissue is very thin at this level.

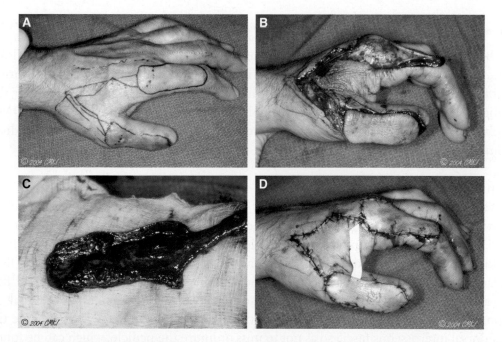

Fig. 20-3 The FDMA flap. **A,** The flap is designed over the index proximal phalanx and MCP joint. **B,** It is elevated and transferred to the dorsal thumb defect. **C,** The neurovascular pedicle is seen with a perivascular soft tissue cuff. **D,** The flap is inset into the dorsal defect, and the donor site is covered with a full-thickness skin graft. (From Christine M. Kleinert Institute for Hand and Microsurgery, Inc., Louisville, Kentucky.)

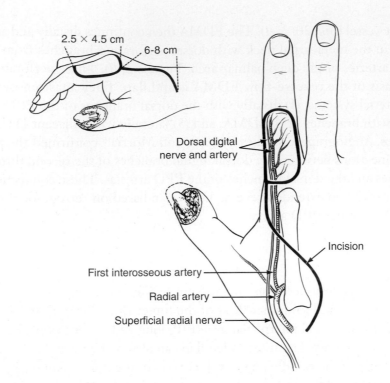

Fig. 20-4   Incision marks are shown in relation to underlying structures. (From Christine M. Kleinert Institute for Hand and Microsurgery, Inc., Louisville, Kentucky.)

A lazy S, or Bruner-type incision, is marked from the head of the second metacarpal bone to the apex of the first interosseous web space (Fig. 20-4). This design allows generous exposure and an en block dissection of the pedicle, without skeletonization and undue risks of vascular damage. Alternatively, a skin bridge can be kept over the pedicle to avoid tunneling the flap during insetting. We prefer to harvest the FDMA flap with a cutaneous bridge over the pedicle to avoid undue pressure on the pedicle from postoperative swelling.

Flap Elevation

Elevation of the FDMA flap begins distally by incising the flap outline over the dorsal proximal phalanx in a radial to ulnar direction, just above the peritenon layer (Fig. 20-5). The lateral skin flaps are raised subdermally to develop a subcutaneous pedicle. A skin bridge is harvested with the subcutaneous pedicle to avoid tunneling the flap. Sensory branches of the radial nerve and one or more subcutaneous veins are identified proximally and included in the pedicle. Dissection is performed from ulnar to radial. As soon as the second metacarpal is reached, the dissection plane deepens to include the first dorsal interosseous fascia so as not to miss or injure the pedicle, which can be found either above or below, or within a groove of the interosseous fascia. This fascia is sharply incised and carefully dissected off the interosseous muscle in an ulnar to radial direction. The FDMA lies just superficial to the first dorsal interosseous fascia, necessitating inclusion of the latter during flap elevation to prevent damage to the pedicle.[20] For this same reason, some authors advocate raising a cuff of first dorsal interosseous muscle in case the FDMA lies deeper. As pedicle dissection continues from distal to proximal and from ulnar to radial, all small perforating branches penetrating the interosseous fascia are coagulated to maximize pedicle length, which can vary from 6 to 8 cm. The pedicle is raised with a generous cuff of subcutaneous fibrofatty tissue without skeletonization. If required, tunneling is performed by undermining the dorsal subcutaneous tissue and skin, and the flap is transferred into the defect without tension, compression, or kinking. The arc of rotation of the FDMA flap allows it to reach the thumb tip, volar second MCP joint, distal antebrachial region, and fifth MCP joint. The donor site is covered with a split- or full-thickness skin graft.

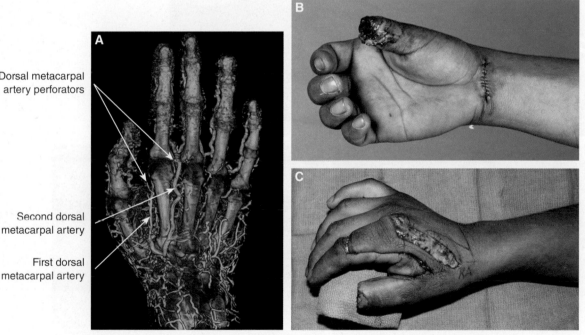

Fig. 20-5 **A,** CT angiogram of the hand shows the FDMA and a large SDMA. **B,** A manual worker crushed his right thumb (dominant hand) in an accident. He had been treated at another institution with a split-thickness skin graft that failed. **C,** An FDMA skin incision was made, preserving a skin bridge overlying the pedicle to avoid tunneling and the flap and any potential pedicle compression, which could lead to venous congestion and/or flap ischemia.

Continued

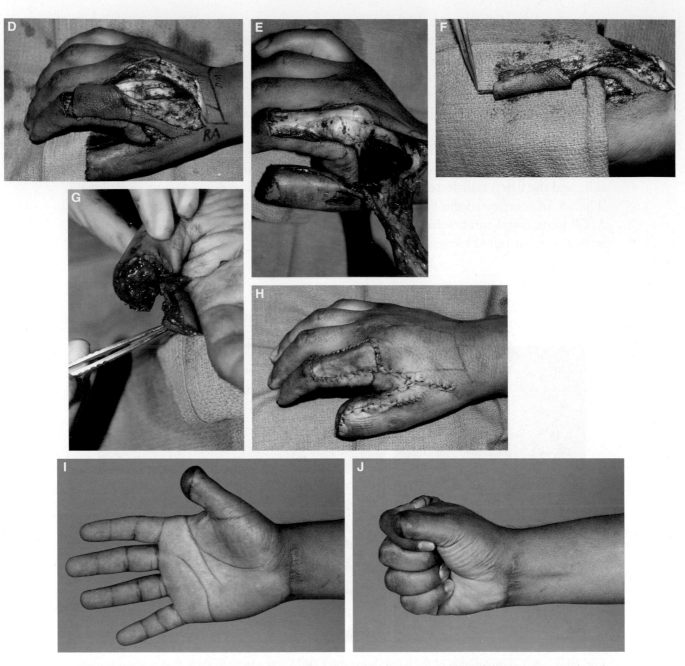

Fig. 20-5, cont'd   D, The FDMA flap was harvested from ulnar to radial and distal to proximal, and a wide flap base was preserved to maximize venous return and arterial inflow. **E,** The FDMA is seen within the harvested flap. The first dorsal interosseous fascia was also harvested to avoid damaging the FMDA. As soon as the ulnar border of the second metacarpal was reached, the dissection was deepened to incorporate the first dorsal interosseous fascia to avoid missing or damaging the FDMA. **F,** The flap can be neurotized by incorporating a dorsal cutaneous branch of the digital nerve. **G,** The dorsal branch of the digital nerve was coapted to the distal stump of the thumb digital nerve. **H-J,** The patient is shown 6 weeks postoperatively.

Pitfalls

The first dorsal interosseous muscle fascia must be included in the flap elevation to avoid inadvertent injury to the FDMA. The pedicle should not be skeletonized and should be raised with a generous cuff of fibrofatty tissue. We keep the base of the flap as wide as possible to preserve venous outflow and arterial perfusion. Postoperative swelling within the tunnel can compress the pedicle and lead to total or partial flap loss. For this reason, we prefer to keep a cutaneous bridge attached to the pedicle and make an incision to reach the defect (Fig. 20-6). This skin bridge is kept intact at its base, and can theoretically improve blood flow through the subdermal plexus to the flap.

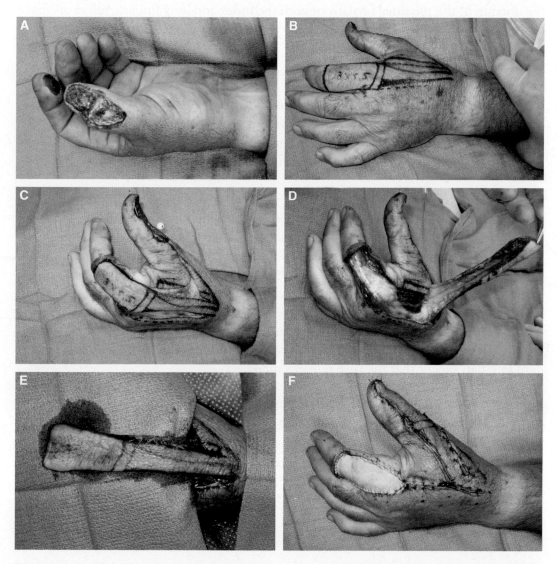

Fig. 20-6 A, Dorsal distal and proximal phalangeal thumb bony and soft tissue defect. **B,** An FDMA flap was designed. The skin bridge extended from the flap and was centered over the pedicle. **C,** The flap was harvested with the skin bridge intact at the base. The communicating incision was made with the defect area. **D,** The flap was harvested with first dorsal interosseous fascia. The FDMA is seen within the flap. **E,** The flap was bleeding bright red blood after release of the tourniquet and before inset. **F,** The flap was inset without tension, with a full-thickness skin graft harvested from the groin.

Modifications

Extended First Dorsal Metacarpal Artery Flap

The extended FDMA flap includes the dorsal skin of the middle phalanx of the index finger up to the DIP joint.[21] The FDMA normally supplies the dorsal skin of the proximal phalanx; any distal extension is considered random and made possible because of the rich dermal-subdermal plexus of the dorsal skin. Flaps as large as 6.5 by 3 cm have been harvested from the dorsal index finger for thumb reconstruction.[22] Gebhard and Meissl[21] have also described successful extension up to the DIP joint for thumb resurfacing with an extended wraparound FDMA flap, which included almost the entire dorsum of the index finger. The FDMA flap can also be extended by including combined skin from the dorsum of the proximal phalanx of both the index and long fingers. Yao et al[23] have harvested a bilobed second web island flap based on the FDMA for reconstruction of circumferential thumb avulsion injuries.

Sensory First Dorsal Metacarpal Artery Flap

The sensory FDMA flap includes a branch of the radial sensory nerve in the flap that is sutured to the recipient injured digital nerve (see Fig. 20-5, *F* and *G*). This flap can be used to cover thumb pulp defects.[24] A preoperative radial sensory nerve block should be performed to assess the sensory innervation of the dorsal proximal phalanx.

Flow-Through Flap

The FDMA can be useful in providing combined dorsal thumb skin coverage and venous outflow in patients with thumb replants and loss of dorsal skin.[6] The distal veins of the FDMA flap are dissected and anastomosed to the dorsal veins of the proximal thumb.

Pseudo-Kite Flap

This flap incorporates the dorsal skin of the first web space and proximal phalanx, and is based on axial flow from the FDMA. The base remains intact and the flap is rotated into the first web after releasing the first space. Elevation is similar to that of the standard kite flap except that the base remains intact.

Second Dorsal Metacarpal Artery Flap

The second dorsal metacarpal artery (SDMA) flap is a reliable sensate flap with a wide arc of rotation. Like the FDMA flap, it serves as a useful and reliable tool for coverage of hand and thumb defects. This flap can be combined with the FDMA island flap to harvest the entire second web space for reconstruction of thumb degloving injuries.[23]

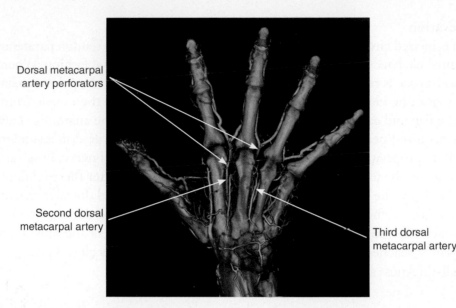

Fig. 20-7 CT angiogram of the hand shows the vascular anatomy of the first, second, and third dorsal metacarpal arteries.

Anatomy

The SDMA generally runs along a line joining the anatomic snuffbox and second web space. In 23 of 29 (79%) cadaveric hands studied by Earley and Milner,[7] the SDMA originated from the dorsal carpal arch (Fig. 20-7). In the remaining six specimens, the SDMA originated from the deep palmar arch, the FDMA, the anterior interosseous artery, or the radial artery. The SDMA passes deep to the extensor digitorum and extensor indicis muscles of the index finger, and superficial to the second dorsal interosseous muscle fascia. As the SDMA reaches the second web space, one or more large perforators can be found between the second and third metacarpal heads in the second intermetacarpal space. These perforators originate from the deep palmar arch and pass dorsally to communicate with the SDMA to supply the dorsal skin. The perforators arise at the level of the metacarpal necks and give off distal branches, which anastomose with the dorsal cutaneous branches of the PPD arteries. These perforator vessels form the basis of the extended SDMA flap and the reverse-flow SDMA flap.

Surgical Technique

Surface Landmarks

The SDMA runs in an oblique line between the anatomic snuffbox and the center of the second web space, between the heads of the second and third metacarpal bones. Depending on the defect's size and location, the flap can be designed over the second intermetacarpal space, over the proximal phalanx of the middle finger, or over the superficial web space. The proximal intersection of the extensor tendons to the index and middle fingers can be considered the pivot point of the flap.[8]

Flap Elevation

The flap is incised circumferentially and dissected off the extensor tendon paratenon of the proximal phalanx. Dissection is performed in a distal to proximal fashion. When the second web space is reached, the communicating perforator from the palmar metacarpal artery must be identified and ligated. An S-shaped incision is then made from the base of the flap and carried proximally over the SDMA toward the anatomic snuffbox until the required pedicle length is obtained. Skin flaps are elevated in a subdermal plane with appropriate superficial veins and branches of the radial nerve. Dissection is deepened along the ulnar aspect of the index extensor tendons. After these tendons are retracted radially, the SDMA can be seen coursing over the second dorsal interosseous muscle and fascia. The SDMA pedicle is dissected from the second dorsal interosseous muscle much like the FDMA (that is, with a generous cuff of fascia and muscle), until the flap safely reaches its intended destination. The donor site is closed primarily or with a full-thickness skin graft.

Pitfalls

As in the dissection of the FDMA flap, the second dorsal interosseous fascia should be included during the elevation of an SDMA flap to avoid inadvertent injury to the SDMA. In addition, the pedicle should not be skeletonized and should be raised with a generous cuff of fibrofatty tissue to minimize risks of venous congestion, vasospasm, and vascular injury.

Modifications

Extended Sensory Dorsal Metacarpal Artery Flap

In 1989, Earley[8] described an extended version of the SDMA flap in which the standard flap design was extended past the PIP joint to include the dorsal skin of the middle phalanx. Variations also included an extended bipennate design, which combined dorsal skin from the middle and index fingers. A second dorsal web flap design was also used for first web space reconstruction.[8]

Sensory Flap

Terminal branches of the radial sensory nerve that innervate the second web space and adjacent dorsal index and middle fingers can be included in the SDMA flap to provide sensation. The course of the sensory radial nerve is similar to that of the SDMA but runs superficial to the extensor tendons. This path becomes a concern when the SDMA is dissected proximally under the extensor tendon to increase pedicle length. Attempts to divide the nerve proximally to increase pedicle length and then perform neurorrhaphy to a recipient digital nerve have been disappointing. To avoid complications, the flap should be transferred with an intact radial sensory branch. This procedure yields two-point discrimination comparable to that of the dorsal second web skin, which is normally approximately 5 to 7 mm.[24]

Double-Pivot Second Dorsal Metacarpal Artery Flap

Described by Karacalar et al[25] in 1996, this modification uses two different pivot points to extend the useful pedicle length of the SDMA flap. The flap is first harvested like the retrograde flow flap described by Quaba and Davison.[13] The SDMA is ligated just distal to the recurrent cutaneous perforator branch, which enters the dorsal skin 1.5 cm proximal to the metacarpal head. The SDMA pedicle is then dissected proximally toward its first main pivot point, which is the origin of the SDMA. The second pivot point corresponds to the recurrent perforator branch of the flap.

Dorsal Metacarpal Artery Perforator Flaps

As described by Quaba and Davison,[13] the DMA flap can be harvested without incorporating the DMA (Fig. 20-8).[26] This flap is based on cutaneous perforators originating

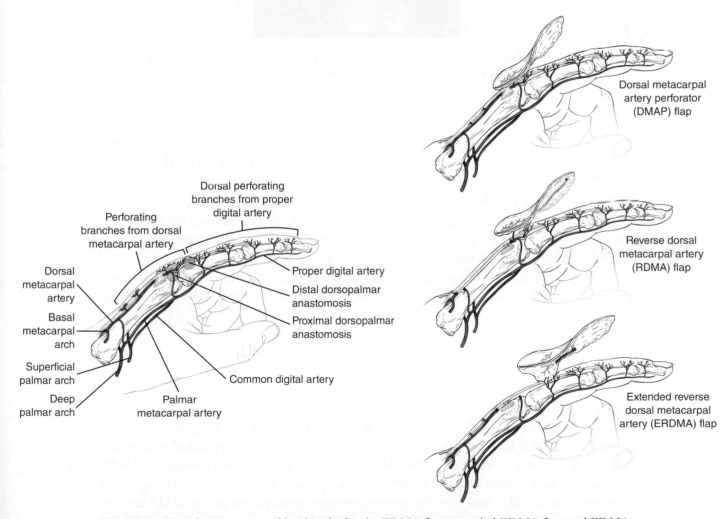

Fig. 20-8 Vascular anatomy and landmarks for the FDMA flap, extended FDMA flap, and FDMA perforator flap. (Modified from Sebastin S, Mendoza R, Chong A. Application of the dorsal metacarpal artery perforator flap for resurfacing soft-tissue defects proximal to the fingertip. Plast Reconstr Surg 128:166e-178e, 2011.)

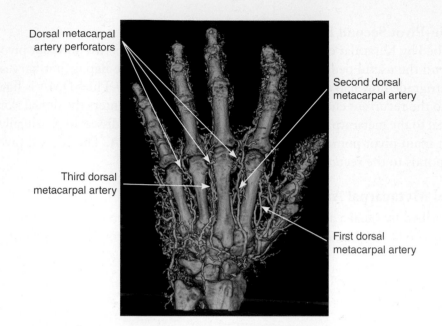

Fig. 20-9   CT angiogram of the hand shows the first, second, and third dorsal metacarpal arteries, and cutaneous perforators to the second, third, and fourth dorsal metacarpal arteries. These perforators form the basis for DMA perforator flaps.

from the DMAs (Fig. 20-9). Flap dissection proceeds from proximal to distal, and is carried above the dorsal interosseous fascia without including the DMA. The dorsal metacarpal artery perforator (DMAP) flap may be raised on the second, third, or fourth intermetacarpal space and is designed as an ellipse, which can extend from the MCP joint to the wrist crease. This cutaneous perforator is very reliable and can almost always be found within the second through fourth intermetacarpal spaces roughly 1 cm proximal to the metacarpal neck. This is in sharp contrast to the third and fourth DMAs, which can sometimes be absent. The flap width and length can vary from 1 to 3.5 cm and from 2 to 9 cm, respectively. The advantages of this perforator-based DMA flap include ease of elevation and thinner coverage for dorsal digital defects.

Anatomy

The DMAP flap blood supply is based on cutaneous perforators derived from the distal portion of the DMA. Four to eight perforators originate along the proximal, middle, and distal thirds of the dorsal metacarpal artery. A dominant cutaneous perforator exists roughly 1.0 to 1.5 cm proximal to the midinterior metacarpal head region and corresponds to the pivot point of the DMAP flap. This flap does not include the DMA, and its vascular supply is based solely on the cutaneous perforator emanating either directly from the DMA or from the communicating branch between the DMA and the palmar metacarpal artery (Figs. 20-10 through 20-12). The perforator can be found just distal to the juncturae tendinae, which allows it to have a longer arc of rotation then the standard DMA flap because of its more distal pivot point.

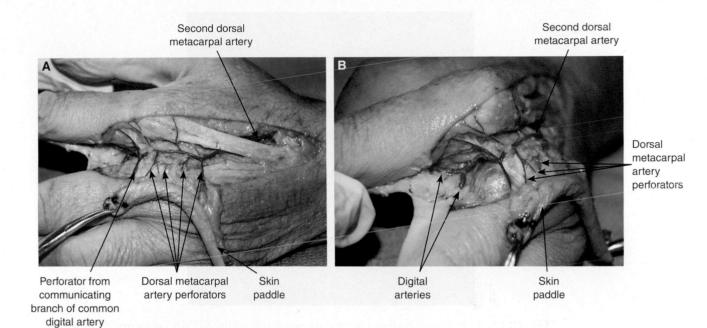

Fig. 20-10 **A,** Red latex injection of the SDMA, DMA, and associated cutaneous perforators. **B,** The SDMA and its associated cutaneous perforators. Note the continuation of the SDMA with the communicating branch and common digital artery.

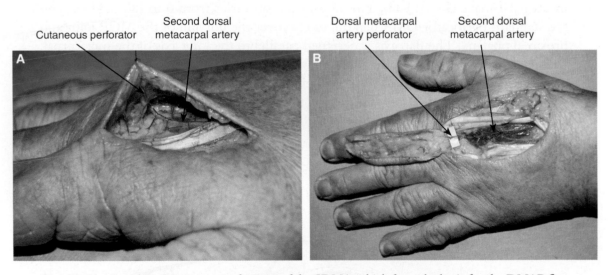

Fig. 20-11 **A** and **B,** Cutaneous perforators of the SDMA, which form the basis for the DMAP flap.

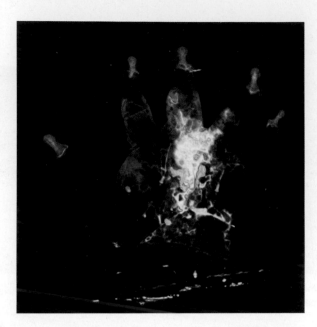

Fig. 20-12   Injection of barium sulfate shows perfusion of the SDMA perforator.

Surgical Technique

Surface Landmarks

The dorsal cutaneous perforator of the DMA is located just distal to the juncturae tendinae and roughly 0.5 to 1 cm proximal to the metacarpal neck within the inter-metacarpal space (Fig. 20-13). The arc of rotation varies from 0 to 180 degrees, and the standard perforator DMA flap can safely cover the dorsum of the MCP joint and proximal phalanx. The flap axis is designed parallel to the long axis of the metacarpal. The proximal flap limit includes the distal wrist crease, whereas the distal limit and tip of the flap ellipse is limited to the intermetacarpal head space (Fig. 20-14).[26] The flap width is based on the dorsal skin laxity and the ability to close the donor site primarily, and usually varies from 1.5 to 3 cm. Wider flaps require a skin graft for the donor site (Fig. 20-15).

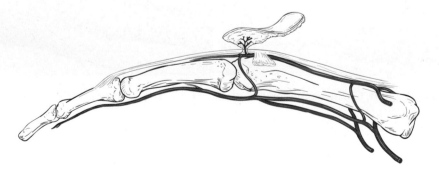

Fig. 20-13   Arterial anatomy of the DMAP flap. The cutaneous perforator of the DMA is located just distal to the juncturae tendinae and roughly 0.5 to 1 cm proximal to the MCP joint.

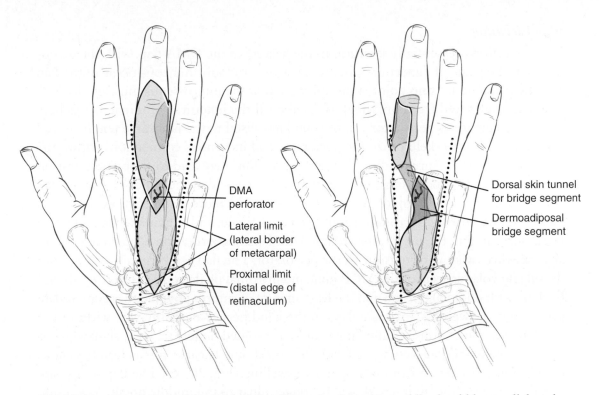

DMA perforator

Lateral limit (lateral border of metacarpal)

Proximal limit (distal edge of retinaculum)

Dorsal skin tunnel for bridge segment

Dermoadiposal bridge segment

Fig. 20-14 Flap design of the DMAP flap. The axis of the skin paddle should be parallel to the axis of the metacarpals. The flap can be harvested in several ways: cutaneous only, cutaneous with an adipofascial bridge, or adipofascial only.(Modified from Sebastin S, Mendoza R, Chong A. Application of the dorsal metacarpal artery perforator flap for resurfacing soft-tissue defects proximal to the fingertip. Plast Reconstr Surg 128:166e-178e, 2011.)

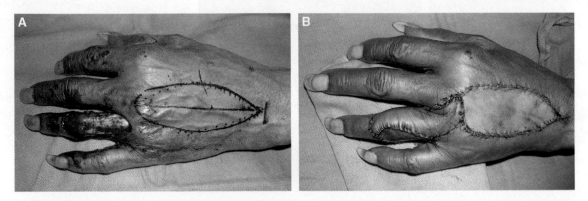

Fig. 20-15 **A** and **B,** A large DMAP flap for nearly circumferential coverage of the proximal phalanx following tumor resection. The donor site has been closed with a full-thickness skin graft harvested from the groin.

Flap Elevation

Flap dissection is essentially identical to the harvest of the DMA flap, with the exception that the plane of dissection initially is between the subcutaneous tissue of the flap and the paratenon. At no point is the epimysium of the interosseous muscles violated. The flap is elevated from proximal to distal until the juncturae tendinae is reached. The flap's cutaneous perforator can be found just distal to the juncturae tendinae, and care is given not to skeletonize the perforator and its venous connections within the subcutaneous tissue surrounding this perforator. This may lead to venous congestion and flap ischemia. Once a cutaneous perforator has been identified, it can be confirmed with handheld pencil Doppler device. At this point, the more distal portion of the skin flap is elevated off the surrounding subcutaneous tissue, and subcutaneous tissue and fascia surrounding the perforator are freed until adequate rotation is possible without any excessive twisting or tension on the perforator. The flap can be used to cover both dorsal and volar aspects of the MCP joint and proximal phalanx. Flap insetting should be done with minimal tension and the least amount of sutures possible to accommodate postoperative swelling. Intrinsic flaps to the hand heal remarkably well without the need for excessive sutures. Tunneling should be avoided under the volar skin, which is less redundant and loose compared with the dorsal skin, because it may lead to venous congestion or ischemia from postoperative swelling (Fig. 20-16). The flap donor site length relative to the digit length will be longer ulnar to the middle finger. As a result, a standard DMAP flap will reach the DIP joint without the need to raise it as an extended flap (Fig. 20-17).

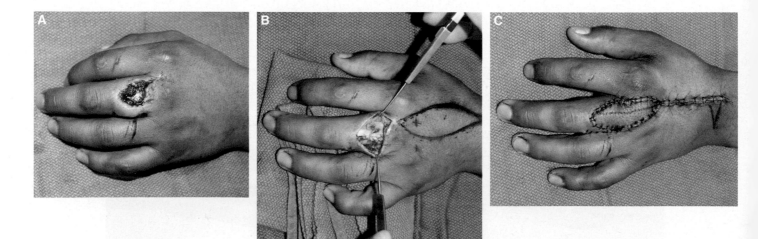

Fig. 20-16 **A,** A dorsoproximal phalanx defect of the middle finger with exposed bone and lacerated extensor tendon. **B,** The wound is shown after debridement and extensor tendon repair. An SDMA perforator flap was designed. The perforator was located with Doppler ultrasound just proximal to the metacarpal neck, between the metacarpal heads. **C,** The flap was inset under minimal tension and provided stable coverage.

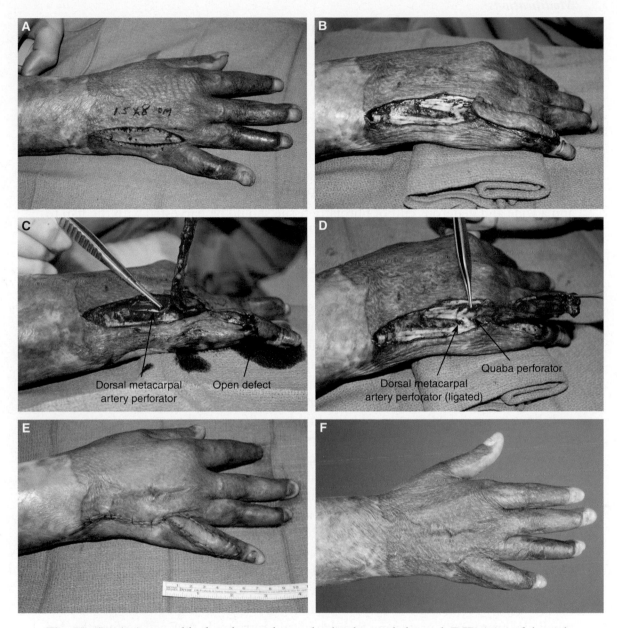

Fig. 20-17 **A,** An unstable dorsal wound over the distal interphalangeal (DIP) joint of the right small finger. A fourth DMAP flap was designed. **B,** The flap was harvested. A cutaneous perforator was located just distal to the juncturae tendinae. **C** and **D,** Sometimes cutaneous perforators will be found along the metacarpal artery and can be ligated until the main perforator distal to the juncturae tendinae is located. Ligation of more proximal perforators will allow a more distal pivot point and flap reach. **E,** The flap was inset with coverage up to the DIP joint and distal phalanx. **F,** The 4-week postoperative result.

Modifications

Extended Dorsal Metacarpal Artery Perforator Flap

Karacalar and Özcan[14] have described a modified version of the DMAP flap. Their flap had an extended arc of rotation and covered the distal phalanx in five patients. It was based on the second and third intermetacarpal spaces and on connections between the dorsal branches of the PPD artery and the terminal branches of the DMA at the level of the proximal phalanx. The largest flap size was 7 by 3 cm. The flap survival rate was 100%. Dissection is similar to that of the DMAP flap but is carried more distally. The DMA cutaneous perforator is ligated, and a pedicle is developed based on connections between the dorsal branches of the digital artery and the terminal cutaneous branches of the DMA over the proximal phalanx. Pedicle skeletonization should be avoided, and a wide and generous cuff of fibrofatty tissue should be harvested with the flap to maximize perfusion. Angiographic studies by Yang and Morris[15] confirm the anatomic basis of this flap modification. This flap allows coverage of more distal defects at the level of the distal phalanx and DIP joint, which could not be treated with a standard reverse flap design (Fig. 20-18).

The standard pivot point for the DMAP flap corresponds to the cutaneous perforator location, which is found within the intermetacarpal space roughly 1 cm proximal to the metacarpal neck. This pivot point allows the flap to reach the proximal phalanx and PIP joint safely but no further. The flap pivot point can be extended by two measures to gain additional flap reach. First, the DMA can be ligated just proximal to the cutaneous perforator so that it does not tether the DMA cutaneous perforator as much and allows more distal flap advancement. In this modification, the cutaneous perforator derives its main blood supply from the dorsal perforating branch of the palmar metacarpal artery. This dorsal perforating branch is equivalent to a communicating branch between the palmar and dorsal metacarpal arteries and is found at the same level as the DMA cutaneous perforator. This modification increases flap reach distally by 5 to 8 mm. Second, a more distal pivot point can be used for more extensive reach to the middle and distal interphalangeal joint. The cutaneous perforator can be ligated, and the flap can be harvested based on retrograde flow through the dorsal branches of the proper digital arteries at the proximal half of the proximal phalangeal level. Multiple connections and linking vessels exist in the subcutaneous tissue between the terminal subcutaneous branches of the DMA, its cutaneous perforator, and the dorsal branches of the digital arteries. By preserving this rich plexus, retrograde flow will perfuse the flap and can significantly increase the distal flap reach by 10 to 15 mm. It is critical to keep the widest pedicle of subcutaneous tissue connected between the distal tip of the flap at the MCP level and the dorsal digital branches over the proximal phalanx. This area of the digit must be intact and not previously injured or else flap loss may result from insufficient retrograde flow. If there is too much tension during flap insetting using the standard pivot point for the perforator DMA flap, then moving the pivot point more distally by one of the measures mentioned previously should be strongly considered.

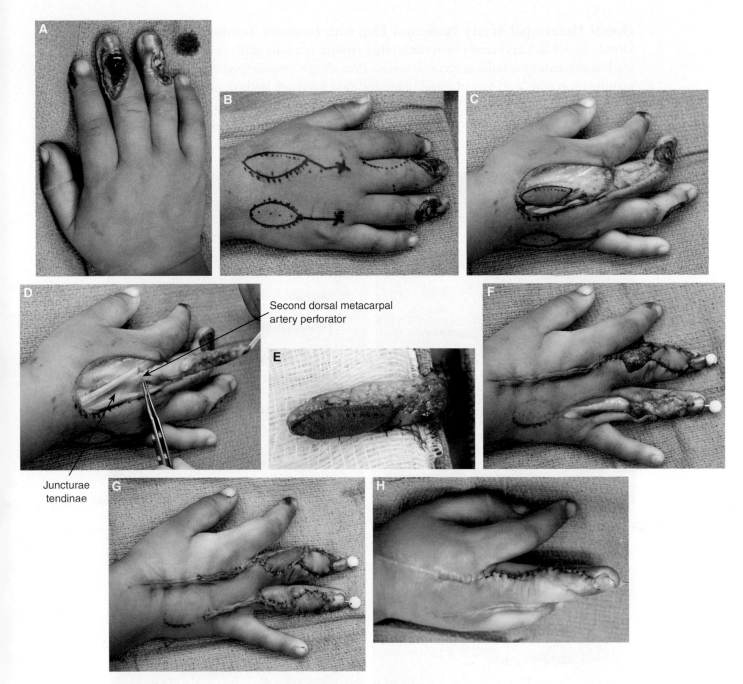

Fig. 20-18   A, This 8-year-old girl had an exposed DIP joint of her right middle and ring fingers caused by a crush avulsion injury. **B,** Second and fourth DMAP flaps were designed. **C,** The SDMAP flap was harvested. A communicating incision was made between the flap pivot point and the defect. **D,** The SDMA perforator can be seen just distal to the juncturae tendinae. **E,** The tourniquet was released to verify flap perfusion before inset. **F** and **G,** The main cutaneous perforator was ligated, and the SDMA cutaneous perforator flap was inset. Vascularity to the flap was maintained through retrograde flow between the dorsal branches of the digital artery and the terminal branches of the SDMAP flap. **H,** The flap was debulked and the skin graft excised 3 months postoperatively.

Dorsal Metacarpal Artery Perforator Flap with Extensor Tendon

Dorsal digital defects caused by trauma often require not only skin coverage or resurfacing but also extensor tendon reconstruction. Providing a vascularized extensor tendon in combination with well-vascularized tissue and skin coverage leads to early rehabilitation and maximal function. The SDMAP flap can be harvested with a portion or all of the extensor indicis proprius for vascularized extensor tendon reconstruction (Fig. 20-19).

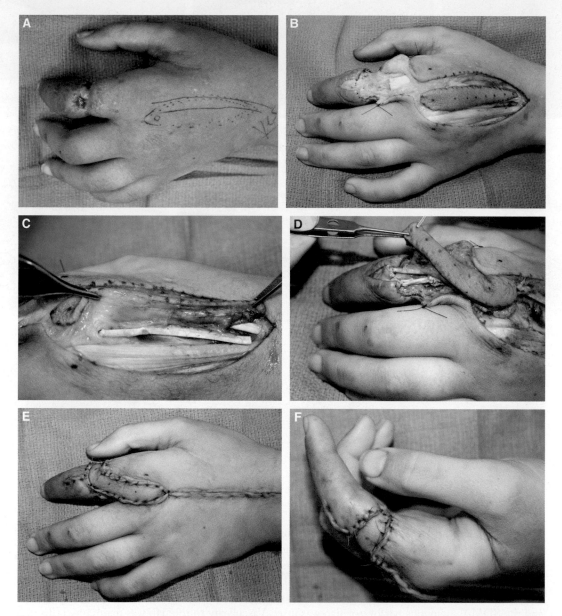

Fig. 20-19   **A,** Left index finger proximal phalanx dorsal defect involving soft tissue and the extensor tendon. A composite SDMAP flap was designed to include a section of the indicis proprius (EIP) extensor tendon. **B,** The flap was harvested. **C,** A section of the EIP tendon was harvested with the flap. Small perforators provide communication between the flap and EIP tendon. **D,** The extensor tendon was repaired, and the flap was rotated. **E** and **F,** The inset flap is shown.

Curved Elliptical Dorsal Metacarpal Artery Perforator Flap

The DMAP flap reach can be extended distally without modifying its standard pivot point location by modifying the flap design only. In this modification, the standard elliptical flap design is converted to a curved elliptical design, which is straightened once the flap is rotated and inset.[26] This modification can yield an additional 8 to 10 mm of length. The proximal flap harvest limit includes the distal dorsal wrist crease, and depending on dorsal skin laxity, flaps wider than 3 cm will most likely require a skin graft for donor site closure (Fig. 20-20).

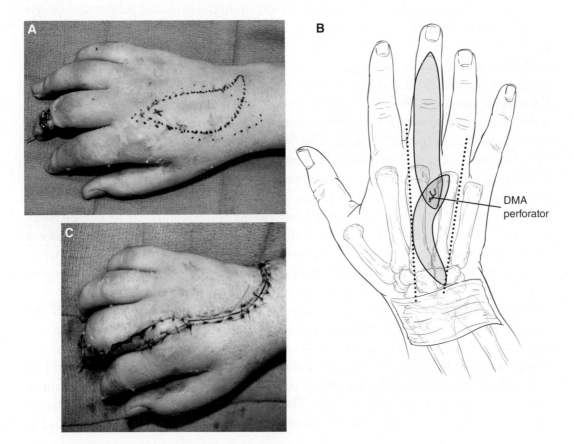

Fig. 20-20 A and **B,** A curved elliptical DMAP flap was designed for this patient. **C,** The flap was inset and the donor site closed. The proximal extent of the flap skin paddle should not cross proximal to the distal wrist crease to maintain adequate blood supply. (**B** modified from Sebastin S, Mendoza R, Chong A. Application of the dorsal metacarpal artery perforator flap for resurfacing soft-tissue defects proximal to the fingertip Plast Reconstr Surg 128:166e-178e, 2011.)

THENAR AND MIDPALMAR PERFORATOR FLAPS

Like the dorsal surface of the hand, the volar surface is a rich source of perforators that are amenable for perforator flap design and harvest. Multiple volar perforators originate from the deep and superficial palmar arches, the superficial palmar branch of the radial artery, the radialis indicis artery, and the princeps pollicis artery. These source arteries can potentially form the basis for local pedicle perforator flaps. Glabrous skin from the thenar and midpalm regions of the volar hand can be used for reconstructing adjacent volar defects with skin of similar color and characteristics. The pedicle perforator thenar flap described by Seyhan[27] is one such example of a versatile volar-based perforator flap of the hand. The flap is based on cutaneous perforators originating from the superficial palmar branch of the radial artery at the intersection of the proximal palmar and thenar crease. Seyhan called this the *keystone area*. It represents a rich source of perforators originating from the connection and confluence of the terminal branch of the superficial palmar arch, superficial palmar radial artery, princeps pollicis artery, and deep palmar arch (Figs. 20-21 and 20-22). Any suitably large perforator from the previously described arteries can be used to design a volar-based pedicle perforator flap. Venous return is supplied by one or two of the venae comitantes that accompany the perforator and by superficial veins in the palm. The flap landmarks include the beginning of the thenar crease distally and the proximal thenar crease proximally, with an extension 2 to 2.5 cm ulnar to the thenar crease. The ulnar border of the flap is harvested first down to the thenar and adductor pollicis fascia. The perforator is then visualized and flow confirmed with a Doppler probe before completing the circumferential flap incision. Like the DMAP flap, the thenar flap perforator should not be skeletonized to preserve venous outflow and prevent arterial vasospasm. The flap is then rotated into place without pedicle kinking or compression. There should be no tension during flap insetting.

Kim et al[28] have also described a radial midpalmar perforator-based island flap. It is based on perforators from the terminal branch of the superficial palmar arch and princeps pollicis artery. The flap is designed on the radial aspect of the midpalm and cutaneous perforators from the terminal branch of the superficial palmar arch that run along the radial border of the second metacarpal. Therefore the flap skin should be designed within this area. The superficial palmar arch connects with the radial palmar digital artery and princeps pollicis artery. The superficial palmar arch and palmar digital artery are ligated to mobilize the flap as an island perforator-based flap (Fig. 20-23).

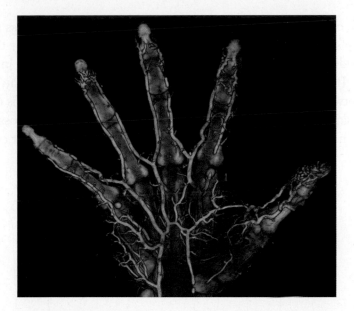

Fig. 20-21   CT angiogram of the hand shows perforators from the superficial palmar arch and superficial palmar branch of the radial artery.

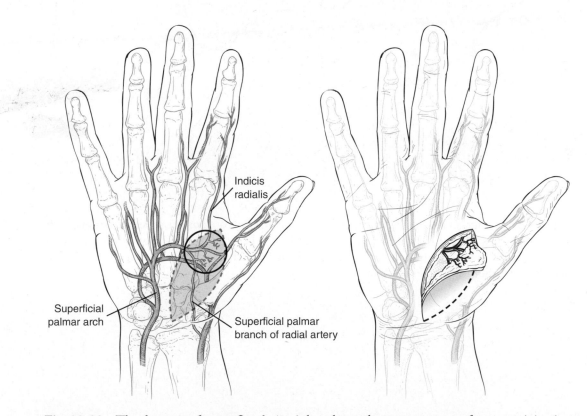

Indicis radialis

Superficial palmar arch

Superficial palmar branch of radial artery

Fig. 20-22   The thenar perforator flap design is based on palmar cutaneous perforators originating from and concentrated at the confluence of the superficial palmar arch, superficial palmar branch of the radial artery, and indicis radialis artery. (Modified from Seyhan T. Reverse thenar perforator flap for volar hand reconstruction. J Plast Reconstr Aesthet Surg 62:1309-1316, 2009.)

The donor site can either be closed primarily or with a split-thickness skin graft, depending on flap size. As with any intrinsic pedicle flap of the hand, any tunneling with potential for pedicle compression should be avoided, and tension-free insetting should be guaranteed. If there are concerns regarding pedicle compression, an opening incision is made between the donor and recipient defects, and the pedicle is covered with a split-thickness skin graft. The donor site is closed primarily whenever possible. Splinting should be continued for 3 to 6 months postoperatively to prevent scar contractures.

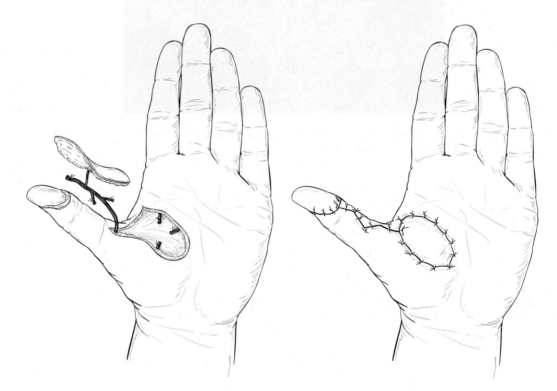

Fig. 20-23   Design and harvest of the midpalmar perforator flap based on the superficial palmar arch for thumb reconstruction. (Modified from Kim KS, Kim ES, Hwang JH, et al. Thumb reconstruction using the radial midpalmar [perforator-based] island flap [distal thenar perforator-based island flap]. Plast Reconstr Surg 125:601-608, 2010.)

DIGITAL ARTERY PERFORATOR FLAPS

Any axial vessel in the hand and digits gives rise to both volar and dorsal perforators, which are amenable to multiple free-style perforator flap designs. Similar to the dorsal metacarpal arteries, the proper digital arteries give rise to multiple cutaneous perforators along their course. The dorsal and volar digital artery cutaneous perforators can therefore form the basis for digital perforator flaps (Fig. 20-24). These flaps can be used as pedicle perforator flaps, V-Y advancement flaps, or rotation flaps based on cutaneous perforators for coverage of small fingertip and distal volar and dorsal digital defects.

Many of the cutaneous digital artery perforators originate from the lateral aspect of the finger distally, forming the basis for the digital artery perforator flap design. The flap is designed as an ellipse and can range from 1 to 2 cm in length and 1 cm in width for a cutaneous flap design, and up to 2 cm in width when used as an adipofascial flap only.[29] Flap elevation is performed superficial to the neurovascular bundle. The perforator closest to the defect is preserved as the flap pedicle and pivot point. The pedicle digital artery perforator flap is then rotated 90 or 180 degrees and inset with minimal tension.

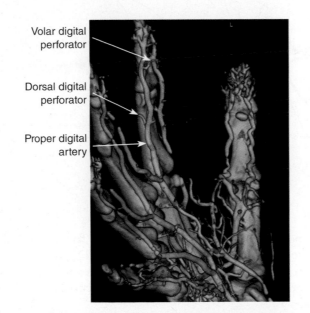

Volar digital
perforator

Dorsal digital
perforator

Proper digital
artery

Fig. 20-24 CT angiogram shows multiple volar and dorsal cutaneous perforators originating from the ulnar and radial digital arteries of the index finger.

If undue pressure on the pedicle is created from primary donor site closure, then the donor site is covered with a skin graft, which can be excised later as needed (Fig. 20-25).

Dorsal digital defects are also amenable to coverage with digital perforator flaps based on dorsal cutaneous perforators from the digital arteries. These perforators are identical to the ones included in cross-finger flaps but are used as island variants for additional flap mobilization (Fig. 20-26). The dorsal digital perforator is identified with Doppler flowmetry, and the flap is designed as a rotation flap or V-Y advancement flap (Figs. 20-27 and 20-28).[30] Flap elevation is carried above the paratenon, and the base of the flap is narrowed carefully once the perforator has been identified to facilitate flap mobilization. A cuff of fibrofatty tissue is retained at the base of the flap and perforator to maximize venous return and arterial perfusion, and to minimize vasospasm. Digital artery perforator flaps present a very useful adjunct to our available digital reconstruction flap. Their flap design can be extremely versatile because of the numerous and varied locations of digital artery perforators. Nevertheless, these flaps can only cover smaller defects and require very meticulous dissection to avoid injuring the perforator.

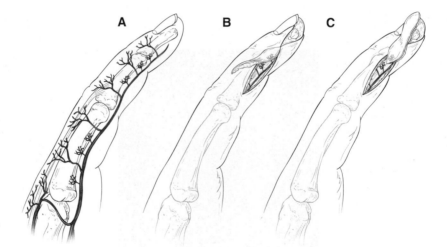

Fig. 20-25   A-C, Design and harvest of a digital artery perforator flap with 180-degree rotation into the defect. The donor site can be closed with a skin graft to avoid pressure over the pedicle and digital artery. (Modified from Mitsunaga N, Mihara M, Koshima I, et al. Digital artery perforator (DAP) flaps: modifications for fingertip and finger stump reconstruction. J Plast Reconstr Aesthet Surg 63:1312-1317, 2010.)

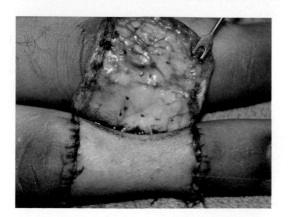

Fig. 20-26   Intraoperative view of a cross-finger flap with dorsal perforators originating from the proper digital artery. These dorsal perforators form the basis for roatation or V-Y advancement dorsal perforator flaps, which can be harvested either as adipocutaneous or adipofascial flaps.

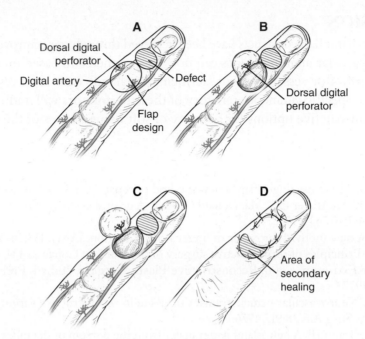

Fig. 20-27 A-D, Design and harvest of the dorsal digital perforator rotation flap. (Modified from Kawakatsu M, Ishikawa K. Dorsal digital perforator flap for reconstruction of distal dorsal finger defects. J Plast Reconstr Aesthet Surg 63:e46-e50, 2010.)

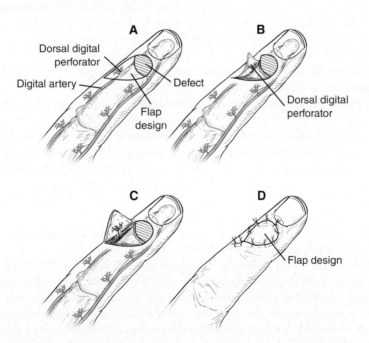

Fig. 20-28 A-D, Design and harvest of the dorsal digital V-Y advancement flap. (Modified from Kawakatsu M, Ishikawa K. Dorsal digital perforator flap for reconstruction of distal dorsal finger defects. J Plast Reconstr Aesthet Surg 63:e46-e50, 2010.)

CONCLUSION

Refinements in hand flap constructs have been achieved through our improved knowledge of the hand's vascular anatomy. Flaps can now be designed and based on constant and identifiable perforator vessels without sacrificing the hand's main axial vessels. Further mapping of the specific cutaneous territory of these perforators will undoubtedly yield improved reconstructive options for a variety of soft tissue defects of the hand.

References

1. Cronin TD. The cross finger flap: a new method of repair. Am Surg 17:419-425, 1951.
2. Kleinert HE, McAlister CG, MacDonald CJ, et al. A critical evaluation of cross finger flaps. J Trauma 14:756-763, 1974.
3. Kutler W. A new method for repair of finger tip amputation. JAMA 133:29-30, 1947.
4. Littler JW. Principles of reconstructive surgery of the hand. In Converse JM, ed. The Hand and Upper Extremity, vol 6. Reconstructive Plastic Surgery, 2nd ed. Philadelphia: WB Saunders, 1977.
5. Littler JW. Neurovascular pedicle transfer of tissue in reconstructive surgery of the hand. J Bone Joint Surg Am 38:917, 1956.
6. Foucher G, Braun JB. A new island flap transfer from the dorsum of the index to the thumb. Plast Reconstr Surg 63:344-349, 1979.

    The authors described an island flap originating from the dorsum of the index finger, performed in 12 patients. The flap was based on the first dorsal metacarpal artery with one or two veins and the terminal branches of the radial nerve. The flap was reliable, with no necrosis. In a single operation, this transfer provides composite resurfacing of the thumb and brings in new blood and nerve supply.

7. Earley MJ, Milner RH. Dorsal metacarpal flaps. Br J Plast Surg 40:333-341, 1987.
8. Earley MJ. The second dorsal metacarpal artery neurovascular island flap. J Hand Surg 14:434-440, 1989.
9. Dautel G, Merle M. Dorsal metacarpal reverse flaps: anatomical basis and clinical application. J Hand Surg 16:400-405, 1991.
10. Dautel G, Merle M. Direct and reverse dorsal metacarpal flaps. Br J Plast Surg 45:123-130, 1992.

    The authors examined the three-dimensional anatomy of vascular systems used for both direct and reverse dorsal metacarpal flaps. Three types of dorsopalmar anastomotic networks were identified at the first and second metacarpal spaces, and in the web space area. These networks were able to supply blood for reverse metacarpal flaps. A series of 12 cases was presented.

11. Foucher G, Bishop AT. Island flaps based on the first and second dorsal metacarpal arteries. Atlas Hand Clin 3:93-107, 1998.
12. Pelissier P, Casoli V, Bakhach J, et al. Reverse dorsal digital and metacarpal flaps: a review of 27 cases. Plast Reconstr Surg 103:159-165, 1999.
13. Quaba AA, Davison PM. The distally-based dorsal hand flap. Br J Plast Surg 43:28-39, 1990.

    The planning and clinical applications of a series of reverse dorsal hand flaps were described. This new flap was based on a direct cutaneous branch of the dorsal metacarpal artery. It is particularly useful in resurfacing web spaces as well as dorsal metacarpal and phalangeal skin defects.

14. Karacalar A, Özcan M. A new approach to the reverse dorsal metacarpal artery flap. J Hand Surg 22:307-310, 1997.

    The authors described harvesting a reverse dorsal metacarpal artery flap based on the vascular connection between the dorsal branch of the proper digital artery and the terminal branches of the dorsal metacarpal artery at the level of the proximal phalanx. Two flaps were raised on the second and three on the third intermetacarpal space. All flaps survived completely and the donor sites were closed by direct approximation.

15. Yang D, Morris SF. Vascular basis of dorsal digital and metacarpal skin flaps. J Hand Surg 26:142-146, 2001.

16. Hirasé Y, Kojima T, Matsuura S. A versatile one-stage neurovascular flap for fingertip reconstruction: the dorsal middle phalangeal finger flap. Plast Reconstr Surg 90:1009-1015, 1992.

17. Endo T, Kojima T, Hirasé Y. Vascular anatomy of the finger dorsum and a new idea for coverage of the finger pulp defect that restores sensation. J Hand Surg 17:927-932, 1992.

18. Chen SL, Chou TD, Chen SG, et al. The boomerang flap in managing injuries of the dorsum of the distal phalanx. Plast Reconstr Surg 106:834-839, 2000.

19. Foucher G, Khouri RK. Digital reconstruction with island flaps. Clin Plast Surg 24:1-32, 1997.

20. Sherif M. First dorsal metacarpal artery flap in hand reconstruction. II. Clinical application. J Hand Surg 19:32-38, 1994.

21. Gebhard B, Meissl G. An extended first dorsal metacarpal artery neurovascular island flap. J Hand Surg 20:529-531, 1995.

22. El-Khatib HA. Clinical experiences with the extended first dorsal metacarpal artery island flap for thumb reconstruction. J Hand Surg 23:647-652, 1998.

23. Yao JM, Song JL, Xu JH. The second web bilobed flap for thumb reconstruction. Br J Plast Surg 49:103-106, 1996.

24. Small JO, Brennen MD. The first dorsal metacarpal artery neurovascular island flap. J Hand Surgery 13:136-145, 1988.

25. Karacalar A, Akin S, Özcan M. The second dorsal metacarpal artery flap with double pivot points. Br J Plast Surg 49:97-102, 1996.

26. Sebastin S, Mendoza R, Chong A. Application of the dorsal metacarpal artery perforator flap for resurfacing soft-tissue defects proximal to the fingertip. Plast Reconstr Surg 128:166e-178e, 2011.

27. Seyhan T. Reverse thenar perforator flap for volar hand reconstruction. J Plast Reconstr Aesthet Surg 62:1309-1316, 2009.

28. Kim KS, Kim ES, Hwang JH, et al. Thumb reconstruction using the radial midpalmar (perforator-based) island flap (distal thenar perforator-based island flap). Plast Reconstr Surg 125:601-608, 2010.

29. Mitsunaga N, Mihara M, Koshima I, et al. Digital artery perforator (DAP) flaps: modifications for fingertip and finger stump reconstruction. J Plast Reconstr Aesthet Surg 63:1312-1317, 2010.

30. Kawakatsu M, Ishikawa K. Dorsal digital perforator flap for reconstruction of distal dorsal finger defects. J Plast Reconstr Aesthet Surg 63:e46-e50, 2010.

Trunk

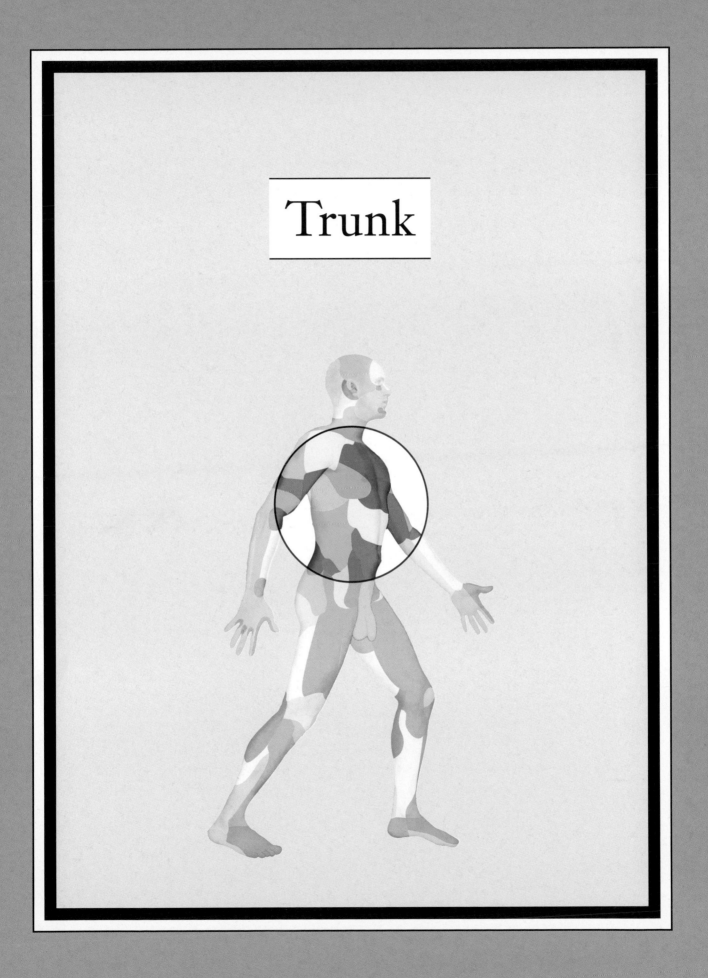

21

Anatomy of the Integument of the Trunk

Christopher R. Geddes
Maolin Tang
Daping Yang
Steven F. Morris

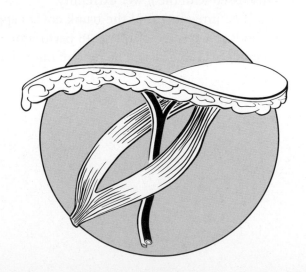

The integument of the trunk is used extensively in reconstructive surgery for flap harvest. Large vascular perforators from 17 source arteries supply the various donor sites of the trunk. Most of these perforators are musculocutaneous, originating from the primary blood supply of the broad superficial muscles in this region. Several large septocutaneous perforators arise from the perimeter of these muscles and from near the joint creases of the extremities, where the skin is tethered to underlying connective tissue. The large septocutaneous perforators are easily distinguishable in angiograms of the integument, because they frequently have a larger diameter and travel greater distances, thus supplying large vascular territories.

The vascular anatomy of the trunk can be represented by the following four regions: chest, abdomen, upper back, and lumbar. The chest region extends from the clavicles to the costal margins and laterally up to the midaxillary line. The abdominal region extends from the costal margin to the iliac crest, the inguinal ligament, and the pubis anteriorly, and is separated from the upper back and lumbar regions by the midaxillary line. The upper back region extends superiorly to a line joining the C7 spinous process with the acromial angle, and inferiorly to the lower margin of the twelfth rib. The lumbar region extends from this inferior boundary of the upper back region to a line joining the two posterior superior iliac spines, and along the iliac crest. The external genitalia (male and female) and perineum are presented separately. The gluteal region is discussed with the lower extremity.

The integument of the trunk covers approximately 30% of the surface area of the body. An average of 122 ± 48 perforators from 17 vascular territories supplies the integument (Table 21-1). The ratio of musculocutaneous to septocutaneous perforators

Table 21-1 Quantitative Data Summary for Cutaneous Vascular Territories of the Trunk

Code	Name of Vascular Territory	Number of Perforators (≥0.5 mm)	Superficial Pedicle Length (mm)	Diameter (mm)	Total Area (cm²)	Area/ Perforator (cm²)	Area of Region (%)	Ratio (MC/ SC)
TCT	Thyrocervical trunk	7 (± 2)	26 (± 14)	0.7 (± 0.2)	170 (± 53)	29 (± 6)	7 (± 2)	4:1
TAA	Thoracoacromial artery	2 (± 1)	24 (± 16)	0.5 (± 0.1)	40 (± 24)	28 (± 14)	2 (± 2)	1:1
ITA	Internal thoracic (mammary) artery	5 (± 2)	30 (± 21)	0.7 (± 0.2)	183 (± 61)	41 (± 16)	8 (± 2)	1:0
LTA	Lateral thoracic artery	1 (± 1)	102 (± 50)	1.4 (± 0.4)	167 (± 70)	139 (± 78)	7 (± 3)	0:1
SEA	Superior epigastric artery	5 (± 1)	25 (± 15)	0.6 (± 0.2)	150 (± 40)	34 (± 9)	6 (± 1)	1:0
DIEA	Deep inferior epigastric artery	5 (± 2)	24 (± 15)	0.7 (± 0.2)	144 (± 55)	33 (± 5)	6 (± 2)	3:1
SIEA	Superficial inferior epigastric artery	1 (± 1)	96 (± 60)	1.2 (± 0.4)	141 (± 106)	114 (± 42)	6 (± 4)	0:1
SCIA	Superficial circumflex iliac artery	1 (± 1)	81 (± 26)	1.0 (± 0.1)	66 (± 20)	52 (± 25)	3 (± 1)	0:1
DCIA	Deep circumflex iliac artery	2 (± 1)	30 (± 14)	0.6 (± 0.1)	87 (± 38)	44 (± 15)	4 (± 2)	1:0
CSA	Circumflex scapular artery	2 (± 1)	53 (± 25)	0.9 (± 0.3)	110 (± 49)	63 (± 42)	5 (± 2)	0:1
TDA	Thoracodorsal artery	3 (± 2)	42 (± 29)	0.9 (± 0.3)	124 (± 66)	54 (± 20)	5 (± 2)	2:1
DPIA	Dorsal branch of posterior intercostal artery	10 (± 3)	27 (± 16)	0.6 (± 0.1)	257 (± 90)	27 (± 10)	11 (± 4)	1:0
LPIA	Lateral branch of posterior intercostal artery	13 (± 5)	28 (± 16)	0.7 (± 0.2)	461 (± 100)	40 (± 16)	19 (± 4)	1:0
LA	Lumbar artery	6 (± 2)	27 (± 12)	0.7 (± 0.1)	157 (± 55)	29 (± 15)	7 (± 3)	1:2

The external pudendal artery, internal pudendal artery, and obturator artery territories were not included in the quantitative analysis for this region. All values are averages, plus or minus the standard deviation for the number, diameter, length, and areas calculated in our series (N = 10). The area of each vascular territory and the area supplied by each perforator were calculated from digital angiograms of the region. (*MC*, Musculocutaneous; *SC*, septocutaneous.)

is 4:1 (Fig. 21-1). The average diameter of and area supplied by a single perforator from the trunk region are approximately 0.7 ± 0.2 mm and 40 ± 15 cm^2, respectively.

The arterial blood supply of the trunk arises from three primary arterial systems: the subclavian/axillary axis, the descending aorta, and the external iliac arteries (Fig. 21-2). Superiorly, branches from the subclavian/axillary axis, including the internal and lateral thoracic, thyrocervical, thoracoacromial, and subscapular arteries, supply the chest, axilla, and part of the upper back. Posteriorly, the descending thoracic and abdominal aorta give off the segmental posterior intercostal, subcostal, and lumbar arteries. Inferiorly, perforators from the epigastric and circumflex iliac branches of the external iliac and common femoral arteries supply the lower abdominal region. The primary vascular supply to the external genitalia and perineum is through perforators from the internal and external pudendal, perineal, and inferior rectal arteries.

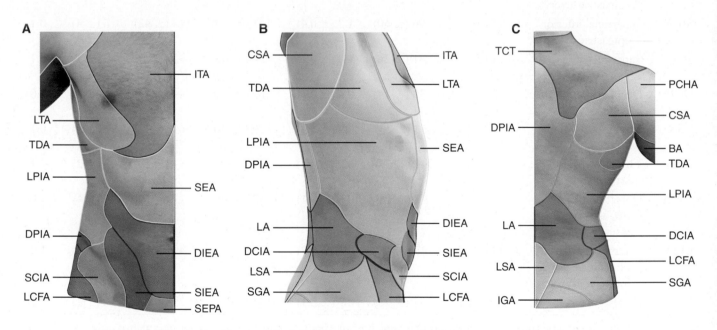

Fig. 21-1 Vascular anatomy of the integument of the trunk. Cutaneous vascular territories are shown in different colors to facilitate identification. **A,** Anterior view of chest and abdominal regions. **B,** Lateral view of the axilla and torso. **C,** Posterior view of the upper back and lumbar regions. (*BA,* Brachial artery; *CSA,* circumflex scapular artery; *DCIA,* deep circumflex iliac artery; *DIEA,* deep inferior epigastric artery; *DPIA,* dorsal branches of posterior intercostal arteries; *IGA,* inferior gluteal artery; *ITA,* internal thoracic [mammary] artery; *LA,* lumbar arteries; *LCFA,* lateral circumflex femoral artery; *LPIA,* lateral branches of posterior intercostal arteries; *LSA,* lateral sacral arteries; *LTA,* lateral thoracic artery; *PCHA,* posterior circumflex humeral artery; *SCIA,* superficial circumflex iliac artery; *SEA,* superior epigastric artery; *SEPA,* superficial external pudendal artery; *SGA,* superior gluteal artery; *SIEA,* superficial inferior epigastric artery; *TCT,* thyrocervical trunk; *TDA,* thoracodorsal artery.)

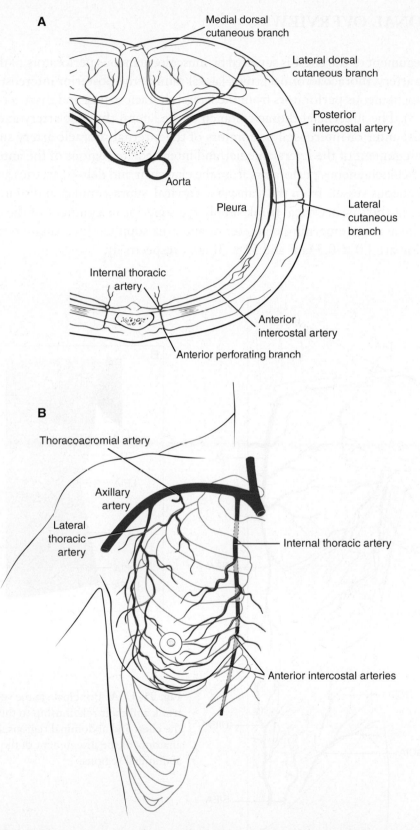

Fig. 21-2   Principal source arteries that supply the integument of the trunk. **A,** Cross section of chest through the sixth intercostal space. **B,** Anterior chest view of right hemithorax.

REGIONAL OVERVIEW
Chest

The integument of the chest is supplied by musculocutaneous perforators of the internal thoracic artery, thoracoacromial artery, lateral rami of the posterior intercostal arteries, and septocutaneous perforators from the lateral thoracic artery and thyrocervical trunk (Fig. 21-3). The superficial thoracic branch of the lateral thoracic artery and the large sequential anterior intercostal perforators of the internal thoracic artery supply most of the integument of the lateral, medial, and intermediate regions of the anterior chest wall. Musculocutaneous perforators from the clavicular and deltoid arteries and variable septocutaneous vessels from the transverse cervical, suprascapular, and supraclavicular branches of the thyrocervical trunk supply the superior integument of the chest (Fig. 21-4). The average emerging diameter of and area supplied by a single perforator in this region are 1.0 ± 0.3 cm^2 and 57 ± 31 cm^2, respectively.

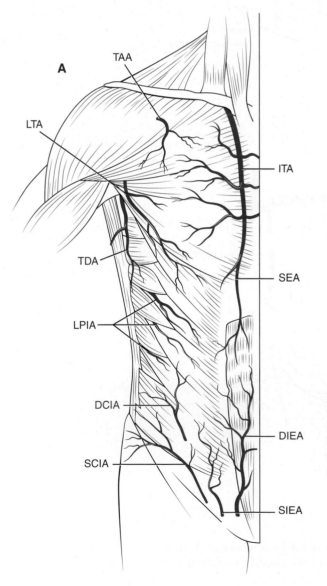

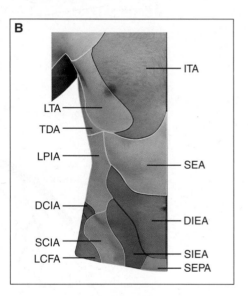

Fig. 21-3   A, Principal source vessels of the trunk and their relationship to the muscles of the chest and abdominal regions. **B,** Vascular anatomy of the integument of the chest and abdominal regions.

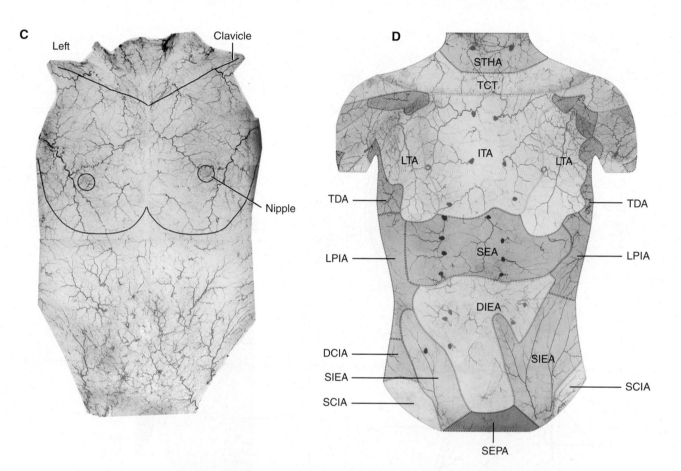

Fig. 21-3, cont'd **C,** Angiogram of the integument of the anterior trunk of a fresh human cadaver specimen injected with lead oxide and gelatin. Lead wires indicate important landmarks, including the clavicles, nipples, and inferior boundary of the pectoralis major muscle. Note the anastomoses between the superficial lateral thoracic artery and the large second internal thoracic artery perforators around the nipple. The abundance of significant (≥0.5 mm) musculocutaneous perforators in the abdominal region from the deep inferior epigastric artery are shown. Lateral to these perforators are the large, vertically oriented superficial inferior epigastric territories. **D,** Angiogram of the integument of the anterior torso of a fresh cadaver specimen injected with lead oxide and gelatin. (Cutaneous vascular territories are shown in different colors to facilitate identification. *DCIA,* Deep circumflex iliac artery; *DIEA,* deep inferior epigastric artery; *ITA,* internal thoracic [mammary] artery; *LCFA,* lateral circumflex femoral artery; *LPIA,* lateral branches of posterior intercostal arteries; *LTA,* lateral thoracic artery; *SCIA,* superficial circumflex iliac artery; *SEA,* superior epigastric artery; *SEPA,* superficial external pudendal artery; *SIEA,* superficial inferior epigastric artery; *STHA,* superior thyroid artery; *TAA,* thoracoacromial artery; *TCT,* thyrocervical trunk; *TDA,* thoracodorsal artery.)

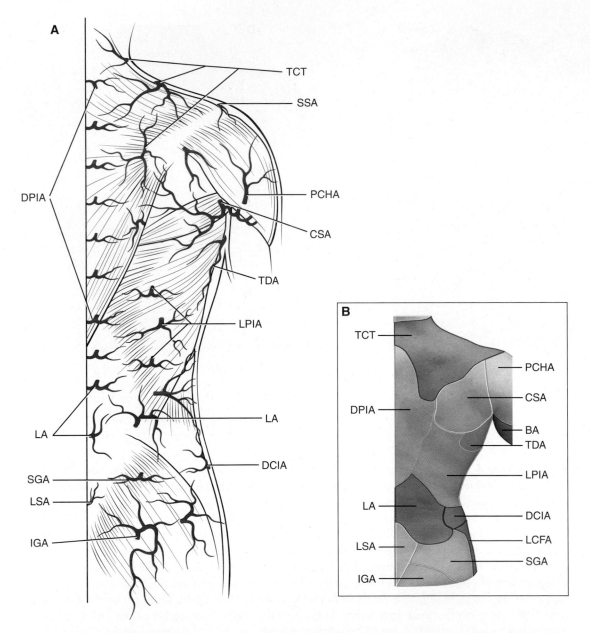

Fig. 21-4   A, Principal source vessels of the trunk and their relationship to muscles of the upper back, shoulder girdle, and lumbar regions. **B,** Vascular anatomy of the integument of the upper back and lumbar regions.

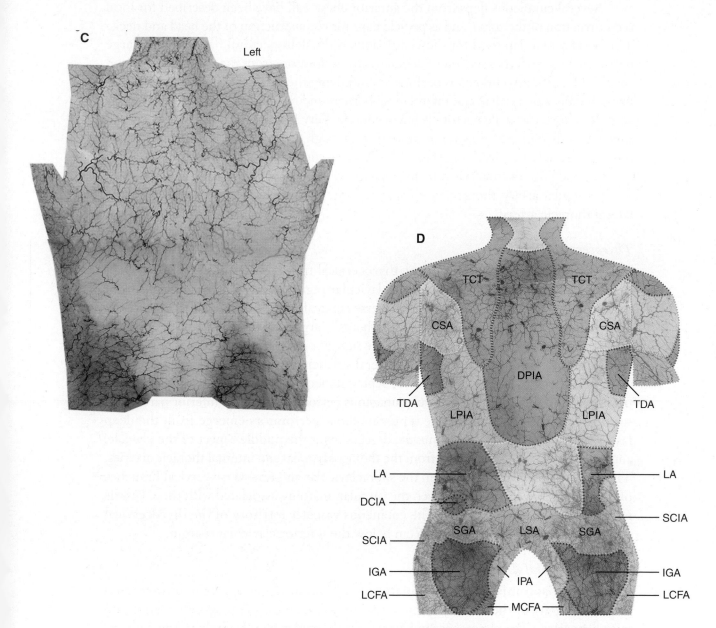

Fig. 21-4, cont'd   C, Angiogram of the integument of the posterior trunk of a fresh human cadaver injected with lead oxide and gelatin. **D,** Angiogram of the integument of the posterior torso of a fresh cadaver injected with lead oxide and gelatin. (Cutaneous vascular territories are shown in different colors to facilitate identification. *BA,* Brachial artery; *CSA,* circumflex scapular artery; *DCIA,* deep circumflex iliac artery; *DPIA,* dorsal branches of posterior intercostal arteries; *IGA,* inferior gluteal artery; *IPA,* internal pudendal artery; *LA,* lumbar arteries; *LCFA,* lateral circumflex femoral artery; *LPIA,* lateral branches of posterior intercostal arteries; *LSA,* lateral sacral arteries; *MCFA,* medial circumflex femoral artery; *PCHA,* posterior circumflex humeral artery; *SCIA,* superficial circumflex iliac artery; *SGA,* superior gluteal artery; *SSA,* suprascapular artery; *TCT,* thyrocervical trunk; *TDA,* thoracodorsal artery.)

Several cutaneous flaps from the anterior chest wall have been described for local reconstruction of the torso, and as pedicle flaps for reconstruction of the head and neck.[1] The best known flap used for these situations is the deltopectoral flap based on large peristernal internal thoracic musculocutaneous perforators from the second intercostal space.[2] The primary cutaneous perforators supplying the integument of the chest arise from the superior, medial, and inferolateral borders and radiate toward the nipple-areola complex above the large pectoralis major muscle. Very few musculocutaneous perforators with a diameter of 0.5 mm or more pass through the belly of the pectoralis major muscle to supply the overlying skin.[1] The primary cutaneous vascular territories of the chest include the thyrocervical trunk, transverse cervical artery, suprascapular artery, dorsal scapular artery, thoracoacromial artery, internal thoracic (mammary) artery, and lateral thoracic artery.

Thyrocervical Trunk

The variability of the anatomy of the thyrocervical trunk makes it difficult to classify the specific vascular supply of the supraclavicular region. The primary branches from the thyrocervical trunk include the transverse cervical artery, suprascapular artery, and dorsal scapular artery. In addition to supplying a large part of the integument of the neck, these rami supply a small region of the superior chest through cutaneous perforators from the thyrocervical trunk and several smaller supraclavicular branches. These arteries give rise to approximately three septocutaneous perforators from the posterior triangle of the neck, and one musculocutaneous perforator from the inferior part of the sternocleidomastoid muscle. The septocutaneous perforators emerge from the deep fascia anterior to the trapezius muscle, descend over the middle aspect of the clavicle, and anastomose with perforators from the thoracoacromial and internal thoracic arteries. These perforators often arise from the supraclavicular and transverse cervical branches of the thyrocervical trunk; however, the vascular anatomy associated with these vessels in this region is often variable. The cutaneous vascular territory of the thyrocervical trunk extends approximately 5 to 6 cm below the inferior clavicular margin.

Thoracoacromial Artery

The thoracoacromial artery originates most commonly as a single branch from the second part of the axillary artery and courses between the pectoralis major and minor muscles.[3] The thoracoacromial artery is the major blood supply to the pectoral muscles, and a secondary supply to the deltoid muscle (anterior head). The artery's trunk descends approximately 1 to 3 cm and gives rise to three primary branches: the pectoral (diameter = 1.7 ± 0.6 mm), clavicular (diameter = 1.1 ± 0.5 mm), and deltoid arteries (diameter = 1.8 ± 0.4 mm). The acromial artery may also be considered a primary branch; however, it commonly originates from the deltoid artery.[1]

Musculocutaneous perforators of the pectoral branch of the thoracoacromial axis are limited to small, inconsistent perforators in the inferolateral and intermediate zones of the pectoralis major muscle. Authors have described several arterial perforators from the pectoral branch of the thoracoacromial artery that wrap around the inferolateral border of the sternocostal head of the pectoralis major muscle to supply the integument[4,5]; however, this finding appears to be inconsistent.[1] Significant perforators (diameter ≥0.5 mm) are more frequently observed emerging from the clavicular and deltoid branches of the thoracoacromial artery. These perforator arteries may be suitable for perforator flap harvest.[1] The clavicular artery perforators appear from either the clavicular head of the pectoralis major muscle as a musculocutaneous perforator, or through the septum between the clavicular and sternocostal heads of the pectoralis major muscle. The average deep pedicle length of the clavicular artery perforators is approximately 6.0 ± 2.1 cm. The dominant perforator from the deltoid branch has an average deep pedicle length of 7.9 ± 2.0 cm and arises from the pectoralis major muscle fibers close to the deltopectoral groove. This branch supplies the integument over the deltoid muscle and is discussed in Chapter 15.

Internal Thoracic (Mammary) Artery

The internal thoracic (mammary) artery is the dominant supply to the integument of the anterior chest through large musculocutaneous perforators that arise from this vessel and its anterior intercostal branches. Of particular importance to the cutaneous supply of this region are the large second, third, and/or fourth (commonly second and fourth) intercostal musculocutaneous perforators. Along with the superficial thoracic artery (and smaller, variable perforators from the thoracoacromial artery), these large perforators contribute to the vascular supply of the breast and form a ring-shaped anastomosis around the nipple-areola complex (see Fig. 21-3, *C*).

In their course to the skin, perforators from the internal thoracic (mammary) artery penetrate the pectoralis major muscle at its fixed attachment to the costal cartilage and ribs and send off nutrient arterial branches to supply the medial aspect of this muscle. The internal thoracic (mammary) artery continues inferiorly to terminate as the superior epigastric and musculophrenic arteries that supply the skin of the superior abdomen.

In our anatomic study, the internal thoracic (mammary) artery gave an average of 5 ± 2 perforators of at least 0.5 mm in diameter that supplied an area of 183 ± 61 cm², or 8% of the integument of the trunk.[1] The average area supplied per perforator was 41 ± 16 cm².

The integument of the chest has traditionally been used for pedicle reconstruction of the head and neck with the deltopectoral flap. However, problems with distal flap necrosis and poor aesthetic results at the donor site have recently limited the use of this procedure. The vascular basis of the deltopectoral flap is the second intercostal perforator. This flap has recently been described as an island flap[6] and as a free flap.[7] Perforator flap dissection in this region involves tracing the vessels through the fibrous insertion of the pectoralis major muscle and through the intercostal space. The deep pedicle length of such a flap is hindered by the vessel's proximity to the ribs. The internal thoracic (mammary) artery is used routinely as a recipient vessel in autologous breast reconstruction with free perforator flaps.

Lateral Thoracic Artery

The lateral thoracic artery arises most commonly as an independent trunk from the third part of the axillary artery. Alternatively, this vessel may stem from the subscapular artery with the thoracodorsal trunk (see Fig. 21-3). The lateral thoracic artery sends large muscular branches to the pectoralis major and serratus anterior muscles, and terminates as a single, large, direct cutaneous branch to the skin overlying the anterior border of the axilla and anterolateral chest. This terminal branch, known as the *superficial thoracic* or *lateral mammary artery*, anastomoses medially with perforators from the internal thoracic artery and is the dominant supply to the lateral half of the breast. This direct cutaneous perforator may also arise as its own trunk from the axillary, subscapular, or thoracodorsal arteries.

The superficial thoracic branch of the lateral thoracic artery has been the basis of several free skin flap descriptions.[8] Despite having a large diameter and distribution in the skin, the proximity of this artery to the breast and the unfavorable nature of the axillary donor site may limit the territory's potential for large perforator flap harvest.

Abdomen

The superior, inferior, and superficial epigastric arteries, lateral intercostal perforators, and deep and superficial circumflex iliac arteries supply the abdominal region. This region has been the focus of numerous anatomic studies as a result of the extensive use of pedicle and free transverse rectus abdominis musculocutaneous (TRAM) flaps and deep inferior epigastric artery perforator (DIEAP) flaps.[9] Flaps from this region tend to have more subcutaneous fat associated with the skin paddle, particularly in obese patients. The vascular territories supplying the integument of the abdominal region include the superior epigastric artery (6%), deep inferior epigastric artery (6%), deep circumflex iliac artery (4%), superficial inferior epigastric artery (6%), superficial circumflex iliac artery (3%), external pudendal artery, and lateral branches of posterior intercostal arteries (19%).

Superior Epigastric Artery

The internal thoracic artery bifurcates at the sixth intercostal space into the musculophrenic artery and superior epigastric artery. The musculophrenic artery follows an oblique course along the inferior costal margin, behind the cartilage of the eighth, ninth, and tenth ribs, giving rise to the lowest anterior intercostal arteries and several small branches to the diaphragm and inferior pericardium. After passing the costal and xiphoid origins of the diaphragm, the superior epigastric artery continues inferiorly along the same line as the internal thoracic artery and may send a large superficial branch (diameter ≥1.0 mm) through the origin of the rectus abdominis muscle to supply the overlying skin. Manchot[10] originally described this branch as the superficial superior epigastric artery. The main trunk of the superior epigastric artery enters the rectus abdominis muscle on its deep surface, approximately 7 cm below the costal margin. The artery subdivides into several branches that arborize further to anastomose inferiorly with the deep inferior epigastric artery, and laterally with terminal branches of the posterior intercostal arteries.

An average of 5 ± 1 musculocutaneous perforators from the superior epigastric artery (diameter $= 0.6 \pm 0.2$ mm) supplied the integument of the superior abdominal region in our series.[1] These vessels often emerged in a zone immediately below the costal margin, up to the first tendinous intersection of the rectus abdominis muscle. Occasionally, these cutaneous perforators pierced the rectus sheath beside the lateral border of the muscle. Perforators from the superior epigastric artery anastomosed with perforators superiorly from the internal thoracic artery, laterally from posterior intercostal vessels, inferiorly from the deep inferior epigastric and superficial inferior epigastric arteries, and medially with the contralateral superior epigastric artery.

When present, the superficial superior epigastric branch of the superior epigastric artery has the potential to provide the vascular basis for a perforator flap donor site from the superior abdominal region. However, similar to the internal thoracic artery, the deep pedicle length is hindered by the proximity of the artery to the sternum and ribs.

Deep Inferior Epigastric Artery

The deep inferior epigastric artery arises deep to the inguinal ligament from the terminal portion of the external iliac artery, usually directly across from the origin of the deep circumflex iliac artery, and rarely as a common trunk with the obturator artery. The vessel ascends between the transversalis fascia and the peritoneum toward the umbilicus until it crosses the linea semilunaris, where it penetrates the rectus sheath and ascends along the posterior surface of the rectus abdominis muscle. The artery travels a variable distance on the deep surface (approximately 10 to 15 cm) before entering the muscle belly. Within the rectus abdominis muscle, the branching pattern of the deep inferior epigastric artery has been classified according to a number of common patterns.[11] Most commonly, the vessel divides into a medial branch that is directed toward the umbilicus, and a more prominent lateral ramus that ascends to the level of the superior tendinous intersection. Both medial and lateral rami have intermuscular anastomotic connections with the superior epigastric artery.

The deep inferior epigastric artery provides predominantly musculocutaneous perforators from the medial and lateral branches. However, the lateral branch also extends beyond the margin of the rectus abdominis muscle to supply the skin through the rectus sheath, anastomosing with the lowest posterior intercostal and subcostal arteries. In our dissection series,[1] there were 5 ± 2 (average) perforators arising from the deep inferior epigastric artery with an emerging diameter of 0.7 ± 0.2 mm. A combined area of 144 ± 55 cm^2 was supplied. The largest population of significant perforators originated from the lateral branch of the deep inferior epigastric artery. These perforators were clustered 4 cm lateral to the umbilicus.

Many studies have examined the suitability of the deep inferior epigastric artery donor site for perforator flap harvest.[9,12-14] Currently, this perforator flap is among the most commonly used, particularly for breast reconstruction.[15-17] The versatility of this large perforator flap has expanded its use for reconstruction of the head and neck,[18] upper extremity,[19] and lower extremity.[20]

Superficial Inferior Epigastric Artery

The superficial inferior epigastric artery is a direct cutaneous perforator artery from the anterior aspect of the common femoral artery. This vessel originates approximately 3 cm below the inguinal ligament as either an independent trunk or together with the superficial circumflex iliac artery.[21] This artery perforates the deep fascia of the femoral triangle almost immediately, and ascends in the subcutaneous tissue superficial to the linea semilunaris. The size of this vessel is often variable; however, it commonly ascends the anterolateral abdominal wall as a large direct cutaneous perforator (diameter ≥1.0 mm) and supplies a significant region of skin.[22]

When a dominant superficial inferior epigastric artery is present, it may reach an external diameter of 2 mm and course approximately 10 cm within the integument before arborizing into terminal medial and lateral branches.[22] These terminal branches anastomose with perforators from the deep epigastric artery and with lateral branches from the posterior intercostal arteries, respectively.

The superficial inferior epigastric artery was the vascular basis for the first reported free flap in the English-language literature.[23] The versatility of this flap has made it useful as a thin flap in hand reconstruction[24,25] and with procedures requiring various amounts of bulk, such as autologous breast reconstruction.[22,26,27]

Superficial Circumflex Iliac Artery

The superficial circumflex iliac artery branches off the lateral side of the common femoral artery (approximately 5 cm below the inguinal ligament) as its own trunk or as a common trunk with the superficial inferior epigastric artery. This vessel is a direct cutaneous artery that supplies a variable territory overlying the hip flexion crease. The artery has two main branches: a superficial branch that is primarily cutaneous and a deep branch that supplies the inguinal muscles, including the superior part of the sartorius muscle near its origin at the anterior superior iliac spine, before emerging as a cutaneous perforator. The territory of the superficial circumflex iliac artery spans the hip flexion crease below the inguinal ligament to the anterior superior iliac spine, where it contributes to a confluence of arterial anastomoses from the superficial inferior epigastric artery (medially), lateral rami of the posterior intercostals and deep circumflex iliac arteries (superiorly), and the ascending branch of the lateral circumflex femoral artery (inferiorly). In the absence of a large cutaneous contribution from the superficial circumflex iliac artery, the adjacent vascular territories supply this region. The primary direct cutaneous perforator of the artery has an emerging diameter of approximately 1.2 mm at the level of the deep fascia.

The groin flap, based on the direct cutaneous perforators from the superficial circumflex iliac artery, has been a workhorse in reconstructive surgery since its description in 1972.[24,28] This flap is a direct cutaneous perforator flap (similar to the neighboring superficial inferior epigastric artery perforator flap) with the advantage of easy dissection as a result of the superficial nature of the source artery. However, like the superficial inferior epigastric artery perforator flap, the superficial circumflex iliac artery perforator flap is subject to variability in the length and caliber of the artery, and has a relatively short, deep pedicle approximately 5 cm long. This short pedicle is usually associated with a small-caliber vessel that requires careful microsurgical technique.[29] The flap donor site provides excellent aesthetic results, scar concealment, and reduces functional loss associated with intramuscular dissection. The superficial circumflex iliac veins are large superficial vessels that can be incorporated into the flap to augment venous drainage and enhance flap survival.[29]

Deep Circumflex Iliac Artery

The deep circumflex iliac artery arises from the distal portion of the external iliac artery, adjacent to the deep inferior epigastric artery. The main trunk courses between the transversus abdominis and internal oblique muscles. Angiograms of the deep tissue show that the deep circumflex iliac artery trunk diverges into ascending and oblique branches at the level of the anterior superior iliac spine. The oblique branch is usually larger in diameter and sends nutrient arteries to the iliac crest and abdominal musculature, and anastomoses with the lumbar, iliolumbar, and posterior intercostal arteries. This branch gives off 2 ± 1 significant musculocutaneous perforators through the external oblique muscle near the midaxillary line. This vessel anastomoses with the iliac branch of the iliolumbar artery posteriorly. In our dissections,[1] we were unable to identify any significant cutaneous perforators from the iliolumbar artery, although smaller branches may terminate in the integument superior to the posterior iliac crest overlying the lumbar triangle. The main trunk of the deep circumflex iliac artery terminates in the deep tissue as a rich intramuscular anastomotic network of muscular branches with the ninth, tenth, and eleventh posterior intercostal and the subcostal arteries in the lateral abdominal wall.

Musculocutaneous perforators from the deep circumflex iliac artery have been used as the basis of an indirect musculocutaneous perforator flap.[30] The deep circumflex iliac artery has also provided numerous other surgical flaps in the region, including a musculocutaneous flap with the external oblique muscle,[31] an adiposal free flap,[32] and a composite osteocutaneous flap with part of the iliac crest for mandibulofacial reconstruction.[30,33]

External Pudendal Arteries

The external pudendal arteries arise as single direct cutaneous branches from the medial aspect of the common femoral artery. There are often numerous external pudendal branches, including superior, middle, and inferior rami that are arranged around the saphenous opening. These vessels supply the integument over the pubic bone and the anterosuperior external genitalia. In males, the distribution of these vessels includes the penis and anterior scrotum. In females, the external pudendal arteries supply the anterior labia majora, anastomosing with the internal pudendal arteries posteriorly. Occasionally these perforators form several true anastomotic vascular arches over the pubic symphysis and supply a midline territory extending up to two thirds of the distance to the umbilicus, anastomosing with the musculocutaneous perforators of the deep inferior epigastric artery superiorly.

Lateral Branches of Posterior Intercostal Arteries

The lateral branches of the posterior intercostal arteries supply musculocutaneous perforators to the lateral lumbar and abdominal regions from the eighth through eleventh arteries and subcostal segmental origins. The posterior intercostal arteries course between transversus abdominis and internal oblique muscles in the lateral trunk region. Musculocutaneous perforators emerge as anterior and posterior rami in one or two longitudinal rows parallel to the anterior border of the latissimus dorsi muscle. The largest of these perforators (diameter ≥1.0 mm) emerges in the chest area where the external oblique muscle meets the serratus anterior and latissimus dorsi muscles in the inferior lateral abdominal region (Fig. 21-5). There is a consistent anteroinferior orientation of the vascular territories of the musculocutaneous perforators from the intercostal arteries that corresponds with the orientation of the deep pedicle.

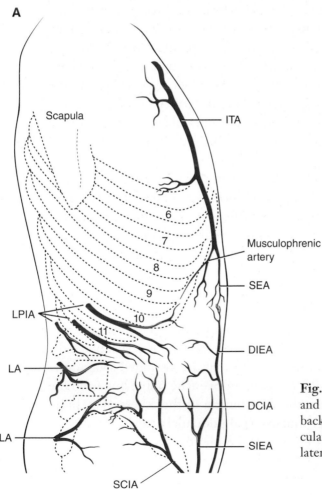

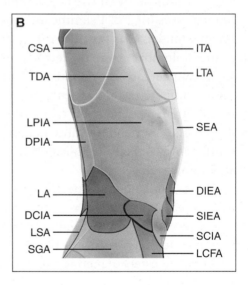

Fig. 21-5   A, Principal source vessels of the trunk and their relationship to the muscles of the upper back, shoulder girdle, and lumbar regions. **B,** Vascular anatomy of the integument of the axilla and lateral trunk regions.

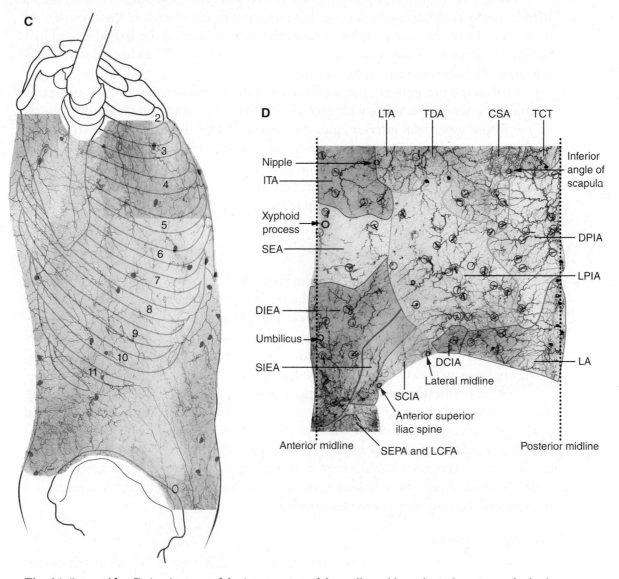

Fig. 21-5, cont'd C, Angiogram of the integument of the axilla and lateral trunk regions of a fresh human cadaver specimen injected with lead oxide and gelatin. The ribs are marked *(2 through 11)* and other major bony structures of the trunk are outlined. **D,** Angiogram of the integument of the torso of a fresh cadaver injected with lead oxide and gelatin. (Cutaneous vascular territories are shown in different colors to facilitate identification. *CSA,* Circumflex scapular artery; *DCIA,* deep circumflex iliac artery; *DIEA,* deep inferior epigastric artery; *DPIA,* dorsal branches of posterior intercostal arteries; *ILA,* iliolumbar artery; *ITA,* internal thoracic [mammary] artery; *LA,* lumbar arteries; *LCFA,* lateral circumflex femoral artery; *LPIA,* lateral branches of posterior intercostal arteries; *LSA,* Lateral sacral artery; *LTA,* lateral thoracic artery; *SCIA,* superficial circumflex iliac artery; *SEA,* superior epigastric artery; *SEPA,* superficial external pudendal artery; *SGA,* superior gluteal artery; *SIEA,* superficial inferior epigastric artery; *TCT,* thyrocervical trunk; *TDA,* thoracodorsal artery.)

The lateral branches of the posterior intercostal arteries supplied an average of 10 to 15 perforators (diameter = 0.7 ± 0.2 mm), and supplied most of the dorsolateral trunk. Approximately five perforators from this system reached the lateral abdominal region. Of particular importance is the subcostal branch, which has been described as the basis of a lateral lumbar perforator flap.[34]

Within the integument, the perforators of the lateral branches of the posterior intercostal artery anastomose with each other. These perforators anastomose anteriorly with the superficial inferior epigastric artery and deep inferior epigastric artery perforators, superiorly with the superficial epigastric artery, and inferiorly with the lumbar, deep, and superficial circumflex iliac arteries. This expansive network of cutaneous anastomoses, the reliability of the deep pedicle, and the abundance of tissue in this loose-skinned region of the abdomen give these vessels a great deal of potential, especially for large skin flap harvest.

Upper Back

The upper back region is supplied predominantly by musculocutaneous perforators of five major source vessels: superiorly by the transverse and deep cervical arteries of the thyrocervical trunk; laterally by branches of the subscapular axis; and medially by perforators of the posterior intercostal arteries. The surface area of this region constitutes approximately 32% of the trunk (12% of the body) and has an average of 24 perforators, each supplying an area of approximately 40 cm².

Several perforator flaps from the upper back region have been reported, including the thoracodorsal artery perforator flap, the septocutaneous circumflex scapular artery perforator flap, and the subcostal artery perforator flap. The vascular territories supplying the integument of the upper back region include the thyrocervical trunk, transverse cervical artery, suprascapular artery, dorsal scapular artery, circumflex scapular artery, thoracodorsal artery, dorsal branches of the posterior intercostal arteries, and lateral branches of the posterior intercostal arteries.

Thyrocervical Trunk

Details regarding the course and deep pedicle of the thyrocervical trunk are discussed in Chapter 10. After reaching the lateral border of the levator scapulae muscle, the transverse cervical artery divides into two muscular branches (superficial and deep) to supply the trapezius muscle. The deep branch, accompanied by its motor nerve, courses deep to the rhomboid muscles and supplies the lower third of the trapezius muscle. The deep branch is usually referred to as the dorsal scapular artery, particularly when it arises as an independent trunk from the axillary artery. This artery sends one or two small musculocutaneous perforators through the trapezius muscle to the dorsal back skin. These perforators anastomose laterally with the dorsal branches of the posterior intercostal arteries, and medially with the large circumflex scapular artery territory. The superolateral component of the vascular territory of the thyrocervical trunk is supplied by perforators from the suprascapular artery branch of the thyrocervical trunk.

The superficial branch of the transverse cervical artery enters the trapezius muscle on its deep surface and divides into ascending and descending rami. The ascending branch supplies the nuchal region. The descending branch, along with branches of the suprascapular branch of the thyrocervical trunk, supplies the lateral aspect of the trapezius muscle. Musculocutaneous perforators from these branches of the thyrocervical trunk emerge from this supraspinous part of the trapezius muscle.

Overall, the thyrocervical trunk sends three to four significant musculocutaneous perforators to nourish the integument of the upper back region. These perforators range from 0.5 to 1.0 mm in diameter. Perforator flaps from the thyrocervical trunk have yet to be described; however, the musculocutaneous perforators over the lateral trapezius muscle are the basis for the lateral trapezius musculocutaneous flap. Harvesting a perforator flap with a long vascular pedicle in this region may be problematic because of the variability of the vascular anatomy associated with the thyrocervical trunk and its branches. Results of several anatomic studies have proposed that the suprascapular flap, in particular, is not practical because of the highly unpredictable nature of the arteries in this region.[35]

Circumflex Scapular Artery

The circumflex scapular artery (diameter = 2.5 mm) originates from the subscapular artery along the lateral border of the scapula. This artery reliably gives a large cutaneous perforator to the skin through the triangular space (between the teres major and minor muscles and the lateral head of the triceps). This cutaneous perforator (diameter = 1.0 to 2.0 mm) divides into two distinctive rami at the level of the deep fascia, or immediately deep or superficial to the fascia. The vessels that result are the transverse (horizontal) branch or scapular cutaneous artery, and a descending (vertical) branch, the parascapular cutaneous artery. In our series,[1] both of these branches had an external diameter of approximately 0.9 ± 0.3 mm and supplied a large area of the upper lateral trunk near the axilla. The superficial pedicle length of the circumflex scapular artery perforators was approximately 53 ± 25 mm, which is significant because the deep pedicle to the subscapular artery is approximately the same length.[36]

Both the scapular flap[37,38] and parascapular flap[39] are based on the direct cutaneous branches of the circumflex scapular artery. This vascular axis is also the basis for the scapular osteocutaneous flap.[40] Traditionally, many of the descriptions of the parascapular and scapular flaps have included the deep fascial layer of connective tissue; however, the results of our anatomic series[1] suggest that the deep fascial plexus is not necessary for survival of the circumflex scapular artery perforator flap.

Thoracodorsal Artery

The thoracodorsal artery is a terminal branch of the subscapular artery. The primary trunk of the thoracodorsal artery enters the deep surface of the latissimus dorsi muscle at the neurovascular hilus, approximately 10 cm inferior to the axillary artery.[41] The artery supplies the superolateral half of the latissimus dorsi muscle to its insertion. Other branches from this artery include muscular branches to the serratus anterior and teres major muscles, and often a large direct cutaneous branch (diameter = 1.0 mm) that supplies the skin over the anterosuperior border of the muscle.

On entering the latissimus dorsi muscle, the thoracodorsal artery divides into a transverse and a descending branch. Normally, the musculocutaneous perforators from the artery originate from the descending branch, which follows the lateral border of the muscle inferiorly. The thoracodorsal artery perforator flap has gained popularity in recent years, particularly for procedures in which a long vascular pedicle, minimal donor site morbidity, and acceptable aesthetic results are needed.[42] This flap has been particularly useful for resurfacing large defects of the trunk and the extremities.[20]

Dorsal Branches of Posterior Intercostal Arteries

The dorsal branches of the posterior intercostal arteries reach the skin as medial and lateral musculocutaneous rami through the erector spinae muscles. The cutaneous territory supplied by these vessels includes an area roughly 5 to 15 cm in width that descends alongside the spinous processes of T3 to T12. In our anatomic series,[1] the average diameter and area supplied by the dorsal branches of these vessels were 0.6 ± 0.2 mm and 257 ± 90 cm², respectively. These perforators could supply flaps used for local reconstruction in the paraspinal region.

Lateral Branches of Posterior Intercostal Arteries

Nine pairs of posterior intercostal arteries arise from the posterolateral aspect of the thoracic aorta; the first and second spaces are supplied by the superior intercostal arteries. In the upper back region, the intercostal arteries travel within the costal groove between the internal intercostal muscles and the innermost layer, the costal pleura. Nutrient musculocutaneous branches from the seventh through eleventh intercostal and subcostal arteries emerge from the costal groove to supply the lower half of the latissimus dorsi muscle. Approximately 10 to 15 significant musculocutaneous perforators emerge from the latissimus dorsi muscle to feed the integument overlying the muscle. The average diameter and area supplied per perforator were 0.7 ± 0.2 mm and 40 ± 16 cm², respectively, in our dissection series.[1]

Cutaneous perforator flaps have been described for the posterior intercostal arteries. Badran et al[43] described the lateral intercostal neurovascular free flap that was called a *neurosensory free flap* at that time. This flap was based on the perforators from the intercostal vessels that have a close relationship with the lateral cutaneous nerves. A pedicle perforator flap has been described for the subcostal artery perforator that sends a musculocutaneous perforator to the skin through the posterior margin of external oblique muscle.[34] Other pedicle flaps, called *narrow pedicle intercostal cutaneous perforator flaps*, have been reported for small injuries of the hands and extremities.[44]

Lumbar Region

The lumbar region is a well-vascularized area that lies between the inferior margin of the ribs and the iliac crest. It is the smallest region in the trunk and makes up only 7% of the trunk surface area. The vascular supply to the integument of this region is primarily from musculocutaneous and septocutaneous perforators from the lumbar arteries. The subcostal and dorsal and lateral intercostal artery perforators may contribute to supply the superior and lateral aspects of the integument of the lumbar region. The vascular territory presented in this region is the lumbar arteries.

Lumbar Arteries

The four lumbar arteries originate from the descending abdominal aorta as paired segmental branches, opposite the bodies of the upper four lumbar vertebral bodies. These vessels send medial and lateral dorsal rami to the integument as septocutaneous perforators between the abdominal muscles and the erector spinae muscles. The lateral branches are large (diameter = 1.0 mm), and supply the integument lateral to the posterior midline. The main trunk of the lumbar arteries perforates the transversus abdominis muscle near the lateral border of the quadratus lumborum muscle. The trunk continues anteriorly and sends musculocutaneous perforators through the internal and external oblique muscles to supply the latissimus dorsi muscle and the integument overlying the thoracolumbar fascia. The lumbar arteries anastomose superiorly with the subcostal artery and posterior intercostal arteries, laterally with the deep circumflex iliac artery, and inferiorly with the iliolumbar, lateral sacral, and superior gluteal arteries.

In our series,[1] the average diameter and area supplied by perforators from the lumbar arteries were 0.7 ± 0.1 and 29 ± 15 cm², respectively. The fourth lumbar artery often gave rise to one or two large cutaneous branches that emerged through or in close proximity to the lumbar triangle and descended over the iliac crest to supply a segment of the superolateral gluteal region.

The lumbar branch of the iliolumbar artery supplies the muscles adjacent to the fifth lumbar vertebral body, because the fifth lumbar artery is usually very small or absent. The iliolumbar artery originates from the internal iliac artery and sends three major branches primarily to the muscles of the iliac fossa. The iliac branch supplies the iliacus muscle and runs parallel to the superior iliac crest, where it anastomoses with the deep circumflex iliac artery. Some authors have reported that this vessel sends perforators into the integument; however, we were unable to locate any significant cutaneous vessels from this source vessel. A pedicle perforator flap has been described based on the lumbar arteries.[45-47] In addition to pedicle flaps, free and sensate lumbar artery perforator flaps are being used for breast reconstruction with anastomosis of the fourth intercostal nerve.[48] Offman et al[49] have documented the vascular anatomy of the lateral flank area.

External Genitalia and Perineum

Surgical reconstruction of the male and female genitalia and perineum necessitates a detailed knowledge of local cutaneous vascular anatomy. This section illustrates the relevant vascular anatomy for both male and female sexes.

The principal vascular territories supplying the external genitalia and perineum are similar for both sexes. Two dominant source arteries and their terminal branches supply the integument of this region: the external pudendal artery with its superior and inferior terminal branches, and the internal pudendal artery with the posterior scrotal branch (male) or the posterior labial branch (female), the septal branch (male), and the dorsal penile artery (male).

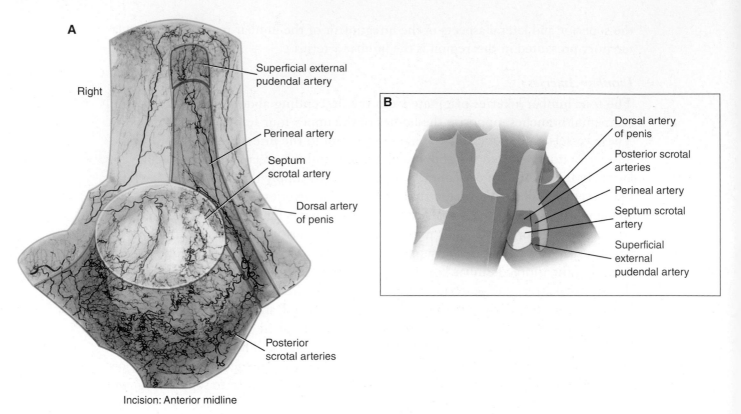

Fig. 21-6   A, Angiogram of the integument of the external genitalia (penis and scrotum) of a male specimen (dorsal midline incision of penis). Note the scrotal boundary and genitocrural fold. **B,** Vascular anatomy of the male external genitalia.

External Pudendal Arteries

Two external pudendal artery branches, the superior (superficial) and inferior (deep) rami, stem from the medial aspect of the common femoral artery, approximately 5 cm below the inguinal ligament. These branches may arise as independent trunks or together as a common trunk. Both vessels course medially and pierce the deep fascia near the saphenous opening where they supply the integument of the superomedial region of the femoral triangle. The superior branch of the external pudendal artery sends an ascending branch that anastomoses with the contralateral artery as a true anastomotic arch overlying the pubic symphysis, and as choke anastomoses with the inferior perforators of the deep inferior epigastric artery in the upper pubic and lower abdominal regions. The descending branch of the superior external pudendal artery supplies the integument of the external genitalia (dorsal shaft of the penis in the male, superior third of the labia majora in the female) along the midline. The inferior ramus supplies the dorsolateral region up to the genitocrural fold (including the anterior scrotal branches in the male and lateral labial branches in the female). Both superior and inferior external pudendal artery branches anastomose with each other, with their contralateral arteries, and with terminal branches of the internal pudendal artery (posterior scrotal or labial arteries) in a dense cutaneous vascular network (Fig. 21-6).

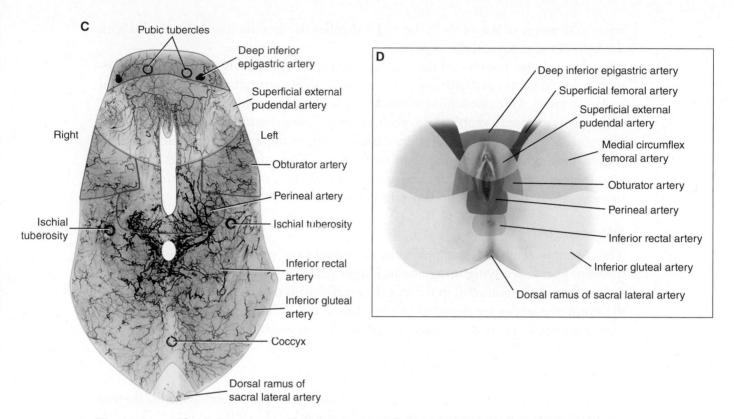

Fig. 21-6, cont'd   C, Angiogram of the integument of the external genitalia and perineum of a female specimen. **D,** Vascular anatomy of the female external genitalia and perineum. (Cutaneous vascular territories are shown in different colors to facilitate identification.)

Internal Pudendal Arteries

The terminal cutaneous branches of the internal pudendal artery supply the posterior aspect of the external male and female genitalia and the perineum. This artery arises as a branch from the internal iliac artery, courses through the greater sciatic foramen, and turns back into the lesser sciatic foramen where it enters the perineal region through the pudendal canal. The inferior rectal branches of the internal pudendal artery supply the anal sphincter and skin surrounding the anus. Several branches of the inferior rectal branches nourish a small medial segment of the integument overlying the gluteus maximus muscle (inferior to the lateral sacral arteries). These branches are extremely difficult to identify in the dense ischiorectal fat and have little clinical relevance for perforator flap harvest.

Further along its course, the internal pudendal artery divides into a superficial and deep branch. The superficial branch (the perineal artery) pierces the urogenital diaphragm near the anterior aspect of the pudendal canal. This artery supplies the urogenital region and the integument of the posterior genitalia through the transverse perineal arteries and posterior scrotal arteries (male) or posterior labial arteries (female). A small segment alongside the scrotal raphe is supplied by perforators of the nutrient vessels to the scrotal septum. The deeper terminal branch of the internal pudendal artery (the artery of the penis in the male) supplies the erectile tissues associated with the bulb of the penis and the vagina.

The vascular anatomy of the integument overlying the shaft of the penis is commonly described as originating from the dorsal penile artery branch of the internal pudendal artery. Our assessment of this anatomy clearly revealed that the dorsal artery of the penis primarily supplied the glans penis and gave rise to few cutaneous vessels.[1] The superior (superficial) and inferior (deep) rami of the external pudendal arteries supplied the skin overlying the shaft of the penis. The exceptions to this pattern of blood supply were the frenulum and prepuce, which were supplied by minute nutrient branches from the deeper dorsal penile vessels (see Fig. 21-6, *A*).

Obturator Artery

The obturator artery rarely supplies any significant cutaneous perforators (diameter = 0.5 mm) to the overlying integument. Larger perforators from the obturator artery appear to be more common in females than males. Insignificant branches arising from the obturator artery are depicted in Fig. 21-6, *C* and *D*. These vessels supply a small area in the upper groin or perineal region of a female cadaver.

References

1. Geddes CR, Tang M, Yang D, Morris SF. An assessment of the anatomical basis of the thoracoacromial artery perforator flap. Can J Plast Surg 11:23-27, 2003.
   The authors reviewed the vascular architecture of the perforators of the thoracoacromial artery through pectoralis major muscle to determine suitability for pedicle or microvascular reconstruction of the head and neck.
2. Bakamjian VY. Total reconstruction of pharynx with medially based deltopectoral skin flap. N Y State J Med 68:2771-2778, 1968.
3. Yang D, Marshall G, Morris SF. Variability in the vascularity of the pectoralis major muscle. J Otolaryngol 32:12-15, 2003.
4. Reid CD, Taylor GI. The vascular territory of the acromiothoracic axis. Br J Plast Surg 37:194-212, 1984.
5. Cormack GC, Lamberty BGH. The Arterial Anatomy of Skin Flaps. London: Churchill Livingstone, 1986.
6. Portnoy WM, Arena S. Deltopectoral island flap. Otolaryngol Head Neck Surg 111:63-69, 1994.
7. Sasaki K, Nozaki M, Honda T, et al. Deltopectoral skin flap as a free skin flap revisited: further refinement in flap design, fabrication, and clinical usage. Plast Reconstr Surg 107:1134-1141, 2001.
8. Agarwal R, Agarwal S, Chandra R. The lateral pectoral flap. J Hand Surg Br 24:542-546, 1999.
9. Koshima I, Soeda S. Inferior epigastric artery skin flaps without rectus abdominis muscle. Br J Plast Surg 42:645-648, 1989.
   An inferior epigastric artery skin flap without rectus abdominis muscle, pedicled on the muscle perforators and the proximal inferior deep epigastric artery, was used in two patients. A large flap without muscle survived on a single muscle perforator.
10. Manchot K. Die Hautarterien des Meslichen Korpers. Leipzig: FCW Vogel, 1889.

11. Boyd JB, Taylor GI, Corlett R. The vascular territories of the superior epigastric and the deep inferior epigastric systems. Plast Reconstr Surg 73:1-16, 1984.

This was a classic study of the vascular anatomy of the anterior abdominal wall. The vascular territories of the superior and deep inferior epigastric arteries were evaluated using dye injection, dissection, and barium radiographic techniques. The dominance of the inferior epigastric artery in supplying the lower abdominal skin and the options for free tissue transfer were comprehensively discussed.

12. Itoh Y, Arai K. The deep inferior epigastric artery free skin flap: anatomic study and clinical application. Plast Reconstr Surg 91:853-863; discussion 864, 1993.

13. Heitmann C, Felmerer G, Durmus C, et al. Anatomical features of perforator blood vessels in the deep inferior epigastric perforator flap. Br J Plast Surg 53:205-208, 2000.

14. Kikuchi N, Murakami G, Kashiwa H, et al. Morphometrical study of the arterial perforators of the deep inferior epigastric perforator flap. Surg Radiol Anat 23:375-381, 2001.

15. Allen RJ, Treece P. Deep inferior epigastric perforator flap for breast reconstruction. Ann Plast Surg 32:32-38, 1994.

16. Blondeel PN, Boeckx WD. Refinements in free flap breast reconstruction: the free bilateral deep inferior epigastric perforator flap anastomosed to the internal mammary artery. Br J Plast Surg 47:495-501, 1994.

17. Blondeel PN. One hundred free DIEP flap breast reconstructions: a personal experience. Br J Plast Surg 52:104-111, 1999.

18. Koshima I, Nanba Y, Tsutsui T, et al. Free perforator flap for the treatment of defects after resection of huge arteriovenous malformations in the head and neck regions. Ann Plast Surg 51:194-199, 2003.

19. Li XJ, Tong J, Wang Y. Combined free toe and free deep inferior epigastric perforator flap for reconstruction of the thumb and thumb web space. J Reconstr Microsurg 16:427-436, 2000.

20. Koshima I, Nanba Y, Tsutsui T, et al. Perforator flaps in lower extremity reconstruction. Handchir Mikrochir Plast Chir 34:251-256, 2002.

21. Taylor GI, Daniel RK. The anatomy of several free flap donor sites. Plast Reconstr Surg 56:243-253, 1975.

22. Williams J, Geddes C, Tang M, et al. Anatomical territory of the superficial inferior epigastric artery. Can J Plast Surg 11:119, 2003.

The variability of the superficial inferior epigastric vessels was described based on anatomic studies using the lead oxide and gelatin injection technique.

23. Daniel RK, Taylor GI. Distant transfer of an island flap by microvascular anastomoses. A clinical technique. Plast Reconstr Surg 52:111-117, 1973.

This classic paper described one of the first free tissue transfers.

24. McGregor IA, Jackson IT. The groin flap. Br J Plast Surg 25:3-16, 1972.

25. Schlenker JD, Atasoy E, Lyon JW. The abdominohypogastric flap: an axial pattern flap for forearm coverage. Hand 12:248-252, 1980.

26. Holmström H. The free abdominoplasty flap and its use in breast reconstruction. An experimental study and clinical case report. Scand J Plast Reconstr Surg 13:423-427, 1979.

27. Hester TR Jr, Nahai F, Beegle PE, et al. Blood supply of the abdomen revisited, with emphasis on the superficial inferior epigastric artery. Plast Reconstr Surg 74:657-670, 1984.

28. O'Brien BM, MacLeod AM, Hayhurst JW, et al. Successful transfer of a large island flap from the groin to the foot by microvascular anastomoses. Plast Reconstr Surg 52:271-278, 1973.

29. Koshima I, Nanba Y, Tsutsui T, et al. Superficial circumflex iliac artery perforator flap for reconstruction of limb defects. Plast Reconstr Surg 113:233-240, 2004.

30. Kimata Y. Deep circumflex iliac perforator flap. Clin Plast Surg 30:433-438, 2003.

31. Taylor GI, Townsend P, Corlett R. Superiority of the deep circumflex iliac vessels as the supply for free groin flaps. Plast Reconstr Surg 64:595-604, 1979.

    The authors presented 16 cases of free transfer of compound flaps from the groin: 11 based on the deep circumflex iliac vessels and 5 based on the superficial circumflex iliac vessels. The vascular basis of free tissue transfers in this region was discussed.

32. Hartrampf CR Jr, Noel RT, Drazan L, et al. Ruben's fat pad for breast reconstruction: a peri-iliac soft-tissue free flap. Plast Reconstr Surg 93:402-407, 1994.

33. Bitter K. Bone transplants from the iliac crest to the maxillo-facial region by the microsurgical technique. J Maxillofac Surg 8:210-216, 1980.

34. Feinendegen DL, Klos D. A subcostal artery perforator flap for a lumbar defect. Plast Reconstr Surg 109:2446-2449, 2002.

35. Kitazawa T, Matsuo K, Moriizumi T, et al. An anatomic examination of the suprascapular flap. Ann Plast Surg 45:405-407, 2000.

36. Shimizu T, Ohno K, Michi K, et al. Morphometric examination of the free scapular flap. Plast Reconstr Surg 99:1947-1953, 1997.

37. Hamilton SG, Morrison WA. The scapular free flap. Br J Plast Surg 35:2-7, 1982.

38. Gilbert A, Teot L. The free scapular flap. Plast Reconstr Surg 69:601-604, 1982.

39. Nassif TM, Vidal L, Bovet JL, et al. The parascapular flap: a new cutaneous microsurgical free flap. Plast Reconstr Surg 69:591-600, 1982.

40. Swartz WM, Banis JC, Newton ED, et al. The osteocutaneous scapular flap for mandibular and maxillary reconstruction. Plast Reconstr Surg 77:530-545, 1986.

41. Angrigiani C, Grilli D, Siebert J. Latissimus dorsi musculocutaneous flap without muscle. Plast Reconstr Surg 96:1608-1614, 1995.

42. Schwabegger AH, Bodner G, Ninkovic M, et al. Thoracodorsal artery perforator (tap) flap: report of our experience and review of the literature. Br J Plast Surg 55:390-395, 2002.

    The thoracodorsal artery perforator (TDAP) flap is indicated in cases where a long vascular pedicle for an appropriate free tissue transfer is necessary, and where aesthetic appearance and minimizing donor site morbidity are important.

43. Badran HA, El-Helaly MS, Safe I. The lateral intercostal neurovascular free flap. Plast Reconstr Surg 73:17-26, 1984.

44. Gao JH, Hyakusoku H, Inoue S, et al. Usefulness of narrow pedicled intercostal cutaneous perforator flap for coverage of the burned hand. Burns 20:65-70, 1994.

45. Ao M, Mae O, Namba Y, et al. Perforator-based flap for coverage of lumbosacral defects. Plast Reconstr Surg 101:987-991, 1998.

46. Roche NA, Van Landuyt K, Blondeel PN, et al. The use of pedicled perforator flaps for reconstruction of lumbosacral defects. Ann Plast Surg 45:7-14, 2000.

47. de Weerd L, Weum S. The butterfly design: coverage of a large sacral defect with two pedicled lumbar artery perforator flaps. Br J Plast Surg 55:251-253, 2002.

48. de Weerd L, Elvenes OP, Strandenes E, et al. Autologous breast reconstruction with a free lumbar artery perforator flap. Br J Plast Surg 56:180-183, 2003.

49. Offman SL, Geddes CR, Tang M, Morris SF. The vascular basis of perforator flaps based on source arteries of the lateral lumbar region. Plast Reconstr Surg 115:1651-1659, 2005.

22

Thoracoacromial Artery Perforator Flap

Geoffrey G. Hallock
Steven F. Morris

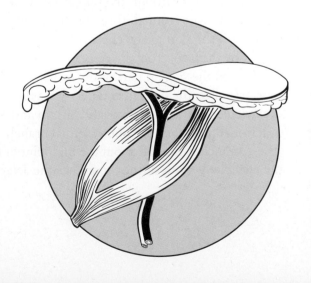

The pectoralis major composite musculocutaneous flap has long been a proven workhorse flap, especially for head and neck reconstruction when based on its dominant pedicle, the thoracoacromial vessels.[1] Its major asset there is avoidance of microsurgery, which is of paramount importance if recipient vessels are nonexistent or unreachable, or if comorbidities preclude such a consideration.[2] Other assets such as capturing the corresponding chest skin territory and attributes as a muscle perforator flap have been relatively neglected, perhaps because of the highly variable and diminutive perforators emanating from the thoracoacromial source vessel, as shown in prior anatomic studies.[3,4] Previous clinical reports have been limited to the inclusion of thoracoacromial perforators with only a minimal intramuscular dissection to form propeller flaps from the chest that are suitable for soft tissue restoration after release of adjacent axillary scar contractures.[5,6] Using the thoracoacromial source vessel itself to provide a longer leash for a pedicle or free thoracoacromial artery perforator (TAAP) flap may make this a more versatile option in certain circumstances.[7]

SURGICAL ANATOMY

The cutaneous vascular supply to the anterior chest region originates primarily from the anterior intercostal or internal mammary vessels medially and from the lateral thoracic artery laterally.[2-4,8] However, there are distinct perforators from the thoracoacromial axis, particularly through the upper portion of the pectoralis major muscle (Fig. 22-1).[3] The perforators from all three of these sources interconnect in an interlacing pattern to nourish the skin of the chest region.

The thoracoacromial artery (source vessel for the TAAP flap) originates as a large trunk from the second part of the axillary artery.[9] Although traditionally stated to have four branches, the deltoid and pectoral branches are the most consistent and largest.[4,9] A clavicular branch has a variable origin and sometimes may not arise from the thoracoacromial trunk itself.[4] The acromial branch almost always is a branch of the deltoid.[4] These branches enter at about the midpoint of the muscle on its undersurface just below the clavicle. Venous outflow parallels the arterial branches.

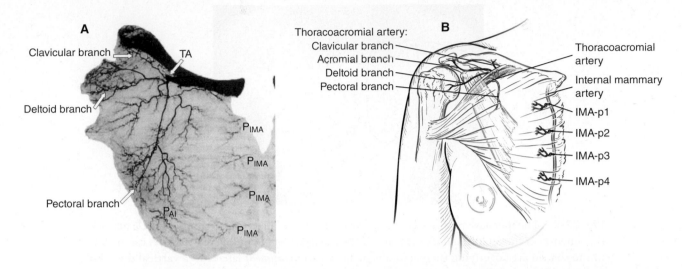

Fig. 22-1 A, A cadaver injection study of the right thoracoacromial axis *(TA)* indicates its major branches. Note filling by capture of adjacent perforators *(P)* of the anterior intercostal *(AI)* and internal mammary arteries *(IMA)*. **B,** The illustration differs in that the acromial branch is a distinct entity arising from the thoracoacromial axis.

The larger deltoid branch supplies the clavicular head of the pectoralis major muscle.[4] The acromial artery is a major branch from which a large direct or musculocutaneous perforator may arise that serves a skin territory overlying the lateral clavicle and deltoid muscle.[3,4] This is a reasonably consistent perforator on which to base a free TAAP flap, although the pedicle will be short and thereby limit reach as a local flap.

The pectoral branch supplies the sternocostal portion of the pectoralis major muscle.[3,4] It quickly divides into three branches (see Fig. 22-1): a lateral branch diverges to join the lateral thoracic artery, and medial and inferior branches at about the fourth intercostal space interconnect with anterior intercostal branches or perforators of the internal mammary artery.[2,3,10] This pattern can be quite variable, but the pectoral branch roughly follows a line drawn from the acromion to the xiphoid process.[9] Numerous small musculocutaneous perforators arise from the pectoral branch proper along this course, but may be inconsistent and unreliable to sustain a muscle perforator flap.[3] The corresponding skin territory of the pectoral branch, as found in selective injection studies, extends lateral to the nipple to beyond the lateral border of the pectoralis major muscle and into the axilla.[4]

SURGICAL TECHNIQUE
Surface Landmarks

Unless CT angiography is available for locating a suitable perforator, handheld audible Doppler ultrasonography may be the best means to identify a perforator from the thoracoacromial axis.[11] The latter's origin is usually just medial to the pectoralis

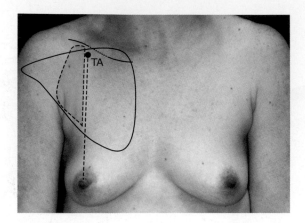

Fig. 22-2   The thoracoacromial axis *(TA)* is located medial to the pectoralis minor muscle just below the junction of the middle and lateral third of the clavicle. Corresponding perforators can be found in the shaded area overlying the pectoralis major muscle *(outlined)* lateral to a vertical line drawn from the TA to the nipple.

minor muscle and below the junction of the middle and lateral thirds of the clavicle (Fig. 22-2).[9,12] The perforator arising from the acromial branch may be found near this point. A free flap may be designed about it using the free-style free flap concept of Wei and Mardini.[13] The pedicle will be short but caliber relatively large, because dissection can include the thoracoacromial trunk itself.

If a local flap with more extensive reach is desirable, capture of a musculocutaneous perforator from the pectoral branch is preferable. A vertical line dropped from the point of origin of the thoracoacromial axis typically intersects the nipple-areola complex (see Fig. 22-1). Audible Doppler is used, searching lateral to this line and above the fourth intercostal space, while proceeding up to the lateral border of the pectoralis major muscle.

Flap Design and Dissection

Once a reasonable perforator is encountered, the potential pedicle length will be the distance from that point to the thoracoacromial axis, the latter serving as the point of local flap rotation. If pedicle length is sufficient to reach to the defect, an appropriately sized flap can be designed (Fig. 22-3). An eccentric design, marked caudally in relation to the perforator, essentially increases the reach of the flap. First, an incision along the lateral border of the flap down to the pectoralis major muscle will allow subfascial dissection below the flap in a medial direction toward the sternum. This must be carefully done with constant vigilance to substantiate the existence of an adequate perforator. If present, the remaining boundaries of the flap are incised; if not, this option must be aborted.

Once deemed suitable, the entire periphery of the flap can be raised to form an island flap based on the chosen perforator. This is followed by tedious intramuscular dissection, with division of muscular side branches as necessary to lengthen the vascular pedicle. Once the undersurface of the muscle is reached, further lengthening along the pectoral branch may require division of pectoralis major muscle fibers if retraction alone does not allow adequate exposure. Cephalad dissection stops once the vascular

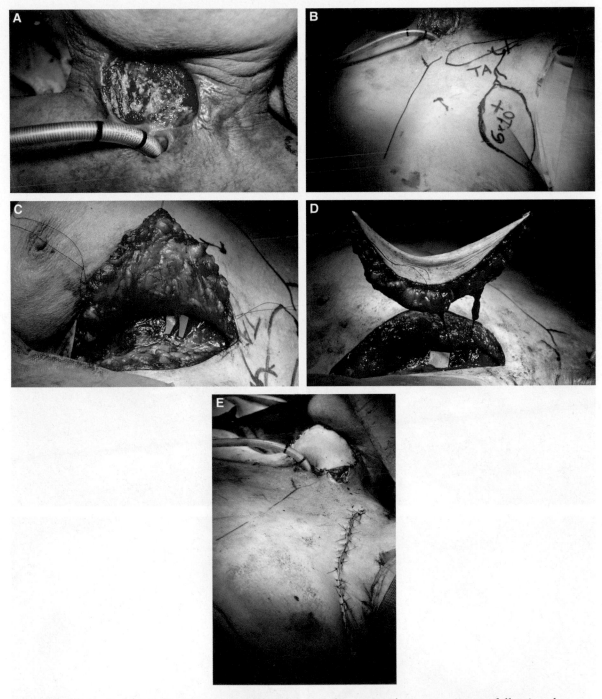

Fig. 22-3   A, An irradiated neck wound with impending carotid exposure is seen following debridement. **B,** The thoracoacromial axis *(TA)* and pectoral branch are marked on the left chest. The perforator *(X)* was detected with an audible Doppler probe. The proposed TAAP flap is designed eccentrically and inferior to this site to increase reach. **C,** Elevation of the lateral border of the flap exposes the perforator coming through the microgrid on the pectoralis major muscle. **D,** An island TAAP flap is also based on the second perforator encountered in line during dissection toward the thoracoacromial axis. **E,** The flap is inset into the neck and the donor site closed directly.

leash is long enough to allow reach to the defect. Bringing the flap under the muscle up to the lower border of the clavicle or through the fenestration that is often present between the clavicular and sternocostal heads gains additional length. This is especially important if the flap is to be transposed to the head and neck. The flap is then inset. Even with wide flaps, direct donor site closure is possible because of chest skin redundancy.

MODIFICATIONS
Chimeric Pectoralis Major Muscle and Thoracoacromial Artery Perforator Flap

A portion of the underlying pectoralis major muscle can be combined when indicated with a TAAP flap to form a chimeric flap (Fig. 22-4).[14] The muscle portion must be circumscribed and based on a separate branch of the chosen thoracoacromial vessel. This branch must be long enough to also allow reach to the defect. Usually, the muscle's malleability facilitates fill; the TAAP flap is inset independently to provide coverage.

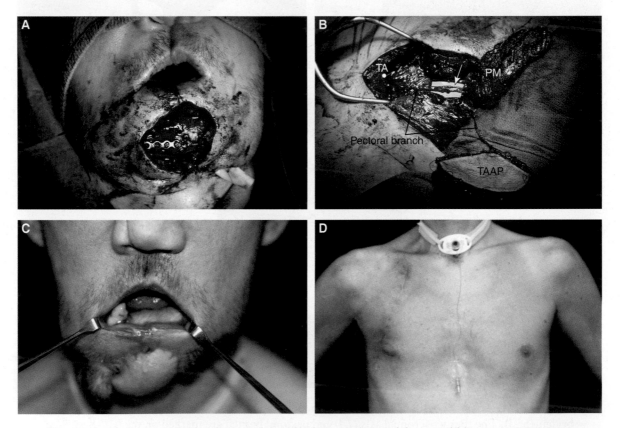

Fig. 22-4 A, Exposed microplates and free fibular transfer used for mandible reconstruction are seen following debridement of a late chin wound breakdown. **B,** A chimeric thoracoacromial artery perforator *(TAAP)* flap and pectoralis major *(PM)* muscle flap from the right chest are harvested, both based on the pectoral branch of the thoracoacromial axis *(TA)*. The independent branch to the PM muscle is indicated by the *white arrow*. The TA *(white dot)* is the point of rotation of this combined flap. **C,** The TAAP flap has restored missing chin skin. The floor of the mouth is composed of calf skin that was transferred with the original free fibular osteoseptocutaneous flap. **D,** On contraction of both pectoralis major muscles, the right anterior axillary fold is diminished because of partial denervation and resection of the pectoralis major muscle.

ADVANTAGES

Position   The patient can be in the supine position for flap harvesting.

Thickness   Because muscle is not included, the perforator flap is much thinner and less bulky than a pectoralis major musculocutaneous flap.

Pedicle Length   As with any muscle perforator flap, the vascular pedicle is longer than the corresponding musculocutaneous flap, because in addition to the length of the included source vessel, the pedicle is extended by the intramuscular distance and extrafascial length traversed by the chosen flap perforator.

Local Flap—Propeller   Intramuscular perforator dissection is minimized to allow rotation of chest skin about that perforator. This advantage has proved valuable for reaching the axilla.[5,6]

Local Flap—Pedicle   Lengthening the vascular pedicle by including the pectoral branch of the thoracoacromial artery facilitates reach to the head and neck in lieu of a free flap. This is especially valuable if neck recipient site vessels have been depleted or are unreachable (see Fig. 22-3).[7]

Donor Site   Thoracic skin redundancy is usually sufficient for direct closure regardless of flap width.

PITFALLS

Anatomic Variation   Although a perforator arising from the acromial branch is relatively consistent and of reasonable caliber, other perforators, especially from the pectoral branch, are usually too diminutive to be reliable.[6]

Pedicled Flap   Use as a local flap where transposition requires a longer vascular leash and usually requires that the pectoral branch be included. Depending on the location of the corresponding musculocutaneous perforator, this may be insufficient to allow reach, especially to head and neck defects. An internal mammary artery perforator flap should then be considered, because it often may be more reliable for transferring the same chest skin territory[8,15] (see Chapter 23).

Free Flap   A small flap based on a perforator of the acromial branch would be the most consistently available option. However, the pedicle will be extremely short.

Breast Disfigurement   Unless the breast is ptotic, reducing breast size or correcting nipple displacement during donor site closure is possible.

Function Preservation   Significant muscle fiber division for pedicle lengthening, or direct injury to either the medial or lateral pectoral motor nerves to the pectoralis major muscle, could result in partial or total denervation[9] (see Fig. 22-4).

References

1. Wei WI, Chan YW. Pectoralis major flap. In Wei FC, Mardini S, eds. Flaps and Reconstructive Surgery. Philadelphia: Saunders Elsevier, 2009.

2. Rikimaru H, Kiyokawa K, Inoue Y, et al. Three-dimensional anatomical vascular distribution in the pectoralis major myocutaneous flap. Plast Reconstr Surg 115:1342-1352, 2005.

3. Geddes CR, Tang M, Yang D, Morris SF. An assessment of the anatomical basis of the thoracoacromial artery perforator flap. Can J Plast Surg 11:23-27, 2003.

   Cadaver injection studies of the thoracoacromial axis demonstrated all musculocutaneous perforators that traverse the pectoralis major muscle. Although some perforators specifically from the thoracoacromial axis were present, these were so-called spent, small vessels with an inconsistent presence. The reliability of a proposed thoracoacromial perforator flap is therefore questioned.

4. Reid CD, Taylor GI. The vascular territory of the acromiothoracic axis. Br J Plast Surg 37:194-212, 1984.

   Excellent ex vivo anatomic injection studies delineated the course of branches of the thoracoacromial axis and corresponding captured skin territories. The deltoid and pectoral branches were the most consistent, with many variations from the classical anatomic descriptions routinely observed.

5. Kosutic D, Krajnc I, Pejkovic B, et al. Thoracoacromial artery perforator 'propeller' flap. J Plast Reconstr Aesthet Surg 63:e491-e493, 2010.

6. Kosutic D. Use of pectoralis major perforators for local "free-style" perforator flap in axillary reconstruction: a case report. Microsurgery 30:159-162, 2010.

   Use of thoracoacromial musculocutaneous perforators with minimal, if any, intramuscular dissection, allowed reliable use of the chest skin overlying the pectoralis major muscle to reach the axilla, if rotated about that perforator as the hub for a propeller flap. Release and coverage of axillary contractures was possible when other skin flap options were unavailable.

7. Hallock GG. The island thoracoacromial artery muscle perforator flap. Ann Plast Surg 66:168-171, 2011.

   Local chest skin flaps based on pectoralis major musculocutaneous perforators and a vascular leash pedicled on the pectoral branch of the thoracoacromial axis can reach head and neck defects. This provides an alternative in lieu of microsurgical tissue transfers, or if the internal mammary artery is deficient or unobtainable.

8. Wong C, Saint-Cyr M, Rasko Y, et al. Three- and four-dimensional arterial and venous perforasomes of the internal mammary artery perforator flap. Plast Reconstr Surg 124:1759-1769, 2009.

9. Serafin D. The pectoralis major muscle flap. In Serafin D, ed. Atlas of Microsurgical Composite Tissue Transplantation. Philadelphia: WB Saunders, 1996.

10. Kiyokawa K, Tai Y, Tanabe HY, et al. A method that preserves circulation during preparation of the pectoralis major myocutaneous flap in head and neck reconstruction. Plast Reconstr Surg 102:2336-2345, 1998.

11. Hallock GG. Attributes and shortcomings of acoustic Doppler sonography in identifying perforators for flaps from the lower extremity. J Reconstr Microsurg 25:377-381, 2009.

12. Hallock GG. The pectoralis major muscle extended island flap for complete obliteration of the median sternotomy wound. Ann Plast Surg 59:655-658, 2007.

13. Wei FC, Mardini S. Free-style free flaps. Plast Reconstr Surg 114:910-916, 2004.

14. Hallock GG. Further clarification of the nomenclature for compound flaps. Plast Reconstr Surg 117:151e-160e, 2006.

15. Neligan PC, Gullane PJ, Vesely M, et al. The internal mammary artery perforator flap: new variation on an old theme. Plast Reconstr Surg 119:891-893, 2007.

23

Internal Mammary Artery Perforator Flap

Peter C. Neligan

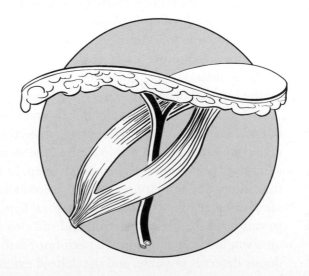

The deltopectoral flap, often referred to by its eponym, the *Bakamjian flap*, was perhaps the first large perforator-based cutaneous flap to come into widespread use. In 1965, Bakamjian[1] described the deltopectoral flap for reconstruction of pharyngoesophageal defects in a two-stage procedure. He described the origin of his flap as follows: "I let the resident take out the tumor, and when I came back in the room, the whole larynx, pharynx, and cervical esophagus were all gone. We used to base this flap out on the shoulder, but it wouldn't have been big enough. Then I remembered those big arteries off the internal mammaries. So I based it medially, and just took the amount of skin I needed. It worked, so we decided to keep on using it." The deltopectoral flap was one of the most commonly used flaps in head and neck reconstruction for many years. Almost 200 articles have been published on this flap from the time of its first description to the present. Before the mid-1970s revolution that shifted toward the use of musculocutaneous and free flaps, the deltopectoral flap had become the principal workhorse for head and neck reconstruction for very good reasons. It can reach superiorly to the level of the zygomatic arch and has sufficient dimensions for virtually any defect of skin and/or mucous membrane throughout the upper aerodigestive tract. The advantages of the flap are its thin, pliable skin with an excellent color match for reconstructing head and neck defects. Furthermore, flap harvest is straightforward. It is used infrequently today in this form because it customarily requires a two-stage procedure: the first is a delaying procedure to capture the territory over the deltoid, and the second is flap elevation and insetting. However, it is still a reliable auxiliary tool in difficult circumstances. The other major disadvantage of the classic Bakamjian flap is the need to use a skin graft on the donor site. This is unsightly, and these days, probably unacceptable; therefore, for practical purposes, this flap has been supplanted by the internal mammary artery perforator (IMAP) flap.

The IMAP flap is based medially and is supplied by perforating branches from the internal mammary artery.[2] The classic dissection of the deltopectoral flap was a subfascial dissection extending to within 2 cm of the sternal border. This incorporates the internal mammary perforators that supply the flap. In Bakamjian's original description, the first four internal mammary perforators were included in the flap. The IMAP flap uses the same vascular supply as the deltopectoral flap; however, the skin paddle can be situated to suit both the reconstruction and the closure. Furthermore, the flap can be raised on a single internal mammary perforator rather than on all four. Direct closure of the donor defect is possible, and the deltoid extension of the classic flap is not required.

ANATOMY OF THE INTERNAL MAMMARY ARTERY

The internal mammary (or thoracic) artery arises from the first part of the subclavian artery. It runs 1 to 2 cm lateral to the edge of the sternum and divides into the deep superior epigastric and musculophrenic arteries between the sixth costal cartilage and the sixth intercostal space. It is accompanied in its distal part by two venae comitantes. These generally merge between the third and fourth intercostal spaces[3,4] to form one internal mammary vein, which ascends to drain into the brachiocephalic vein. At each thoracic segment, the internal mammary artery gives off a number of branches. Posteriorly, there is a mediastinal or pericardial branch; medially, a sternal branch; and laterally, an anterior intercostal branch and a branch to the pectoralis major muscle. The anterior intercostal branch anastomoses with the posterior intercostal branch from the thoracic aorta. The internal mammary artery commonly has a diameter of 1 to 2 mm, measured at the level of the fourth costal cartilage, and its accompanying vein is 2 to 3 mm.[3,5-9] When there are two internal mammary veins, the medial vein tends to be larger.[10] The internal mammary vessels tend to be larger on the right side[7,11] (Fig. 23-1).[9]

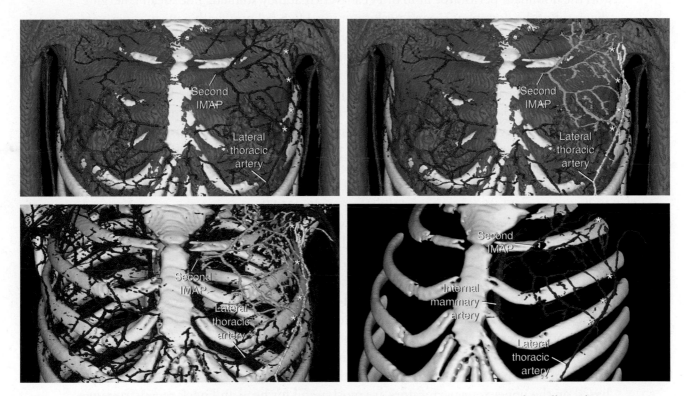

Fig. 23-1 Three-dimensional angiogram of the internal mammary system. Note the collateralization of territories distally. (*IMAP,* Internal mammary artery perforator.) (From Gillis JA, Prasad V, Morris SF. Three-dimensional analysis of the internal mammary artery perforator flap. Plast Reconstr Surg 128:419e-426e, 2011.)

ANATOMY OF THE PERFORATOR

A cutaneous perforating branch passes through the intercostal muscles and the medial fibers of the pectoralis major to supply the overlying skin in a segmental manner. This cutaneous perforating branch, or IMAP, is given off by the internal mammary artery in the first 5 to 6 intercostal spaces.

The perforator pedicle usually consists of 1 artery and 1 vein, with an accompanying nerve, the anterior cutaneous branch of the corresponding intercostal nerve. The second perforator is most often the largest in both sexes, generally 0.8 mm.[2] In females, the third and fourth perforators also tend to be large because they contribute to the arterial supply of the breast. However, the internal mammary perforators have been shown to vary in size and dominance among patients and from side to side.[1,12,13] Daniel et al[12] and Palmer and Taylor[13] found that there was a single dominant perforator in 85% of cases, which was at least twice the size of any other perforator, whereas in the other 15%, there was codominance, with two perforators of equal size. The diameter of the dominant perforator is 0.5 to 1.2 mm, and that of the accompanying vein is 1.5 to 3.2 mm.[14,15] Morris et al[9] found that the second internal mammary artery perforator was the dominant perforator in 10 of 14 cadavers that they studied. The mean emerging diameter of the dominant second perforator was 1.0 ± 0.4 mm, with a mean superficial length of 51.8 ± 16.1 mm on angiograms of the latex-injected and lead oxide–injected cadavers. The mean distance from the sternal margin to the point of emergence from the internal mammary artery was 7 ± 1.4 mm. Their three-dimensional reconstructions demonstrated anastomoses between the dominant perforator and the lateral thoracic artery (see Fig. 23-1). This was corroborated by Frey et al,[16] who also commented on flap dimensions. They found that the IMAPs supplied the skin of the ventromedial thorax and breast from the clavicle to the skin of the cranial abdominal wall in a sequential order. The mean size of all injected skin areas was 84 ± 54 cm^2 (13 by 7 cm). The biggest detected skin dimensions were 16 by 9 cm on average for the second IMAP (area 138 ± 41 cm^2). The mean external diameter of the IMAP was 1.3 ± 0.5 mm (range 0.4 to 2.9 mm). The mean dissectible length was 8.3 ± 3.6 cm (range 3 to 17 cm). The largest diameter was found for the second IMAP, with a mean of 1.6 ± 0.5 mm (range 0.9 to 2.3 mm).

In our cadaver injection studies, the second and third perforators were reliably the largest, although based on our clinical experience, the first and fourth can be of sufficient size to carry an IMAP flap. The fifth perforator was small. However, Daniel et al[12] and Palmer and Taylor[13] reported that any of the first six intercostal spaces could contain a perforator 1 mm or larger in diameter. An IMAP flap could therefore be based on any of these perforators, provided that the accompanying vein was adequate. Flaps based on the upper four perforators are most useful for head and neck reconstruction; however, flaps based on the fifth, sixth, or seventh perforators can be used for other indications, including chest wall reconstruction. After the fifth rib, there is a "conjoint" costal cartilage, which becomes much more difficult to dissect and may limit the dissection of the lowermost perforator.

ANGIOSOMAL TERRITORY

The consistency of the angiosomal territory for all perforators may result from the high degree of arterial interconnection within the chest skin, notably, the mammary branch of the second perforator, which forms a medial arcade between the second, third, and fourth perforators.[12] In our cadaver injection studies, the limits of the flap are the sternal midline to the anterior axillary line, and the clavicle to the level of the xiphisternum. Palmer and Taylor[13] also noted that few significant vessels cross the midline of the chest. In contrast to this midline watershed zone of the chest, the superficial epigastric angiosomal territory crosses the midline by 5 cm in the abdomen.[17] This may be a reflection of the need for a sternal blood supply. In its lateral half, the IMAP territory overlaps the territory of the acromiothoracic angiosome, as demonstrated by Reid and Taylor[18] (Fig. 23-2).

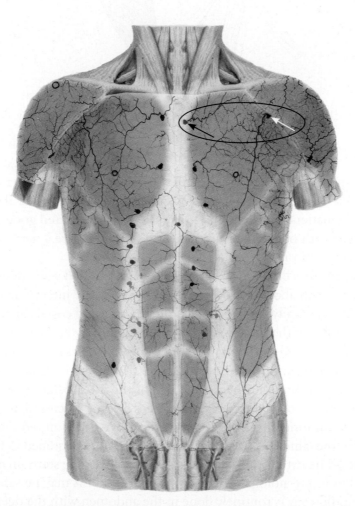

Fig. 23-2 Injection study of the anterior torso. In this specimen, major perforators of the internal mammary artery arose bilaterally through the second and fourth intercostal spaces. An IMAP flap based on the second perforator *(black arrow)*, designed to capture the adjacent territory of the thoracoacromial axis *(white arrow)* and deltoid region, would correspond to the classic deltopectoral flap. (Anatomic study courtesy Steve F. Morris, MD.)

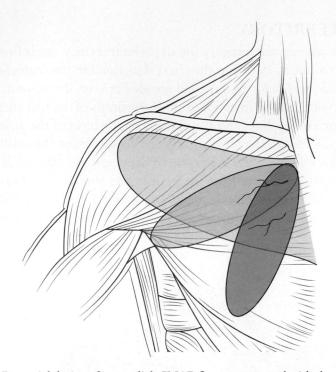

Fig. 23-3 Potential designs for a pedicle IMAP flap as compared with the classic deltopectoral flap.

Fig. 23-3 shows various designs of the IMAP flap that can be carried on a single perforator. When used as a pedicle flap, it is quite usual for the IMAP flap to maintain its sensation. The patient shown in Fig. 23-4 subjectively reported good flap sensation. This is consistent with our findings in cadaveric studies, where a nerve frequently accompanied the perforator.

The IMAP flap has limitations that need to be considered when designing the flap. The flap will not reach above the jawline reliably unless the internal mammary artery is mobilized. This generally requires removing one or more costal cartilages. The dissection is very similar to that required for internal mammary exposure in microsurgical breast reconstruction, and microsurgical experience is necessary for safe dissection of the perforators. Mobilization of the root pedicle (that is, the internal mammary artery itself) necessitates dividing the anterior branch of the intercostal nerve, which results in an insensate flap. According to injection studies already discussed, it cannot be harvested across the midline of the chest. However, Boyd et al[17] noted that flaps can be safely elevated in the clinical situation well beyond the limits outlined in fresh cadaveric injection studies. The extent to which blood can pass over the sternum and supply the contralateral skin in physiologic situations is unclear, but it may be safe to raise flaps that cross the midline, as is routinely done in the abdomen with the deep inferior epigastric artery perforator (DIEAP) flap. We have not done this, nor can we comment on how far across the midline the flap can be dissected and remain viable. Intraoperative fluorescent angiography is a useful tool to help resolve such clinical dilemmas.[19]

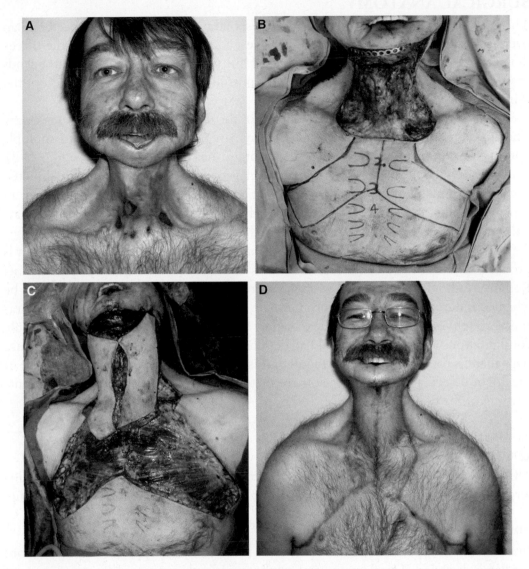

Fig. 23-4 **A,** A patient who had previous mandibulectomy and bilateral neck dissections with radiation therapy now had unstable skin. **B,** Local rotation IMAP flaps were designed based on the second intercostal perforator. **C,** The flaps were rotated in propeller fashion into the neck. The donor defects were closed directly. **D,** Postoperative appearance. (**A, B,** and **D** from Vesely M, Murray DJ, Novak CB, Gullane PJ, Neligan PC. The internal mammary artery perforator flap: an anatomical study and a case report. Ann Plast Surg 58:156-161, 2007.)

SURGICAL ANATOMY

The potential territory of the IMAP flap corresponding to that of the deltopectoral flap overlaps three angiosomes of the anterior chest and shoulder. As shown in the three-dimensional chest wall angiogram in Fig. 23-1, the internal mammary perforator sends branches in an oblique direction so that it is possible to modify the orientation of the skin paddle if necessary.

This means that the classic orientation of the deltopectoral flap is not necessary when the flap is raised purely as an internal mammary perforator flap. There are multiple options for skin paddle design once the perforator has been identified (see Fig. 23-3). The relatively large size of the internal mammary perforators, their laterally directed orientation, and abundant distal collateralization, which can routinely be captured, all explain the efficacy in harvesting this unusually large cutaneous flap. The distal collateralization of these vessels can be appreciated in the angiogram (see Fig. 23-1). Other flap designs follow the course of other internal mammary perforators, if desired. It is probably best not to consider these new flaps as deltopectoral flaps by another name. Rather, we should remember how much more versatile this vascular territory can be when considered in terms of angiosomes. The internal mammary artery sends perforators through each intercostal space to supply the overlying skin. This allows multiple configurations and many potential flap designs. Such designs make it possible to raise flaps that have all the desired attributes of this region, and may allow direct closure of the donor defect. This is in contrast to the deltopectoral flap, which requires traditional grafting of the donor site (see Fig. 23-2).

SURGICAL TECHNIQUE
Positioning

Although the supine position is preferable, access to the IMAP flap and its specific intercostal perforator is possible with the patient in a lateral position with the flap side up.

Surface Landmarks and Flap Design

Internal mammary artery perforators can be located with Doppler flowmetry before the flap is designed. The flap can be planned as an island incorporating one or more of these perforators and customized in a manner that includes the most suitable skin for reconstruction and facilitates direct donor site closure. Preoperative CT angiography can be a useful adjunct for flap planning, because it can help determine the best IMAP based on size.

IMAP Flap Dissection

If uncertainty exists as to which IMAP to use, the pedicle or pedicles can be approached from the medial direction. In this way, the size of the IMAPs can be evaluated and the best vessel or vessels chosen. The flap can then be designed based on this decision and raised from distal to proximal. The pectoralis fascia can be included with the flap, depending on the reconstructive requirements. As dissection approaches the sternal border, the internal mammary perforators can be seen entering the deep surface of the flap. At this point a decision is made as to which perforator or perforators are going to perfuse the flap. If the flap is being used as a propeller flap, the standard techniques for propeller flaps apply (that is, the perforator is dissected to its source vessel, the internal mammary artery, and then rotated into the defect). Skeletonization of the perforating vessels demands meticulous intramuscular dissection through the pectoralis major and intercostal muscles back to the internal mammary artery. Alternatively, the pedicle can be divided and transferred as a true perforator free flap using supermicrosurgical techniques. The third alternative is to dissect the perforator down to the internal mammary vessels and mobilize them. This maneuver provides a longer and larger-caliber vascular leash, as Sasaki et al[5] showed with the IMAP free flap, and similarly provides a longer pedicle if the flap is being pedicled (Fig. 23-5). Removing costal cartilages proximally allows further dissection of the internal mammary vessel and greatly increases the arc of rotation of the flap.

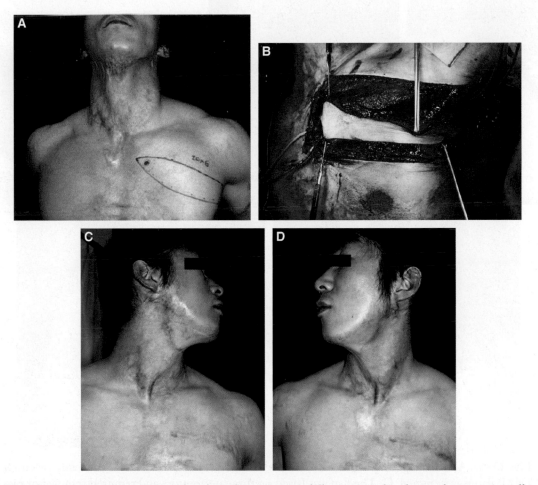

Fig. 23-5 A, A patient presented with neck contracture following gasoline burns that were initially treated with skin grafts. A bipedicle Siamese IMAP free superthin flap (see Chapter 78) was designed on the anterior chest. A cutaneous branch of the lateral thoracic vessels was used laterally, and an internal mammary perforator *(black dot)* medially. **B,** The thin flap was raised on the chest, attached at either end by its respective vascular perforators. **C** and **D,** Both facial vessels were used as the recipient site for the respective pedicles. Aesthetic coverage after contracture release was excellent because of the extreme thinness of the flap and good color match after microsurgical transfer. The flap was narrow enough for primary donor site closure. (**A, B,** and **D** from Ogawa R, Hyakusoku H. Bipedicled free super-thin flap harvesting from the anterior chest. Plast Reconstr Surg 113:1299-1300, 2004.)

MODIFICATIONS
Esophageal Replacement
Because of the remarkable length of the IMAP flap, it can be tubed to replace the cervical esophagus in its entirety, with an extension superiorly reaching as far as the nasopharynx. Placing the axis of the flap beside the sternum allows the incorporation of several perforators. Using the previously described technique of costal cartilage removal and internal mammary mobilization, the flap can be tunneled up into the neck and the donor site closed directly (Fig. 23-6).

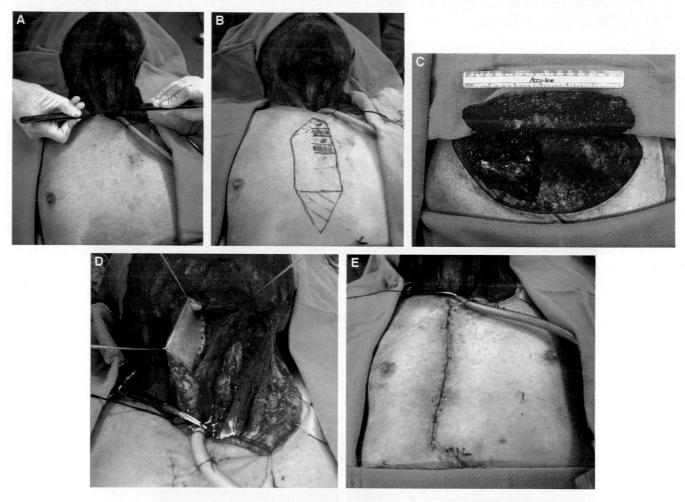

Fig. 23-6   A, Pharyngoesophagectomy was performed on this patient. **B,** A vertically oriented IMAP flap was designed. **C,** The flap was based on three perforators and required removal of two costal cartilages. **D,** It was pedicled into the neck and used to close the pharyngoesophageal defect. **E,** Final closure of the donor defect.

PITFALLS

- The major pitfalls associated with harvesting this flap relate to the technical issues of perforator dissection. If costal cartilages are to be removed, it is important to dissect the perforator first so that removal of the cartilage does not inadvertently injure the vessel. By having it under direct vision, such injury can be avoided.
- Judicious patient selection is needed if nipple shift or distortion is a concern and if presternal scarring is likely to be poor.
- Using this flap in women requires careful assessment, because breast displacement may occur.

References

1. Bakamjian VY. A two-stage method for pharyngoesophageal reconstruction with a primary pectoral skin flap. Plast Reconstr Surg 36:173-184, 1965.

2. Vesely M, Murray DJ, Novak CB, Gullane PJ, Neligan PC. The internal mammary artery perforator flap: an anatomical study and a case report. Ann Plast Surg 58:156-161, 2007.

   The authors described the anatomic basis for the internal artery mammary perforator (IMAP) flap in this cadaveric study and presented a clinical case report. The IMAP flap is based on a single or double perforator of the internal mammary artery that is included in the pedicle for added length. It provides a very useful source of local tissue with skin of good texture and color for head and neck reconstruction and, being muscle free, is thin. With preservation of the anterior cutaneous branch of the intercostal nerve, the flap has the potential to be sensate. A large area can be covered, particularly if bilateral flaps are raised. The donor site can be closed directly. In selected patients, it offers an excellent option for use in head and neck reconstruction and should be considered as an alternative to the deltopectoral and pectoralis major flaps.

3. Arnez ZM, Valdatta L, Tyler MP, et al. Anatomy of the internal mammary veins and their use in free TRAM flap breast reconstruction. Br J Plast Surg 48:540-545, 1995.

4. Ninković M, Anderl H, Hefel L, et al. Internal mammary vessels: a reliable recipient system for free flaps in breast reconstruction. Br J Plast Surg 48:533-539, 1995.

5. Sasaki K, Nozaki M, Honda T, et al. Deltopectoral skin flap as a free skin flap revisited: further refinement in flap design, fabrication, and clinical usage. Plast Reconstr Surg 107:1134-1141, 2001.

   The deltopectoral skin flap is an axial flap and can therefore be fashioned as a free skin flap. Although color and texture of the skin are well suited for facial resurfacing, the structural features of inconsistent thickness of the skin, the short vascular pedicle, minute caliber of the nutrient vessel, and donor site morbidity often preclude the use of this flap for this purpose. The authors reported on the deltopectoral skin flap fabricated as a free skin flap transferred by means of a microsurgical technique in 27 patients over 13 years. The anterior perforating branches of the internal mammary vessels were the primary nutrient vessels of the flap in seven instances. The external caliber of this artery varied between 0.6 and 1.2 mm (average 0.9 mm). The accompanying vein varied between 1.5 and 3.2 mm (average 2.3 mm). Coaptation of these vessels with those in the recipient site was technically difficult. Thrombosis occurred at the anastomotic site in three patients, requiring reoperation; two flaps were saved. Flap failure was drastically reduced in the remaining 20 patients by including a segment of the internal mammary vessel when fabricating the vascular pedicle. The size of the internal mammary arterial segment averaged 2.1 mm, and the average size of the accompanying vein was 2.9 mm. The problem of bulk was managed by surgical defatting/thinning of the flap at the time of flap fabrication and transfer. A V-Y skin flap advancement technique for wound closure was used in eight patients.

6. Dupin CL, Allen RJ, Glass CA, et al. The internal mammary artery and vein as a recipient site for free-flap breast reconstruction: a report of 110 consecutive cases. Plast Reconstr Surg 98:685-689; discussion 690-692, 1996.

7. Feng LJ. Recipient vessels in free-flap breast reconstruction: a study of the internal mammary and thoracodorsal vessels. Plast Reconstr Surg 99:405-416, 1997.

8. Schwabegger AH, Milomir N. Internal mammary artery and vein. Plast Reconstr Surg 100:1360-1361, 1997.

9. Gillis JA, Prasad V, Morris SF. Three-dimensional analysis of the internal mammary artery perforator flap. Plast Reconstr Surg 128:419e-426e, 2011.

10. Arnez ZM, Khan U. The internal mammary artery and vein as a recipient site for free-flap breast reconstruction. Plast Reconstr Surg 100:1359-1360, 1997.

11. Hefel L, Schwabegger A, Ninković M, et al. Internal mammary vessels: anatomical and clinical considerations. Br J Plast Surg 48:527-532, 1995.

12. Daniel RK, Cunningham DM, Taylor GI. The deltopectoral flap: an anatomical and hemodynamic approach. Plast Reconstr Surg 55:275-282, 1975.

13. Palmer JH, Taylor GI. The vascular territories of the anterior chest wall. Br J Plast Surg 39:287-299, 1986.

14. Harii K, Omori K, Omori S. Free deltopectoral skin flaps. Br J Plast Surg 27:231-239, 1974.

15. Taylor GI, Daniel RK. The anatomy of several free flap donor sites. Plast Reconstr Surg 56:243-253, 1975.

16. Schmidt M, Aszmann OC, Beck H, Frey M. The anatomic basis of the internal mammary artery perforator flap: a cadaver study. J Plast Reconstr Aesthet Surg 63:191-196, 2010.

   The perforating branches of the internal mammary artery have recently been described as recipient vessels for free tissue transfer breast reconstruction. However, reports on perforator flaps based on these vessels are rare. The aim of this study was to investigate the vascular basis of the internal mammary artery perforator (IMAP) flap and to describe the location and size of the individual flaps. The IMAPs of 10 fresh female cadavers were injected with methylene blue solution. The location and size of the labelled skin area were observed. Finally, the arterial perforators were dissected, and the length, diameter, and distance of the lateral sternal border to the perforation point were recorded. The IMAPs supplied the skin of the ventromedial thorax and breast from the clavicle to the skin of the cranial abdominal wall in a sequential order. The mean size of all injected skin areas was 84 ± 54 cm² (13 by 7 cm). The biggest detected skin dimensions were 16 by 9 cm on average for IMAP 2 (area 138 ± 41 cm²). The mean external diameter of the IMAP was 1.3 ± 0.5 mm (range 0.4 to 2.9 mm). The mean dissectible length was 8.3 ± 3.6 cm (range 3 to 17 cm). The largest diameter was found for IMAP 2 with a mean of 1.6 ± 0.5 mm (range 0.9 to 2.3 mm). The study demonstrated a reliable anatomy of the IMAP flap. Based on these results, different clinical applications exist for the individual IMAP flaps. The flaps based on IMAP 1 or 2 may be rotated cranially for tracheostoma or anterior neck reconstruction. The flaps based on IMAP 4 supplying the skin of the inframammary fold could be used for reconstruction of the contralateral thoracic wall or breast. The harvest site of IMAP 1 and 2 can be closed directly if the width of the flap is less than 6 cm. The IMAP 4 harvest site could be closed via a reduction mammaplasty technique, thus minimizing donor site morbidity.

17. Boyd JB, Taylor GI, Corlett R. The vascular territories of the superior epigastric and the deep inferior epigastric systems. Plast Reconstr Surg 73:1-16, 1984.

18. Reid CD, Taylor GI. The vascular territory of the acromiothoracic axis. Br J Plast Surg 37:194-212, 1984.

19. Liu DZ, Mathes DW, Zenn MR, Neligan PC. The application of indocyanine green fluorescence angiography in plastic surgery. J Reconstr Microsurg 27:355-364, 2011.

24

Superior Epigastric Artery Perforator Flap

Tetsuji Uemura
Geoffrey G. Hallock

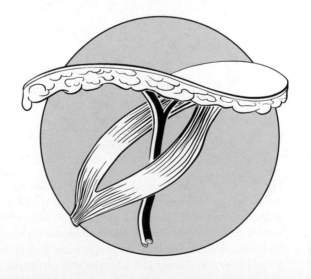

The concept of deep fascia perforators providing circulation to the integument has been understood since at least the time of Manchot.[1] Perforator-based flaps were first introduced by Kroll and Rosenfield,[2] and Koshima et al[3] are generally credited for coining the name "perforator flap." Coincidentally, Koshima and Soeda[4] carried out a seminal clinical series of periumbilical flaps without muscle that relied on perforators of the deep inferior epigastric vessels. This region quickly became widely used as the donor site of choice for autogenous tissue breast reconstruction.[5] Injection studies by Taylor and Palmer[6] demonstrated that the deep inferior epigastric artery enters the rectus abdominis muscle on its posterior surface at the level of the arcuate line. There

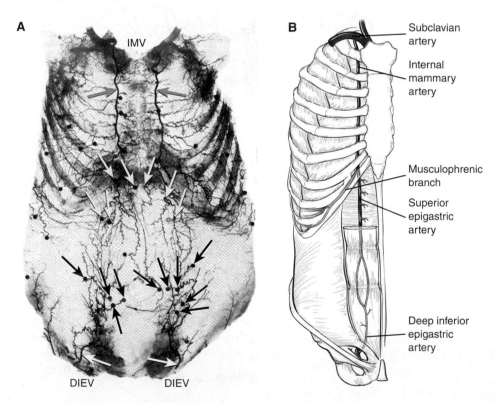

Fig. 24-1 A, Angiogram of an abdomen showing the well-known periumbilical perforators *(black arrows)* of the deep inferior epigastric vessels *(DIEV, white arrows)* and the perixiphisternal perforators *(yellow arrows)* of the superior epigastric vessels, which are the terminus of the internal mammary vessels *(IMV, orange arrows)*. **B,** A schematic representation highlights the unusual origin, course, and terminus of the deep inferior epigastric arteries within the rectus abdominis muscle. (**A** adapted from Taylor GI, Palmer JH. The vascular territories (angiosomes) of the body: experimental study and clinical applications. Br J Plast Surg 40:113-141, 1987.)

it usually, almost immediately, divides into medial and lateral trunks and then gives off a series of cutaneous perforators, especially in the periumbilical area (Fig. 24-1). These are the basis for the deep inferior epigastric artery perforator (DIEAP) flap.[5]

The DIEAP flap has been so dominant in the realm of perforator flaps that its carrier's classification as a type III muscle, according to the schema of Mathes and Nahai,[7] has often been overlooked. By definition then, the rectus abdominis muscle actually has a dual system of dominant source vessels and is unique in that each enters the muscle at opposite extremes. The superior epigastric artery is the often-forgotten pedicle, which enters the rectus abdominis muscle at the costal margin. Similar to its counterpart—the deep inferior epigastric artery—it gives off a series of perforators that pass through the rectus muscle to supply the skin of the upper abdomen.[8] Taylor and Palmer[6] demonstrated this in their injection studies.

The superficial epigastric artery perforators have been recognized for a long time as the means of circulation to the vertical rectus abdominis musculocutaneous flap[8,9] and the horizontally oriented thoracoepigastric flap.[8,10] I (G.G.H.) first reported on the possibility of a "true" perforator flap based only on the perforators of the superior epigastric vessels.[11] In my (T.U.) cadaver series,[12] I better described the specific surgical anatomy of these perforators, with more clinical applications as a local pedicle flap for the anterior chest wall and upper abdominal wall reconstruction. Hamdi and colleagues[13] also reported their clinical experiences with the superior epigastric artery perforator (SEAP) flap, extolling the added advantage of multidetector-row CT angiography to better identify preoperatively the location of these perforators and thereby simplify flap design.

ANATOMY

The internal mammary artery bifurcates under the costal cartilage of the sixth rib to give rise to the superior epigastric artery and the musculophrenic artery.[8,13] Behind the seventh costal cartilage, the superior epigastric artery pierces the posterior rectus sheath and enters the medial posterior surface of the rectus abdominis muscle.[13] At the costal margin, this artery often gives off its first large perforator that is sometimes called the *superficial superior epigastric artery*. This perforator is from the deep system and therefore has no similarity to the superficial inferior epigastric artery. The superior epigastric artery then arborizes within the rectus abdominis muscle and continues caudally to meet a corresponding member of the deep inferior epigastric artery, forming choke anastomoses or sometimes a true arterial connection at or about the level of the midpoint between the xiphisternum and umbilicus.[6]

In all specimens of my (T.U.) preserved cadaver study,[12] I consistently found on either side of the midline at least one adequate musculocutaneous perforator from the superior epigastric artery that penetrated the upper anterior rectus sheath. The range was one to three perforators at a mean distance of 35 mm (range 10 to 82 mm) from midline, and a mean distance of 26 mm (range 12 to 50 mm) from the inferior costal margin. In other anatomic dissections, Hamdi and colleagues[13] found superior epigastric artery perforators to be 1.5 to 6.5 cm lateral to the midline and 3 to 16 cm below a horizontal line centered at the junction of the sternum and xiphoid. They found that there are usually at least two significant musculocutaneous perforators larger than 1.0 mm in diameter through each of the paired rectus abdominis muscles.[13] Mah et al[14] corroborated these findings, explaining that if a horizontal line is drawn midway between the xipohid and umbilicus, superior epigastric artery perforators will most likely be found within the medial half of the muscle above this line, with most in a perixiphisternal location. They also found that most of these perforators were musculocutaneous, but occasionally a direct or circummuscular perforator coursed around the medial border of the rectus abdominis muscle.

SURGICAL TECHNIQUE
Patient Positioning

Usually a local SEAP flap is chosen to close a contiguous chest or abdominal defect. Both the donor and recipient site are best accessed with the patient in a supine position.

Surface Landmarks

The tip of the xiphoid is usually palpable. A vertical line drawn from this point to the umbilicus marks the midline of the abdomen. A parallel line through the nipple roughly approximates the linea semilunaris or lateral border of the rectus abdominis muscle. The costal margins represent the superior border of the abdomen. A horizontal line midway between the xiphoid and umbilicus completes a near-trapezoid region for each hemi-abdomen, within which the superior epigastric artery perforators are found (Fig. 24-2).

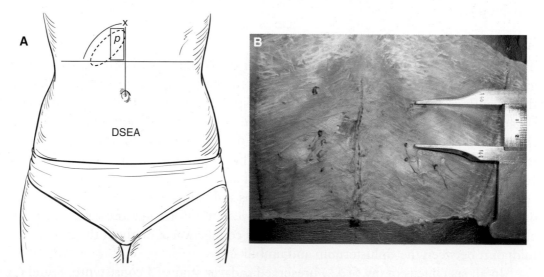

Fig. 24-2   A, Superior epigastric artery perforators are located within a rectangle bounded by the midline of the abdomen and the medial half of the rectus abdominis muscle, superiorly by the costal margin, and inferiorly by a horizontal line through the midpoint of a line drawn from the xiphoid *(x)* to the umbilicus. The preferred axis of an SEAP flap *(dashed lines)* is oriented somewhat transversely about the designated perforator *(p)* and parallel to the costal margin. **B,** Perforators identified in preserved cadavers. *(DSEA, Deep superior epigastric artery.)*

Flap Design

Accurate preoperative identification of a pertinent superior epigastric artery perforator facilitates appropriate flap design. Hamdi et al[13] and Mah et al[14] have shown that multidetector-row CT readily accomplishes this objective. Alternatively, acoustic Doppler sonography suffices for locating a perforator in the epigastric region (see Fig. 24-2). Flap dimensions must match those of the defect. Saint-Cyr et al[15] suggest that for all trunk flaps a transverse orientation captures the maximum number of adjacent perforasomes; however, for the SEAP flap, an axis parallel to the costal margin may be preferred, and a vertical (Fig. 24-3) or any other orientation may even be possible, depending on the size of the flap. The flap's boundaries must encompass the chosen perforator and may cross the midline, but extreme caution is required because there may be little vascular crossover, as with the DIEAP flap.

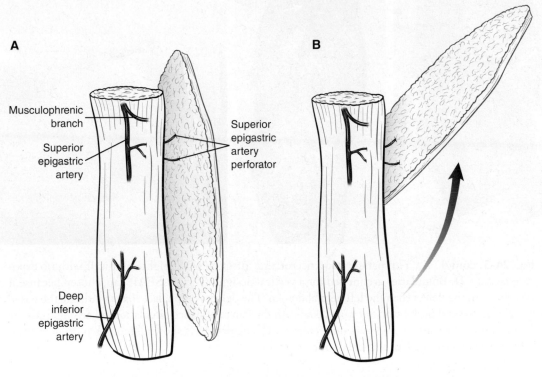

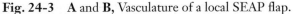

Fig. 24-3   A and B, Vasculature of a local SEAP flap.

Continued

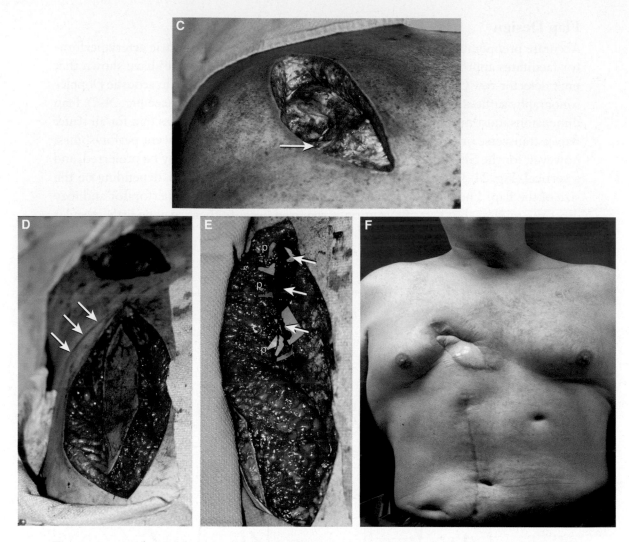

Fig. 24-3, cont'd   C, This patient had a necrotizing infection of the right chest wall, with rib exposure *(arrow).* **D,** Boundaries are incised for a vertical design of a right SEAP flap, chosen because it was closer to the defect than the left hemiabdomen. The defect is cephalad. *Arrows* indicate the costal margin. **E,** Several perforators *(p)* were taken with the flap to enhance circulation, all arising from the superior epigastric artery source pedicle *(arrows).* **F,** The patient is shown 6 months postoperatively. Note the right paramedian vertical donor site scar.

Flap Dissection

An exploratory incision down to the anterior rectus sheath is made along part of the cephalic border of the flap to confirm the location of the chosen perforator. A suprafascial dissection continues until one or more superior epigastric artery perforators are identified to ensure the accuracy of the preoperative markings and/or allow redesign of the flap boundaries as necessary. All remaining edges of the flap can then be incised down to the abdominal wall fascia. The anterior rectus sheath is opened carefully above and below the chosen perforator, and retracted to expose its course over and into the rectus abdominis muscle. If additional pedicle length is needed, the muscle is split along the corresponding intramuscular septum to allow intramuscular dissection of the perforator with coagulation or ligation of muscle side branches. This dissection proceeds toward the costal margin, excluding muscle and fascia, until an island flap based on the given perforator can be advanced or rotated into the defect. Taking a slightly longer pedicle than necessary helps avoid excessive twisting, tension, or compression of the vascular pedicle as the flap is inset to cover the lower half of the anterior chest wall or the epigastric area of the abdomen.

ADVANTAGES

The SEAP flap may become the method of choice for closing the epigastric area (see Chapter 63), because it is a local flap, and the rectus abdominis muscle will remain relatively intact. This minimizes the risk of hernia, retains blood flow to the subcutaneous layer of the remaining donor site, and retains the muscle as a flap option for this region, if needed later.

MODIFICATIONS
Free Flap

Similar to the DIEAP flap, the SEAP flap can be used as a microsurgical tissue transfer. However, the superior epigastric vessels have a much smaller caliber than the deep inferior epigastric vessels.[16] Because pedicle dissection usually stops at the costal margin, a much shorter pedicle must be anticipated. An upper abdominal scar at the donor site will be more conspicuous than, for example, a DIEAP flap that can be better hidden by clothing.

Propeller Flap

If a reasonable perforator is available, a perforator-pedicle propeller SEAP flap can be rotated 90 to 180 degrees about the perforator to close an adjacent defect.[17] Although any anterior rectus sheath or muscle dissection may thereby be totally avoided, it may be safer to cut the fascia just around the vessel to avoid kinking or compression of the perforator after rotation.

PITFALLS
Vertical Dimensions

Mah et al[14] found no superior epigastric perforators below a horizontal line through the midpoint of a line drawn from the xiphoid to the umbilicus. That area represents the watershed between the superior and deep inferior epigastric territories and may be unreliable.

Horizontal Dimensions

Tai and Hasegawa[10] reported that an abdominal flap with a transverse axis may be extended to the posterior axillary line, but Mah et al[14] had several cases of flap tip necrosis when the flap extended beyond the anterior axillary line. Once the costal margin is reached, the next adjacent perforasome arises from intercostal perforators that may be variably captured.

Donor Site Closure

Not only is a skin graft not aesthetically acceptable in the upper abdomen, graft take may be compromised if ribs or abdominal wall fascia are exposed. Primary donor site closure is always preferable. The design of the SEAP flap can have any shape and be oriented in any direction; however, the means to achieve proper donor site closure often determines the optimal design.

Internal Mammary Artery Absence

Bilateral obliteration of the internal mammary arteries is not uncommon, especially when used for cardiac revascularization. Extensive dissection of the superior epigastric artery pedicle could devascularize the chosen perforator, but flow may remain if collaterals from intercostals or the deep inferior epigastric vessels are not disturbed.

CONCLUSION

The reliable vascular territory of the SEAP flap extends vertically from the costal margin to the midpoint of a line connecting the umbilicus and xiphoid, and laterally to the anterior axillary line. Capture of the contralateral hemiabdomen may be variable and unreliable, which is often true with the DIEAP flap. A local SEAP flap can be used for midchest and abdominal wall reconstructions, often preserving the workhorse pectoralis major and rectus abdominis muscles for future considerations. Harvesting the SEAP flap is easy, quick, minimally invasive, and preserves the integrity and function of the abdominal wall musculature and fascia.

References

1. Manchot C. The Cutaneous Arteries of the Human Body. New York: Springer-Verlag, 1983.
2. Kroll SS, Rosenfield L. Perforator-based flaps for low postrior midline defects. Plast Reconstr Surg 81:561-566, 1988.
3. Koshima I, Moriguchi T, Fukuda H, Soeda S, et al. Free, thinned, paraumbilical perforator-based flaps. J Reconstr Microsurg 7:313-316, 1991.
4. Koshima I, Soeda S. Inferior epigastric artery skin flaps without rectus abdominis muscle. Br J Plast Surg 42:645-648, 1989.
5. Allen RJ, Treece P. Deep inferior epigastric perforator flap for breast reconstruction. Ann Plast Surg 32:32-38, 1994.
6. Taylor GI, Palmer JH. The vascular territories (angiosomes) of the body: experimental study and clinical applications. Br J Plast Surg 40:113-141, 1987.
7. Mathes SJ, Nahai F. Classification of the vascular anatomy of muscles: experimental and clinical correlation. Plast Reconstr Surg 67:177-187, 1981.
8. Moon HK, Taylor GI. The vascular anatomy of rectus abdominis musculocutaneous flaps based on the deep superior epigastric system. Plast Reconstr Surg 82:815-829, 1988.
9. Sakai S, Takahaski H, Tanabe H. The extended vertical rectus abdominis myocutaneous flap for breast reconstruction. Plast Reconstr Surg 83:1061-1067, 1989.
10. Tai Y, Hasegawa HA. A transverse abdominal flap for reconstruction after radical operations for recurrent breast cancer. Plast Recontr Surg 53:52-54, 1974.

11. Hallock GG. The superior epigastric (RECTUS ABDOMINIS) muscle perforator flap. Ann Plast Surg 55:430-432, 2005.

Although musculocutaneous perforators from the deep superior epigastric artery were known to exist, they had never been used in a clinical example as a perforator flap. In this single case report, an SEAP flap with a vertical axis was used to cover exposed ribs of the anterior chest wall.

12. Uemura T. Superior epigastric artery perforator flap: preliminary report. Plast Reconstr Surg 120:1e-5e, 2007.

In cadaver dissections, at least one major deep superior epigastric artery perforator was found to pierce the anterior rectus sheath in each hemiabdomen. Clinical examples of SEAP flaps with a vertical or horizontal axis were used to close chest and abdomen wounds.

13. Hamdi M, Van Landuyt K, Ulens S, et al. Clinical applications of the superior epigastric artery perforator (SEAP) flap: anatomical studies and preoperative perforator mapping with multidetector CT. J Plast Reconstr Aesthet Surg 62:1127-1134, 2009.

The authors used the deep SEAP flap to close difficult chest wounds. Multidetector-row CT angiography was used to preoperatively identify the requisite perforator to facilitate an exact flap design. Intraoperatively, all perforators were confirmed as predicted.

14. Mah E, Rozen WM, Ashton MW, et al. Deep superior epigastric artery perforators: anatomical study and clinical application in sternal reconstruction. Plast Reconstr Surg 123:1719-1723, 2009.

Anatomic studies of perforators of the deep superior epigastric artery showed that they most commonly arise through the medial half of the rectus abdominis muscle in a region extending from the costal margin to a horizontal line passing through the midpoint of a line drawn from the xiphoid to umbilicus. Most of these perforators were found in the perixiphisternal area. An SEAP flap with a transverse axis, similar to that of a thoracoepigastric flap, was used to cover lower median sternotomy wounds. Only the portion of the flap medial to the anterior axillary line was found to be reliable.

15. Saint-Cyr M, Wong C, Schaverien M, et al. The perforasome theory: vascular anatomy and clinical implications. Plast Reconstr Surg 124:1529-1544, 2009.

16. Canales FL, Furnas H, Glafkides M, et al. Microsurgical transfer of the rectus abdominis muscle using the superior epigastric vessels. Ann Plast Surg 24:534-537, 1990.

17. Woo KJ, Pyon JK, Lim SY, et al. Deep superior epigastric artery perforator 'propeller' flap for abdominal wall reconstruction: a case report. J Plast Reconstr Aesthet Surg 63:1223-1226, 2010.

25

Deep Inferior Epigastric Artery Perforator Flap

Phillip N. Blondeel

Rossella Sgarzani

Colin M. Morrison

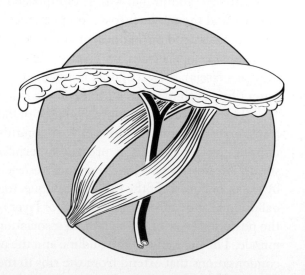

The deep inferior epigastric artery perforator (DIEAP) flap arose as a refinement of the conventional myocutaneous lower abdominal flap. The myocutaneous perforators of the inferior epigastric vessels were described[1] soon after the first transverse rectus abdominis musculocutaneous (TRAM) flap was performed for breast reconstruction by Holmström and Robbins.[2,3] In 1989 Koshima and Soeda[4] reported the first clinical application of the inferior epigastric artery perforator flap. They demonstrated that it was possible to harvest the same amount of lower abdominal skin and fat as in the TRAM flap, without sacrificing the rectus abdominis muscle. Koshima et al[5] then reported 13 other cases with free, thin, paraumbilical perforator-based flaps. Later Pennington et al[6] used an anastomosis between the distal end of the ipsilateral pedicle and the contralateral pedicle to augment the blood supply of a free TRAM flap. Allen and Treece[7] reported 22 successful breast reconstructions with the DIEAP free flap, and Blondeel[8] and Blondeel and Boeckx[9] improved the understanding of the flap and popularized its use for autologous breast reconstruction.

Although commonly used for breast restoration to provide a soft, naturally shaped, long-lasting result, these qualities make the DIEAP flap ideal for covering a variety of soft tissue defects.

ANATOMY

The anterior abdominal wall is composed of skin, superficial fascia, the abdominal muscles and their aponeuroses, preperitoneal fat, transversalis fascia, and peritoneum. The skin is lax and only adherent at the linea alba and umbilicus. The superficial fascia consists of a superficial fatty layer (Camper's fascia) and a deeper membranous layer (Scarpa's fascia). Scarpa's fascia is attached to the medial half of the inguinal ligament. Laterally it is continuous with the fascia lata of the thigh.

The abdominal wall muscles consist of the paired external oblique, internal oblique, transversus abdominis, and rectus abdominis. In 83% of patients, a small triangular muscle, the pyramidalis, is present superficial to the rectus abdominis.[10] The rectus sheath is a fibrous envelope that encloses each muscle. The anterior layers are formed by the aponeurosis of the external oblique, together with the anterior half of the internal oblique aponeurosis. The posterior layer of the internal oblique aponeurosis forms the posterior layer of the sheath, in association with the aponeurosis of the transversus muscle. The linea alba in the midline and the paired linea semilunaris laterally are fascial condensations that extend from the ribs to the pubis. Beneath the lower quarter of the rectus abdominis muscle, the posterior layer of the rectus sheath is absent. The lower border of this sheath is called the *linea semicircularis* or *arcuate line.* The deep inferior epigastric artery arises from the external iliac artery, just above the inguinal ligament, and approaches the rectus abdominis muscle from its lateral side. The artery is accompanied by two venae comitantes and forms an excellent pedicle for free microvascular transfer. Milloy et al[11] found that the inferior epigastric artery ascends anterior to the linea semicircularis on the posterior surface of the rectus abdominis muscle and enters its substance in the middle third (78%), lower third (17%), or upper third (5%).

The anatomy of the deep inferior epigastric artery system is very variable.[12,13] The average pedicle length is 10.3 cm, and the average vessel diameter is 3.6 mm. Normally it divides into two branches, with a dominant lateral branch in most patients (54%). However, if the deep inferior epigastric artery does not divide, it has a central course (28%) with multiple small branches to the muscle and centrally located perforators. If the medial branch is dominant (18%), flow appears to be significantly lower than in a central system or in patients with a dominant lateral branch.[14]

Blondeel et al[14] found two to eight large (0.5 mm diameter or larger) perforators on each side of the midline. The majority of these perforators emerged from the anterior rectus fascia in a paramedian rectangular area 2 cm cranial and 6 cm caudal to the umbilicus, and 1 to 6 cm lateral to the umbilicus. Anatomic symmetry was rarely encountered (Fig. 25-1). The closer a perforator is to the midline, the better the blood supply to the most remote part of the flap on the contralateral side, because one choke vessel less has to be transgressed. However, the lateral perforators are often dominant and easier to dissect, because they run more perpendicularly through the muscle. The sensory nerve that runs with these perforating vessels is also often much larger. The medial perforators provide better perfusion of the flap, but they have a longer intramus-

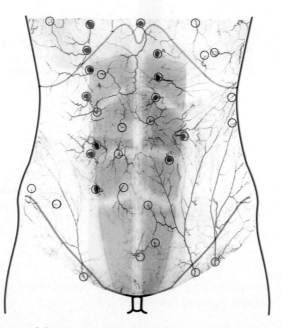

Fig. 25-1 This angiogram of the integument of the abdomen shows direct perforators *(blue circles)* and indirect perforators *(red circles).*

cular course, requiring more elaborate dissection with extensive longitudinal splitting of the muscle. An alternative is to extend the design of the flap to include more tissue from the flank and even from the craniolateral buttock area. If one is uncertain as to whether or not enough volume can be transferred, the perforators can be dissected on both sides (Siamese flap).[9]

Preference is also given to perforators that pass through the rectus abdominis muscle at the level of the tendinous intersections. At this point, the perforators are frequently large and have few muscular side branches. The distance from the subcutaneous fat to the deep inferior epigastric vessels is also shorter, simplifying this most delicate part of the dissection.[15]

As a result, the design of a DIEAP flap is made over the most centrally located and largest lateral perforator located by preoperative CT scan investigation, if sufficient abdominal subcutaneous fat tissue is available and zone IV can be discarded. At the origin of the perforator, several nerves are encountered.

Although there is no constant anatomy, mixed segmental nerves run underneath or through the muscle from laterally. They split into a sensate nerve running with the perforator into the flap and a motor nerve crossing on top of the deep inferior epigastric vessels distal to the bifurcation of the perforator, into the medial part of the rectus abdominis muscle[16] (Fig. 25-2).

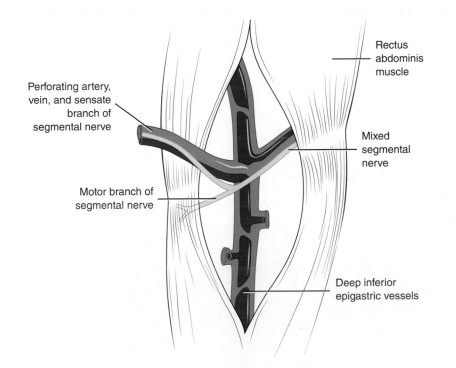

Fig. 25-2   This lateral view of the left rectus abdominis muscle shows typical anatomy observed during the dissection of a lateral perforator of a DIEAP flap.

Motor nerves enter the posterior surface of the rectus abdominis with the lateral-row perforators,[17] arising from the lateral trunks of the deep inferior epigastric artery (DIEA), and penetrate the rectus muscle slightly more medial than the perforating vessels. Any dissection to the lateral half of the rectus abdominis muscle risks damage to these nerves and creates the potential for rectus muscle denervation. Medial-row perforators are not related to these motor nerves; therefore their dissection is less risky.

Rozen et al[18] used intraoperative nerve stimulation to study the distribution of motor nerves supplying the rectus abdominis muscle. According to their results, motor nerves can be divided into type 1 and type 2 nerves. Type 1 nerves are small and innervate small, longitudinal strips of rectus muscle, with significant overlap between adjacent territories. Therefore they can be sacrificed without affecting function. Type 2 are single, large nerves at the level of the arcuate line. These supply the entire width and length of rectus muscle and may contribute to donor site morbidity if sacrificed.

The most variable anatomic alterations occur in this area and should always be anticipated. The superficial inferior epigastric artery originates 2 to 3 cm below the inguinal ligament directly from the common femoral artery (17%), or from a common origin with the superficial circumflex iliac artery (48%). It then passes superiorly and laterally in the femoral triangle, deep to Scarpa's fascia, and crosses the inguinal ligament at the midpoint between the ASIS and the pubic tubercle. Above the inguinal ligament, the superficial inferior epigastric artery pierces Scarpa's fascia and lies in the superficial subcutaneous tissue. During its course, the artery lies deep and parallel to the superficial inferior epigastric vein, which drains directly into the saphenous bulb.[19] It is the largest vein draining the skin paddle of the DIEAP flap and is located below the dermal plexus but above Scarpa's fascia, midway between the ASIS and pubic symphysis. Harvesting an elliptical skin island transects this vein, redirecting the venous drainage through the smaller perforating veins. Connections between the superficial epigastric vein and the deep inferior epigastric system exist in every patient, but substantial medial branches crossing the midline have been found to be absent in 36% of cases.[20,21] In these flaps, venous connections are only present through the subdermal capillary network. This explains why the portion of a flap farthest from the midline may suffer from venous congestion and why the presence of this problem is so variable and unpredictable.

The lymphatic drainage of the DIEAP flap can be divided into a superficial and a deep system. The superficial collectors are located directly underneath the reticular dermis. Deep cuts performed during deepithelialization may injure this system. The superficial collectors drain to the superficial lymph nodes in the groin. The deep system drains the deep structures of the abdominal wall (the muscles and fascia) and is located in close proximity to the arteries and veins. Careful dissection of the vascular pedicle avoids iatrogenic damage to this lymphatic vasculature. The deep system drains to the inferior epigastric artery and then to the deep iliac nodes.[22]

SURGICAL TECHNIQUE

The fundamental principle in raising a DIEAP flap is to center the flap over identi-fied main muscular perforators and not on the midline, as in a TRAM flap. The final dimensions, shape, and position of the flap are determined by the size of the flap that needs to be harvested, keeping in mind that the perforators in the lower abdomen run predominantly cranially and laterally after they pierce the anterior rectus fascia, and the area most distant from the vascular pedicle (zone IV) is frequently poorly vascularized. However, the final design of a DIEAP flap should be symmetrical over the midline to facilitate aesthetic donor site closure (Fig. 25-3).

Ideally, a medial, distally located perforator with multiple branches and a large accompanying vein should be selected. This type of perforator ensures that the great-est number of branches are included in the DIEAP flap and decreases the distance of dissection between the perforator and the deep inferior epigastric vessels. If a large flap is required, two or three perforators in the same perimysial plane can be dissected to increase blood flow.

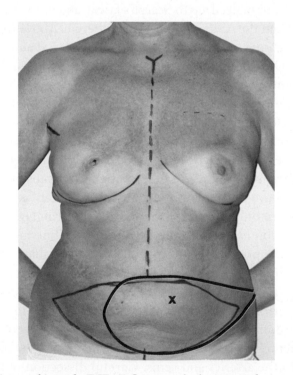

Fig. 25-3   Preoperative marking of a DIEAP flap over the largest perforator *(x)*. A symmetrical and elliptical skin island *(black line)* will be harvested, but the tissues farthest away from the perforator *(zone IV)* will be discarded. To harvest a larger flap, more tissue is taken from the lateral parts of the abdomen, and even the flanks *(red line)*.

Planning

Before surgery a CT scan of the lower abdominal wall is performed. Multidetector-row helical CT rapidly delineates an anatomic area of interest, giving excellent resolution and low-artifact rating. It takes less than 10 minutes to perform and is well tolerated by patients. This has become the modality of choice for identifying abdominal wall perforators.[23-25] The surgeon can interpret the images before and during surgery and correlate preoperative and intraoperative findings (Figs. 25-4 and 25-5).

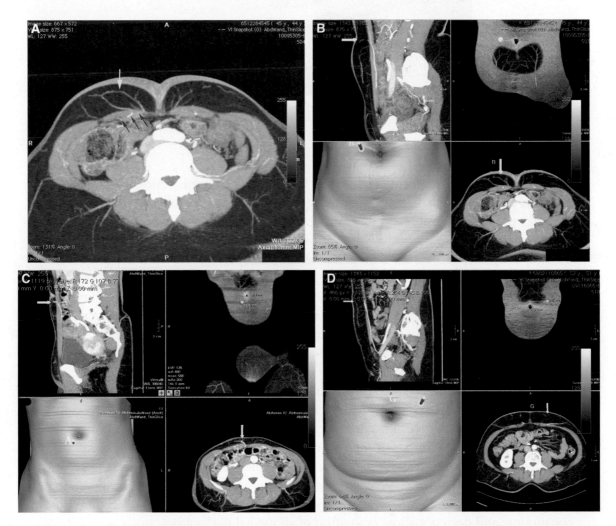

Fig. 25-4   A, This transverse CT angiographic image at the level of the umbilicus shows multiple anterior and posterior perforators of the lower torso. They are grouped in the posterior intercostal perforators, the lateral intercostal perforators, and the anterior perforators of the deep inferior epigastric artery. Direct shunts between different perforators are visible *(yellow arrow)*. The intramuscular and submuscular course of the deep inferior epigastric artery is also shown *(blue arrows)*. **B,** Different views and three-dimensional skin surface identification of the same perforator. The sagittal view *(top right)* shows the course of the vessel through the rectus abdominis muscle. The perforator is located with reference to the umbilicus in a coronal plane. **C,** Similar views of a large pararectal perforator turning around the medial edge of the right rectus abdominis muscle. **D,** Similar views of a perforator emerging from the central portion of the rectus abdominis muscle but turning sharply laterally, immediately after piercing the deep fascia. Such perforators will only vascularize the lateral part of the ipsilateral half and provide very little or no flow across the midline.

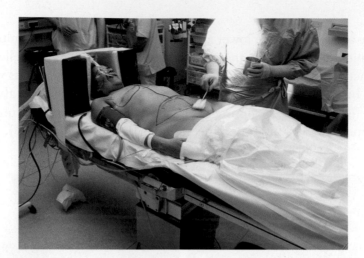

Fig. 25-5   This patient is positioned for a DIEAP flap for secondary breast reconstruction.

The scanning is performed in conjunction with the administration of intravenous contrast medium and allows evaluation of the donor vessels. Information collected includes the exact location and intramuscular course of vessels from their origin, the caliber of the perforators, and identification of the dominant vessel (see Fig. 25-4, *A*). The radiologist describes the emergence of the main perforators from the deep fascia as points on a 1 cm grid system *(x, y)* based on the umbilicus (see Fig. 25-4, *B*).

Delineating the relative dominance of the deep and superficial systems allows the surgeon to consider different options preoperatively. Not only can this modality be used to select suitable patients preoperatively, but also operative times are reduced by a mean of 21% with the obvious associated cost benefits.[26]

The disadvantages of multidetector-row helical CT lie in the x-ray dosage and intravenous contrast media, with the resultant risk of anaphylaxis. The x-ray dose, albeit significant, is less than a conventional liver CT scan and can be combined with staging or preoperative chest investigations to reduce the overall exposure. The use of MR imaging to avoid the high x-ray dose is promising, but needs further sophistication.[27]

Duplex Doppler and the unidirectional Doppler probe are considered a second choice, because CT scanning provides superior precision. Moreover, the unidirectional Doppler probe requires expertise, often generates false-positive signals, can be time consuming, and does not allow evaluation of all medial perforators.

Patient Positioning

The patient is placed in a supine position with the arms beside the trunk. Two intravenous lines, an indwelling urinary catheter, and antithrombotic stockings are applied. A warming blanket helps keep the patient's core body temperature at 37° C (98.6° F). A protective case is placed around the head to protect both the face and anesthetic tubing from compression by the surgeons' elbows. Two electrocautery units are installed for separate use by both teams.

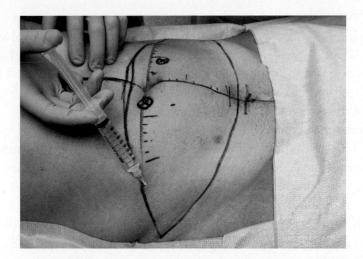

Fig. 25-6 The skin is marked preoperatively, and lidocaine and epinephrine are injected subcutaneously at the incision lines (except for the area around the superficial epigastric vein).

Preoperative Marking

The abdomen is marked with the patient under general anesthesia in the operating room. A 1 cm grid system based on the umbilicus is marked. The emergence of the most dominant perforators from the deep fascia is identified by the CT scan and recorded on the abdomen.

A fusiform skin island is drawn on the abdomen, similar to the one used for breast reconstruction with a free TRAM flap, but the bulk of the flap is centered over the selected perforator. Although the size and shape may vary slightly, the borders of a DIEAP flap arc generally located at the level of the suprapubic crease, the umbilicus, and both anterior superior iliac spines, but the flap may be extended laterally to the midaxillary lines (see Fig. 25-3). A DIEAP flap generally measures 12 to 15 cm high and 30 to 45 cm wide. However, the tension of the donor site following closure should be estimated, because this ultimately limits the size of the flap that can be harvested. A horizontal line is drawn just above the umbilicus, and another one is marked 12 to 15 cm below this. At a level 4 cm below the umbilicus, the lateral limits of the flap are marked 15 to 23 cm on either side of midline (Fig. 25-6). The amount of subcutaneous fat present in the flanks is assessed; this can be included in the flap if required. All the outer markings are connected by a continuous line placed in natural skin creases.

Operative Procedure

The proposed incision lines are infiltrated with a dilute solution of local anesthetic and epinephrine (40 ml 1% xylocaine with 1:100,000 epinephrine in 40 ml sterile water), except in the region of the superficial epigastric veins (see Fig. 25-6). Three separate stab incisions are then placed around the umbilicus and connected with the aid of skin hooks. The umbilicus is incised circumferentially down to the fascia.

While making the inferior incision, care is taken to preserve the superficial epigastric veins. The preoperative CT angiogram provides good information on their size and location. If the venous drainage of the flap is insufficient or thrombosis of the perforating vein or veins occurs after the anastomosis, the superficial epigastric veins can be used as an additional venous conduit. Two or three veins may be present, but they commonly unite further down the abdominal wall. The veins are dissected over a length of 2 to 3 cm and ligated with clips to make them easily retrievable later if needed (Fig. 25-7). If the caliber of the superficial epigastric artery is large enough, a skin island similar to the DIEAP flap can be harvested on these two vessels.

The incisions are continued down to the fascia. Beveling is avoided unless extra volume is required, because this may later lead to a depressed scar in the lower abdomen. Laterally, however, the flap may be beveled to include more fat and reduce residual dog-ears.

Dissection of the vascular pedicle of a DIEAP flap can be divided into three different technical stages: suprafascial, intramuscular, and submuscular. The most demanding stage is the intramuscular dissection of the vascular pedicle. Complete muscle relaxation is necessary until donor site closure is obtained.

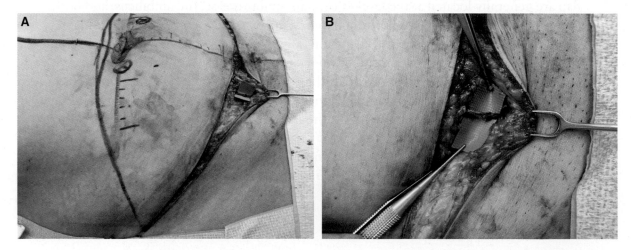

Fig. 25-7 A and **B,** The superficial epigastric vein is isolated and dissected over a short distance.

Suprafascial Dissection

Dissection begins laterally in the flanks and progresses medially with the aid of cutting and coagulating diathermy. The skin and subcutaneous fat are lifted off the external oblique fascia up to the lateral border of the rectus abdominis muscle. At this point dissection proceeds more cautiously as the perforators are identified. Gentle traction on the flap helps provide good exposure of the vessels.

Before starting the suprafascial dissection, an elastic hook can be positioned on the superior border of the superior incision to mark the vertical bearing of the most dominant perforator identified by the CTA scan. The dissection can progress rapidly to the preselected perforator, with ligation of the more laterally positioned perforators (Fig. 25-8).

If CT data are not available, the surgeon can try to visualize as many perforators as possible before selecting the largest one. This method needs some expertise, can be time consuming, and does not allow evaluation of all medial perforators.

If the caliber of one vessel is estimated to be insufficient, an adjacent perforator located on the same vertical line can also be dissected. The abdominal wall muscles must be relaxed at all times and the perforating vessels kept moist with normal saline solution. No antispasmodic agents are routinely used. When dissecting a perforator from the lateral side, it is important to realize that a side branch may be located more medially. Extra care must be taken when dissecting the full circumference of a vessel,

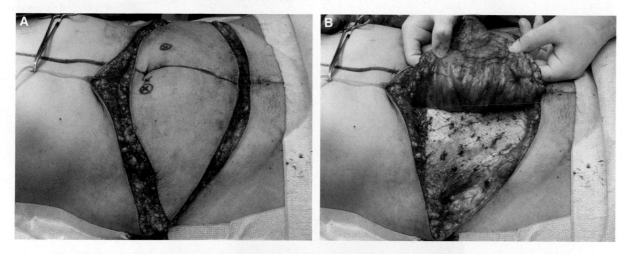

Fig. 25-8   A, The elastic retractor in the upper edge of the upper incision indicates the approximate positioning of the dominant perforator in a lateral to medial direction. **B,** The surgeon is close to the perforator and should dissect more slowly and meticulously.

but complete dissection helps prevent vessel damage when raising the flap from the contralateral side (Fig. 25-9). Next, the connective tissue cuff enclosing the perforator is incised circumferentially at the level of the deep fascia, exactly at the edge of the gap through the fascia to enter the loose connective tissue layer encircling the vessels (Fig. 25-10).

The anterior rectus fascia is then incised with scissors following the direction of the rectus abdominis muscle fibers at the rim of the tiny gap in the fascia through which the perforating vessel passes (Fig. 25-11, *A*). If more than one perforator is dissected, the different gaps can be connected with each other (Fig. 25-11, *B*). A small cuff of fascia may be left around the perforator if the vessel is small or the surgeon's experience is limited.

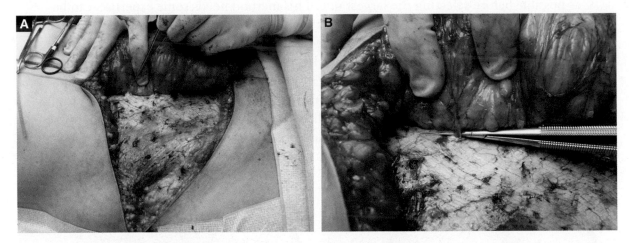

Fig. 25-9   **A,** Two perforators are identified on the same vertical line. **B,** In a first step, the upper perforator is freed circumferentially between the fat and the deep fascia.

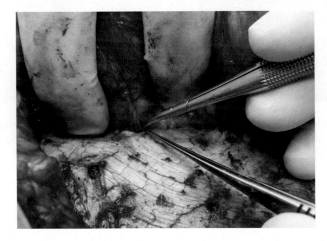

Fig. 25-10   The connective tissue cuff around the perforator is incised circumferentially at the level of the deep fascia to enter the loose connective tissue layer encircling the vessels.

Lifting the fascia helps mobilize the perforator, which can be freed by blunt dissection, gently pushing away the loose connective tissue. The perforator can be adherent to the deep surface of the anterior rectus fascia for a variable distance before it plunges into the muscle. The division of the fascia is continued superiorly for 3 to 4 cm and inferiorly to the lateral border of the rectus abdominis muscle in an oblique line toward the inguinal ligament (Fig. 25-12, *A*). At this point the division of the fascia is directed medially in the direction of the fibers of the external oblique muscle. This avoids a continuous area of weakness of the lower abdominal wall, because the fascia is closed on top of the rectus abdominis muscle (Fig. 25-12, *B*). The muscle is undermined over a short distance, just to expose the most caudal part of the deep inferior epigastric ar-

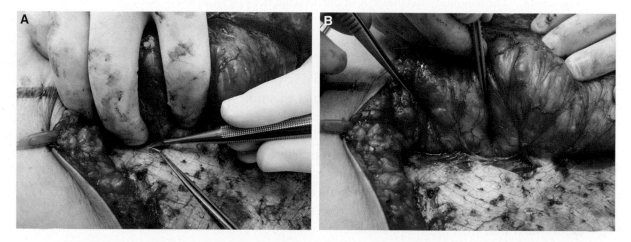

Fig. 25-11 **A** and **B,** The deep fascia is incised following the direction of the muscle fibers both cranially and distally, connecting multiple perforators if necessary.

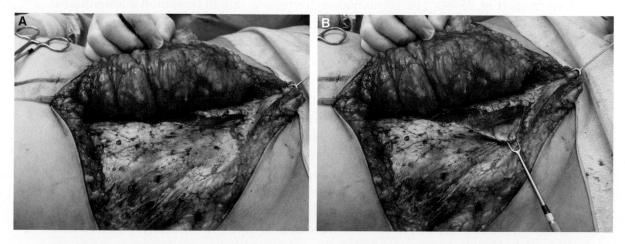

Fig. 25-12 **A,** The deep fascia is incised further caudally, remaining about 1 to 1.5 cm medial to the lateral border of the rectus abdominis muscle. **B,** By lifting and retracting the lateral part of the deep fascia, the lateral border of the muscle and the retromuscular fat pad can be visualized.

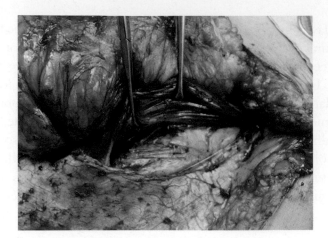

Fig. 25-13   The continuity and integrity of the deep inferior epigastric artery and vein are visually inspected.

tery and vein and check its integrity (Fig. 25-13). If these vessels are harmed or severely scarred, one might abandon the dissection at this time and, to avoid losing precious time, harvest the contralateral pedicle.

It is advisable to fully complete the DIEAP flap dissection on one side before progressing to the other. This allows a contralateral DIEAP flap or TRAM flap—a life boat—to be performed if the perforator is inadvertently damaged. The vessels must be protected at all stages, and complete muscle relaxation is necessary until donor site closure is obtained. As dissection progresses, the DIEAP flap should be secured to the abdominal wall with the aid of staples.

Intramuscular Dissection

Before dissecting between the muscle fibers, it is crucial to once again free the perforator circumferentially at the level of the loose connective tissue layer between the muscle and deep fascia (Fig. 25-14). The rectus abdominis muscle should be split in a longitudinal direction in the perimysial plane through which the perforating vessel traverses. Splitting the muscle fibers makes dissection easier as the vessel becomes larger (Fig. 25-15). By deroofing the perforator and the main axial vessel in and below the muscle, the course of the vessels become clear, and previously injured, more distal vessels can be excluded (Fig. 25-16). Wider exposure will facilitate dissection enormously. When the course of the perforator is clear, the vessels can be dissected circumferentially (Fig. 25-17).

The perforator is again liberated by blunt dissection, staying close to the vessel at all times as it remains covered by a thin layer of loose connective tissue. As a general rule, if resistance to dissection is encountered, a side branch or a nerve will be identified. Different muscular branches must be ligated with care. Hemoclips are placed or bipolar coagulation is done 1 to 2 mm away from the main vessel so that if a clip inadvertently comes off, it can easily be replaced. Moreover, the ligated branch can be used to hold the pedicle. This technique avoids damage and spasm of the main perforating vessel.

Placing a vessel loop around the vascular pedicle helps retract the vessels without any unnecessary tension. It is important that the vessel loop is held by hand and not

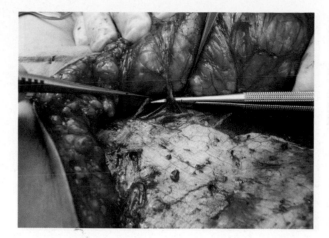

Fig. 25-14   Dissection continues around the perforator, freeing it just below the deep fascia.

Fig. 25-15   Splitting the muscle fibers in the plane of the perforator or perforators provides wide exposure and facilitates dissection. Perfect hemostasis must be maintained.

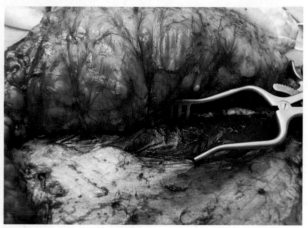

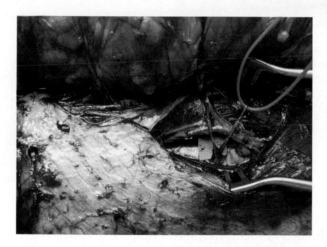

Fig. 25-16   Deroofing allows exact identification of the course of the vessels. Motor nerves are liberated and kept intact.

Fig. 25-17   Circumferential dissection around the perforator frees it completely.

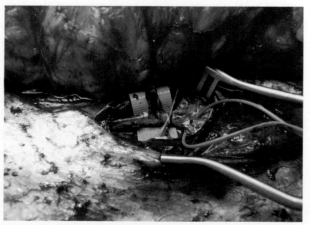

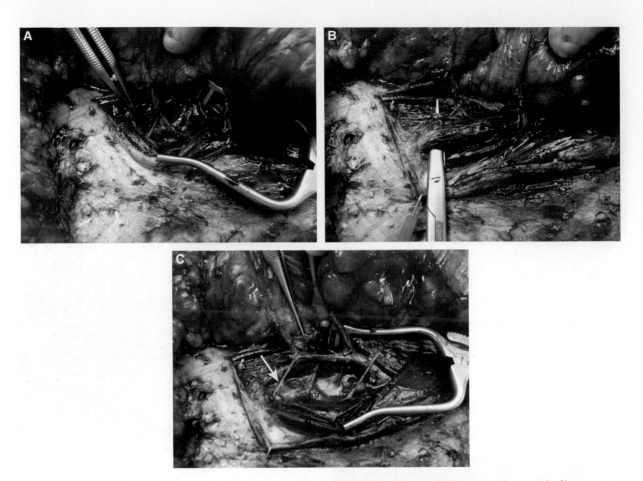

Fig. 25-18   A, The second, more cranial perforator is freed in the same fashion. **B,** The muscle fibers between both perforators are transected at the level of the nearest tendinous inscription, allowing the muscle to be more easily resutured after the flap and its pedicle are removed. This transection provides very wide exposure and easy access to the final part of the dissection. **C,** Motor nerves *(arrow)* running between two perforators and above the deep inferior epigastric artery need to be cut. If they are large, they can be resutured after harvest.

with a surgical instrument to have proper tactile feedback of the applied traction. All the side branches are ligated with bipolar coagulating diathermy and small hemoclips to the origin of the perforator on the axial branch of the deep inferior epigastric vessel at the posterior surface of the rectus abdominis muscle.

If two perforators in the same perimysial plane have been selected, the rectus abdominis muscle must be widely separated. If the perforators run in two adjacent perimysial planes, some fibers may have to be cut (Fig. 25-18). However, transection of large parts of the rectus abdominis muscle should be avoided.

Once the course of the perforator is known, a sensory nerve branch running intimately with the vessels can be identified, especially with lateral perforators. The sensory branch most commonly splits off the mixed segmental nerve at the level of the lateral branch of the deep inferior epigastric artery. Mixed segmental nerves can enter the rectus abdominis muscle at very variable locations, from 1 cm medial to its lateral

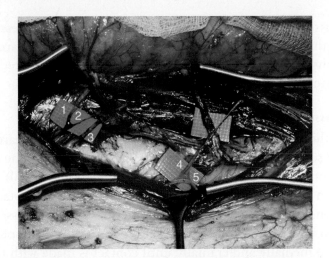

Fig. 25-19 The deep inferior epigastric artery perforators of the right rectus abdominis muscle are dissected, exposing two lateral perforators and the axial deep inferior epigastric vessels. After the nerves are dissected off the vessels, the following nerve branches can be identified. *1*, Mixed motor-sensory nerve crossing over the vessels and running superficially in the muscle, probably joining a more medial perforator nearby; *2*, Pure sensory branch joining the most cranial perforator; *3*, Motor or mixed nerve passing underneath the vessels. This one can easily be preserved; *4*, Motor nerve crossing over the vessels distal to the lowest perforator. This nerve can also be preserved; *5*, Recurrent motor branch innervating the lateral part of the muscle.

border on the anterior surface to two thirds medial to the lateral border on the posterior surface. These mixed nerves are accompanied by segmental blood vessels. In the distal third of the rectus abdominis muscle, these vessels anastomose with the most lateral vascular axis of the rectus muscle, which is often the lateral branch of the deep inferior epigastric vessels. The mixed nerves run oblique and anterior to the deep inferior epigastric vessels in most individuals and split into a sensory and motor branch at variable distances. At the point where the segmental nerves cross the deep inferior epigastric artery, motor branches often split into a medial branch and lateral or recurrent branch that innervates the lateral part of the rectus muscle. When harvesting a muscle-sparing TRAM flap, all of these motor nerves will be cut, thereby denervating large parts of the rectus abdominis muscle (Fig. 25-19). The pure sensory branches join with the perforating vessels and run together to the skin. When dissecting the perforator vessels of the rectus abdominis muscle, as reported previously, the sensory branch of the segmental nerves can easily be visualized and dissected over a length of 3 to 9 cm.

During dissection all motor nerves crossing from lateral to medial over the vascular axis should be dissected for a few centimeters and preserved (see Fig. 25-19). Many motor or mixed sensory/motor nerves run very close (mostly anterior, but not exclusively) to the lateral branch of the deep inferior epigastric artery and vein. They need to be lifted off by staying very close to the epineurium to avoid any damage to the vessels. Vasa nervorum may bleed for a moment. Occasionally, the nerve runs between the artery and the vein. In those cases, it needs to be cut and resutured. By liberating the nerves, the muscle can be retracted and split more, obtaining better exposure. At the end of the dissection, when the pedicle is divided distally, the vessels can easily be passed underneath the intact motor nerves. When two perforators are dissected and a motor branch runs between those two perforators, the nerve will need to be cut. Once the flap is harvested, it can be resutured.

Submuscular Dissection

The distolateral border of the rectus abdominis is raised. Special care is taken not to injure the mixed segmental nerves entering the muscle laterally. The lateral border is freed cranially until a large segmental nerve is observed (Fig. 25-20). Mobilizing this nerve laterally can increase exposure. The plane posterior to the distal rectus abdominis muscle is opened, exposing the main deep inferior epigastric vessel. Side branches of the main stem are ligated, and the dissection continues by retracting the rectus abdominis muscle medially and cranially until contact is made with the surgical field of intramuscular dissection. A vessel loop positioned around the axial vessels during the intramuscular dissection can be pulled through to ensure that all adhesions of the pedicle are released (see Fig. 25-20).

The length of the pedicle can be tailored to meet the needs of different recipient sites or the demands of the flap's shape. The more distal the perforator's location in the flap, the further the deep inferior epigastric vessels need to be dissected into the groin. Frequently, however, the pedicle can be transected at the lateral border of the rectus abdominis muscle. At this level, there is sufficient pedicle diameter and length for a safe microsurgical anastomosis. Furthermore, the first and most distal muscular branch of the deep inferior epigastric artery can be preserved, ensuring proper vascularization of the distal part of the muscle (see Fig. 25-20).

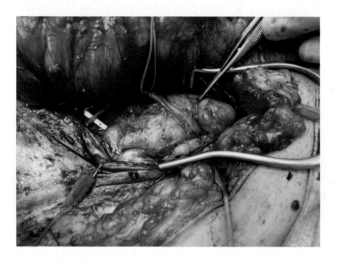

Fig. 25-20 The intramuscular dissection is connected to the submuscular dissection and continued caudally. Care is taken not to cut the segmental nerves at the lateral border of the muscle *(yellow bar)*. Dissection proceeds down to the first medial muscular branch of the deep inferior epigastric artery *(forceps)*. If more length is needed, one can continue down to the iliac vessels.

If one is certain that the blood flow through the deep inferior epigastric vessel is sufficient, the remainder of the flap can be raised. In cases of midline scars, or when a large flap is needed, the same vascular dissection can be performed on the contralateral side. Otherwise, all remaining perforators are ligated, the umbilicus is released, and the entire skin flap is raised. The pedicle is finally transected when the recipient vessels have been prepared. A hemoclip can be placed on the lateral vena comitans to help orient the pedicle.

After the pedicle is divided, the flap is turned over and the vessels placed carefully onto its undersurface. One has to be meticulous about the position of the pedicle, because it tends to rotate very easily, especially if only one perforator has been harvested. The flap is then weighed, photographed, and transferred. The ischemia time is noted. The flap is placed on moist gauze at the recipient site to prevent desiccation and stapled to the surrounding skin for security. The flap may be rotated to facilitate microsurgery, provided this is noted and the rotation reversed at the end of the procedure.

Donor Site Closure and Fashioning the Umbilicus

Because no fascia has been resected, primary tension-free closure of the fascia with a running nonabsorbable 1-0 mattress suture is always possible. The upper skin flap is undermined with cutting diathermy to the level of the xiphoid and costal margin. Care is taken not to cut the cranial superior epigastric perforators, because they guarantee the blood flow to the abdominoplasty flap, together with the lateral intercostal perforators. Two suction drains are placed at the upper and lower margins of the skin flaps and exit suprapubically on each side of the midline.

Three 4-0 absorbable stitches are positioned between the subcutaneous layer of the umbilicus and the deep fascia (at 3, 6, and 9 o'clock positions). These are left in place with the needle and will be tied only after a third passage through the subcutaneous layer of the abdominal wall in the final umbilicus position. The operating table is put in a flexed position to facilitate closure of the anterior abdominal wall. After a temporary midline closure, the position of the umbilicus is marked on the anterior abdominal wall, and a 2 to 2.5 cm vertical line is drawn and incised.

The abdominoplasty flap is thinned at the site of the new umbilicus by progressive trimming of the subcutaneous fat 3 cm around the new site of the umbilicus. In particular, the upper part is thinned aggressively. The umbilicus is then passed through the defect and inset, and the three absorbable stitches are tied. One more absorbable suture is placed at the 12 o'clock position, only approaching the dermis of the abdominoplasty flap skin and the dermis of the umbilicus. The skin is closed with continuous 5-0 nonabsorbable suture.

Scarpa's fascia is approximated with interrupted 2-0 absorbable sutures with particular attention to medial advancement of the wound edges of the abdominoplasty flap to reduce the dog-ears in the flanks. Finally, interrupted 3-0 sutures are placed intradermally to evert the skin edges, and a skin adhesive is applied. No further abdominal dressing is needed.

CASE EXAMPLES
Deep Inferior Epigastric Artery Perforator Flap for Bilateral Breast Reconstruction

This 61-year-old woman consulted for a bilateral secondary autologous breast reconstruction. Seven years earlier she had undergone a modified radical mastectomy of her left breast for treatment of a pT3N1M0 lobular carcinoma, followed by chemotherapy and radiation therapy (Fig. 25-21, *A*). Four years later, a multifocal invasive lobular carcinoma pT2N1M0 was diagnosed on the right side. This was treated by a modified radical mastectomy, followed by chemotherapy and radiation therapy. Three years later, after an uneventful oncologic follow-up, she consulted for bilateral reconstruction. Bilateral free DIEAP flaps were performed (Fig. 25-21, *B*). No postoperative complications occurred. Six months postoperatively, a bilateral nipple reconstruction was performed through a modified CV flap. Three months later, a bilateral tattoo of the areolar area and nipple were performed (Fig. 25-21, *C* and *D*).

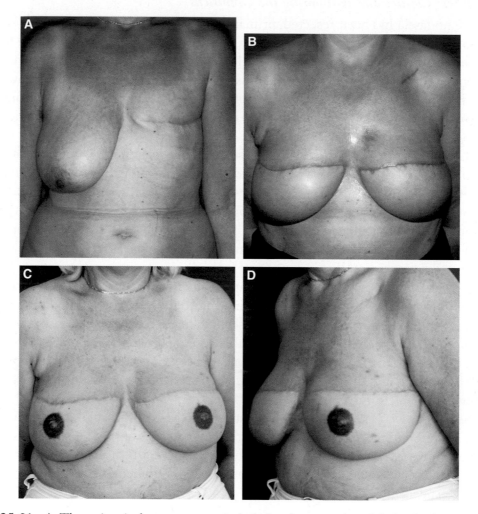

Fig. 25-21 A, The patient is shown preoperatively, before her second modified radical mastectomy. She presented for a secondary bilateral reconstruction 3 years after the second mastectomy. **B,** She is shown after bilateral DIEAP flap transfer and before nipple-areola complex reconstruction. **C** and **D,** Her final result is shown 1 year postoperatively, after nipple-areola reconstruction.

Deep Inferior Epigastric Artery Perforator Flap for Lymphedema

This 40-year-old woman presented with severe lymphedema of her right lower leg after a major degloving injury of her right upper leg and knee. Before arriving at our clinic, she had undergone multiple corrective procedures at and around the knee but was left with significant soft tissue loss in the anterior, lateral, and posterior thigh area (Fig. 25-22, *A* through *C*). Additionally, she had developed peripheral lymphedema of her right leg, distal to the lesion. A resurfacing procedure was performed with a bilateral DIEAP flap, both pedicles being connected to the superficial femoral vessels (Fig. 25-22, *D*). Together with the DIEAP flap, the superficial lymph nodes of the left groin were transferred, vascularized by the superficial circumflex iliac vessels. The lymph nodes were positioned in a subcutaneous plane, on the inner side of the knee directed toward the popliteal fossa. The superficial circumflex iliac artery and vein were anasto-

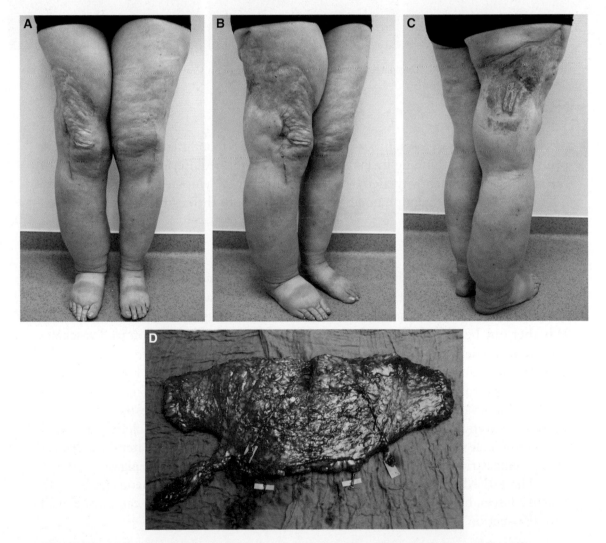

Fig. 25-22 A-C, The patient is shown preoperatively, after a degloving injury of the right upper thigh. She had lymphedema of the right leg and foot. **D,** A bilateral (Siamese-type) DIEAP flap, together with the superficial lymph nodes, is vascularized by the superficial circumflex iliac artery and vein.

Continued

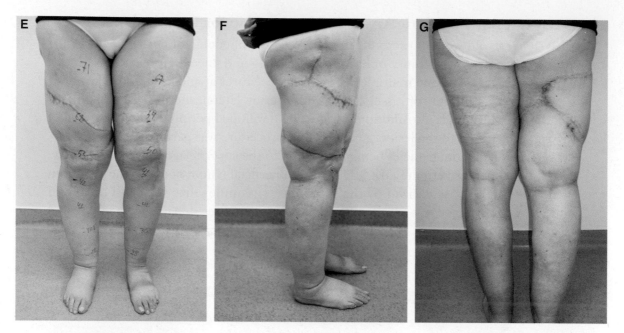

Fig. 25-22, cont'd   E-G, The patient is shown after undergoing a skin-tightening procedure and liposuction for flap-thinning.

mosed in the popliteal fossa. In a secondary procedure 6 months later, a skin-tightening procedure and flap thinning by liposuction were performed. Residual lymphedema of the foot was subsequently treated by two additional distal lymphovenous anastomoses. The DIEAP flap with lymph node transfer solved both the aesthetic and functional problems in this case.

MODIFICATIONS

The basic design of the DIEAP flap can be modified to accommodate a variety of soft tissue defects and recipient sites. The shape of the skin paddle can be oriented in an oblique or horizontal direction. The main problem is defining the size of the skin paddle. Whether one believes in the perforasome theory[28,29] or a more randomized vascularization of the dermal plexus,[30,31] it is still impossible to determine preoperatively the exact territory that will be safely vascularized by one single perforator. Intraoperatively, additional information on tissue perfusion can be obtained using laser-induced fluorescence of indocyanine green,[32,33] especially if very large flaps are harvested or aberrant vascular anatomy is suspected. If there is any doubt, we recommend including a second vascular pedicle (contralateral deep inferior epigastric artery or ipsilateral superficial inferior epigastric artery, superficial circumflex iliac artery, or superior epigastric artery).

The DIEAP flap may also be thinned by trimming the subcutaneous fat beneath Scarpa's fascia, but this can be dangerous and an equally good result can be achieved with liposuction of the flap 6 months after surgery.

The length of the vascular pedicle can also be altered. A perforator flap without a deep inferior epigastric vessel and with a very small perforator anastomosis can be used in select patients. The flap elevation time is shortened, and there are many small recipient vessels throughout the body to which the perforator can be anastomosed.[34]

As mentioned previously, in each DIEAP flap a pure sensory branch of the tenth or eleventh intercostal nerve that innervates the rectus abdominis muscle may be isolated.[16] This branch is fairly large and joins the perforating vessels where they pierce the anterior rectus fascia. It can be mobilized by retrograde dissection through the muscle to the point at which it joins its motor branch. It is then anastomosed to a suitable donor nerve at the recipient site, providing cutaneous sensation to the flap.

Moreover, if a very large DIEAP flap has been harvested, the arterial input may be supercharged by an additional anastomosis with the ipsilateral or contralateral superficial inferior epigastric artery or with the contralateral deep inferior epigastric vessels. In extreme cases, the superficial circumflex iliac vessels can be included to provide better vascularization of the lateral tips of the flap.

In case of venous congestion the venous outflow may be supercharged by an additional anastomosis with the ipsilateral or contralateral superficial inferior epigastric vein, or any vein from the deep or superficial system that is large enough to be anastomosed.

The two venae comitantes of the pedicle are often connected by a common branch. In case of venous congestion, it is also possible to anastomose the ipsilateral superficial inferior epigastric vein to the second vein of the pedicle to provide the superficial system with an outflow through the first vein of the pedicle.

In cases of midline scars, or when a large flap is needed and one is uncertain as to whether or not enough volume can be transferred on one perforator, the vascular dissection can be performed on both sides (Siamese flap).[9]

The DIEAP flap can also be transferred in conjunction with a lymph node flap to treat arm lymphedema.[35,36] A number of superficial lymph nodes from the groin, surrounding the superficial circumflex vessels, are harvested in conjunction with the DIEAP flap on its contralateral side. Though this is a conjoint flap, both flaps cannot survive on the contralateral perforators of the deep inferior epigastric artery only. The deep inferior epigastric artery of the DIEAP flap is anastomosed to the internal mammary artery, and either the superficial inferior epigastric artery or the superficial circumflex iliac artery of the contralateral side is anastomosed to one of the axial recipient vessels (lateral thoracic, serratus branch, thoracodorsal vessels, or large lateral intercostal vessels).

The vascular territory of the DIEAP flap can be supercharged or extended by creating conjoint flaps. Perforator or direct cutaneous flaps from neighboring vascular territories can be taken together with a DIEAP flap in one big skin paddle if very large surfaces need to be covered. Obviously, the feeding vessels and their perforators will need to be dissected as well, and multiple vessels will need to be anastomosed either to the same recipient vessel or to different recipient vessels, according to the anatomy of the recipient site.

PITFALLS AND RISK FACTORS

The dissection of a DIEAP flap has a steep learning curve, involving a very specific dissection technique of the perforating vessels. As long as dissection is performed close to the vessels in a plane of loose connective tissue surrounding the pedicle, side branches and crossing nerves can be easily identified and preserved. Dissection through other planes will cause excessive bleeding and slow the surgeon down. Two golden rules must be applied in any type of perforator flap surgery: the field must be bloodless and exposure must be wide. A common mistake is to be misled by eagerness to follow the perforator vessels into the deep tissues in a small hole. Muscle, septum, or other tissues through which the perforators travel should be opened widely to obtain a clear overview and control bleeding.

A number of technical considerations are important in planning and executing the dissection. The wrong choice of perforator can lead to disastrous complications. With the help of a CT scan and direct intraoperative visualization, the most important perforator can be identified. Any unusual course along the length of the perforator, such as rounding the medial or lateral edge of the rectus abdominis muscle, must be considered. Dominance of the superficial system should be recognized at the beginning of the flap harvest, when the lower edge of the flap is incised. In these cases, a superficial inferior epigastric artery perforator (SIEAP) flap should be harvested.

During pedicle dissection, vessels should not be overstretched. The use of vessel loops is limited to the actual dissection. These should not be left in place, because they can accidentally come under traction in a later phase of the operation.

Side branches should be ligated at a distance of 2 to 3 mm away from the pedicle. When a vascular clip or a ligating suture is placed too close to the main pedicle, it can interrupt the arterial or venous flow. Care should be taken during the motor nerve dissection. Excessive traction or crushing of the nerve can permanently affect its function.

In case of a free flap, torsion of the pedicle can easily occur during flap transfer. Exact orientation with the help of vascular clips can help prevent this problem. Following anastomosis, kinking of the pedicle can be avoided by placing the pedicle in smooth curves once shaping is completed. When shaping the fat, excessive defatting can lead to areas of partial flap necrosis or fat necrosis. Delayed defatting with liposuction is a safer procedure. Poorly vascularized areas, such as zone IV, should be resected during the initial procedure to reduce postoperative complications.

In inexperienced hands, DIEAP flap dissection will require a longer operating time than a conventional myocutaneous flap. After a number of cases, operating time will decrease and be comparable to myocutaneous flap harvesting, or even shorter if a limited pedicle length is needed.[26,34]

Abdominal scarring is probably the most important risk factor for raising a DIEAP flap. It can cause major problems when dissecting perforators and epigastric vessels. Intramuscular scarring is not always diagnosed on preoperative ultrasound and can spread out farther than suspected from the place and length of a previous incision.

Smoking is considered a relative contraindication to a raising a DIEAP flap. Our impression is that in smokers the area most distant from the vascular pedicle (zone IV) is less well perfused, with prolonged vascular spasm. Smokers who request elective delayed reconstructions are asked to stop smoking at least 3 months before becoming a candidate for surgery. This is an additional way to test the patient's motivation. A nonmotivated patient and a poor general medical condition are the only absolute contraindications.

CONCLUSION

The DIEAP flap has become the workhorse not only for breast reconstruction but also for reconstructing large surface defects on the torso and proximal parts of the limbs. The key feature in the preoperative phase is to identify the artery of the dominant perforator by CT or MRI. This provides exact information on the size and position of the vessel on the abdominal wall. Additionally, it gives important information on the three-dimensional structure and branching of the perforator vessel.

Every surgeon needs to develop his or her own surgical style during training and while progressing through the learning curve. Independent of a surgeron's surgical technique, easy and successful exposure of the perforator vessel within the rectus abdominis muscle can be obtained by following three easy principles: (1) Obtain wide exposure by splitting the muscle following the direction of the muscle fibers, (2) stay close to the perforator vessel within the loose connective tissue layer that surrounds it, and (3) maintain a bloodless field by systematically ligating or clipping the side branches. Excessive traction on the vessels must be avoided; it is the most common reason for thrombosis caused by tearing of the intima.

Venous drainage occurs through either the deep or superficial system. Dominance may only become apparent after anastomosing the donor vessels to the recipient vessels. One needs to be flexible and, therefore, prepared to change the intraoperative plan and provide extra drainage by connecting an additional vein. Arterial grafts are ideal for bridging venous connections, but supplementary microsurgical anastomoses can be avoided by systematically leaving some extra length of the superficial epigastric vein at the beginning of the procedure. Critical inspection and careful positioning of the pedicle of the flap just before closing is the most crucial step to avoid early postoperative flow problems.

References

1. Boyd JB, Taylor GI, Corlett R. The vascular territories of the superior epigastric and the deep inferior epigastric systems. Plast Reconstr Surg 73:1-16, 1984.
2. Holmström H. The free abdominoplasty flap and its use in breast reconstruction. An experimental study and clinical case report. Scand J Plast Reconstr Surg 13:423-427, 1979.
3. Robbins TH. Rectus abdominis myocutaneous flap for breast reconstruction. Aust N Z J Surg 49:527-530, 1979.
4. Koshima I, Soeda S. Inferior epigastric artery skin flaps without rectus abdominis muscle. Br J Plast Surg 42:645-648, 1989.
5. Koshima I, Moriguchi T, Soeda S, et al. Free thin paraumbilical perforator-based flaps. Ann Plast Surg 29:12-17, 1992.
6. Pennington DG, Nettle WJ, Lam P. Microvascular augmentation of the blood supply of the contralateral side of the free transverse rectus abdominis musculocutaneous flap. Ann Plast Surg 31:123-126; discussion 126-127, 1993.
7. Allen RJ, Treece P. Deep inferior epigastric perforator flap for breast reconstruction. Ann Plast Surg 32:32-38, 1994.

8. Blondeel PN. One hundred free DIEP flap breast reconstructions: a personal experience. Br J Plast Surg 52:104-111, 1999.

9. Blondeel PN, Boeckx WD. Refinements in free flap breast reconstruction: the free bilateral deep inferior epigastric perforator flap anastomosed to the internal mammary artery. Br J Plast Surg 47:495-501, 1994.

10. Van Landuyt K, Hamdi M, Blondeel P, et al. The pyramidalis muscle free flap. Br J Plast Surg 56:585-592, 2003.

11. Milloy FJ, Anson BJ, McAfee DK. The rectus abdominis muscle and the epigastric arteries. Surg Gynecol Obstet 110:293-302, 1960.

12. Heitmann C, Felmerer G, Durmus C, et al. Anatomical features of perforator blood vessels in the deep inferior epigastric perforator flap. Br J Plast Surg 53:205-208, 2000.

13. Kikuchi N, Murakami G, Kashiwa H, et al. Morphometrical study of the arterial perforators of the deep inferior epigastric perforator flap. Surg Radiol Anat 23:375-381, 2001.

14. Blondeel PN, Beyens G, Verhaeghe R, et al. Doppler flowmetry in the planning of perforator flaps. Br J Plast Surg 51:202-209, 1998.

15. Vandevoort M, Vranckx JJ, Fabre G. Perforator topography of the deep inferior epigastric perforator flap in 100 cases of breast reconstruction. Plast Reconstr Surg 109:1912-1918, 2002.

16. Blondeel PN, Demuynck M, Mete D, et al. Sensory nerve repair in perforator flaps for autologous breast reconstruction: sensational or senseless? Br J Plast Surg 52:37-44, 1999.

17. Rozen WM, Ashton MW, Murray AC, et al. Avoiding denervation of rectus abdominis in DIEP flap harvest: the importance of medial row perforators. Plast Reconstr Surg 122:710-716, 2008.

18. Rozen WM, Ashton MW, Kiil BJ, et al. Avoiding denervation of rectus abdominis in DIEP flap harvest II: an intraoperative assessment of the nerves to rectus. Plast Reconstr Surg 122:1321-1325, 2008.

19. Taylor GI, Daniel RK. The anatomy of several free flap donor sites. Plast Reconstr Surg 56:243-253, 1975.

20. Blondeel PN, Arnstein M, Verstraete K, et al. Venous congestion and blood flow in free transverse rectus abdominis myocutaneous and deep inferior epigastric perforator flaps. Plast Reconstr Surg 106:1295-1299, 2000.

21. Carramenha e Costa MA, Carriquiry C, Vasconez LO, et al. An anatomic study of the venous drainage of the transverse rectus abdominis musculocutaneous flap. Plast Reconstr Surg 79:208-217, 1987.

22. Felmerer G, Muehlberger T, Berens von Rautenfeld D, et al. The lymphatic system of the deep inferior epigastric artery perforator flap: an anatomical study. Br J Plast Surg 55:335-339, 2002.

23. Masia J, Clavero JA, Larranaga JR, et al. Multidetector-row computed tomography in the planning of abdominal perforator flaps. J Plast Reconstr Aesthet Surg 59:594-599, 2006.

24. Masia J, Larranaga J, Clavero JA, et al. The value of the multidetector row computed tomography for the preoperative planning of deep inferior epigastric artery perforator flap: our experience in 162 cases. Ann Plast Surg 60:29-36, 2008.

> The authors presented a preoperative abdominal wall study conducted using a multidetector scanner in 162 women who had undergone breast reconstruction with abdominal perforator flaps. The scanner provided valuable preoperative information enabling identification of the most suitable perforator for its caliber, location, course, and anatomic relationships. Once located, the surgeon could proceed directly to its dissection during surgery, making it a faster and safer technique.

25. Rozen WM, Garcia-Tutor E, Alonso-Burgos A, et al. Planning and optimising DIEP flaps with virtual surgery: the Navarra experience. J Plast Reconstr Aesthet Surg 63:289-297, 2010.

26. Uppal RS, Casaer B, Van Landuyt K, et al. The efficacy of preoperative mapping of perforators in reducing operative times and complications in perforator flap breast reconstruction. J Plast Reconstr Aesthet Surg 62:859-864, 2009.

   The effects of preoperative perforator mapping on various aspects of perforator flap surgery were studied. They concluded that it can reduce operative times and facilitate selection of the most reliable perforators. By ensuring good flap perfusion, preoperative mapping reduces length of stay (contributing to savings for the hospital), complications such as postoperative fat necrosis, and delayed healing. This study found that operative times were shortest after CT scanning compared with duplex perforator mapping.

27. Greenspun D, Vasile J, Levine JL, et al. Anatomic imaging of abdominal perforator flaps without ionizing radiation: seeing is believing with magnetic resonance imaging angiography. J Reconstr Microsurg 26:37-44, 2010.

28. Rozen WM, Ashton MW. Re: The perforasome theory: vascular anatomy and clinical implications. Plast Reconstr Surg 125:1845-1846, 2010.

29. Saint-Cyr M, Wong C, Schaverien M, et al. The perforasome theory: vascular anatomy and clinical implications. Plast Reconstr Surg 124:1529-1544, 2009.

   The authors investigated the three- and four-dimensional arterial vascular territory of a single perforator, known as a perforasome, in major clinically relevant areas of the body. Direct and indirect linking vessels play a critical part in perforator flap perfusion, and every clinically significant perforator has the potential to become either a pedicle or free perforator flap.

30. Tregaskiss AP, Goodwin AN, Acland RD. The cutaneous arteries of the anterior abdominal wall: a three-dimensional study. Plast Reconstr Surg 120:442-450, 2007.

   The authors examined the vascular anatomy of the abdominal integument to determine why the rate of complications is significant in some series and how they may be prevented. The unpredictable orientation and course of deep inferior epigastric artery perforators indicates that the blood supply of abdominal perforator flaps may often be more random than axial. This accounts for much of the ischemia-related morbidity observed with flaps based on these perforators.

31. Tregaskiss AP, Goodwin AN, Bright LD, et al. Three-dimensional CT angiography: a new technique for imaging microvascular anatomy. Clin Anat 20:116-123, 2007.

32. Holm C, Mayr M, Hofter E, et al. Assessment of the patency of microvascular anastomoses using microscope-integrated near-infrared angiography: a preliminary study. Microsurgery 29:509-514, 2009.

33. Holm C, Mayr M, Hofter E, et al. Perfusion zones of the DIEP flap revisited: a clinical study. Plast Reconstr Surg 117:37-43, 2006.

34. Koshima I, Inagawa K, Urushibara K, et al. Paraumbilical perforator flap without deep inferior epigastric vessels. Plast Reconstr Surg 102:1052-1057, 1998.

35. LoTempio M, Studinger R, Vaisille C, et al. Lymph node transplantation in breast reconstruction using perforator flaps. Cancer Res 69(Suppl 24), abstract no. 3112, 2009.

   The authors introduced a treatment for breast reconstruction that combines the DIEAP flap with lymph node transplantation for lymphedema.

36. Tobbia D, Semple J, Baker A, et al. Experimental assessment of autologous lymph node transplantation as treatment of postsurgical lymphedema. Plast Reconstr Surg 124:777-786, 2009.

26

Superficial Inferior Epigastric Artery Perforator Flap

Milomir Ninkovic
Charlotte Holm

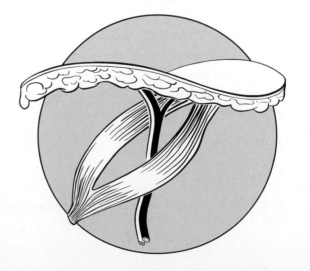

The first mention of the superficial epigastric artery perforator (SIEAP) flap* was by John Wood[1] in 1863, who used an SIEAP pedicle flap to correct a severe burn contracture of the forearm of an 8-year-old girl. Describing the blood supply to the lower abdomen, Wood stated: "The largest and most important of these are the superficial epigastric vessels proceeding from the common femoral across Poupart's ligament, upward and inward toward the umbilicus . . ." The SIEAP pedicle flap was applied by Shaw and Payne[2] and by Barfred[3] for forearm coverage. Antia and Buch[4] appear to be the first to have used the SIEAP flap as a free flap for reconstructing a soft tissue deficiency of the face. This flap was applied as an abdominal dermofat graft by direct anastomosis of blood vessels. Daniel and Taylor[5] and Boeckx et al[6] also used it as a free flap.

The SIEAP flap has been described for different reconstructions, including abdominal wall, head and neck, limb, and vaginal.[7-9] For breast reconstruction, use of the true *abdominoplasty*/SIEAP flap has been reported in a limited number of patients. Grotting[10] first described this flap for immediate breast reconstruction in 1991. In 1994 Volpe et al[11] showed the versatility of the SIEAP flap for breast reconstruction. This flap was reported to be transplanted successfully between identical twins for breast reconstruction in 1995 by Hartrampf et al.[12] Arnez et al[13,14] described using an SIEAP flap to reduce donor site morbidity in breast reconstruction.

An SIEAP flap could be an ideal flap for breast reconstruction because of both the donor site morbidity and the quality and volume of the tissue (Fig. 26-1). However, the flap has never been very popular because of its variable vascular anatomy, insufficient pedicle length, small vessel diameter, and insufficient blood supply for the complete lower abdominal region. Compared with other flaps such as the transverse rectus abdominis musculocutaneous (TRAM) or deep inferior epigastric artery perforator (DIEAP) flaps, which are harvested from the same donor site, the SIEAP flap is rarely used for breast reconstruction.

---

*Although there is no consensus whether the superficial inferior epigastric artery flap is truly a perforator flap, it is designated here as the SIEAP flap.

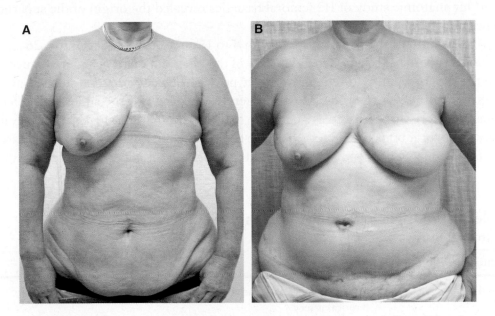

Fig. 26-1 A, This woman was seen for breast reconstruction. She is a typical candidate for reconstruction using an SIEAP flap. **B,** She is shown postoperatively.

ANATOMY

The blood supply of the abdominal wall is complex, with major contributions from the superficial circumflex iliac artery, deep circumflex iliac artery, superior and deep inferior epigastric arteries, external oblique perforators, and the superficial inferior epigastric artery. Many authors believe that the latter represents the key to a complete understanding of the blood supply of the abdominal wall, and is its single most important source of blood.[11,15,16] This artery can supply almost the entire hemiabdomen. The region runs from the inguinal ligament upward to the caudal border of the pectoralis muscle (sparing a triangle limited by the anterior axillary line, the caudal border of the pectoralis muscle, and the last caudal rib) and medially to the lateral border of the contralateral rectus abdominis muscle. Using the SIEAP flap for a free tissue transfer, we have increased the vascular territory by anastomosing a contralateral superficial vein to support perfusion of the most medial part of the lower abdominal flap pedicle on the superficial inferior epigastric artery.

As a result of repeated investigations of the blood supply of the lower abdominal wall, we conclude that the primary vascular source of the lower abdomen is still unclear. The superficial inferior epigastric artery pedicle was reported to be missing in 35% of the cadavers in a study with 100 dissections.[17] In two clinical studies, the pedicle was missing in 13%[18] and 40%.[19] Because of this variability, the superficial inferior epigastric artery is not always responsible for the dominant blood supply to the suprafascial abdominal wall.

Our anatomic study of 112 femoral triangles revealed the origin of the superficial epigastric artery in all cases (Table 26-1).

The length of the pedicle varied from 8 to 15 cm (mean 12.5 cm) (Fig. 26-2). An additional superficial vein was found in 75% of the cases and was situated more medially than the superficial inferior epigastric artery pedicle. The contralateral superficial vein was present 100% of the time. Most frequently, the origin of the superficial inferior epigastric artery was observed as a common pedicle with the superficial circumflex iliac artery (47%) or it branched directly from the common femoral artery (36.5%). The artery had its origin from the deep femoral artery together with the superficial circumflex iliac

Table 26-1   Origin of the Superficial Inferior Epigastric Artery From Anatomic Study

Occurrence Rate	Origin
47.0%	Common pedicle with the superficial circumflex iliac artery from the femoral artery
36.5%	Directly from the common femoral artery
12.0%	From the deep femoral artery together with the superficial circumflex iliac artery
2.5%	Directly from the external pudendal artery or the inferior epigastric artery
2.0%	Directly from the deep femoral artery

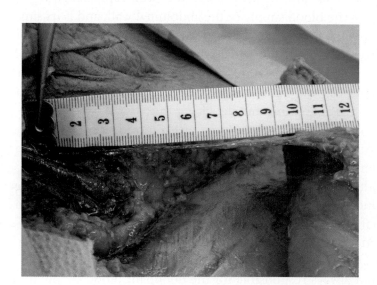

Fig. 26-2   The length of the superficial inferior epigastric artery varied from 8 to 15 cm in our study.

artery in 12% of the cases, from the external pudendal artery and the inferior epigastric artery in 2.5%, and directly from the deep femoral artery in 2%. Regardless of its origin, the superficial inferior epigastric artery arose approximately 1 to 3 cm inferior to the inguinal ligament. The vessel traversed through the femoral sheath and fascia cribrosa and turned superiorly to course anterior to the inguinal ligament. It ascended between the membranous and fatty layers of the superficial fascia, and usually reached as high as the area of the umbilicus. This artery supplied blood to the superficial lymph nodes, superficial fascia, and the skin in the area covered. The diameter of the vessel ranged from 0.4 to 2.6 mm (mean 1.2 mm).

Most books and papers describe the position of the superficial inferior epigastric artery pedicle as approximately midway between the superior iliac crest and the pubis. However, our anatomic study and clinical experience have shown that the pedicle lies slightly more laterally (Fig. 26-3). If neither pedicle is usable because of the small vessel caliber, the sole superficial vein must be dissected and preserved bilaterally. Using these veins could make the venous drainage safer, especially when using the contralateral SIEAP pedicle or a DIEAP flap for reconstructing a large breast or covering huge soft tissue defects. The anatomic study and clinical experience have shown a different anatomic pattern for each case. The dominance of blood supply from the most superficial to the deepest layer must be determined during surgery. For lower abdominal flaps, the SIEAP flap should be dissected on both sides. If these vessels are not suitable for microvascular transfer, deep perforators of the DIEAP or TRAM flap are used.

The SIEAP flap is based on direct perforators that pierce only the deep fascia. Discussion still exists over whether the SIEAP flap is a true perforator flap, because the pedicle does not perforate the muscle or intermuscular septum.

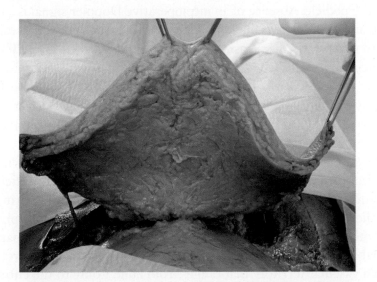

Fig. 26-3 The vascular pedicle of an SIEAP flap is dissected.

SURGICAL TECHNIQUE
Surface Landmarks

The SIEAP flap can be designed in different ways, according to the reconstructive requirements. The flap can be a pedicle or free flap, and it can be created in a transverse (horizontal), vertical, or oblique fashion. By staggering the inferior ends of the incisions and undermining to achieve mobility for closure of the angles, it is possible to rotate the base through an arc of 180 degrees.

If an SIEAP flap is used as a pedicle flap, the arc of rotation and amount of translation depend on the origin and length of the pedicle. The flap is most commonly designed with a transverse (horizontal) orientation. In this case, it extends from the ipsilateral superior iliac spine to the lateral border of the rectus muscle on the contralateral side, and from the level of the umbilicus to the level of the pubic tubercle. The advantage of this design is that the donor site is closed as in an abdominoplasty procedure.

The patient should be in a standing position when preoperative markings are drawn. For identification of the superficial inferior epigastric vessels, the midpoint between the anterior iliac spine and pubic tubercle is marked. Often the superficial inferior epigastric artery pedicle can be found lateral to this point.

Vascular Anatomy

The origin of the superficial inferior epigastric vessels is found 1 to 3 cm below the inguinal ligament. The pedicle pierces the cribriform fascia one finger's width beneath the inguinal ligament and ascends in the subcutaneous tissue to the level of the umbilicus. The exact location of the artery can be confirmed by Doppler ultrasound or a duplex color investigation. Only the surgical dissection itself at the level of the inguinal ligament confirms the presence and caliber of the pedicle. In my clinical experience, the caliber of the pedicle is sufficiently large if the Doppler signal is strong enough after dissection of the pedicle. Absence of an intraoperative Doppler signal is a contraindication for using an SIEAP flap. If the Doppler signal is present but very weak, papaverine can be used to release vascular spasms. The vessels are checked 15 to 20 minutes later to evaluate the viability of the flap.

Objective intraoperative algorithms based on the size of the superficial inferior epigastric artery pedicle have been previously proposed, and they suggest that an SIEAP flap can be raised if the caliber of the artery is at least 1.5 mm at the level of the abdominal incision.[20]

Even if a sufficient pedicle is found, however, another problem with the SIEAP flap is the variability of the vascular territory provided by the superficial epigastric pedicle. As demonstrated by our in vivo perfusion measurements, confirmed by studies using CTA, there is substantial variability in the superficial inferior epigastric artery angiosome, both among patients and between the two sides of a single patient.[21,22] The strongly variable branching pattern of the superficial inferior epigastric artery is responsible for a vascular territory that ranges from zone I only to the entire abdominal flap, including zone IV.[20] In most patients, however, the perfusion pattern should be regarded as purely hemiabdominal, and harvesting should not be extended across the midline. A recent anatomic study using three- and four-dimensional computed angiography compared the perfusion of an SIEAP flap with that of a DIEAP flap based on a lateral row perforator.[23] This study proposed that the flow in an SIEAP flap is mediated through communication with the perforators of the deep inferior epigastric artery and occurs by means of recurrent flow through the subdermal plexus up to the abdominal midline.[23] The varying vascular territory was attributable to differences in linking vessels across the midline. Based on our personal experience and intraoperative perfusion measurements, the interindividual variability in the superficial inferior epigastric artery angiosome is important, and it should always be considered when planning a transfer of the lower abdominal flap on the superficial epigastric artery. Intraoperative perfusion measurements using indocyanine green angiography (ICGA) may be useful, especially if the contralateral half of the flap is needed for reconstruction.

Preoperative imaging of the individual superficial inferior epigastric artery anatomy, including the presence, size, location, and branching pattern, is another important tool that helps the surgeon choose the most suitable pedicle for tissue transfer. It is our clinical experience that the contribution of each individual system to the perfusion of the lower abdomen is inversely related: When the superficial system is strongly developed, the perforators from the deep epigastric system are mostly of diminutive size, and vice versa. Such reciprocal relationships between adjacent vascular systems were described in 1936 by Salmon[24] and referred to collectively as the *law of equilibrium.*

Markings for the SIEAP flap for breast reconstruction follow the standard abdominoplasty pattern. The SIEAP flap needs to be planned according to skin and volume requirements, keeping in mind that only half of the lower abdominal region has adequate blood perfusion. Rather than taking too much tissue across the midline, a more lateral design is recommended (but no farther laterally than the lateral border of the contralateral rectus abdominis muscle). In some patients, a prominent superficial inferior epigastric vein is visible through the abdominal skin, making identification of the superficial inferior epigastric artery easier.

After the skin is incised, and under loupe magnification, the superficial epigastric vein is identified lying very superficially and medially. Dissection is continued more laterally and deeply, but superficial to Scarpa's fascia, to find the superficial inferior epigastric artery pedicle. If sufficient flow is confirmed by Doppler sonography, the pedicle dissection is continued to the femoral vein and artery to obtain sufficient vessel length and diameter. If the diameter of the artery is too small at the level of the femoral artery, it is possible to take a patch of the femoral artery to increase the vessel diameter.

Two veins drain a unilateral SIEAP flap. One is a superficial vein, which is medial and superficial to the superficial inferior epigastric artery pedicle and always has a large diameter. The other vein is a vena comitans (there are one or two together with the artery). The venae comitantes should have an acceptable diameter for microvascular anastomosis. If it becomes apparent that the superficial inferior epigastric artery on one side of a lower abdominal flap has an inappropriate diameter or length, the contralateral artery should be explored in the same way. The superficial vein should always be dissected and preserved. It can serve as a lifeboat to increase venous drainage or as alternative venous drainage if thrombosis of the deep venous system occurs. The vascular anatomy of each side is usually different. Appropriate superficial inferior epigastric arteries on both sides were found only once in a personal series of 105 dissections of lower abdominal flaps.

The incisions of the flap edges are completed to the level of the external oblique fascia, from which the entire flap can be harvested in the plane superficial to the aponeurosis of the abdominal muscles. The dominant lateral- or medial-row perforators from the deep epigastric system are to be preserved above the abdominal fascia on either side. After these perforators are clamped, the vascular territory of the superficial inferior epigastric artery is estimated, either by clinical inspection or objective perfusion assessments (such as ICGA), which are more precise. The contribution of the deep inferior epigastric system to the perfusion of the abdominal ellipse can be estimated by removing the microclamps after complete staining of the superficial inferior epigastric artery vascular territory has occurred. The surgical technique is then modified accordingly.

Considering the substantial variability of the superficial inferior epigastric artery angiosome, preserving both vascular systems before deciding on the surgical technique seems to be a rational modification of the original technique, which offers the deep epigastric system as a surgical alternative if the vascular territory offered by the superficial system is insufficient for reconstruction.[21]

An SIEAP flap is harvested similar to an abdominoplasty flap (Fig. 26-4). In a very thick panniculus the superficial system might not be sufficiently developed in the deepest portions below Scarpa's fascia. The transition from the superficial to deep system can be observed as a shift in colors from normal gold-red (as seen in a nicely perfused superficial fat part of the flap) to a dark yellow color (indicating a less well perfused, deeper area of the flap). Therefore trimming the deepest fat layer, deep to Scarpa's fascia, is recommended. Care must be taken around the entrance of the superficial inferior epigastric artery pedicle. If neither pedicle is satisfactory, the deep inferior epigastric vessel system needs to be harvested as a DIEAP or TRAM flap.

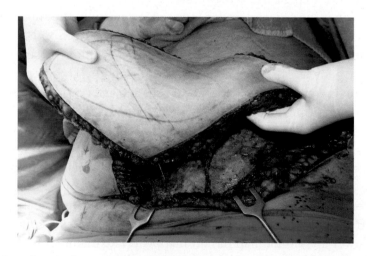

Fig. 26-4   This patient is shown intraoperatively. Notice the lateral superficial inferior epigastric artery and medial superficial inferior epigastric vein.

Neighboring Anatomic Structures

Because of the vascular variability, the surgeon needs to have sufficient flexibility to create a different flap nearby or in the same region. In breast reconstruction, the use of the DIEAP or TRAM flap may be an option.[14,25]

One important vascular system involves the deep inferior epigastric artery. This artery leaves the external iliac artery immediately above the inguinal ligament, ascends obliquely along the medial margin of the deep inguinal ring, and runs forward in the extra peritoneal tissue (forming the lateral umbilical fold). In passing medially, it pierces the transversalis fascia and enters the rectus sheath. Above the level of the umbilicus, the artery's terminal divisions form an anastomosis with branches of the superior epigastric artery. This anastomosis varies in its degree of development.[26]

One study has shown that the course of the deep inferior epigastric artery has marked variability from one case to another and from one hemiabdominal side to the other in the same case.[27] Segmental branches of the deep epigastric system pass upward and outward into the neurovascular plane of the abdominal wall, where they anastomose with the terminal branches of the lower six intercostal arteries and the ascending branch of the deep circumflex iliac artery. This anastomosis consists of multiple, narrow choke vessels.[28] There are similar connections between the superior and the deep inferior epigastric arteries within the rectus abdominis muscle, well above the level of the umbilicus. Many perforating arteries pass through the anterior rectus sheath, but the highest concentration of the major perforators is in the paraumbilical area. The vessels are terminal branches of the deep inferior epigastric artery. They feed into a subcutaneous vascular network that radiates from the umbilicus like spokes of a wheel. Choke connections exist with adjacent territories: inferiorly with the superficial inferior epigastric artery, inferolaterally with the superficial circumflex iliac artery, and superiorly with the superior epigastric artery. The dominant connections exist superolaterally with the lateral cutaneous branches of the intercostal arteries.[28]

The second important vascular system is the superficial circumflex iliac artery and vein. In our anatomic study (see Table 26-1), the superficial inferior epigastric artery had a common origin with the superficial circumflex iliac artery from the femoral artery in 47% of all dissected femoral triangles. This common origin is the most suitable surgical option for raising the SIEAP flap. The superficial circumflex iliac artery can be included in an SIEAP flap to increase the blood supply and allow a larger flap to be harvested, if necessary.

MODIFICATIONS
Breast Reconstruction

The SIEAP flap could be the flap of first choice for breast reconstruction in overweight or obese women. In these patients, the vessel diameter is enlarged because of the vascular requirements of the thick fat layer in the lower abdominal region. One hemiabdomen or less is often enough for breast reconstruction. The flap dissection is straightforward, and the blood supply of the ipsilateral lower abdominal region is excellent. The SIEAP flap is often very valuable in bilateral breast reconstruction. One breast may be reconstructed with the SIEAP flap and the second with the DIEAP flap, thereby reducing donor site morbidity, operating time, and length of hospital stay.

To reconstruct a very large breast or to cover a large surface defect, the entire lower abdominal flap with all four zones could be used if the SIEAP flap is combined with a second pedicle of the DIEAP flap. In immediate breast reconstruction, the superficial epigastric vessels are sutured to the thoracodorsal artery and vein. The perforators of the deep inferior epigastric vessels are sutured to the internal mammary vessels or, on occasion, to the second or third intercostal perforator of the internal mammary artery. In secondary breast reconstruction, the internal mammary vessels are used. If two pedicles are anastomosed (SIEAP-DIEAP), one artery may be anastomosed to the proximal end of the divided internal mammary artery, and the second artery (the artery of the long DIEAP pedicle) may be anastomosed to the distal end of the internal mammary artery. The veins of both pedicles may be anastomosed to both venae comitantes of internal mammary vessels (if they are available) or to a branching intercostal vein.

In thin women with a small contralateral breast, the SIEAP flap can be used for breast reconstruction if only a small amount of tissue is needed, and if the diameter of the superficial inferior epigastric artery is appropriate.

Other Reconstructions

The SIEAP flap can be employed for other reconstructive purposes. It can be used to correct contour deformities, augment soft tissue, or to fill dead space and cavities. Romberg's disease (progressive hemifacial atrophy) and hemifacial microsomia with soft tissue deficiency can be treated with an SIEAP flap. The SIEAP flap has appropriate volume to restore contour deformities in the face and has sufficient pedicle length for microsurgical anastomosis. The vascular pedicle can be anastomosed to the superficial temporal vessels. The deepithelialized flap can then be tailored, positioned, and sutured to give appropriate fullness and symmetry to the face. A thoracic cavity can be filled easily using an SIEAP flap, which offers both volume as a filling material and a huge skin island for soft tissue coverage. Therefore thoracic wall reconstruction is a good indication for a free SIEAP flap.

PITFALLS

The anatomy of the abdominal wall blood supply is very variable; therefore preoperative investigations using duplex color sonography or CTA (Fig. 26-5) are extremely useful when planning a free flap dissection from the lower abdominal region. If the vascular pedicle of the SIEAP flap has an appropriate diameter at the level of the lower abdominal incision and a good Doppler signal, pedicle dissection has to continue to the femoral vessels. In this region dissection could present some difficulties, because the vessels branch in this area and the pedicle passes near the lymph nodes. Nevertheless,

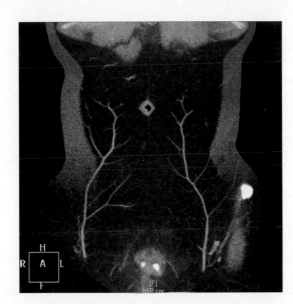

Fig. 26-5   This preoperative CTA image shows the superficial inferior epigastric system.

this dissection significantly increases the length of the pedicle and the diameter of the vessel. Continuing down to the femoral vessels is the most important step in dissecting an SIEAP flap. If the diameter of the superficial epigastric artery seems too small, a patch of femoral artery can facilitate microvascular anastomosis. However, if the diameter of the vessels on one side seems to be too small, or if a superficial inferior artery cannot be found, the contralateral side must be dissected. The anatomy of the lower abdominal vessels is not symmetrical, and the superficial epigastric artery is usually well developed only on one side. The superficial epigastric vein is present on both sides, and is always adequate for microvascular anastomosis.

If the superficial epigastric vessels have inappropriate diameters or are absent, dissection in the lower abdominal region can continue by harvesting a DIEAP flap or a TRAM flap. If a larger size and volume is needed for the SIEAP flap, the contralateral superficial epigastric vein may be dissected. Additional microvascular anastomosis of this vein significantly improves perfusion across the abdominal midline, making it possible to enlarge the SIEAP flap. By including one perforator of the deep inferior epigastric artery, all zones of the lower abdominal free flap can be included in the flap for coverage of a huge defect. Obviously, this maneuver involves microsurgical anastomosis of two pedicles, but it offers the advantage of a safer blood supply, making fat or skin necrosis less likely. Dissection of more than one vascular system and intraoperative selection of the most appropriate pedicle or pedicles for tissue transfer are critical components of modern reconstructive breast surgery. They help optimize blood supply, thereby reducing donor site morbidity to a minimum.

References

1. Wood J. Extreme deformity of the neck and forearm. Med Chir Trans 46:151, 1863.
2. Shaw D, Payne R. One staged tubed abdominal flap. Surg Gynecol Obstet 83:205, 1946.
3. Barfred T. The Shaw abdominal flap. Scand J Plast Reconstr Surg 10:56-58, 1976.
   > *The results of using 28 abdominal Shaw flaps (tubed axial pattern flaps based on the inferior superficial epigastric artery and vein) were reported.*
4. Antia NH, Buch VI. Transfer of an abdominal dermo-fat graft by direct anastomosis of blood vessels. Br J Plast Surg 24:15-19, 1971.
5. Daniel R, Taylor GI. Distant transfer of an island flap by microvascular anastomoses. A clinical technique. Plast Reconstr Surg 52:111-117, 1973.
6. Boeckx WD, de Coninck A, Vanderlinden E. Ten free flap transfers: use of intraarterial dye injection to outline a flap exactly. Plast Reconstr Surg 57:716-721, 1976.
7. Stern HS, Nahai F. The versatile superficial inferior epigastric artery free flap. Br J Plast Surg 45:270-274, 1992.
   > *A series of 27 successful SIEAP free flaps were analyzed for a number of clinical and surgical variables. The anatomy and surgical technique of the flap were detailed, and its advantages and disadvantages relative to other free flaps used for soft tissue contour were considered. The authors analyzed a variety of recipient sites as well as details of the vascular pedicle and its constancy.*
8. Stevenson TR, Hester TR, Duus EC, et al. The superficial inferior epigastric artery flap for coverage of hand and forearm defects. Ann Plast Surg 12:333-339, 1984.
   > *This article discussed using the skin of the lower abdomen as a flap for wounds of the distal upper extremity. Its versatility in positioning and viability were also presented.*
9. Chen ZJ, Chen MY, Chen C, et al. Vaginal reconstruction with an axial subcutaneous pedicle flap from the inferior abdominal wall: a new method. Plast Reconstr Surg 83:1005-1012, 1989.
   > *A new method of vaginal reconstruction was reported. The left inferior abdominal wall flap with the subcutaneous pedicle containing superficial epigastric blood vessels and/or the superficial circumflex iliac vessel and the external pudendal vessels and their branches were raised and passed through an immediate extraperitoneal tunnel to be the artificial vagina.*
10. Grotting JC. The free abdominoplasty flap for immediate breast reconstruction. Ann Plast Surg 27:351-354, 1991.
    > *Dr. Grotting presented his experience using a free flap from the low abdominal wall, based on the superficial inferior epigastric artery and vein, for immediate breast reconstruction. This procedure results in total sparing of the rectus abdominis muscle and may be applicable in thinner women with smaller breasts who cannot spare the larger ellipse of the TRAM flap.*
11. Volpe AG, Rothkopf DM, Walton RL. The versatile superficial inferior epigastric flap for breast reconstruction. Ann Plast Surg 32:113-117, 1994.
    > *Eight superficial inferior epigastric flaps were used to reconstruct seven breasts in six patients. This article discussed the flap's advantages. A cadaver was used to illustrate its clinical territory.*
12. Hartrampf CR, Beckenstein MS, Sherbert D, et al. Successful transplantation of abdominal tissue between identical twins for breast reconstruction. Presented at the Annual Meeting of the American Society of Plastic and Reconstructive Surgeons, Montreal, Quebec, Oct 1995.
13. Arnez ZM, Khan U, Pogorelic D, et al. Breast reconstruction using the free superficial inferior epigastric artery (SIEA) flap. Br J Plast Surg 52:276-279, 1999.
    > *The authors reported their experience with five tissue transfers based on the superficial inferior epigastric vessels. The anatomy was reviewed as well as techniques and limitations.*

14. Arnez ZM, Khan U, Pogorelic D, et al. Rational selection of flaps from the abdomen in breast reconstruction to reduce donor site morbidity. Br J Plast Surg 52:351-354, 1999.

    This paper presented an approach for harvesting the lower abdominal wall tissue to reduce donor site morbidity, primarily by keeping the musculature of the abdominal wall intact.

15. Hester TR Jr, Nahai F, Beegle PE, et al. Blood supply of the abdomen revisited, with emphasis on the superficial inferior epigastric artery. Plast Reconstr Surg 74:657-670, 1984.

    The authors discussed angiographic confirmation of multiple communications between the superficial inferior epigastric artery and other major sources of abdominal wall blood supply. Experience using the SIEAP flap as a pedicle and microsurgical transfer was described.

16. Taylor I. Discussion of Hester TR Jr, Nahai F, Beegle PE, Bostwick J III. Blood supply of the abdomen revisited, with emphasis on the superficial inferior epigastric artery. Plast Reconstr Surg 74:657-666; discussion 667-670, 1984.

17. Semple JL. Retrograde microvascular augmentation (turbocharging) of a single-pedicle TRAM flap through a deep inferior epigastric arterial and venous loop. Plast Reconstr Surg 93:109-117, 1994.

    The authors presented their technique using a single-pedicle TRAM flap with a transmidline retrograde microvascular loop anastomosis of the deep inferior epigastric artery and vein. Turbocharging allowed increased blood flow to the remote areas of the flap as well as augmented venous outflow. In addition, the abdominal wall donor site was similar to that of a single pedicle.

18. Timmons MJ. Landmarks in the anatomical study of the blood supply of the skin. Br J Plast Surg 38:197-207, 1985.

    This paper reviews achievements of previous investigators who studied the anatomy of the blood supply of the skin.

19. Taylor GI, Caddy CM, Watterson PA, et al. The venous territories (venosomes) of the human body: experimental study and clinical implications. Plast Reconstr Surg 86:185-213, 1990.

    The venous architecture of the integument and underlying deep tissues was studied in six total-body fresh human cadavers and in a series of isolated regional studies of the limbs and torso. Results were discussed in detail, and the clinical implications were presented with particular reference to the design of flaps, the delay phenomenon, venous free flaps, the pathogenesis of flap necrosis, the muscle pump, varicose veins, and venous ulceration.

20. Spiegel AJ, Khan FN. An intraoperative algorithm for the use of the SIEA flap for breast reconstruction. Plast Reconstr Surg 120:1450-1459, 2007.

21. Holm C, Mayr M, Höfter E, et al. Interindividual variability of the SIEA angiosome: effects on operative strategies in breast reconstruction. Plast Reconstr Surg 122:1612-1620, 2008.

    The vascular territory of the superficial inferior epigastric artery was evaluated intraoperatively using ICGA in 25 patients undergoing SIEAP flap surgery. The results of the perfusion measurements are discussed.

22. Rozen WM, Chubb D, Grinsell D, et al. The variability of the superficial inferior epigastric artery (SIEA) and its angiosome: a clinical anatomical study. Microsurgery 30:386-391, 2010.

    This was a clinical anatomic study of 500 hemiabdominal walls in 250 consecutive patients undergoing preoperative CTA before autologous breast reconstruction. The presence, size, location, and branching pattern of the superficial inferior epigastric artery were assessed in each case. Its anatomy was found to be highly variable, and larger vessel diameters correlated with a decrease in diameter of ipsilateral deep inferior epigastric artery perforators.

23. Schaverien M, Saint-Cyr M, Arbique G, et al. Arterial and venous anatomies of the deep inferior epigastric perforator and superficial inferior epigastric artery flaps. Plast Reconstr Surg 121:1909-1919, 2008.

    In 10 DIEAP flaps harvested from fresh cadavers and 2 abdominoplasty specimens, three- and four-dimensional angiography and venography were used to evaluate the microvascular anatomy and perfusion of DIEAP and SIEAP flaps.

24. Salmon M. Artères de la Peau. Paris: Masson, 1936.

25. Blondeel N, Vanderstraeten GG, Monstrey SJ, et al. The donor site morbidity of free DIEP flaps and free TRAM flaps for breast reconstruction. Br J Plast Surg 50:322-330, 1997.

> *This study was undertaken to demonstrate that the DIEAP flap can provide the advantages of autologous breast reconstruction with lower abdominal tissue, and avoid the abdominal wall complications of the TRAM flap. Eighteen patients underwent DIEAP flap breast reconstruction. Results were compared with those of 20 patients who received free TRAM flaps and 20 control subjects. The authors' data demonstrate that the free DIEAP flap can limit surgical damage to the rectus abdominis and oblique muscles.*

26. Cormack G, Lamberty B. The Arterial Anatomy of Skin Flaps. Edinburgh: Churchill Livingstone, 1994.

27. El-Mrakby HH, Milner RH. Bimodal distribution of the blood supply to lower abdominal fat: Histological study of the microcirculation of the lower abdominal wall. Ann Plast Surg 50:165-170, 2003.

> *Fat necrosis is a common postoperative complication in TRAM flap breast reconstruction. A histologic quantification of the blood supply to the lower abdominal fat was undertaken to define this problem further.*

28. Boyd JB, Taylor GI, Corlett R. The vascular territories of the superior epigastric and the deep inferior epigastric systems. Plast Reconstr Surg 73:1-16, 1984.

> *The vascular territories of the superior and deep inferior epigastric arteries were investigated by dye injection, dissection, and barium radiographic studies. Based on these studies, the relative merits of the superior and deep inferior epigastric arteries with respect to local and distant tissue transfer using various elements of the abdominal wall were discussed in detail.*

27

Deep Circumflex Iliac Artery Perforator Flap With Iliac Crest

Yoshihiro Kimata

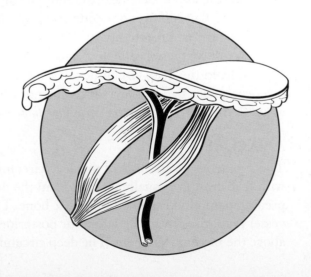

Microvascular free tissue transfer techniques have become the most reliable method for reconstructing the mandibular bone after trauma or ablative surgery for malignant tumors. The iliac crest is an excellent donor site for mandibular reconstruction because of its width, length, and high vascularity. The iliac crest is also well suited to a simultaneous, two-team approach for head and neck reconstruction. However, if the defect extends to the intraoral mucosa with mandibular bone, a skin flap combined with vascularized bone is preferred. In such cases, the iliac crest osteocutaneous free flap can be used, as described by Taylor et al.[1]

Reported disadvantages of this flap include the tenuous vascular supply to the skin unless a significant number of perforators are included with the flap. Furthermore, a soft tissue shroud incorporated to reduce tractive and shearing forces can compromise vessel patency and flap viability.[2,3] Also, if a cuff of abdominal musculature is left attached to the flap to include many perforators, the increased thickness of the subcutaneous tissue makes the flap too bulky for reconstruction of intraoral defects. On the basis of the ascending branches of the deep circumflex iliac artery, Ramasastry et al[4] resolved these problems by using the internal oblique muscle with the iliac crest to resurface mucosal defects of the oral cavity.[2]

A second, additional soft tissue flap has sometimes been used for intraoral reconstruction, including a radial forearm flap, lateral arm flap, or jejunal graft. Kimata et al[5] described the use of an anterolateral thigh flap for this purpose. However, the addition of a second flap requires a second series of microsurgical anastomoses and increases operative time and morbidity.

To resolve these problems, Safak et al[6] investigated musculocutaneous perforators derived from the deep circumflex iliac artery and suggest that the volume of the iliac osteocutaneous flap can be reduced by not using a muscle cuff. They refer to the flap as a *deep circumflex iliac artery perforator flap with iliac crest.*[7,8]

ANATOMY

The cutaneous perforators of the deep circumflex iliac artery perforator (DCIAP) flap with iliac crest are usually derived from the deep circumflex iliac artery, which is the predominant blood supply of the iliac bone. The deep circumflex iliac artery is a large vessel that arises from the lateral or posterior surface of the external iliac artery, just above the inguinal ligament. The deep circumflex iliac artery passes obliquely upward, parallel to the inguinal ligament, toward the anterior superior iliac spine (ASIS). Approximately 1 cm medial to the ASIS (after giving off an ascending branch that supplies the internal oblique muscle), the deep circumflex iliac artery pierces the transversalis fascia and passes along the inner lip of the iliac crest. At the midpoint of the crest beyond the ASIS, the artery pierces the transverse abdominis muscle and anastomoses with the iliolumbar arteries.

In its course along the inner lip of the iliac crest, the deep circumflex iliac artery gives off several small perforators that penetrate the transverse abdominis, internal oblique, and external oblique muscles. These perforators supply the skin in an area extending 1 to 3 cm above the iliac crest and 6 cm posterior to the ASIS[7] (Fig. 27-1)[8]. Taylor et al[9] investigated the size and number of these perforators in 10 patients undergoing abdominal lipectomy. From three to nine (average 6.5) small musculocutaneous perforators emerged from the deep circumflex iliac artery through the abdominal muscles in an area extending 2.5 cm above and 6 cm posterior to the ASIS. In each case, at least one dominant perforator (up to 1 mm in diameter) was present. Safak et al[6] described anatomic variations of the branching pattern of perforators derived from the deep circumflex iliac artery. In 70% of their dissections, the artery gave rise to a series of small perforators (0.3 to 0.5 mm in diameter) that penetrated the abdominal muscles to supply the overlying skin. In the remaining 30%, a dominant perforator (averaging 1.5 mm in diameter and 6 cm in length) and several smaller perforators were identified.

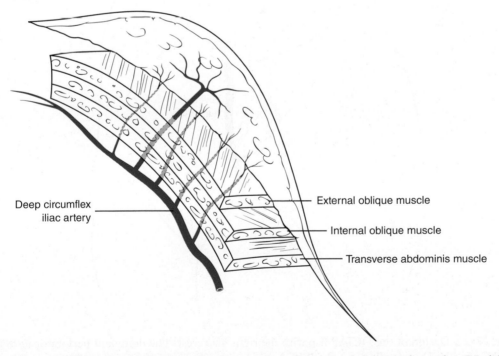

Deep circumflex iliac artery

External oblique muscle

Internal oblique muscle

Transverse abdominis muscle

Fig. 27-1 Location of the deep circumflex iliac artery perforators and abdominal muscles. (Modified from Kimata Y. Deep circumflex iliac perforator flap. Clin Plast Surg 30:433-438, 2003.)

When no dominant perforator is present, the vascular supply to the cutaneous skin is tenuous unless several small perforators are included in the flap. However, small perforators are difficult to dissect from the abdominal musculature. Therefore the DCIAP flap can be elevated safely only if dominant perforators (more than 1 mm in diameter) are present. In my previous study, a dominant perforator (approximately 1 mm) was found in 5 (50%) of 10 cases, using flaps 10 to 17 cm long, 4 to 8 cm wide, and 10 to 25 mm thick.[7,8]

SURGICAL TECHNIQUE

The skin incision is made from the upper border of the skin flap, and the flap is elevated toward the iliac crest immediately above the external oblique muscle (Figs. 27-2 and 27-3). During this procedure, the dominant perforator (at least 1 mm in diameter) and several small perforators are identified as they emerge from the external oblique muscle. Because the dominant vessel is able to supply the skin flap independently, the small perforators are sacrificed. The dominant perforator is then dissected free from the

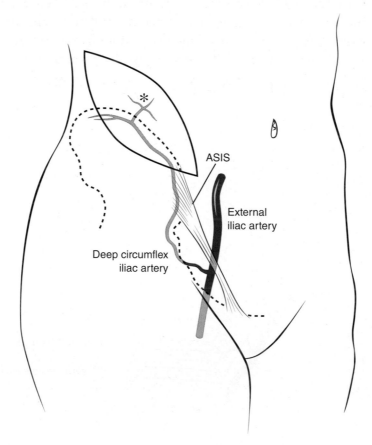

Fig. 27-2   Design of the DCIAP flap with the right iliac crest. The dominant perforator *(asterisk)* is identified by Doppler flowmetry. *(ASIS,* Anterior superior iliac spine.)

abdominal musculature to the parent deep circumflex iliac artery with careful ligation of the numerous small branches. Leaving a small cuff of abdominal muscle attached to the perforator helps protect it from damage. After the dominant perforator is isolated, the inferior border of the skin is incised and the DCIAP flap is elevated from the iliac crest. The bone and deep circumflex iliac artery are harvested in the usual manner.

In some cases, the diameter of the dominant perforator is too small and complicates dissection from the abdominal muscles during the previously described skin incision. When this occurs, the osteocutaneous flap should be elevated in the usual manner, or a second free flap should be elevated as a cutaneous flap. If no perforators are identified with Doppler flowmetry, other free flaps should be considered for intraoral reconstruction.

The donor site is closed by approximating the transverse abdominis muscle and transversalis fascia to the iliacus muscle and inguinal ligament. The external oblique muscle and fascia are then sutured to the tensor fascia lata and gluteus medius muscles and fascia. The skin and subcutaneous tissue are closed in layers.

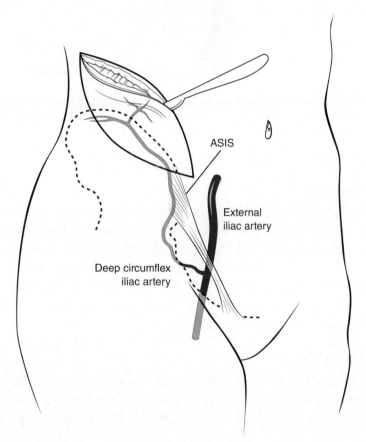

Fig. 27-3 The first skin incision is made from the upper border of the skin flap. (*ASIS*, Anterior superior iliac spine.)

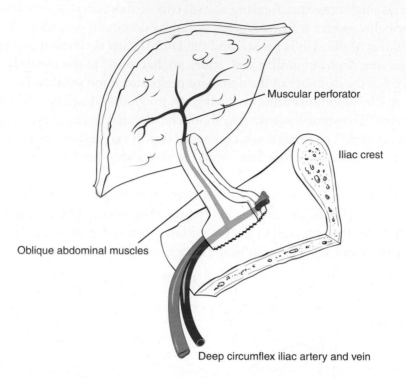

Muscular perforator

Iliac crest

Oblique abdominal muscles

Deep circumflex iliac artery and vein

Fig. 27-4 The DCIAP flap with iliac crest is elevated. A small cuff of abdominal muscle is attached to the dominant perforator. (Modified from Kimata Y. Deep circumflex iliac perforator flap. Clin Plast Surg 30:433-438, 2003.)

Surface Landmarks

Before surgery, the presence and location of the dominant perforator of the deep circumflex iliac artery are investigated with a Doppler flowmeter. The perforator is usually 1 to 3 cm above the iliac crest and 6 cm posterior to the ASIS. A skin flap is designed that includes the perforator and has a central long axis along the upper border of the anterior part of the iliac crest[8] (Fig. 27-4). If the perforators are not detected with a Doppler flowmeter, a cutaneous flap with iliac crest should be elevated in the usual manner, or a second flap must be considered.

MODIFICATIONS

Instead of elevating a second free cutaneous flap from another area when no dominant perforator is found, a better choice may be to elevate a groin flap. The cutaneous territory of the groin flap overlaps that of the DCIAP flap. Furthermore, the groin flap

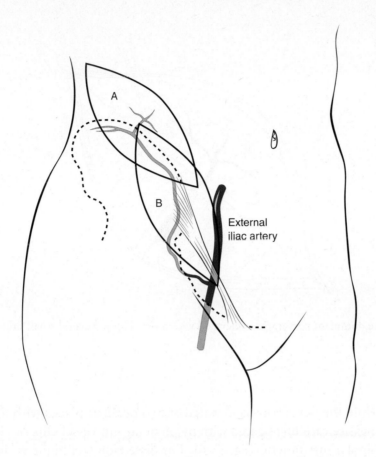

Fig. 27-5   Design of the DCIAP flap *(A)* and the groin flap *(B)*.

can be designed and elevated using the incision of the upper border of the DCIAP flap (Fig. 27-5). Therefore, if the dominant perforator is found to be too small when the incision is made at the upper border of the DCIAP flap, a groin flap can be elevated as a second free flap with additional microsurgical procedures.

Because the blood supply to the iliac crest courses along its medial aspect, the bicortical or unicortical segment of an iliac bone may be harvested with a DCIAP flap. The iliac crest and several muscular attachments to the outer cortex of the iliac bone are preserved when only the inner surface of the iliac bone is harvested with the DCIAP flap.

PITFALLS
Because the dominant perforators pass through the abdominal muscles, a slightly more complicated procedure is necessary to dissect them. To confirm the course of the dominant perforator in the abdominal muscles, the muscles immediately above the perforator are incised sharply.

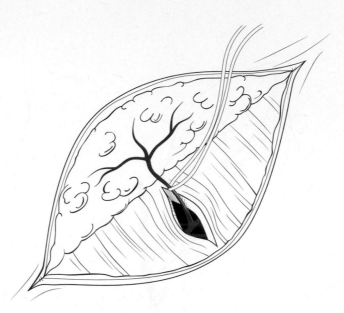

Fig. 27-6   The dominant perforator is elevated with a vessel loop. Several small branches are carefully ligated.

Then, while the perforator is elevated at two or three places with a vessel loop, several branches are carefully ligated with nylon or an autovessel clip, or electrocoagulated with a bipolar instrument (Fig. 27-6). The dissection technique is similar to that used for the musculocutaneous perforator of an anterolateral thigh flap.[5]

CASE EXAMPLE

This 53-year-old man had a squamous cell carcinoma of the left gingiva that involved the left mandible. A composite resection with neck resection was carried out. Simultaneously, a 4 by 10 cm DCIAP flap involving the right iliac crest was designed and elevated. The dominant perforator (approximately 1 mm in diameter) was dissected with a small cuff of muscle[7] (Fig. 27-7). The origin of the DCIAP was isolated, and a 3 by 6.5 cm section of the iliac crest was harvested.

The DCIAP flap with iliac crest was transferred to the mandibular defect. Both the transferred cutaneous portion and the bone portion of the flap survived in their entirety, and the patient was subsequently fitted with tissue-borne dentures[7] (Figs. 27-8 and 27-9).

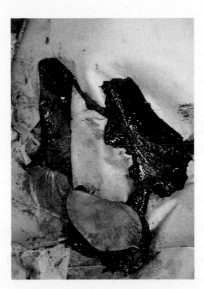

Fig. 27-7 The DCIAP flap with iliac crest is elevated before the pedicle is harvested. (Reprinted from Br J Plast Surg, Volume 54, Kimata Y, Uchiyama K, Sakuraba M, et al. Deep circumflex iliac perforator flap with iliac crest for mandibular reconstruction, pages 487-490, copyright 2001, with permission from Elsevier.)

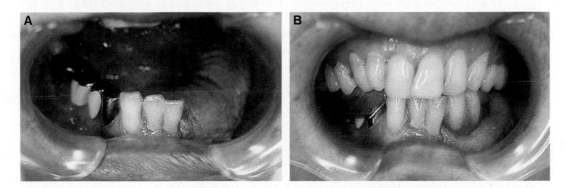

Fig. 27-8 **A,** Intraoral appearance after reconstruction of the left mandibular bone. **B,** Intraoral appearance with tissue-borne dentures. (Reprinted from Br J Plast Surg, Volume 54, Kimata Y, Uchiyama K, Sakuraba M, et al. Deep circumflex iliac perforator flap with iliac crest for mandibular reconstruction, pages 487-490, copyright 2001, with permission from Elsevier.)

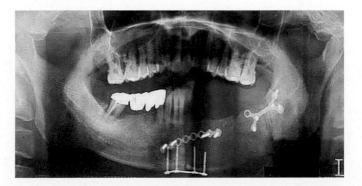

Fig. 27-9 Panoramic radiograph of the reconstructed mandible. (Reprinted from Br J Plast Surg, Volume 54, Kimata Y, Uchiyama K, Sakuraba M, et al. Deep circumflex iliac perforator flap with iliac crest for mandibular reconstruction, pages 487-490, copyright 2001, with permission from Elsevier.)

References

1. Taylor GI, Townsend P, Corlett R. Superiority of the deep circumflex iliac vessels as the supply for free groin flaps: clinical work. Plast Reconstr Surg 64:745-759, 1979.

2. Urken ML, Vickery C, Weinberg H, et al. The internal oblique-iliac crest osseomyocutaneous free flap in oromandibular reconstruction. Arch Otolaryngol Head Neck Surg 115:339-349, 1989.

   The authors reported the use of the internal oblique–iliac crest osteomusculocutaneous microvascular free flap in 20 patients for oromandibular reconstruction. The internal oblique muscle, based on the ascending branches of the deep circumflex iliac artery and vein, was used to resurface mucosal defects of the oral cavity and pharynx.

3. Taylor GI, Corlett RJ. Microvascular free transfer of a compound deep circumflex groin and iliac crest flap to the mandible. In Strauch B, Vasconez LO, Hall-Findlay EJ, eds. Grabb's Encyclopedia of Flaps, vol 1. Boston: Little Brown, 1990.

4. Ramasastry SS, Granick MS, Futrell JW. Clinical anatomy of the internal oblique muscle. J Reconstr Microsurg 2:117-122, 1986.

5. Kimata Y, Uchiyama K, Ebihara S, et al. Versatility of the free anterolateral thigh flap for reconstruction of head and neck defects. Arch Otolaryngol Head Neck Surg 123:1325-1331, 1997.

   The authors discussed techniques to minimize the problems of confirmation and perforator dissection in anterolateral thigh flaps. They concluded that this flap can be used to successfully repair a variety of large defects of the head and neck.

6. Safak T, Klebuc MJ, Mavili E, et al. A new design of the iliac crest microsurgical free flap without including the "obligatory" muscle cuff. Plast Reconstr Surg 100:1703-1709, 1997.

   The authors discussed incising a small collar of abdominal muscle around the pedicle, obviating the need for the previously customary 2.5 cm protective muscle cuff.

7. Kimata Y, Uchiyama K, Sakuraba M, et al. Deep circumflex iliac perforator flap with iliac crest for mandibular reconstruction. Br J Plast Surg 54:487-490, 2001.

8. Kimata Y. Deep circumflex iliac perforator flap. Clin Plast Surg 30:433-438, 2003.

9. Taylor GI, Townsend P, Corlett R. Superiority of the deep circumflex iliac vessels as the supply for free groin flaps: experimental work. Plast Reconstr Surg 64:595-604, 1979.

28

Superficial Circumflex Iliac Artery Perforator Flap

Isao Koshima
Takumi Yamamoto
Mitsunaga Narushima
Makoto Mihara

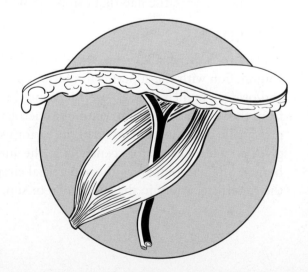

The rapid evolution of perforator flap techniques means that musculocutaneous and fasciocutaneous flaps based on major vessels are increasingly being replaced by flaps based on smaller perforators. Such perforator-based flaps allow muscle, fascia, and major vessels to be preserved without compromising the size of the skin territory harvested or the safety of the flap. The major driving force behind the development of perforator flaps has been the reduction of donor site morbidity. The concept of musculocutaneous perforator flaps also can be applied to conventional axial pattern flaps, such as a groin flap. The superficial circumflex iliac artery perforator (SCIAP) flap is based on a single perforator vessel branching off the superficial circumflex iliac artery (SCIA) and a small segment of the SCIA.

The advantages of the SCIAP flap are that (1) it is not necessary to dissect the SCIA system back to the femoral artery, as required with the groin flap; (2) only the dominant perforator and a short length of the pedicle are required to nourish the flap; (3) flap elevation time is short; (4) primary defatting or thinning of the flap is possible; (5) it is possible to harvest a pure adipose flap without skin to correct volume deficits; (6) donor site morbidity is minimal and in a concealed area; and (7) the associated cutaneous superficial circumflex iliac vein is available as an additional venous drainage system. The main disadvantage of the SCIAP flap is that supermicrosurgery is necessary to dissect and anastomose the small, short-pedicle vessels to recipient vessels of the same size. This is a versatile flap that can be used to reconstruct a diverse range of defects.[1-3]

ANATOMY

The SCIA is the smallest superficial branch of the femoral artery and arises near or in conjunction with the superficial inferior epigastric artery. The vessel has a superficial and/or deep branch (Fig. 28-1). If present, the superficial branch is often short, arising from the femoral artery and running superolaterally (Fig. 28-2). This branch is located proximally over the deep fascia of the sartorius muscle and distally in the fatty tissue. It gives off a few perforators centrally in the anteromedial groin region. The superficial branch often accompanies the superficial circumflex iliac vein, which runs parallel to the superficial artery in the subdermal or superficial layer of fatty tissue.

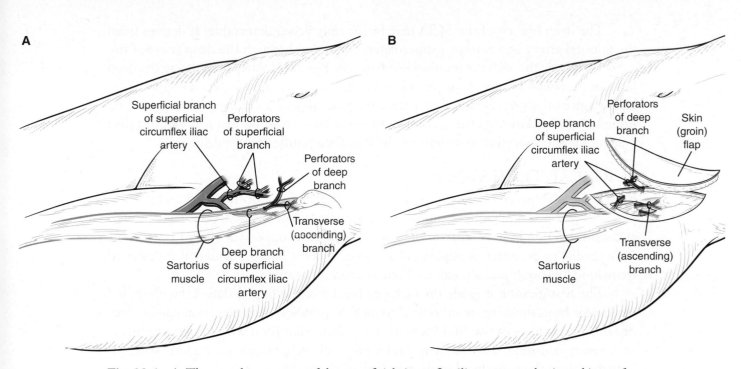

Fig. 28-1   A, The vascular anatomy of the superficial circumflex iliac artery and vein and its perforators. **B,** Elevation of the SCIAP flap on the deep branch of the superficial circumflex iliac artery.

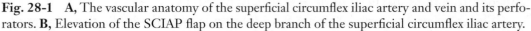
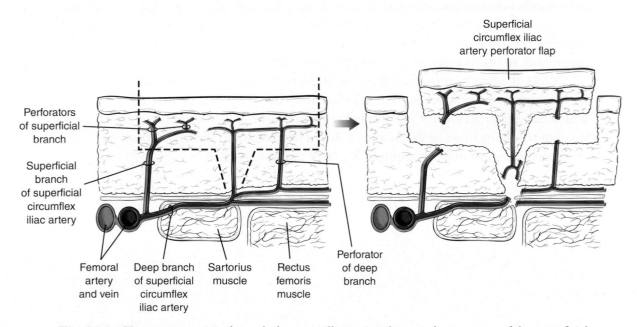

Fig. 28-2   Transverse section through the groin illustrating the vascular anatomy of the superficial circumflex iliac artery and vein and its perforators in relation to the SCIAP flap. The flap is based on the deep branch of the superficial circumflex iliac artery.

The deep branch of the SCIA may be the only vessel detectable. It derives from the femoral artery and runs in a superolateral direction beneath the deep fascia of the sartorius muscle through the inguinal ligament (see Fig. 28-2). After penetrating the deep fascia at the lateral border of the sartorius muscle, the deep branch enters the suprafascial layer to give off several perforators in the anterolateral portion of the groin region. The branches to the skin sometimes connect to perforators from the deep circumflex iliac system, the superior gluteal system, or the lateral circumflex femoral system.

SURGICAL TECHNIQUE

Preoperative Doppler examination helps confirm the course of the SCIA and localize perforators. The dominant perforator of the deep branch of the SCIA is usually located at the intersection of the course of the artery and a line dropped vertically from a point 3 cm medial to the anterior superior iliac spine. When a flap is planned, it is designed to include this point and a portion of skin over the iliac spine.

The first incision is made through one border of the flap to detect the identified perforator from the deep or superficial branch. Suprafascial flap elevation commences distally. Perforators of the SCIA system are readily identified with loupe magnification. Once identified, the dominant perforator is dissected down to the level where it branches from the superficial or deep branch of the SCIA.

The associated superficial circumflex iliac vein is included in the flap as a venous drainage system, because the venae comitantes of the SCIA are sometimes quite small (less than 0.5 mm in diameter). After dissection of the perforator and SCIA system, the other border of the flap is incised, and the flap is elevated as an island flap. If necessary, thinning is carried out at this stage, using scissors to defat the underside of the flap and taking care to protect the area around the perforator.

Once the flap is completely free, the SCIA and venae comitantes are ligated, along with a length of the superficial circumflex iliac vein. The free groin perforator flap, with a dominant perforator and a small segment of the SCIA system, is transferred to the donor site. In most cases the donor defect can be closed directly, although a split-thickness skin graft may be required if a large flap is harvested.

MODIFICATIONS
Flap Thinning

A conventional groin flap with thick fatty tissue cannot easily be thinned by removing significant fatty tissue in a single stage, because the superficial circumflex artery pedicle runs subfascially or in the deep layer of the fatty tissue. The total artery must be preserved throughout the axis of the groin flap, otherwise thinning may lead to partial necrosis. For this reason, thinning the groin flap has not become popular. However, thinning an SCIAP flap is much easier, because only a short length of the SCIA (3 cm) and the main perforator running perpendicularly into the flap are involved.

Groin Adipose Perforator Flap

The deep adipose tissue around the SCIA can be vascularized by a single perforator. An adipose flap can therefore be raised that is sufficient for facial atrophy augmentation or autologous breast augmentation. Both the DIEAP and SCIAP adipose flap donor sites are scarcely discernible after direct closure, with minimal contour deformity.

Combined Thigh–Superficial Circumflex Iliac Artery Perforator Flap

The perforators of the superficial circumflex iliac vessels and those of the lateral circumflex femoral system (LCFAP) or superficial femoral system (SFAP) can be used in conjunction to reconstruct larger defects, such as cervical skin defects involving the pharyngoesophagus. Although apparently similar to Siamese flaps (two or more flaps with a double vascular pedicle anastomosed separately to one or more recipient vessels), this combined flap consists of two adjacent flaps that are simultaneously elevated with their individual pedicles that are then anastomosed as a bridge flap (the pedicle of one flap is anastomosed to the distal end or main side branch of the pedicle of the other flap). This combined flap is unique in that the skin territory of the main flap, the anterolateral or anteromedial thigh flap, is extended with an additional vascular anastomosis between the vascular pedicle of the neighboring SCIAP flap and the distal end of the axial lateral circumflex femoral or superficial femoral system. The bridge flap therefore only has a single source vessel.

The advantages of the combined flap are (1) simultaneous elevation of the flaps during tumor resection and (2) more certain vascularization of a large flap.

Combined Vascularized Iliac Bone–Superficial Circumflex Iliac Artery Perforator Flap

In most cases, the deep circumflex iliac artery (DCIA) provides branches to the iliac crest and oblique abdominal muscles, and perforators to the overlying skin. Sometimes the DCIA perforators are absent and a dominant SCIA system takes over the blood flow for that area. If it is the intention to harvest a vascularized iliac osteocutaneous DCIA flap and the DCIA perforators are absent, skin necrosis will occur. To prevent this major complication, the skin island should be supercharged by anastomosing the SCIA and vein to the ascending branch of the DCIA and vein.

CASE EXAMPLES
Combined Thigh–Superficial Circumflex Iliac Artery Perforator Flap

This 74-year-old man with a laryngeal carcinoma underwent a total laryngectomy and a left radical neck dissection.[4] Despite extensive postoperative radiation therapy, the tumor recurred, with invasion of the cervical esophagus (Fig. 28-3, *A* and *B*). One year after the primary surgery, the hypopharynx, cervical esophagus, and irradiated anterior portion of cervical skin were resected.

To reconstruct this extremely large defect, a combined thigh-groin flap was harvested, measuring 30 by 10 cm (Fig. 28-3, *C*). The patient was placed supine on the operating table, and a flap was designed to encompass the thigh and groin perforators and the superficial circumflex iliac vessels outlined longitudinally on the anterior aspect of the thigh and groin. Initially, the lateral border of the flap was incised and the skin flap elevated subfascially to identify the perforators and the superficial circumflex iliac vessels. The perforators were dissected through the lateral or medial intermuscular septum of the thigh and the superficial circumflex iliac vessels through the inguinal ligament. Once the pedicles were securely dissected, the whole flap was elevated as one unit. The proximal end of the SCIA was transected, and then the proximal level of the lateral circumflex femoral vessels was transected.

The central portion of the combined flap was deepithelialized with a dermatome, and the flap was folded over so that the epithelialized surface was external (Fig. 28-3, *D*). The distal portion of the anterior thigh flap was rolled into a tube with the cutaneous surface inward to create an esophageal-type conduit. The prefabricated flap was then transferred into the prepared defects. The rolled tube was interposed into the esophageal gap, and a nasogastric tube was inserted. The groin portion of the combined flap was used to cover the anterior cutaneous cervical defect, and the deepithelialized central portion of the flap was coapted tightly to the caudal hypopharynx.

Vascular anastomoses were established between the transverse cervical vessels and the lateral circumflex femoral vessels, and between the muscle branch (to the vastus lateralis) of the descending branch of the lateral circumflex femoral system and the superficial circumflex iliac vessels (Fig. 28-3, *E*). An additional venous anastomosis was performed between the distal end of the descending branch and the external jugular vein. The donor defect was closed with a meshed, split-thickness skin graft (Fig. 28-3, *F*).

The postoperative course was uneventful, with no complications such as infection, flap necrosis, or fistula formation (Fig. 28-3, *G*). The gastric feeding tube was removed 4 months after surgery, after patency of the reconstructed esophagus was confirmed on a barium swallow series (Fig. 28-3, *H*). Eighteen months after reconstruction, the patient continued to complain of slight dysphagia from resection of the hypopharynx, but there was no evidence of carcinoma recurrence and no problem with the neoesophagus itself. Ambulation in the donor leg was normal.

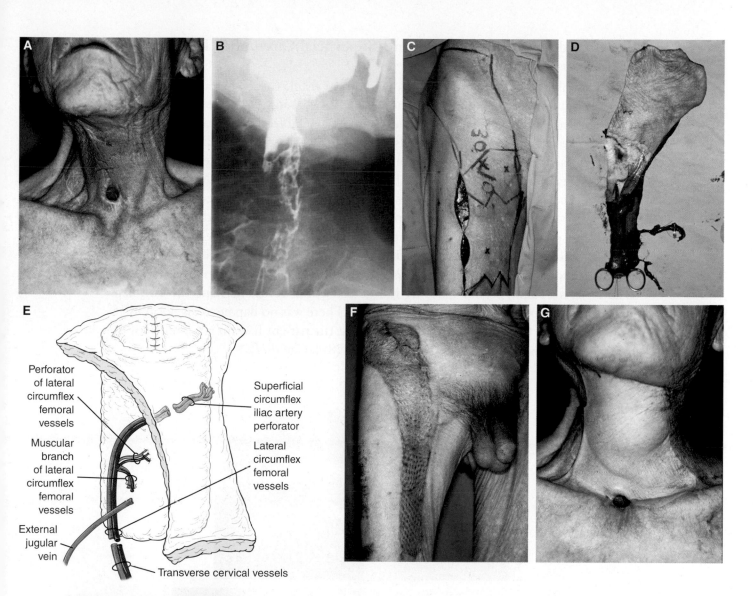

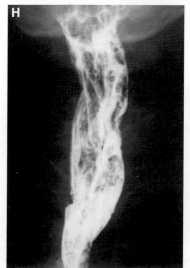

Fig. 28-3 **A,** This 74-year-old man had recurrent laryngeal carcinoma that invaded his cervical esophagus and irradiated anterior cervical skin. **B,** A preoperative barium swallow investigation revealed the severity of the esophageal stenosis. **C,** A combined anterior thigh and groin flap was outlined on the anterior aspect of the right thigh. When the first incision was made through the lateral border of the flap, the superficial circumflex iliac vessels and the main perforator from the descending branch of the lateral circumflex femoral system were identified. **D,** The central portion of the flap was deepithelialized and folded over. The anteromedial thigh flap was rolled longitudinally to form the new esophagus, and the flap was inset. **E,** The reconstruction. **F,** A split-thickness mesh skin graft was used to close the donor site. **G** and **H,** The patient is shown 6 months postoperatively. A barium swallow series confirmed the patency of the esophagus. (**A-D** and **F-H** from Koshima I, Yamamoto H, Moriguchi T, et al. Extended anterior thigh flaps for repair of massive cervical defects involving pharyngoesophagus and skin: an introduction to the "mosaic" flap principle. Ann Plast Surg 32:321-327, 1994; **E** adapted from same source.)

Combined Vascularized Iliac Bone–Superficial Circumflex Iliac Artery Perforator Flap

This 58-year-old man presented with a mandibular fistula caused by radiation necrosis after irradiation for a mandibular carcinoma (Fig. 28-4, *A* and *B*).[5] After a wide resection that included scarred skin and osteomyelitis of the mandible, the left transverse cervical vessels were exposed as recipient vessels (Fig. 28-4, *C*). A vascularized iliac osteocutaneous flap was elevated from the left groin region based on the DCIA vessels (Fig. 28-4, *D*). However, during the procedure it became apparent that the DCIA perforator was missing, because there was no bleeding from the skin island of the osteocutaneous flap. The SCIA vessels could, however, be retrieved in the same skin island. After transferring the vascularized bone flap to the prepared recipient side, the DCIA vessels were anastomosed to the left transverse cervical vessels. The SCIA vessels were anastomosed to the ascending branch of the DCIA vessels to prevent loss of the skin island (Fig. 28-4, *E* and *F*). As a result, dermal bleeding was detected after revascularizing the skin flap.

The postoperative course was uneventful. There was no flap necrosis, local infection, or salivary fistulas. Ten years after surgery, the patient had no recurrence of the carcinoma or absorption of the iliac bone (Fig. 28-4, *G* and *H*).

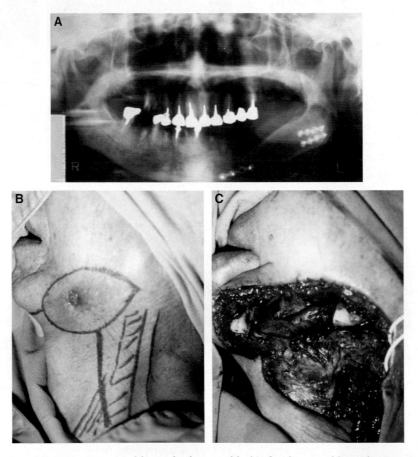

Fig. 28-4   A and **B,** This 58-year-old man had a mandibular fistula caused by radiation necrosis after irradiation for a mandibular carcinoma. **C,** The affected bone and skin were resected.

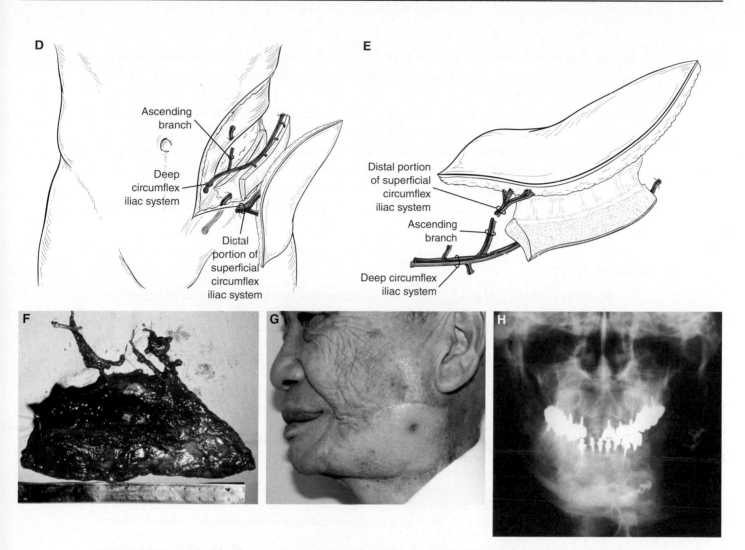

Fig. 28-4, cont'd   D, The vascularized iliac osteocutaneous flap was elevated with the DCIA and vein from the left groin region. **E,** The SCIA and vein were anastomosed to the ascending branch of the DCIA and vein to prevent necrosis of the skin flap. The DCIA and vein were anastomosed to the left transverse cervical vessels. **F,** The pedicle of the SCIAP flap shows the combined iliac bone vascularized by the DCIA and vein. **G,** Ten years postoperatively, the patient has normal cheek contours. **H,** Conventional radiography shows no absorption of the vascularized bone graft. (**A-C** and **F** and **G** from Koshima I, Nanba Y, Tsutsui T, et al. Sequential vascularized iliac bone graft and a superficial circumflex iliac artery perforator flap with a single source vessel for established mandibular defects. Plast Reconstr Surg 113:101-106, 2004; **D** and **E** adapted from same source.)

PITFALLS

The major disadvantage of the SCIAP flap is the need to learn supermicrosurgery techniques to be able to plan, dissect, and anastomose the smaller, shorter perforator vessels. Based on our results, the essential pedicle of a groin flap is not the SCIA itself but a dominant perforator of the superficial or deep branch of the SCIA system, and this perforator is responsible for the vascular territory of the groin flap. We found that one dominant perforator and a short length of the deep branch is enough to nourish a relatively large groin flap. A perforator groin flap differs from a conventional groin flap in that it includes only a short distal segment of the SCIA system and a single perforator, whereas a conventional groin flap employs the whole length of the SCIA system, including the superficial and/or deep branches.[6-11] Therefore, when a large flap is required, perforators of both branches should be harvested, and when a small or adipose flap is needed, a perforator from either branch can be used. The perforator is located approximately two fingerbreadths medial to the anterior superior iliac spine.[12] The perforator of the deep branch of the SCIA emerges from beneath the deep fascia to continue more superficially, whereas the distal portion of the deep branch enters the sartorius muscle. Clinical localization is a useful adjunct to investigation with the Doppler probe.

References

1. Koshima I, Nanba Y, Nagai A, et al. Penile reconstruction with bilateral superficial circumflex iliac artery perforator (SCIP) flaps. J Reconstr Microsurg 22:137-142, 2006.
2. Koshima I, Nanba Y, Tsutsui T. Superficial circumflex iliac artery perforator flap for reconstruction of limb defects. Plast Reconstr Surg 113:233-240, 2004.
3. Yoo KW, Shin HW, Lee HK. A case of urethral reconstruction using a superficial circumflex iliac artery. Arch Plast Surg 39:253-256, 2012.
4. Koshima I, Yamamoto H, Moriguchi T, et al. Extended anterior thigh flaps for repair of massive cervical defects involving pharyngoesophagus and skin: an introduction to the "mosaic" flap principle. Ann Plast Surg 32:321-327, 1994.
5. Koshima I, Nanba Y, Tsutsui T, et al. Sequential vascularized iliac bone graft and a superficial circumflex iliac artery perforator flap with a single source vessel for established mandibular defects. Plast Reconstr Surg 113:101-106, 2004.
6. McGregor IA, Jackson IT. The groin flap. Br J Plast Surg 25:3-16, 1972.
   This was the original description of the groin flap, the first axial pattern flap in common use.
7. Smith PJ, Foley B, McGregor IA, et al. The anatomical basis of the groin flap. Plast Reconstr Surg 49:41-47, 1972.
8. O'Brien BM, McLeod AM, Hayhurst JW, et al. Successful transfer of a large island flap from the groin to the foot by microvascular anastomoses. Plast Reconstr Surg 52:271-278, 1973.
9. Harii K, Ohmori K, Torii S, et al. Free groin skin flaps. Br J Plast Surg 28:225-237, 1975.
10. Taylor GI, Daniel RK. The anatomy of several free flap donor sites. Plast Reconstr Surg 56:243-253, 1975.
11. Acland RD. The free iliac flap: a lateral modification of the free groin flap. Plast Reconstr Surg 64:30-36, 1979.
    By moving the outline of the free groin flap laterally so that the medial margin lies lateral to the underlying femoral triangle, a uniformly slender flap with a long vascular pedicle is obtained. The anatomic findings, a method for safe dissection of the superficial circumflex iliac vessels, and the results of 18 clinical cases were presented.
12. Chuang DC, Colony LH, Chen HC, et al. Groin flap design and versatility. Plast Reconstr Surg 84:100-107, 1989.
    The authors discussed newer designs of several flaps, including the use of the two-fingerbreadth rule for the groin flap and the combined sartorius-cutaneous groin flap.

29

Circumflex Scapular Artery Perforator Flap

Patricio Andrades
Geoffrey G. Hallock

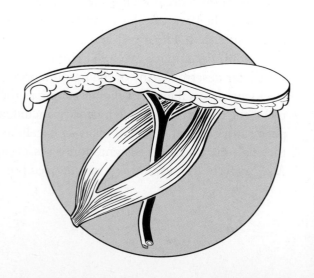

The subscapular vascular tree reaches an abundance of potential soft tissue flaps and is even a reservoir for vascularized bone grafts.[1-3] The circumflex scapular vessels are typically the first major branch. As early as 1889, Manchot[4] was well aware that the latter's terminal cutaneous twigs exited the triangular space to supply a skin territory overlying the scapula (Fig. 29-1). Because the circumflex scapular vessels first had to traverse the septum between the teres major and teres minor muscles before reaching the integument, Nakajima et al[5] considered this to be a septocutaneous type of deep fascia perforator. The skin flap nourished by this solitary circumflex scapular perforator has been classified as a type B fasciocutaneous flap, according to the schema of Cormack and Lamberty.[6] This perforator passes directly from the circumflex scapular source vessel without penetrating any other tissues except the deep fascia; therefore it is a direct perforator. Any flap variations encompassing the supplied territory of the dorsal thoracic fascia[7] could also be called *direct perforator flaps.*[8]

Manchot[4] depicted the branches of the circumflex scapular perforator to be radiating outward from the hub of the triangular space, similar to the spokes of a wheel (see Fig. 29-1). Later, clinically pragmatic studies of the circulation to the dorsal trunk by Saijo[9] and dos Santos[10] accentuated the horizontal branch of the circumflex scapular artery hub, and what is now known as the *scapular flap* was predicted to be a potential free flap donor site. In 1979, Gilbert and Teot[11] performed the first free scapular flap in Paris. Soon thereafter, flaps based on all the other branches were performed, beginning with the parascapular flap based on the descending cutaneous branch, described by Nassif et al.[12] The ascending scapular flap,[13-15] incorporating an ascending branch, and an inframammary extended circumflex scapular flap, using an anterior branch,[16] were later described. Any of the permutations or combinations of these dorsal thoracic fasciocutaneous flaps are reliable as long as the specific tributary of the direct perforator of the circumflex scapular artery is included, and overlapping territories of adjacent perforators are captured.[7] This is an excellent cutaneous free flap donor site, because the anatomy is very consistent, donor vessel caliber is large, and pedicle length is long. A segment of the scapula as a vascularized bone graft can also be included, making this an extremely versatile donor site for almost all types of reconstruction—whether the upper[17] or lower [15,18,19] extremity or even the mandible or maxilla.[2,20-22] As a local pedicle flap, it can extend as far as the side of the face, posterior scalp, anterior chest, upper arm, axilla, or shoulder, with a range mirroring that of the more familiar latissimus dorsi muscle.[13,23] However, because no specific dominant cutaneous nerve innervates this entire area, all of these flaps are relatively insensate.[10,24,25]

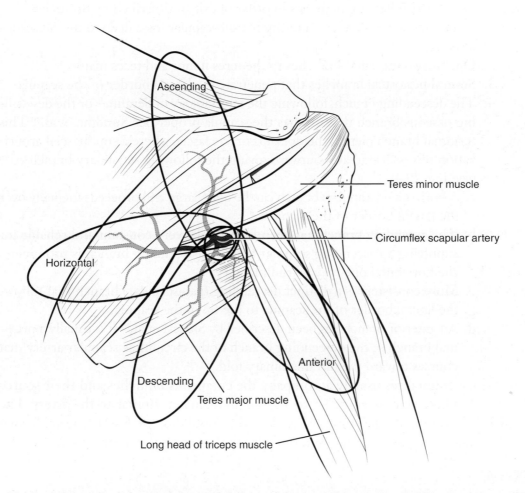

Fig. 29-1 The cutaneous perforator of the circumflex scapular artery exits the triangular space bounded above by teres minor, below by teres major, and laterally by the long head of the triceps muscle. The four possible dorsal thoracic fascia flaps, as outlined, are based and oriented along the axis of a distinct and usually consistent tributary: anterior (inframammary extended circumflex scapular flap); ascending (ascending scapular flap); descending (parascapular flap); and horizontal (scapular flap).

ANATOMY
Vascular

The cutaneous blood supply to the dorsal trunk has been most recently described by Hwang et al,[7] complementing many previous investigators.[9-11,26-28] Typically, the subscapular artery originates from the third part of the axillary artery, then quickly divides into thoracodorsal and circumflex scapular branches. The circumflex scapular artery proceeds toward the lateral border of the scapula to emerge through the triangular space bordered by the teres minor muscle superiorly, the teres major muscle inferiorly, and the triceps muscle laterally (see Fig. 29-1). During this course, the circumflex scapular artery gives off the following branches in order of exit, as described by Strauch[29]:

1. The infrascapular branch, entering the subscapular fossa deep to the subscapularis
2. One or two muscular branches to the teres minor and teres major
3. Several periosteal branches that penetrate the lateral border of the scapula
4. The descending branch, following the terminology of Serafin,[25] or the descending osseous branch that reaches the scapula proper per Sundine et al.[30] This terminal branch pierces the dorsal thoracic fascia, where a suprafascial arborization of vessels radiates outward giving the following secondary branches [4,16] (see Fig. 29-1):
   a. A horizontal (scapular) branch can be quite large and proceeds medially over the lateral border of the scapula.
   b. The ascending branch has been found to be very constant and reliable for supplying an ascending scapular flap. If an ascending branch is prominent, the horizontal one may be rudimentary.[14]
   c. More consistent is a distinct descending (parascapular) branch that follows the lateral border of the scapula to the tip of the scapula.
   d. An anterior branch has been described by Siebert et al.[16] It is usually a proximal branch of the descending branch of the circumflex scapular artery that courses toward the inframammary fold.

Two venae comitantes usually accompany the cutaneous branches and their source artery.[31,32] These veins average 1.5 to 4.5 mm in diameter, similar to the artery. The pedicle length from the subscapular vessels to the dorsal thoracic fascia can vary from 6 to 14 cm and be further lengthened if the subscapular vessels themselves are included.[25]

Nerve

The cutaneous innervation of the upper lateral region of the back is through branches of the cervical plexus, dorsal nerve roots, and circumflex nerves. There is no single, independent, dominant nerve that would permit harvest of a sensate flap.[10]

Bone

The blood supply to the scapula is from multiple sources arising from the subscapular axis.[30] The lateral border can be sustained by periosteal branches of the descending osseous branch of the circumflex scapular artery.[17,30,33] The angle of the scapula is similarly vascularized; but is also nourished by the angular branch of the thoracodorsal artery, though less consistently.[30] Nevertheless, recent anatomic and clinical studies have shown that this angular branch is a constant vessel on which free tissue transfer of the scapular angle may be reliably based.[34,35] The medial border of the scapula can rely on fascial attachments from the overlying dorsal thoracic fascia through musculoperiosteal branches to the bone.[21,30,31,36,37]

SURGICAL TECHNIQUE

Surface Landmarks

The design of any of the major dorsal thoracic fascia flaps must be oriented about a central axis that corresponds to the course of the named tributary. The base of the flap will usually encompass the triangular space where the cutaneous perforator pierces the deep fascia. This point can be somewhat variable and can be found anywhere along the lateral border of the middle third of the scapula. Serafin[25] stated that the approximate location of the triangular space is at the lateral scapular border, two fifths the distance inferiorly on a line connecting the midportion of the spine of the scapula to the inferior angle. The triangular space may also be found by applying the following formula:

$$D1 - (D - 1)/2$$

where D1 is the location of the perforator measured from the midpoint of the scapular spine, and D is the distance between the midpoint of the spine and the tip of the scapula. Generally, the perforator may be better localized preoperatively by audible Doppler sonography.[38]

Specific Vascular Anatomy

Scapular Flap

The important bony landmarks are most easily marked with the patient in the upright position. The nearly horizontal axis of this flap that corresponds to the horizontal branch of the circumflex scapular perforator is drawn, beginning where that perforator, as identified with acoustic Doppler sonography, emerges through the triangular space, and then parallels the spine of the scapula. The flap may extend from the midaxillary line medially to the vertebral column, or even to the contralateral side. The vertical boundaries extend from the scapular spine above to the angle of the scapula below. If the cutaneous flap does not exceed 7 to 12 cm in width, direct closure of the donor site remains possible.[25,39] This limitation can be avoided with an adipofascial flap.

With the patient in a prone or lateral decubitus position, dissection starts by incising to, but not including, the underlying muscular aponeurosis. The flap can be elevated in a retrograde fashion toward the pedicle, either from medial to lateral or superior to inferior. However, elevation should always proceed toward the triangular space to permit identification of any vascular anomalies and ensure accurate retention of the correct vascular pedicle to the flap. It is not unusual for the cutaneous perforator to exit the triangular space extremely laterally or medially. Thus it is worth repeating that great care must always be taken to precisely identify the location of the perforator once the lateral border of the scapula has been accessed, regardless of the approach. Only after the location of the cutaneous perforator is confirmed should the remaining flap boundaries be raised, because they can always be altered as necessary. The vascular pedicle is then carefully dissected back through the triangular space by retracting the triceps, teres major, and teres minor muscles. The branches to the teres minor, teres major, infraspinatus, and infrascapular muscles must be ligated and transected to obtain a 6 to 9 cm vascular pedicle length. When a longer pedicle is required, a tunnel is bluntly dissected under the teres minor muscle. If necessary a 5 cm axillary incision may be made for better exposure of the subscapular vessels. Once the thoracodorsal artery and vein are ligated, a maximum pedicle length of 11 to 14 cm is possible.

Parascapular Flap

The parascapular flap should be raised with the same precautions described for the scapular flap. However, its axis of orientation follows the *descending branch* of the circumflex scapular artery, which roughly parallels the lateral border of the scapula[36] (Fig. 29-2). Whereas the superior margin of the flap at the least must correspond to the level of the pedicle at the triangular space, the inferior tip of the flap can sometimes reach the angle of the scapula. Nassif[40] has devised a formula to estimate the potential maximum flap length, which varies directly with the height of the patient, as follows:

$$\text{Maximum length of flap (cm)} = 16.5 \times \text{Height (m)}$$

If a longer cutaneous flap is necessary, a possible solution is a conjoined flap with a portion of the underlying latissimus dorsi muscle attached to supplement vascularization.[41]

After widely undermining the trunk,[12] direct donor site closure is still possible for a parascapular flap up to 15 cm wide. Another precaution is that the requisite descending branch commonly arises from the circumflex scapular source vessels *before* reaching the triangular space as a separate perforator. A more important concern is that, in some cases, this separate perforator descends to exit below (rather than above) the teres major muscle.[14,28] For these reasons, the suggestion by Nassif[40] to always raise this flap in a retrograde fashion is sage advice to permit visualization of these anomalies as they are encountered. If the cutaneous branch exits below the teres major muscle, then that muscle may need to be split to gain the desired pedicle length. However, for the conventional anatomic situation, further pedicle dissection would follow that described for a scapular flap.

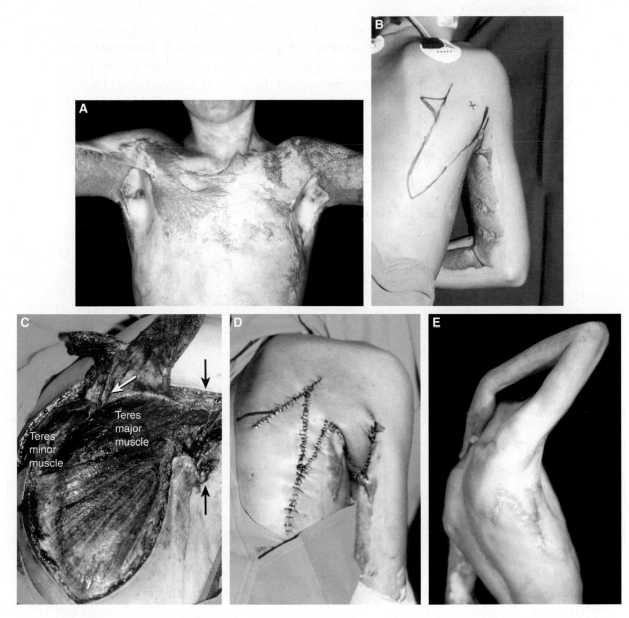

Fig. 29-2 Local parascapular flap. **A,** This patient demonstrates bilateral limitation of arm abduction and elevation caused by burn scar contractures of the posterior axillary webs. **B,** Before releasing the right axilla, the circumflex scapular artery perforator was identified at site *x* with acoustic Doppler sonography. A peninsular parascapular flap, with its long axis paralleling the lateral border of the scapula, was outlined around this perforator. A medial dart made this a bilobed flap to facilitate direct closure of the donor site, which can be problematic in the presence of rigid burn scars. **C,** The descending branch of the circumflex scapular artery perforator is seen on the undersurface of the flap entering its base *(white arrow)* as it emerges through the triangular space. Note the wide separation of the burn scar defect after release of the posterior axillary web contracture *(between black arrows)*. **D,** Flap inset with the major parascapular lobe spanning the axilla. The minor dart was used to release tension on the closure of the major lobe donor site, thereby allowing direct closure of the entire donor site. **E,** Postoperatively the patient was able to completely elevate and abduct the right arm.

Ascending Scapular Flap

The ascending scapular flap is relatively thin compared with the thickness of the scapular or parascapular flaps.[13-15] This flap variation is designed and raised in a fashion similar to the scapular flap, except that the skin ellipse must be drawn vertically with its lateral border medial to a line extending from the apex of the axilla to the acromion. The medial border of this flap must be drawn lateral to a line that extends from the axilla to the root of the neck on the side of the donor site. Its upper limit is the anterior border of the upper trapezius muscle. Inferiorly, the flap must be based over the triangular space to capture the requisite branch of the circumflex scapular perforator. Direct closure is possible if the width of the flap does not exceed 10 cm.

Inframammary Extended Circumflex Scapular Flap

Beginning at the identified point of the circumflex scapular cutaneous perforator in the triangular space, the longitudinal axis of this flap lies within the inframammary fold. The length of the flap is reliable up to the anterior axillary line, but may sometimes be stretched to reach the level of the nipple.[16] A retrograde dissection is suggested (as with the parascapular flap), because the anterior branch to this flap is usually a proximal branch of the descending branch of the circumflex scapular artery perforator, which itself is occasionally anomalous.[16]

MODIFICATIONS

All permutations of dorsal thoracic fascia flaps can consist of fascial, adipofascial, or fasciocutaneous variations, either alone or in combination with each other or with any of the other muscle or osseous flaps in this region that are dependent on the subscapular axis.[1-3,42]

Pedicle Perforator Flap

Although the technical descriptions enumerated here have emphasized the approach as if for a microsurgical transfer as a free flap, all variations of circumflex scapular artery perforator flaps can also be used as local island or peninsular flaps.[13,23] Depending on the branch chosen, the arc of rotation extends to the posterior trunk, shoulder, axilla, and lateral thoracic wall. Most simply, the fixed point of rotation is at the triangular space, where the perforator pierces the dorsal thoracic fascia (see Fig. 29-2). This point can be extended back to the axillary vessels to increase reach and lessen the risk of pedicle twisting; but such a maneuver requires a more meticulous dissection.

Expanded Flap

Both pretransfer and posttransfer tissue expansion of the skin of the dorsal thoracic region have been reported.[43,44] Usually this expansion has been performed to permit direct closure of the donor site in lieu of skin grafting. With pretransfer expansion, the potential flap size can also be augmented, a procedure that is probably related to invoking the delay phenomenon to reliably capture adjacent perforator territories.[44] In addition, unavoidable flap thinning occurs, which may be advantageous. Any expander envelopes must be positioned well away from the triangular space to avoid damage to the cutaneous perforator and limit scarring or fibrosis that could make identification of tissue planes difficult during subsequent pedicle dissection.

Vascularized Bone

The lateral border of the scapula below the triangular space, when captured as an osteofascial flap, is the most reliable source of flat, straight, corticocancellous scapular bone because of direct musculoperiosteal communications with the descending osseous branch of the circumflex scapular artery. The length of the lateral scapular border (from the glenoid fossa to the inferior angle) ranges from 10 to 14 cm, and the thickness of the lateral border is 0.7 to 1.2 cm. The midportion of the scapula is quite thin (0.2 cm), making it ideal for palatal or orbital floor reconstruction.[29] The descending osseous branch is the terminus of the circumflex scapular vessels[33] and must be preserved with the osseous flap during its elevation.[18,22,30]

The medial scapula can also be transferred as a vascularized bone graft. However, this graft requires maintenance of connections with some form of a dorsal thoracic fascia flap, because circulation to the bone in this variation is always indirectly through tenuous fascial connections.[21,33] Whether transferring the lateral or medial border of the scapula, it is important to protect the angle of the scapula to preserve function and minimize the risk of winging of the scapula.[33]

To improve bone viability or in cases of increased bone requirements, the inferior angle of the scapula may be incorporated based in the angular branch of the thoracodorsal vessels. Deraemaecker et al[45] first described the free transfer of the inferior angle of the scapula based on a vessel they named the "angular branch." Later, Coleman and Sultan[46] described a bipedicle osteocutaneous scapular flap in which the inferior angle of the scapula was transferred with the lateral margin of the scapula to reconstruct multiple bony defects. Allen et al[47] described the "latissimus-bone flap," in which the inferior angle of the scapula was included in a traditional latissimus dorsi muscle flap. This modification demonstrates the great versatility of the subscapular system of flaps.

Combined Flaps

If a very large cutaneous flap is needed, the realm of all tributaries of the circumflex scapular cutaneous perforator can be assimilated to capture almost the entire dorsal thoracic fascia, or to be an even larger conjoined flap, if that would include a perforator from an adjacent territory.[48] A very long conjoined perforator megaflap can also provide extreme reach, possibly remaining attached at one end, similar to a local flap, but requiring supercharging of a second perforator at the opposite extreme (Fig. 29-3).[49] Conversely, each circumflex scapular artery perforator flap subtype can be raised as an independent flap, or taken as multiple flaps joined together only by their common source vessel, the circumflex scapular artery, as *chimeric flaps.*[19,49,50] Similarly, if also based on their common subscapular axis as a chimeric flap, the latissimus dorsi and/or serratus anterior muscles (Fig. 29-4), and/or the scapula as a vascularized bone graft using either the angular branch of the thoracodorsal system or the descending osseous branch of the circumflex scapular artery, can be added with any of these cutaneous flaps for unrestricted flap insetting with an almost unlimited array of reconstructive alternatives.[14,37,51]

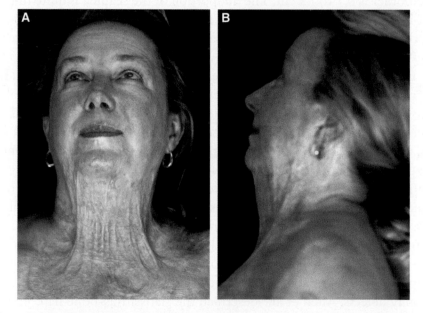

Fig. 29-3   Local supercharged conjoined dorsal thoracic perforator flap. **A** and **B,** This patient had anterior neck and upper chest burn scar contracture.

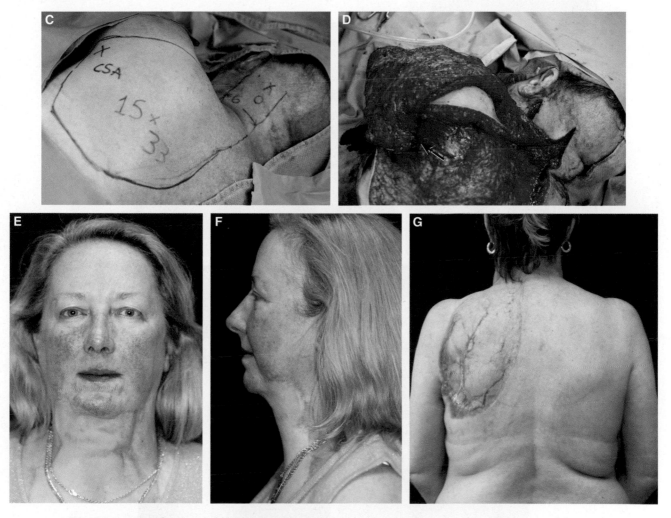

Fig. 29-3, cont'd C, A left dorsal thoracic megaflap was designed to remain attached at the posterior neck to capture the transverse cervical artery perforator at point *x*, with the circumflex scapular artery *(CSA)* perforator found at *x* near the left axilla. **D,** The undersurface of the elevated flap is shown just before rotation to the anterior neck, with circumflex scapular vessels seen exiting the triangular space *(arrow)*. This will supercharge the flap after microanastomoses to the right facial vessels. **E** and **F,** The patient is shown postoperatively. Her neck contracture is released, and her aesthetic appearance is improved by this independent branch–based type of indigenous conjoined perforator flap. (See Chapter 3 for flap classifications.) **G,** Postoperatively the donor site remains unsightly.

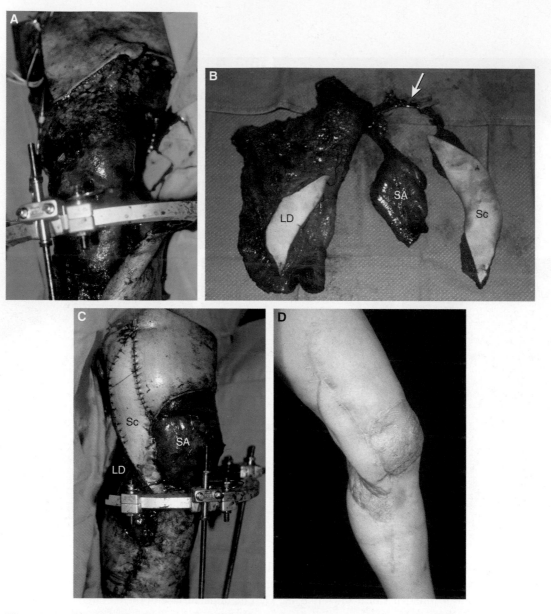

Fig. 29-4   Chimeric free scapular flap. **A,** This patient had an extensive soft tissue degloving injury and fracture of the left knee. **B,** A chimeric free flap is shown, composed of latissimus dorsi *(LD)* musculocutaneous, serratus anterior *(SA)* muscle, and a scapular *(Sc)* flap. The separate vascular pedicles converge to the subscapular vessels *(arrow)*. **C,** The flaps were independently inset, with the latissimus dorsi flap covering the popliteal area, the serratus anterior muscle over the patella, and the scapular flap along the medial thigh. **D,** The result is shown postoperatively.

PITFALLS
Positioning
None of the dorsal thoracic flaps can be harvested with the patient in the supine position.

Donor Site Aesthetics
A large cutaneous flap leaves a donor site scar that may be difficult to conceal and may require a skin graft for closure (see Fig. 29-3). The result may be aesthetically displeasing. The scar created with the inframammary extended circumflex scapular flap, at least in women, is hidden under the breast fold.[16]

Perforator Location
The exact point at which the circumflex scapular cutaneous perforator penetrates along the lateral border of the scapula can be variable. This site must always be precisely identified before incising all flap boundaries, and especially island flaps, so that boundary adjustments will still be possible.

Descending Branch Anomalies
The cutaneous tributary to the parascapular flap is commonly anomalous. Although this tributary is occasionally a separate branch exiting the triangular space, it may exit beneath the teres major muscle.[14,28] Nassif[40] recommends a retrograde dissection of the parascapular flap as a precaution that would allow earlier identification of this variation.

Bone Flaps
Of the lateral and medial scapular bone flaps, the lateral flap is more reliable because of constant direct musculoperiosteal communications with vessels from the descending osseous branch of the circumflex scapular artery.[20,32,36] The medial scapular bone flap must retain dorsal fascial connections, which can make harvest and insetting cumbersome. However, a longer pedicle extending across the width of the scapula would be possible with the medial bone flap.[36]

Source Vessel Origin
The origin of the circumflex scapular vessels is normally from the subscapular system. Occasionally, the artery or vein, or both, may arise directly from the axillary vessels.[27] This will make various forms of combined flaps from this region more difficult to execute.

CONCLUSION

The circumflex scapular artery is the first major branch of the well-known subscapular axis. Its cutaneous terminus passes in the septum between the teres major and teres minor muscles so that this can be considered a septocutaneous perforator. After piercing the deep fascia, branches radiate like the spokes of a wheel about this direct perforator to supply the dorsal thoracic fascia. Although variations in caliber are frequent, a horizontal branch reliably supplies the scapular flap and a descending branch the parascapular flap, thus named because its axis parallels the lateral border of the scapula. The latter can be combined as a vascularized bone flap, if desired. The vascular pedicle can be extended deep into the axilla to obtain a long pedicle of large caliber, if needed, making this a versatile donor site for either a free flap or a local flap with a long range and large arc of rotation.

References

1. Hallock GG. Permutations of combined flaps using the subscapular system. J Reconstr Microsurg 13:47-54, 1997.

   The subscapular axis is the ultimate source vessel for multiple muscle, bone, and cutaneous flaps from the dorsal thoracic region. These can be combined to yield dozens of local or free flap combinations; yet the latter still require but a single microastomosis to supply all flaps if they are kept intact with this common source vessel.

2. Sano K, Hallock GG, Ozeki S, et al. Devastating massive knee defect reconstruction using the cornucopian chimera flap from the subscapular axis: two Case Reports. J Reconstr Microsurg 22:25-32, 2006.

3. Girod A, Nadaud F, Mosseri V, et al. Use of chimeric subscapular artery system free flaps for soft-tissue reconstruction of the oral cavity and oropharynx: advantages and donor-site morbidity. Plast Reconstr Surg 124:445e-446e, 2009.

4. Manchot C. The Cutaneous Arteries of the Human Body. New York: Springer-Verlag, 1983.

5. Nakajima H, Fujino T, Adachi S. A new concept of vascular supply to the skin and classification of skin flaps according to their visualization. Ann Plast Surg 16:1-17, 1986.

6. Cormack GC, Lamberty BG. A classification of fascio-cutaneous flaps according to their patterns of vascularisation. Br J Plast Surg 37:80-87, 1984.

7. Hwang JH, Hwang K, Bang SI, et al. Reliability of vascular territory for a circumflex scapular artery-based flap. Plast Reconstr Surg 123:902-909, 2009.

   The authors performed fresh cadaver injection studies to evaluate the cutaneous vascular territories of the circumflex scapular artery and the area supplied by perforators from neighboring anatomic vascular territories. They defined safe limits for designing circumflex scapular artery perforator flaps.

8. Hallock GG. Direct and indirect perforator flaps: the history and the controversy. Plast Reconstr Surg 111:855-866, 2003.

9. Saijo M. The vascular territories of the dorsal trunk: a reappraisal for potential flap donor ites. Br J Plast Surg 31:200-204, 1978.

   Basic anatomy of the vascular territories of the dorsal trunk in cadaver injection studies demonstrated that two main groups of vessels were source vessels: the subscapular and the posterior intercostal systems. Branches of the circumflex scapular artery, which is a main trunk of the subscapular artery, terminated within the skin overlying the scapula. Based on these observations, the scapular flap was correctly predicted as a potential free flap donor site.

10. dos Santos LF. The vascular anatomy and dissection of the free scapular flap. Plast Reconstr Surg 73:599-603, 1983.

11. Gilbert A, Teot L. The free scapular flap. Plast Reconstr Surg 69:601-604, 1982.

12. Nassif TM, Vidal L, Bovet JL, et al. The parascapular flap: a new cutaneous microsurgical free flap. Plast Reconstr Surg 69:591-600, 1982.

13. Maruyama Y. Ascending scapular flap and its use for the treatment of axillary burn scarcontracture. Br J Plast Surg 44:97-101, 1991.

14. Ohsaki M, Maruyama Y. Anatomical investigations of the cutaneous branches of the circumflex scapular artery and their communications. Br J Plast Surg 46:160-163, 1993.

    From dissections of the scapular region in cadavers, the authors noted that the cutaneous branches of the circumflex scapular artery distributed flow to three distinct areas by ascending, horizontal, and descending branches. The ascending branch was consistently present—the basis for a reliable ascending scapular flap.

15. Sawaizumi M, Maruyama Y, Kawaguchi N. Vertical double flap design for repair of wide defects of the lower limb, using combined ascending scapular and latissimus dorsi flaps. J Reconstr Microsurg 11:407-414, 1995.

16. Siebert JW, Longaker MT, Angrigiani C. The inframammary extended circumflex scapular flap: an aesthetic improvement of the parascapular flap. Plast Reconstr Surg 99:70-77, 1997.

    This flap variation incorporating the dorsal thoracic fascia has a central axis proceeding from the inframammary fold to the circumflex scapular perforator arising from the triangular space. The donor site scar is well hidden within the inframammary fold, and avoids widening and hypertrophy seen with the more traditional parascapular and scapular flap designs.

17. Datiashvili RO, Shibaev EY, Chichkin VG, et al. Reconstruction of a complex defect of the hand with two distinct segments of the scapula and a scapular fascial flap transferred as a single transplant. Plast Reconstr Surg 90:687-694, 1992.

18. Sekiguchi J, Kobayashi S, Ohomori K. Use of the osteocutaneous free scapular flap on the lower extremities. Plast Reconstr Surg 91:103-112, 1993.

19. Koshima I, Soeda S. Repair of a wide defect of the lower leg with the combined scapular and parascapular flap. Br J Plast Surg 38:518-521, 1985.

20. Swartz WM, Banis JC, Newton D, et al. The osteocutaneous scapular flap for mandibular and maxillary reconstruction. Plast Reconstr Surg 77:530-545, 1986.

21. Thoma A, Archibald A, Payk I, et al. The free medial scapular osteofasciocutaneous flap for head and neck reconstruction. Br J Plast Surg 44:477-482, 1991.

22. Ugurlu K, Özçelik D, Haclkerim S, et al. The combined use of flaps based on subscapular vascular system for unilateral facial deformities. Plast Reconstr Surg 106:1079-1089, 2000.

23. Yanai A, Nagata S, Hirabayashi S, et al. Inverted-U parascapular flap for the treatment of axillary burn scar contracture. Plast Reconstr Surg 76:126-129, 1985.

24. Barwick WJ, Goodkind DJ, Serafin D. The free scapular flap. Plast Reconstr Surg 69:779-785, 1982.

25. Serafin DG. The scapular flap. In Serafin, ed. Atlas of Microsurgical Composite Tissue Transplantation. Philadelphia: WB Saunders, 1996.

26. Kim PS, Gottlieb JR, Harris GD, et al. The dorsal thoracic fascia: anatomic significance with clinical applications in reconstructive microsurgery. Plast Reconstr Surg 79:72-80, 1987.

27. Rowsell AR, Davies DM, Eisenberg N. The anatomy of the subscapular-thoracodorsal arterial system: study of 100 cadaver dissections Br J Plast Surg 37:574-576, 1984.

    The circumflex scapular artery is a branch of the subscapular artery in 97% of cadavers, and otherwise a direct branch of the axillary artery. The thoracodorsal artery is a branch of the subscapular artery in 94% of cases. Therefore, if a combined flap is planned that must rely on both of these vessels, on rare occasions there may not be a common source vessel.

28. Cormack GC, Lamberty BG. The anatomical vascular basis of the axillary fascio-cutaneous pedicled flap. Br J Plast Surg 36:425-427, 1983.

      Cadaver injection studies of the dorsal thoracic fascia outlined the fascial plexus in this area, with an axiality paralleling the course of the branches of the direct perforator of the circumflex scapular artery. Musculocutaneous perforators ran almost perpendicular to the deep fascia and passed directly to the subcutaneous plexus, with minimal contributions to the level of the deep fascia. This study confirmed that if a skin flap, in general, is to be raised with inclusion of the deep fascia with the expectation that this alone will increase reliability and safe length:breadth ratios, this must not be done randomly, but planned according to the anatomic vascular basis of that plexus and a knowledge of the direction in which it runs.

29. Strauch B, Yu HL. Back. In Strauch B, Yu HL, eds. Atlas of Microvascular Surgery: Anatomy and Operative Approaches, 2nd ed. New York: Thieme, 2006.

30. Sundine MJ, Sharobaro VI, Ljubic I, et al. Inferior angle of the scapula as a vascularized bone graft: an anatomic study. J Reconstr Microsurg 16:207-211, 2000.

      Injection studies of the subscapular artery showed that two branches of this axis converged on the angle of the scapula: (1) the well-known angular branch that arises from the thoracodorsal artery and (2) the descending osseous branch of the circumflex scapular artery. The latter is always present, whereas the angular artery was not found in some dissections. The descending osseous branch is also larger in caliber and has a greater number of periosteal branches.

31. Aharinejad S, Dunn RM, Fudem GM, et al. The microvenous valvular anatomy of the human dorsal thoracic fascia. Plast Reconstr Surg 99:78-86, 1997.

      Microvenous valves of the dorsal thoracic fascia may have a role in improving hemodynamics in chronic venous insufficiency after transfer of a scapular flap. These valves are similar in structure to valves of the lower extremity.

32. Imanishi N, Nakajima H, Aiso S. Anatomical relationship between arteries and veins in the scapular region. Br J Plast Surg 54:419-422, 2001.

33. Serafin DG. The scapular osteocutaneous flap. In Serafin DG, ed. Atlas of Microsurgical Composite Tissue Transplantation. Philadelphia: WB Saunders, 1996.

      The descending [sic osseous] branch is the terminus of the circumflex scapular artery and originates after the last muscle branch, usually the infrascapular branch, which courses between the infraspinatus muscle and scapula. It provides direct musculoperiosteal communications to the lateral scapula. Transfer of a medial scapula osseous segment requires a fasciocutaneous attachment, so that will be less well vascularized than the lateral segment.

34. Dolderer JH, Kelly JL, McCombe D, et al. Maxillofacial osseous reconstruction using the angular branch of the thoracodorsal vessels. J Reconstr Microsurg 26:449-454, 2010.

35. Seneviratne S, Duong C, Taylor GI. The angular branch of the thoracodorsal artery and its blood supply to the inferior angle of the scapula: an anatomical study. Plast Reconstr Surg 104:85-88, 1999.

      Eighty-one cadaveric dissections were performed, revealing the consistent presence of the thoracodorsal artery and four vascular patterns of origin of the angular branch. Selective India ink perfusion studies demonstrated a reliable supply to the inferior angle of the scapula to the extent of 6 cm of the vertebral margin and 3 cm of the lateral margin.

36. Serafin DG. The parascapular flap. In Serafin DG, ed. Atlas of Microsurgical Composite Tissue Transplantation. Philadelphia: WB Saunders, 1996.

37. Fairbanks GA, Hallock GG. Facial reconstruction using a combined flap of the subscapular axis simultaneously including separate medial and lateral scapular vascularized bone grafts. Ann Plast Surg 49:104-108, 2002.

38. Hallock GG. Attributes and shortcomings of acoustic Doppler sonography in identifying perforators for flaps from the lower extremity. J Reconstr Microsurg 25:377-381, 2009.

39. Urbaniak JR, Koman LA, Goldner RD, et al. The vascularized cutaneous scapular flap. Plast Reconstr Surg 69:772-778, 1982.

The rule of twos is helpful in approximating the outline of the scapular flap. The medial flap border may extend to within 2 cm of the spinous process of the vertebrae, the lateral border may extend to 2 cm superior to the posterior axillary crease, the inferior border may extend to 2 cm superior to the inferior edge of the scapula, and the superior border to 2 cm inferior to the spine of the scapula.

40. Nassif TM. The parascapular flap (discussion). In Serafin DG, ed. Atlas of Microsurgical Composite Tissue Transplantation. Philadelphia: WB Saunders, 1996.

41. Hallock GG. The combined parascapular fasciocutaneous and latissimus dorsi muscle conjoined free flap. Plast Reconstr Surg 121:101-107, 2008.

42. Hallock GG. Metachronous flaps from the same subscapular axis. Plast Reconstr Surg 109:2424-2430, 2002.

43. Hallock GG. Dorsal thoracic fasciocutaneous flap salvage of the failed transverse rectus abdominis musculocutaneous flap. Ann Plast Surg 29:257-260, 1992.

44. Russell RC, Khouri RK, Upton J, et al. The expanded scapular flap. Plast Reconstr Surg 96:884-895, 1995.

Pretransfer tissue expansion of the scapular region creates a flap with greater surface area, reduces flap thickness or bulk, and permits primary donor closure. This is a tedious process that cannot be done on an emergent basis. Inelasticity of the transferred flap can be a detriment.

45. Deraemaeker R, Tienen CV, Lejour M, et al. The serratus anterior-scapular free flap: a new osteomuscular unit for reconstruction after radical head and neck surgery [abstract]. In Proceedings of the Second International Conference on Head and Neck Cancer, Boston, MA, July/Aug 1988.

46. Coleman JJ III, Sultan MR. The bipedicled osteocutaneous scapula flap: a new subscapular system free flap. Plast Reconstr Surg 87:682-692, 1991.

47. Allen RJ, Dupin CL, Dreschnack PA, et al. The latissimus dorsi/scapular bone flap (the "latissimus/bone flap"). Plast Reconstr Surg 94:988-996, 1994.

48. Hallock GG. Branch-based conjoined perforator flaps. Plast Reconstr Surg 121:1642-1649, 2008.

49. Hallock GG. The complete nomenclature for combined perforator flaps. Plast Reconstr Surg 1720-1729, 2011.

50. Hallock GG. Further clarification of the nomenclature for compound flaps. Plast Reconstr Surg 117:151e-160e, 2006.

51. Bakhach J, Peres JM, Scalise A, et al. The quadrifoliate flap: a combination of scapular, parascapular, latissimus dorsi and scapula bone flaps. Br J Plast Surg 49:477-481, 1996.

30

Dorsal Scapular Artery Perforator Flap

Claudio Angrigiani
Filip B. Stillaert

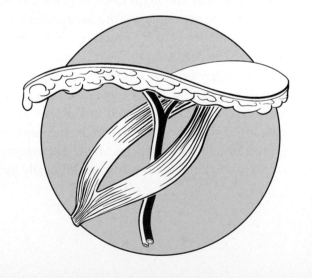

The back is a frequently used donor site for flaps, because it can provide thin, pliable tissue with minimal bulk. The resulting scar is inconspicuous. The dorsal scapular artery perforator (DSAP) flap is a safe and reliable method for transferring skin and subcutaneous tissue from the back to the anterior neck, face, and thoracic wall. The vessels provide a good possibility of raising an island flap from the back and transferring it to the anterior chest, neck, or face without microvascular anastomosis—in other words, as a distant island flap. Unfortunately, this is not an easy flap, because of possible anatomic variations. However, we believe it is worthwhile to attempt because of the advantages it offers. Microvascular anastomosis and the technical requirements for free tissue transfer are not required. There is minimal morbidity at the donor site, because the trapezius muscle is completely spared, preserving full shoulder motion. The donor area is frequently closed directly, resulting in an inconspicuous scar.

The DSAP flap is nourished by the cutaneous branches of the superficial branch of the dorsal scapular artery perforators of the dorsal scapular artery and vein. These perforators are consistently present[1-3] (Fig. 30-1).

A 25 by 12 cm flap raised on these vessels can be harvested with a long pedicle (15 to 16 cm) and tunneled under the main portion of the trapezius, levator scapulae, and omohyoid muscles to reach the anterior thoracic wall, cheek, and neck[4] (Fig. 30-2).

Traditionally, it was thought that the superficial branches of the transverse cervical artery and vein (the main vascular pedicle of the trapezius muscle) perfuse this cutaneous area (the upper part of the back), which was raised in the so-called lower trapezius musculocutaneous flap. Several reports indicate the contribution of the dorsal scapular artery to the perfusion of the trapezius musculocutaneous flap.[5,6] The authors of these reports suggest that this branch be included in the lower trapezius musculocutaneous flap to ensure flow to the most distal part of the flap. We believe this technique could be done only if the omohyoid and levator scapulae muscles are sectioned to incorporate the dorsal scapular pedicle, which runs underneath these muscles. If it is included in a conventional lower trapezius flap, it is necessary to section its origin at the rhomboid muscle, blocking its flow. It is anatomically included in the flap, but not functionally.

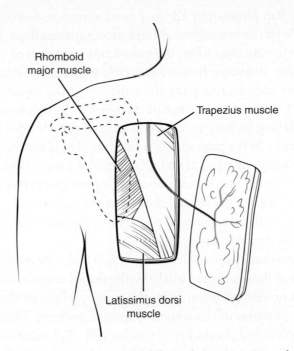

Rhomboid
major muscle

Trapezius muscle

Latissimus dorsi
muscle

Fig. 30-1 The dorsal scapular perforator island flap. The trapezius muscle is split, and the rhomboidei can be observed.

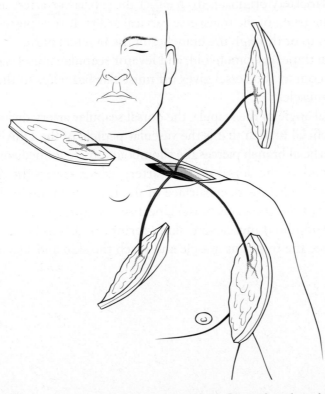

Fig. 30-2 The arc of rotation of the DSAP flap with its long leash.

The perforator flap philosophy allowed us to eliminate or reduce to a minimum the volume of muscle in the conventional musculocutaneous flaps. In this manner, we can create a true perforator flap when the cutaneous branches of the dorsal scapular flap have an appropriate diameter. In some cases there are several cutaneous perforators through the trapezius muscle, following the pathway of the superficial branch of the dorsal scapular artery at the deep surface of the muscle. In this situation, we prefer to perform a muscle-sparing technique, raising a strip of muscle containing the vascular pedicle with its branches. It is a time-saving procedure that does not increase morbidity.

The part of the integument (skin and subcutaneous tissue) raised in the DSAP flap is also fed by the intercostal cutaneous branches or perforators (especially the second, fifth, seventh, and ninth); the horizontal branch of the superficial circumflex scapular system (scapular flap); and the superficial posterior scapular through the main portion of the trapezius (at the superior part).

It has been shown that it is possible to raise a skin and subcutaneous island from the medial back with blood flow provided solely by the dorsal scapular cutaneous branches. This island receives no contribution from the main pedicle of the trapezius muscle and spares the main function of the trapezius muscle entirely. Thus shoulder motion is completely preserved and morbidity is minimized. A clinical series that involved 45 patients demonstrated that the dorsal scapular artery perforator flap is an alternative for anterior chest, anterior neck, and head reconstruction.

ANATOMY

The dorsal scapular artery originates from either the subclavian artery as an independent branch or from the trunk of the transverse cervical artery. It runs posteriorly and almost horizontally, deep to or through the branches of the brachial plexus.[7-9] The artery then courses under the trapezius, omohyoid, and levator scapulae muscles on top of the rib cage. During its course, the vessel gives off muscular branches to the omohyoid and levator scapulae muscles.

At the medial angle of the scapula, the dorsal scapular artery divides into two main branches: a superficial branch that is the vascular pedicle of the DSAP flap and a deep branch. The superficial branch pierces the rhomboid muscle immediately after its origin from the main trunk of the dorsal scapular artery, which covers the rhomboid at that point, and appears under the deep surface of the trapezius muscle. The branch runs on the deep belly of the trapezius muscle, perfuses that muscle, and gives off several branches to the rhomboid muscle and skin (perforators). These cutaneous branches (perforators) pierce the trapezius muscle and reach the skin and subcutaneous tissue.

The dorsal scapular artery perforators are normally located approximately 6 cm inferior to the superomedial angle of the scapula, and 1 to 2 cm medial to the lateral border of the trapezius muscle (Fig. 30-3). According to the Dubreuil Chambardell compensation law, in some cases there are several cutaneous branches of equal size, and sometimes there are one or two of larger diameter than the other ones. We found up to six small to moderate cutaneous branches. In this situation, it is preferable to incorporate a strip of trapezius muscle, including all branches instead of performing a true perforator flap (as shown in the cadaveric surgical demonstration on p. 584) similar to a muscle-sparing technique. When a large perforator is present, a true perforator flap can be safely performed. This was the case in 9 of 45 cases.

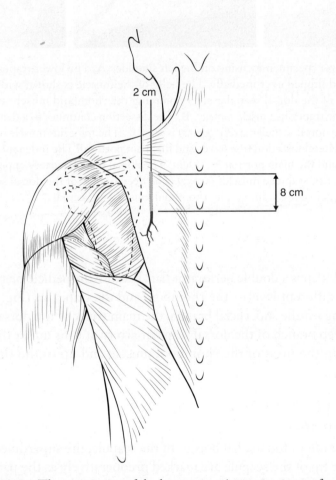

Fig. 30-3 The emergence of the lower trapezius cutaneous perforator.

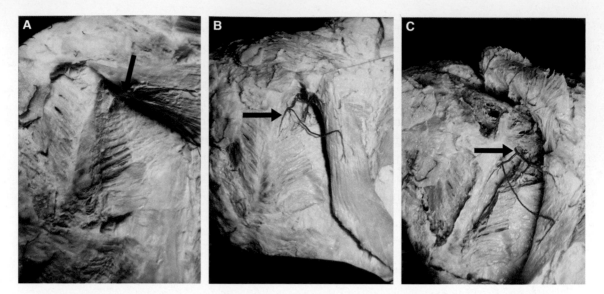

Fig. 30-4   Cadaver specimen focusing on the left shoulder. **A,** The lower trapezius muscle is transected distally and flipped over medially. The belly of the muscle is shown with the superficial or muscular branch of the dorsal scapular artery piercing the rhomboid muscle and attached to the undersurface of the trapezius muscle *(arrow).* **B,** The dissection continues to a deeper level where the deep branch of the dorsal scapular artery *(arrow)* is seen. **C,** The trapezius muscle has been completely elevated from its lateral insertion (the lower and the main portion). The independent vascularization of the lower part and the main portion is evident. The dorsal scapular artery appears from under the omohyoid and levator scapulae muscles *(arrow).* The deep branch of the dorsal scapular artery runs on the medial border of the scapula. The rhomboid muscle is resected.

The DSAP flap is a double perforator flap, because the pedicle pierces two different muscles at two different levels—the rhomboid and the trapezius (Fig. 30-4).

After giving off the superficial branch, the main trunk of the dorsal scapular artery becomes the deep branch of the dorsal scapular artery. It runs under the medial border of the scapula in the mass of the rhomboid muscle and up to the tip of the scapula, which it perfuses.

SURGICAL TECHNIQUE
Surface Landmarks

The skin projection of the medial border of the scapula, the superomedial angle of the scapula, and the tip of the scapula are marked preoperatively as the patient stands with arms at the side of the body. The spinous processes of the vertebrae are also marked to indicate the midline. A line drawn between the spine of the scapula and the spinous process of the tenth thoracic vertebra indicates the approximate location of the lateral border of the trapezius muscle. A point is marked 2 cm medial to the lateral border of the trapezius muscle at the level of the middle of the scapula. This point represents the emergence of the cutaneous perforator through the trapezius muscle and must be included in the flap design (see Fig. 30-5, *H*). The cutaneous perforator can be identified preoperatively with a Doppler probe, though this is not routinely done.

A 20 by 20 cm skin paddle can be safely harvested on this perforator. The flap design may be oriented in any direction. Most commonly we use a vertical design or a minimal external oblique design for better closure of the donor area.

Vascular Anatomy and Flap Elevation

The skin is incised along the margins of the flap. Under loupe magnification, dissection is performed superficial to the deep fascia up to the lateral border of the trapezius muscle. The cutaneous perforator is identified and deeply dissected to the main trunk of the superficial dorsal scapular artery through the trapezius muscle. Gentle elevation of the edge of the trapezius muscle allows identification of the superficial dorsal scapular artery. The artery runs on the deep surface of the trapezius muscle from the point where it pierces the rhomboid muscle. Care must be taken when the trapezius muscle is elevated, because the superficial dorsal scapular artery pierces the rhomboid muscle at variable levels. Most frequently, the vessel is seen piercing the rhomboid muscle at the level of the superomedial angle of the scapula, or even several centimeters inferior to that point.

The superficial dorsal scapular artery is liberated from the belly of the trapezius muscle with blunt dissection. Muscle branches are ligated, and the cutaneous perforator is dissected free. Dissection is continued through the rhomboid muscle. The deep branch (or main trunk) of the dorsal scapular artery is identified, ligated, and sectioned. The levator scapulae, omohyoid, and trapezius muscles are held with a long retractor to help create the tunnel. It is possible to observe the dorsal scapular artery running on top of the rib cage through the areolar tissue. The muscle branches to the omohyoid and levator scapulae muscles are ligated and sectioned. The origin of the dorsal scapular artery is visible at the end of this tunnel. A long cannula is passed through this tunnel superior to (above) the pedicle until the tip of the cannula contacts the deep surface of the skin of the supraclavicular area. A skin incision is made at this level, and the tunnel is then completed. The flap is passed through the tunnel and left there temporarily, wrapped in moist gauze. Even large flaps (25 by 25 cm) are easily tunneled without sectioning the muscles.

The donor area is closed directly or with a skin graft. The wound is draped, and the patient is turned to a dorsal decubitus position. The flap is easily mobilized because of its long vascular pedicle. The flap is inset in the corresponding site and sutured in place.

CASE EXAMPLE

This 49-year-old man with cavum oris cancer had an extensive soft tissue defect (Fig. 30-5, *A*). He had been treated initially with a pectoralis major flap and adjuvant radiation therapy. An extensive wound dehiscence developed postoperatively, and he was referred to our department for further treatment. The mandible was exposed intraorally. The entire anterior cervical region was scarred from radiation therapy.

Flaps were required for three areas: (1) coverage and reconstruction of the anterior cervical region, (2) coverage of the exposed mandible intraorally, and (3) soft tissue coverage of the extensive defect overlying the neurovascular structures in the neck. A free TRAM flap was designed with two skin paddles—one small skin paddle to cover the mandible and a larger skin paddle to reconstruct the anterior cervical region (Fig. 30-5, *B* and *C*). The rectus muscle was used to cover the neurovascular structures and restore bulk within the neck. Anastomoses were performed to the internal mammary vessels (Fig. 30-5, *D*). The immediate postoperative result is shown in Fig. 30-5, *E*.

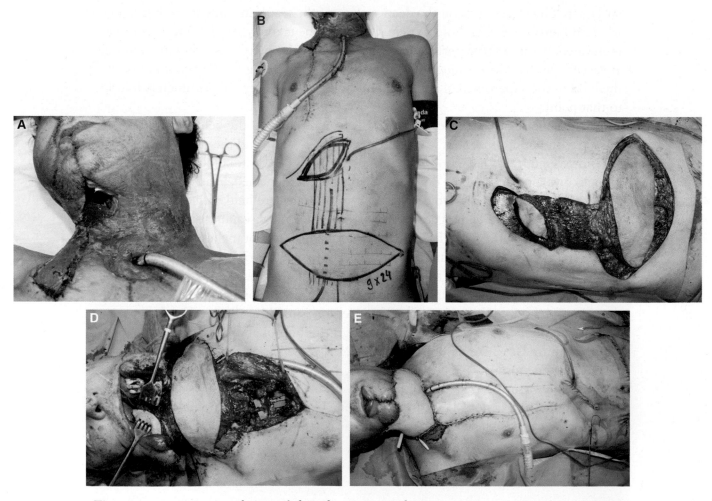

Fig. 30-5 **A,** Extensive soft tissue defect after treatment for cavum oris cancer. **B** and **C,** A TRAM flap with two skin paddles was performed. **D,** The early reconstruction is shown. **E,** The patient is shown immediately after surgery.

Two months postoperatively, the patient presented with wound breakdown at the mandibular angle caused by previous radiation treatment (Fig. 30-5, *F* and *G*). A pedicle DSAP flap was chosen to cover the remaining defect (Fig. 30-5, *H*). The cutaneous perforators can easily be identified with a subfascial dissection (Fig. 30-5, *I*). With the trapezius muscle lifted up, the superficial dorsal scapular artery can be identified (Fig. 30-5, *J*). One can dissect between the fibers of the trapezius muscle or harvest a small piece of the muscle around the perforator. Once the flap is completely freed, a tunnel is created cranially underneath the trapezius muscle up to the defect (Fig. 30-5, *K*). Once in place, the flap can be molded to cover the defect (Fig. 30-5, *L*).

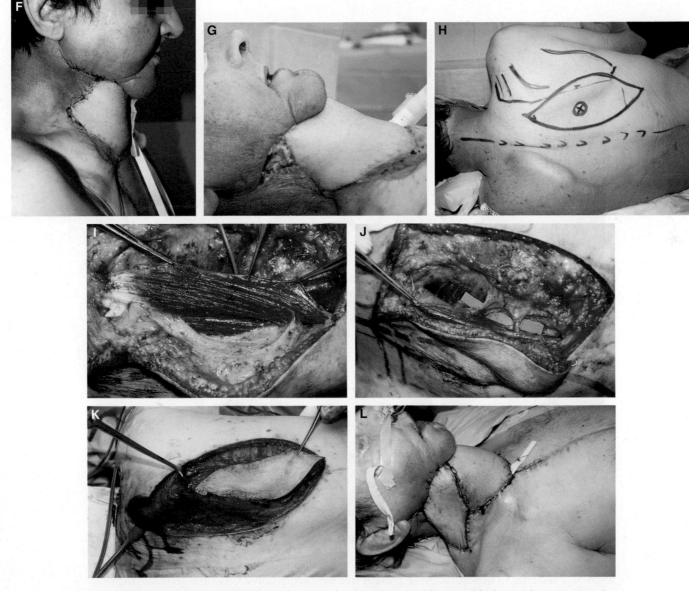

Fig. 30-5, cont'd **F** and **G,** The wound has broken down at the mandibular angle, exposing the vessels. **H,** The DSAP flap was designed preoperatively. **I,** The perforators were identified. **J,** The submuscular superficial dorsal scapular artery was isolated. **K,** A submuscular tunnel was created under the trapezius muscle. **L,** The patient is shown immediately postoperatively.

MODIFICATIONS

The medial border and the tip of the scapula can be included as a vascularized bone by harvesting the deep branch of the dorsal scapular artery. This branch also gives off a cutaneous branch, making it possible to raise an independent skin island, which is useful when lining and skin coverage are necessary.

The deep branch of the dorsal scapular artery is easily identified in the mass of the rhomboid muscle as one follows the superficial branch to the point where it pierces this muscle. The deep branch is dissected inferiorly through the muscle. Several bone branches to the medial border of the scapula are observed. A predetermined bone segment or the complete medial border of the bone can be harvested[10] (Fig. 30-6).

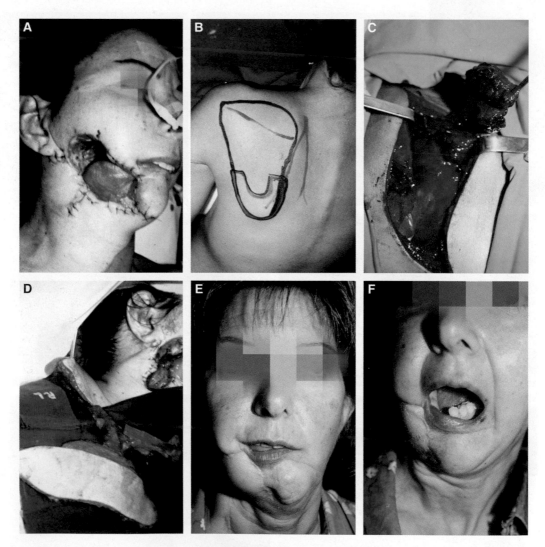

Fig. 30-6   A, This patient developed a full-thickness defect on her right cheek after a mandibular tumor was resected. Complete failure of a fibular free flap occurred. **B-D,** A dorsal scapular cutaneous (double-padded) flap with an osseous component from the medial border of the scapula was elevated and tunneled to the anterior part. **E,** Skin and mucosa were closed, and bone was reconstructed. **F,** Opening of the mouth is acceptable in the immediate postoperative period.

PITFALLS

It is important to perform a gentle elevation of the lateral border of the trapezius muscle. The superficial branch of the dorsal scapular artery travels from the rhomboid muscle, which it pierces, to the belly of the trapezius muscle, where it attaches. If the trapezius muscle is pulled strongly, the artery will be stretched near its emergence from the rhomboid muscle.

The cutaneous perforator of the superficial branch of the dorsal scapular artery may pierce the rhomboid muscle at different levels, including the lateral border of the muscle. Therefore careful dissection is essential until the vessel is directly observed.

References

1. Salmon M. Les artères des muscles du tronc. Paris: Masson, 1933.
2. Haas F, Pierer G, Weiglein A, et al. The lower trapezius muscle island flap. Anatomic principles and clinical relevance. Handchir Mikrochir Plast Chir 31:15-20, 1999.

    A dissection study was carried out to examine characteristics of the subclavian artery and its branches, vessel diameter at different levels, the course of the pedicle under the levator scapulae muscle, the arc of rotation of the island flap, and the variations of the segmental intercostal branches to the lower part of the trapezius muscle. Based on results, a new nomenclature for the branches of the subclavian artery, a proper pedicle definition, and a technique for safe flap elevation are possible.

3. Tan KC, Tan BK. Extended lower trapezius island myocutaneous flap: a fasciomyocutaneous flap based on the dorsal scapular artery. Plast Reconstr Surg 105:1758-1763, 2000.

    The lower trapezius island musculocutaneous flap in head and neck reconstruction has often been limited or discouraged by reports of significant failure rates. The authors examined the vascular anatomy and clinical use of the extended lower trapezius musculocutaneous flap based solely on the dorsal scapular artery system.

4. Angrigiani C, Grilli D, Karanas YL, et al. The dorsal scapular island flap: an alternative for head, neck, and chest reconstruction. Plast Reconstr Surg 111:67-78, 2003.

    A cadaveric and clinical study was performed to evaluate the anatomy of the dorsal scapular vessels and their vascular contribution to the skin, fascia, and muscles of the back. The authors concluded that the dorsal scapular vessels provide a reliable blood supply to the skin of the medial back, making it a versatile flap to use as an island flap. They recommend this versatile island pedicle flap as an alternative to microvascular free tissue transfer for reconstructing defects in the head, neck, and anterior chest.

5. Netterville JL, Wood DE. The lower trapezius flap. Vascular anatomy and surgical technique. Arch Otolaryngol Head Neck Surg 117:73-76, 1991.

    The blood supply to the skin provided by the dorsal scapular artery was studied. A surgical technique using the lower trapezius flap, including the dorsal scapular artery, was described. This technique significantly extends the usefulness of the lower trapezius flap, decreasing the morbidity caused by division of the upper portion of the trapezius muscle during flap harvest.

6. Weiglein AH, Haas F, Pierer G, et al. Anatomic basis of the lower trapezius musculocutaneous flap. Surg Radiol Anat 18:257-261, 1996.

    The arterial supply of the lower trapezius muscle was examined. The authors concluded that the lower trapezius musculocutaneous flap merits consideration in head and neck reconstruction.

7. Huelke DF. A study of the transverse cervical and dorsal scapular arteries. Anat Rec 103: 233-245, 1958.
8. Daseler EH, Anson BJ. Surgical anatomy of the subclavian artery and its branches. Surg Gynecol Obstet 108:149-174, 1959.

9. Cormack GC, Lamberty BGH. The Arterial Anatomy of Skin Flaps. New York: Churchill Livingstone, 1994.

10. Krespi YP, Oppenheimer RW, Flanzer JM, et al. The rhombotrapezius myocutaneous and osteomyocutaneous flaps. Arch Otolaryngol Head Neck Surg 114:734-738, 1988.

The rhombotrapezius flap in head and neck reconstruction was studied. The authors described a flap that provides bulk for augmenting facial defects. The flap includes the trapezius and rhomboid muscles and offers a longer pedicle with a greater arc of rotation. It may include the medial border of the scapula when bone is necessary.

31

Thoracodorsal Artery Perforator Flap

Koenraad Van Landuyt

Colin M. Morrison

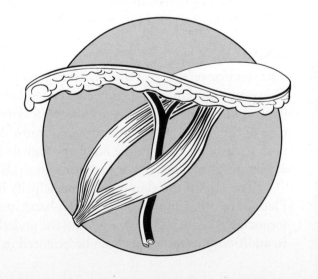

The use of cutaneous flaps from the lateral thoracic region date back to the early years of microsurgery[1] and include the thoracodorsal skin flap,[2] free lateral thoracic flap,[3] and axillary flap.[4,5] These flaps are based on the lateral thoracic artery, the superficial or accessory lateral thoracic artery, or the cutaneous branch of the thoracodorsal artery.[6] However, the anatomic variation in the location and size of these vessels made them unreliable as free flaps, but the subaxillary pedicled flap[7] and the lateral thoracic region flap[8] did regain some interest as pedicle procedures.

The constant anatomic location and size of the thoracodorsal artery[9,10] made the latissimus dorsi musculocutaneous flap a workhorse of reconstructive surgery.[11] Various methods were developed to split the muscle either longitudinally or transversely[12,13] to reduce donor site morbidity and flap bulk. Some authors also described extending the skin island as a fasciocutaneous flap based on the musculocutaneous perforators of the thoracodorsal artery or expanding the muscle to augment its reconstructive capabilities.[14,15] Despite harvesting the entire muscle, significant donor site morbidity following a latissimus dorsi flap has not been well demonstrated.[16] However, conceptually, a flap that leaves the underlying muscular component intact seems more likely to have less of an aesthetic and functional deficit.

In 1995 Angrigiani et al[17] first described the use of a cutaneous island of the latissimus dorsi flap based on a single perforator of the thoracodorsal artery for lower extremity reconstruction. Since then the thoracodorsal artery perforator (TDAP) flap has also been described for reconstructing the head and neck, trunk, and extremities.[18-23]

ANATOMY

The vascular territory of the TDAP flap essentially overlies the latissimus dorsi muscle. However, the skin island can be extended beyond the anterior border of the muscle, depending on the musculocutaneous perforators of the thoracodorsal artery. An advantage of the TDAP flap is that the perforator does not need to be centered to reliably perfuse this flap, though the number of reliable perforators is considerably less than in a deep inferior epigastric artery perforator (DIEAP) or anterolateral thigh (ALT) flap.

The size of the skin island is principally limited by the need for primary closure. Flaps of up to 25 by 14 cm have been harvested without significant problems. Seroma formation is reduced, because none of the underlying latissimus dorsi muscle is sacrificed. In addition, the skin island can be oriented in different directions, depending on the reconstructive needs or preferred direction of the scar. One of the possible flap designs includes a bilobed flap with a smaller ellipse oriented transversely to aid in closure of the larger vertical ellipse, after the flap is rotated 90 degrees.

The skin territory is large, because perforators in this area are spaced widely apart, creating larger angiosomes and increasing the vascular territory of this flap.[24] The neighboring territories include the lateral thoracic artery and, anteriorly, the superficial or accessory thoracic artery. The lateral cutaneous branches of the intercostals also anastomose with these. Posteriorly, the perforators from the costal groove segment of the intercostals and the lumbar artery perforators dominate. Cranially, the TDAP flap extends to the region of the scapular and parascapular flaps, based on the circumflex scapular artery. According to the dynamic perfusion theory of Taylor and Palmer,[25] parts of these territories can also be included in the TDAP flap.

SURGICAL TECHNIQUE
Surface Landmarks

The patient is placed in a lateral decubitus position with the arm abducted 90 degrees at the shoulder and flexed 90 degrees at the elbow. The anterior border of the latissimus dorsi muscle is palpated and marked. To include all potential cutaneous perforators of the thoracodorsal artery, the anterior boundary of the flap should lie in front of the latissimus dorsi, at the level of the vascular hilus. This is located approximately 8 cm below the axillary crease. The flap is designed as a vertical ellipse over the latissimus dorsi. Its width depends on the recipient site requirements and the desire for primary donor site closure. Flaps of up to 14 by 25 cm have been safely raised based on a single perforator.

The design of the TDAP flap can be modified depending on whether free or pedicled transfer of tissue is required. A free TDAP flap should be based on the thoracodorsal pedicle, but a local flap can be based on the intercostal, serratus, or capillary perforators.[26] In the latter instance, the tissue is often rotated as a propeller, as opposed to being transposed.

Some authors have recommended preoperative duplex or Doppler imaging to help identify perforators.[27] Unfortunately, the superficial vascular landmarks are not as constant as those of the abdomen, where perforators can be centered on the umbilicus. This makes it more difficult to preoperatively plan a grid on which to mark the exit points of these perforators, in comparison to a DIEAP flap. In addition, after their exit from the latissimus dorsi, the perforators run posteriorly on top of the muscle fascia for a variable distance (2 to 6 cm). This can be misleading when attempting to identify the exact exit point of the perforator from the muscle if using a handheld Doppler probe. Moreover, most of the perforators tend to exit over the course of the descending branch of the thoracodorsal artery, which can lead to false positive results when using Doppler sonography for identification.

The initial incision of a TDAP flap is at the anteroinferior border of the skin island, allowing identification of the anterior border of the latissimus dorsi muscle and adjustment of the anterior border of the flap accordingly.

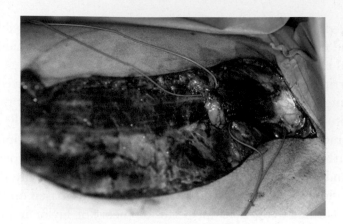

Fig. 31-1   Superficial thoracic vessels contour the anterior border of the latissimus dorsi muscle.

Vascular Anatomy

The main perforators normally lie in a row overlying the course of the descending branch of the thoracodorsal artery.[28] As previously mentioned, the perforator does not need to be centrally located to perfuse the TDAP flap. Dissection proceeds posteriorly and superiorly in the loose areolar tissue plane between the latissimus dorsi muscle fascia and the overlying fat. As the dissection proceeds more proximally, care should be taken not to overlook a cutaneous branch of the thoracodorsal artery, either as a direct branch (or the superficial thoracic artery of Manchot) or as a perforator emerging around the anterior border of the latissimus dorsi muscle (Fig. 31-1).

Once a suitable perforator has been selected (one artery and two venae comitantes), it is dissected through the underlying muscle to the main vascular trunk. Perforators are contained within a fatty layer to allow excursion during muscular contraction. As a result, they can be readily freed from the surrounding muscle fibers by dissecting close to the vascular pedicle using a combination of loupe magnification ligation, clipping, and/or bipolar coagulation of the various muscular branches. No attempt should be made to harvest the flap as a muscle-sparing procedure, because this causes capillary oozing and bleeding that will obscure the course of the perforator through the muscle, making vessel damage more likely.

Where two or more suitable perforators are found, perforator selection depends on the required pedicle length. A perforator positioned more distally on the muscle allows a longer pedicle length, but also necessitates a longer dissection time. Some of the more distal perforators can originate from the intercostal vessels, and this should be determined as early as possible in the procedure. This is done by releasing the anterior border of the latissimus dorsi muscle and inspecting its undersurface (Fig. 31-2).

Once the complete intramuscular pathway has been dissected, the thoracodorsal pedicle is harvested in a routine fashion. The total pedicle length depends on the location of the perforator on the muscle, the intramuscular course of the vessel, and the length of the thoracodorsal pedicle itself. Dissecting the thoracodorsal perforator and the axial vessels provides a pedicle length of 14 to 18 cm.

The posterior rami of the lateral cutaneous branches of the intercostal nerves enter the skin together with the perforators but tend to run more posteriorly and in a deeper plane, directly on top of the muscle (Fig. 31-3). To harvest a sensate flap, one or more

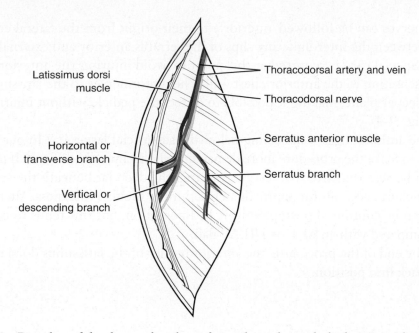

Fig. 31-2 Branches of the thoracodorsal vessels are shown beneath the latissimus dorsi muscle.

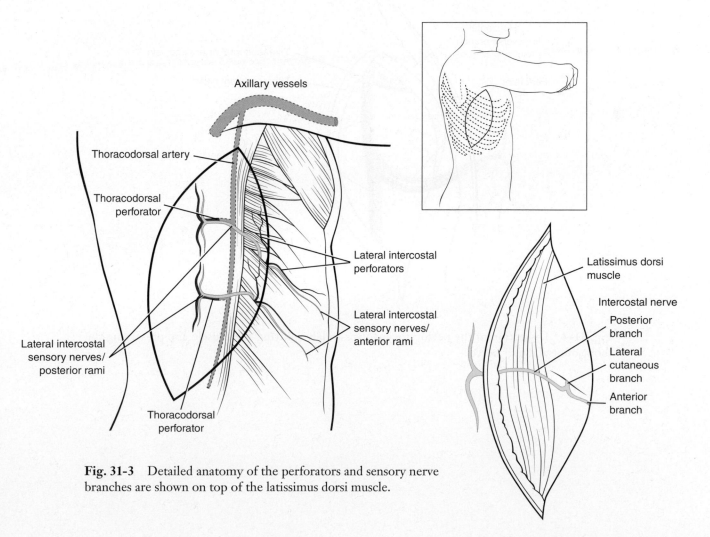

Fig. 31-3 Detailed anatomy of the perforators and sensory nerve branches are shown on top of the latissimus dorsi muscle.

of these nerves can be followed anteriorly to their origin from the lateral cutaneous branch, between the interdigitating slips of the serratus anterior and external oblique muscles. Special care is required at this point to avoid injuring the anterior rami to preserve sensation to the anterior chest wall. The motor nerves to the latissimus dorsi run in a deeper plane, making it possible to dissect the pedicle without injuring these nerves (Fig. 31-4).

Some authors suggest dissecting below the superficial fascia.[29-31] In our opinion, this tends to make the procedure more demanding and technically difficult. If necessary, tissue can be removed after harvest by resecting the deep fat beneath the superficial fascia, which can account for approximately a third of the flap thickness. Alternatively, the flap can be contoured postoperatively by liposuction, but this tends to be less effective compared with an ALT or DIEAP flap.

At the end of the procedure, the anterior border of the latissimus dorsi muscle is sutured back into position.

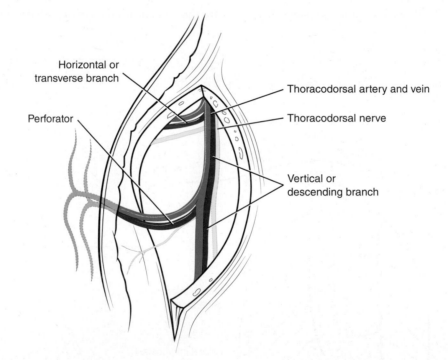

Horizontal or transverse branch

Perforator

Thoracodorsal artery and vein

Thoracodorsal nerve

Vertical or descending branch

Fig. 31-4   Dissection of the perforator involves widely splitting the muscle and preserving the thoracodorsal motor nerve.

Neighboring Anatomic Structures

In some patients, extra venous outflow can be achieved by incorporating the lateral thoracic vein, which descends more anteriorly on the lateral thoracic wall. This vein gives off branches that connect with the intercostal veins, running in conjunction with the posterior rami of the lateral cutaneous branches of the intercostal nerves. The lateral thoracic vein continues on the anterolateral chest wall and forms a subcutaneous network with the superficial epigastric vein. Unfortunately, it rarely drains directly into the thoracodorsal pedicle. Most often it finishes separately from the axillary vein, requiring an additional microvascular anastomosis.

MODIFICATIONS

In addition to harvesting the TDAP flap as a free flap, it is also possible to raise a pedicle flap with either a transversally or longitudinally oriented skin island. As a pedicle flap, the skin island does need to be passed between the muscle fibers, requiring a larger muscular split. However, it is still usually possible to harvest the flap without significantly injuring the motor nerves (Fig. 31-5).

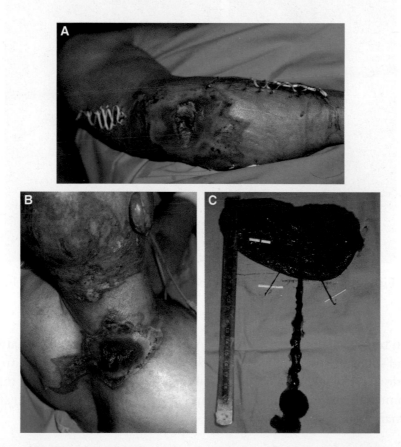

Fig. 31-5 A and **B,** This patient had a high-voltage burn with entry and exit points at the right elbow and neck. **C,** A free TDAP flap covered the elbow, and a pedicle TDAP flap was placed in the neck defect.

Continued

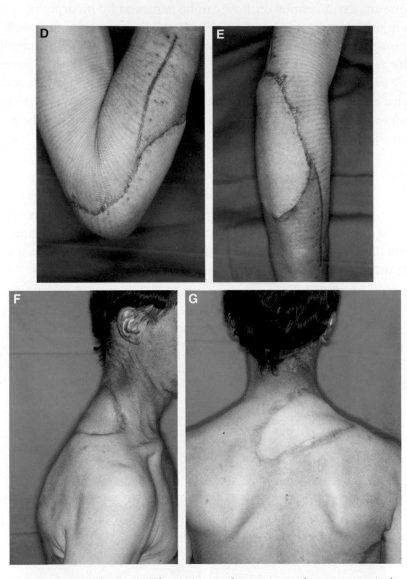

Fig. 31-5, cont'd   D-G, The patient is shown 6 months postoperatively.

When transversely oriented, the TDAP flap takes advantage of a natural fold in the skin and subcutaneous tissue of the back, a similar skin paddle design to the classic latissimus dorsi musculocutaneous flap used for breast reconstruction. In this instance, the anteromedial corner of the TDAP flap is positioned at the lateral extent of the inframammary crease.

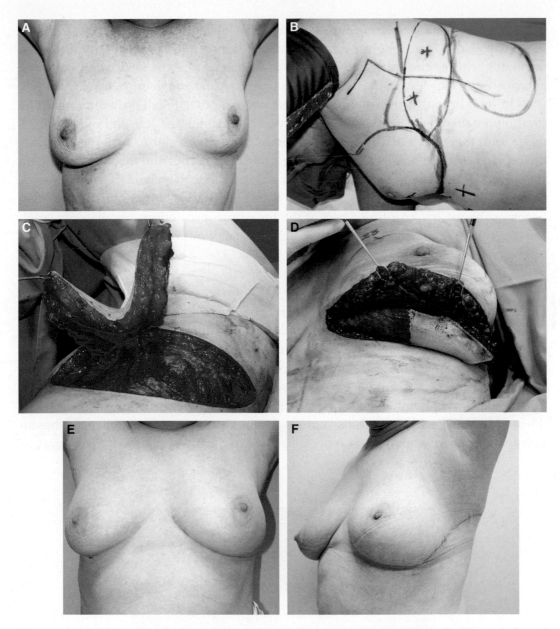

Fig. 31-6 A, This patient is shown before surgery to correct breast asymmetry. **B,** The main lateral intercostal and thoracodorsal perforators *(red Xs)* were located by Doppler sonography. **C** and **D,** The flap was harvested and positioned. **E** and **F,** She is shown 3 months postoperatively.

The main indications for a transversely oriented TDAP flap are in breast surgery,[32] either for partial breast reconstruction after ablative surgery or autologous augmentation for hypoplasia or congenital deformity of the breast (Fig. 31-6). Another good indication is simultaneous breast augmentation and mastopexy for postbariatric surgery patients.

A longitudinally oriented skin island reaches the distal third of the upper arm and elbow, the neck, shoulder, and upper back area.

As with a scapular-parascapular flap, the TDAP flap can also be harvested as a bi-lobed flap, with a large longitudinal and a smaller transversely oriented skin island that facilitates primary closure after 90 degrees of rotation. Since the pivot point lies more anteriorly, the flap reaches further into the anterior axilla and deltopectoral groove.

In total breast reconstruction, the dissection approach is slightly different. The maximum size of the TDAP flap is determined by pinching the skin and subcutaneous tissue folds together. The flap is then harvested from a posterior to anterior direction, the primary incision being made at the inferoposterior border and then proceeding on the surface of the latissimus dorsi muscle. It is much easier to include the muscle fascia, with dissection similar to that of the SGAP flap. The anterior border of the TDAP flap becomes the medial or inferior part of the breast reconstruction. The flap can reach the superolateral, inferolateral, and inferomedial quadrants of the breast. All the scars can be concealed by a brassiere.

ADVANTAGES

One of the biggest advantages of the TDAP flap is the combination of tissues that can be incorporated by the thoracodorsal pedicle.[33-36] A compound flap can be created with (1) a split latissimus dorsi muscle component,[37] including the descending branch, (2) the serratus muscle[38] or thoracodorsal fascia[39] component, including the serratus branches (Fig. 31-7), (3) the anterior margin of the scapula, including the angular branch,[40] or (4) scapular or parascapular skin flaps, including the circumflex scapular pedicle.[41,42] The perforator itself, through its suprafascial and intramuscular course, also has an independent range of motion of approximately 4 to 6 cm.

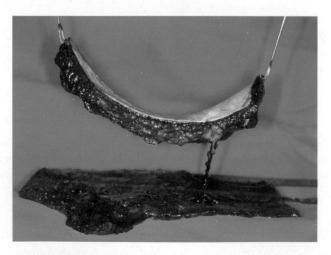

Fig. 31-7   A compound TDAP flap can be created with a serratus muscle and/or thoracodorsal fascia component.

PITFALLS

Considering the size of the latissimus dorsi muscle and in comparison to other perforator flaps, the TDAP flap has far fewer suitable perforators, making it anatomically slightly less reliable. It is also more difficult to identify the perforators preoperatively, making this flap slightly riskier for less experienced surgeons.[43] It is, therefore, essential to identify a large perforator in a suitable location before continuing with the dissection. After dissection, the vessel is prone to spasm, which can make size evaluation difficult. The perforator should ideally incorporate two discernible veins and an artery.

After a suitable perforator is identified, the intramuscular dissection is straightforward. It is essential to stay close to the vessel and ligate, clip, or coagulate even the smallest side branch at a safe distance from the main pedicle. We emphasize that including muscle in the dissection of the perforator is particularly dangerous, because it leads to capillary oozing, obscuring the course of the perforator, its side branches, and associated nerves.

The more distal the perforator branch from the descending branch of the thoracodorsal vessels, the longer the pedicle. On the other hand, the smaller the perforator, the longer its intramuscular course, and the more likely it is to be an intercostal rather than a thoracodorsal perforator. Traction on the perforator should be avoided at all costs, and continuous irrigation with warm saline helps prevent vessel desiccation and spasm.

After the vascular anastomosis and flap inset, a brisk capillary refill can often be observed. This is most likely from reperfusion edema. Perforator flaps can survive in low-flow conditions. Venous outflow problems, such as those resulting from thrombosis of the venous anastomosis, can easily be masked in the early postoperative period, when the flap will survive by oozing from its wound edges. Prolonged bleeding, a bluish tinge, swelling of the flap, or a drop in skin temperature with preserved microcirculation should alert the surgeon to reexplore the flap.

Low venous output also allows flap salvage after late venous thrombosis by applying leeches. In contrast to more bulky perforator flaps, such as the DIEAP, where major fat necrosis can be expected after venous congestion and salvage by revision surgery is required, with the TDAP flap, leeches can be a valuable alternative to more heroic procedures.

The cosmetic result depends on the orientation of the flap. A longitudinally oriented flap can leave a rather unattractive scar, although it is partially hidden on the lateral chest wall by the upper limb. In female patients, primary closure of a large donor site under tension can temporarily displace the nipple-areola complex laterally. If the flap is transversely oriented, the donor site scar can be hidden by a brassiere, but can still cause a contour deformity if harvested unilaterally. Nevertheless, this is not nearly as unsightly as a traditional musculocutaneous latissimus dorsi flap.

References

1. Taylor GI, Daniel RK. The anatomy of several free flap donor sites. Plast Reconstr Surg 56:243-253, 1975.
2. de Coninck A, Vanderlinden E, Boeckx W. The thoracodorsal skin flap: a possible donor site in distant transfer of island flaps by microvascular anastomosis. Chir Plast (Berlin) 3:283-291, 1976.
3. Harii K, Torii S, Sekiguchi J. The free lateral thoracic flap. Plast Reconstr Surg 62:212-222, 1978.
4. Baudet J, Guimberteau JC, Nascimento E. Successful clinical transfer of two free thoraco-dorsal axillary flaps. Plast Reconstr Surg 58:680-688, 1976.

   Two cases were presented using a new flap from the axilla, based on the thoracodorsal artery and vein. In the first case, the flap was used to cover an extensive exposure of the dura mater. In the second case, it was transferred to cover a large area of skin loss in the knee with joint involvement. Further investigation was necessary to accurately ascertain the possibilities and the limits of this flap.

5. de Coninck A, Boeckx W. Autotransplants using vascular microsutures. Acta Chir Belg 74:581-586, 1975.
6. Maxwell GP, Stueber K, Hoopes JE, et al. A free latissimus dorsi myocutaneous flap: case report. Plast Reconstr Surg 62:462-466, 1978.
7. Chandra R, Kumar P, Abdi SH, et al. The subaxillary pedicled flap. Br J Plast Surg 41:169-173, 1988.
8. Bhattacharya S, Bhagia SP, Bhatnagar SK, et al. The lateral thoracic region flap. Br J Plast Surg 43:162-168, 1990.
9. Bartlett SP, May JW Jr, Yaremchuk MJ, et al. The latissimus dorsi muscle: a fresh cadaver study of the primary neurovascular pedicle. Plast Reconstr Surg 67:631-636, 1981.
10. Rowsell AR, Davies DM, Eisenberg N, et al. The anatomy of the subscapular-thoracodorsal arterial system: study of 100 cadaver dissections. Br J Plast Surg 37:574-576, 1984.
11. Cabanie H, Garbe JF, Guimberteau JC, et al. Anatomical basis of the thoracodorsal axillary flap with respect to its transfer by means of microvascular surgery. Anat Clin 2:65-73, 1980.
12. Godina M. The tailored latissimus dorsi free flap. Plast Reconstr Surg 80:304-306, 1987.
13. Rowsell AR, Godfrey AM, Richards MA, et al. The thinned latissimus dorsi free flap: a case report. Br J Plast Surg 39:210-212, 1986.
14. Spinelli HM, Fink JA, Muzaffar AR. The latissimus dorsi perforator-based fasciocutaneous flap. Ann Plast Surg 37:500-506, 1996.

   The authors described a new and useful extension of the latissimus dorsi musculocutaneous unit that consists of a fasciocutaneous segment based on musculocutaneous perforators from the thoracodorsal artery. The vascular anatomy of the flap was described and illustrated, and clinical cases were presented.

15. Elliot D, Lewis-Smith PA, Piggot TA, et al. The expanded latissimus dorsi flap. Br J Plast Surg 41:319-321, 1988.
16. Russell RC, Pribaz J, Zook EG, et al. Functional evaluation of latissimus dorsi donor site. Plast Reconstr Surg 78:336-344, 1986.
17. Angrigiani C, Grilli D, Siebert J, et al. Latissimus dorsi musculocutaneous flap without muscle. Plast Reconstr Surg 96:1608-1614, 1995.

   The authors described raising the cutaneous island of the latissimus dorsi musculocutaneous flap based on only one cutaneous perforator.

18. Guerra AB, Metzinger SE, Lund KM, et al. The thoracodorsal artery perforator flap: clinical experience and anatomic study with emphasis on harvest techniques. Plast Reconstr Surg 114:32-41, 2004.
19. Guerra AB, Lyons GD, Dupin CL, et al. Advantages of perforator flaps in reconstruction of complex defects of the head and neck. Ear Nose Throat J 84:441-447, 2005.
20. Oritiz CL, Mendoza MM, Sempere LN, et al. Versatility of the pedicled thoracodorsal artery perforator (TDAP) flap in soft tissue reconstruction. Ann Plast Surg 58:315-320, 2007.

21. Ayhan S, Tuncer S, Demir Y, et al. Thoracodorsal artery perforator flap: a versatile alternative for various soft tissue defects. J Reconstr Microsurg 24:285-293, 2008.

22. Lee SH, Mun GH. Transverse thoracodorsal artery perforator flaps: experience with 31 free flaps. J Plast Reconstr Aesthet Surg 61:372-379, 2008.

23. Bidros RS, Metzinger SE, Guerra AB. The thoracodorsal artery perforator-scapular osteocutaneous (TDAP-SOC) flap for reconstruction of palatal and maxillary defects. Ann Plast Surg 54:59-65, 2005.

24. Heitmann C, Guerra A, Metzinger SW, et al. The thoracodorsal artery perforator flap: anatomic basis and clinical application. Ann Plast Surg 51:23-29, 2003.
    The authors detailed the vascular anatomy of the thoracodorsal artery and its cutaneous perforator vessels in 20 fresh cadavers.

25. Taylor GI, Palmer JH. The vascular territories (angiosomes) of the body: experimental study and clinical applications. Br J Plast Surg 40:113-141, 1987.

26. Koshima I, Narushima M, Mihara M, et al. New thoracodorsal artery perforator (TAPcp) flap with capillary perforators for reconstruction of upper limb. J Plast Reconstr Aesthet Surg 63:40-45, 2010.

27. Kim JT. Latissimus dorsi perforator flap. Clin Plast Surg 30:403-431, 2003.

28. Mun GH, Lee SJ, Jeon BJ. Perforator topography of the thoracodorsal artery perforator flap. Plast Reconstr Surg 121:497-504, 2008.

29. Kim JT, Koo BS, Kim SK, et al. The thin latissimus dorsi perforator-based free flap for resurfacing. Plast Reconstr Surg 107:374-382, 2001.

30. Hyakusoku H, Gao JH. The "super-thin" flap. Br J Plast Surg 47:457-464, 1994.

31. Lin CT, Huang JS, Hsu KC, et al. Different types of suprafascial courses in thoracodorsal artery skin perforators. Plast Reconstr Surg 121:840-848, 2008.

32. Van Landuyt K, Hamdi M, Blondeel P, et al. Autologous breast augmentation by pedicled perforator flaps. Ann Plast Surg 53:322-327, 2004.
    A technique was described for autologous breast augmentation based on perforator flaps of the lateral chest wall. The advantages, disadvantages, and indications were also presented.

33. Hallock GG. Permutations of combined free flaps using the subscapular system. J Reconstr Microsurg 13:47-54, 1997.
    The advantages of transferring the latissimus dorsi and serratus anterior muscle flaps simultaneously and with other combined flaps were discussed.

34. Van Landuyt K, Blondeel P, Monstrey S, et al. Clinical experience with the thoracodorsal perforator flap. Presented at the Ninth Annual European Association of Plastic Surgeons Meeting, Verona, Italy, May 1998.

35. Van Landuyt K, Blondeel P, Monstrey S, et al. Chimera perforator flaps in extremity reconstruction. Presented at the Eleventh Annual European Association of Plastic Surgeons Meeting, Berlin, Germany, June 2000.

36. Van Landuyt K, Hamdi M, Blondeel P, et al. The chimera principle in the thoracodorsal artery perforator flap. Presented at the Inaugural Congress of the World Society for Reconstructive Microsurgery, Taipei, Taiwan, Oct/Nov 2001.

37. Cavadas PC, Teran-Saavedra PP. Combined latissimus dorsi-thoracodorsal artery perforator free flap: the "razor flap." J Reconstr Microsurg 18:29-31, 2002.

38. Schwabegger AH, Hussl H, Rainer C, et al. Clinical experience and indications of the free serratus fascia flap: a report of 21 cases. Plast Reconstr Surg 102:1939-1946, 1998.

39. Colen LB, Pessa JE, Potparic Z, et al. Reconstruction of the extremity with the dorsal thoracic fascia free flap. Plast Reconstr Surg 101:738-744, 1998.

40. Seitz A, Papp S, Papp C, et al. The anatomy of the angular branch of the thoracodorsal artery. Cells Tissues Organs 164:227-236, 1999.

41. Wu WC, Chang YP, So YC, et al. The combined use of flaps based on the subscapular vascular system for limb reconstruction. Br J Plast Surg 50:73-80, 1997.

42. Chen HC, El-Gammal TA, Chen HH, et al. Economy of donor site incisions: multiple free flaps of the subscapular family for extensive extremity wounds and bilateral foot defects. Ann Plast Surg 41:28-35, 1998.

43. Schwabegger AH, Bodner G, Ninković M, et al. Thoracodorsal artery perforator (TAP) flap: report of our experience and review of the literature. Br J Plast Surg 55:390-395, 2002.

Suggested Readings

Angrigiani C, Grilli D, Siebert J. Latissimus dorsi musculocutaneous flap without muscle. Plast Reconstr Surg 96:1608-1614, 1995.

This was the original article describing the possibility of raising the skin island over the latissimus dorsi muscle independent of this muscle, based on one single musculocutaneous perforator coming off the thoracodorsal pedicle. The anatomic study in 40 fresh cadavers located the main perforator consistently about 8 cm below the axillary crease and about 2 to 3 cm beyond the anterior border of the latissimus dorsi. More perforators were found further down, overlying the descending branch of the thoracodorsal artery. Five clinical cases were also presented.

Cormack GC, Lamberty BG. The Arterial Anatomy of Skin Flaps, 2nd ed. Philadelphia: Churchill Livingstone, 1994.

This comprehensive volume on the vascular territories of the human body and different arterial pedicles supplying the skin is essential reading for understanding and planning skin flaps.

Hallock GG. Permutations of combined free flaps using the subscapular system. J Reconstr Microsurg 13:47-54, 1997.

The author described his clinical experience with a variety of compound (chimera)-type flaps based on the subscapular/thoracodorsal system, stressing the possible indications and advantages.

Heitmann C, Guerra A, Metzinger SW, et al. The thoracodorsal artery perforator flap: anatomic base and clinical application. Ann Plast Surg 51:23-29, 2003.

The authors presented findings on the vascular anatomy of the thoracodorsal artery and its cutaneous perforator vessels, based on 20 fresh cadavers dissections.

Kim JT. Latissimus dorsi perforator flap. Clin Plast Surg 30:403-431, 2003.

In this amply illustrated overview article with clinical cases the author discussed his reliance on preoperative Doppler and color duplex imaging for identifying perforators (which is contrary to our practice), the possibility of thinning the flap, and advantages over the scapular/parascapular flap.

Kim JT, Koo BS, Kim SK. The thin latissimus dorsi perforator based free flap for resurfacing. Plast Reconstr Surg 107:374-382, 2001.

The authors described their technique of dissecting the flap above the superficial fascia to further reduce flap thickness.

Russell RC, Pribaz J, Zook EG, et al. Functional evaluation of latissimus dorsi donor site. Plast Reconstr Surg 78:336-344, 1986.

The authors reviewed cosmetic and functional results at the donor site in 24 patients who had free or pedicle muscle and musculocutaneous latissimus dorsi flap procedures for a variety of problems. All patients had a contour deformity and a scar, depending on the amount of skin taken. Most patients had mild to moderate shoulder weakness with loss of shoulder range of motion, which improved with the recruitment of synergistic motor units.

Schwabegger AH, Bodner G, Ninkovic M, et al. Thoracodorsal artery perforator (TAP) flap: report of our experience and review of the literature. Br J Plast Surg 55:390-395, 2002.

The authors reported their initial experience with the TDAP flap, including a high failure rate.

Serafin DG. Atlas of Microsurgical Composite Tissue Transplantation. Philadelphia: Saunders, 1996.

Spinelli HM, Fink JA, Muzaffar AR. The latissimus dorsi perforator based fasciocutaneous flap. Ann Plast Surg 37:500-506, 1996.

A technique was described for extending the range of the traditional latissimus dorsi flap by isolating its skin island on its perforators and turning it over after deepithelialization.

32

Intercostal and Lumbar Artery Perforator Flaps

Vani Prasad

Steven F. Morris

Geoffrey G. Hallock

Phillip N. Blondeel

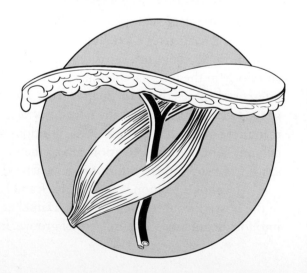

Intercostal Artery Perforator Flap

Perforator flaps based on both the anterior and posterior intercostal artery perforators have been described by several authors.[1-5] These are most often based on the dorsal rami and lateral branches of the posterior intercostal artery. Esser[6] first suggested using intercostal vessels to supply a skin flap in 1931. In 1974, Dibbell[7] described a neurovascular sensory island flap of abdominal skin, based on the tenth intercostal neurovascular bundle. Daniel et al[8] further developed the concept of sensory skin flaps for coverage of pressure ulcers and raised a musculocutaneous intercostal neurovascular island flap based on the lateral branches of the posterior intercostal arteries. Kerrigan and Daniel[9] studied in detail the anatomy of the lower (seventh through eleventh) posterior intercostal arteries. In 1984, Badran et al[10] described the first neurovascular free flap based on the lateral branch of the posterior intercostal artery and demonstrated that intercostal flaps could be raised without delay and without any muscle in the flap, thus creating a true intercostal perforator flap. The first free perforator flap based on the musculocutaneous perforators was performed inadvertently while attempting to harvest a thoracodorsal artery perforator (TDAP) flap.[11] Intercostal artery perforator flaps can be used as pedicle or free flaps.

ANATOMY
Posterior Intercostal Vessels

The first two intercostal spaces are supplied by the superior intercostal arteries, branches of the subclavian artery. The nine paired posterior intercostal arteries arise posteriorly from the descending aorta, anastomose with the anterior intercostal vessels, and terminate anteriorly in the internal mammary artery or deep superior epigastric artery, supplying intercostal spaces three through eleven. The branch that runs along the lower border of the twelfth rib is called the *subcostal artery*. The right intercostal arteries are longer than those on the left because of the position of the aorta on the left side of the vertebral column. The standard relationship of the neurovascular structures in the intercostal space from superior to inferior is vein, artery, and nerve (Fig. 32-1).

Manchot,[12] Salmon,[13] and Cormack and Lamberty[14] described the vascular anatomy of the posterior intercostal arteries. Daniel et al[8] divided posterior intercostal arteries into four segments: vertebral, costal groove, intermuscular, and rectus (Fig. 32-2). The

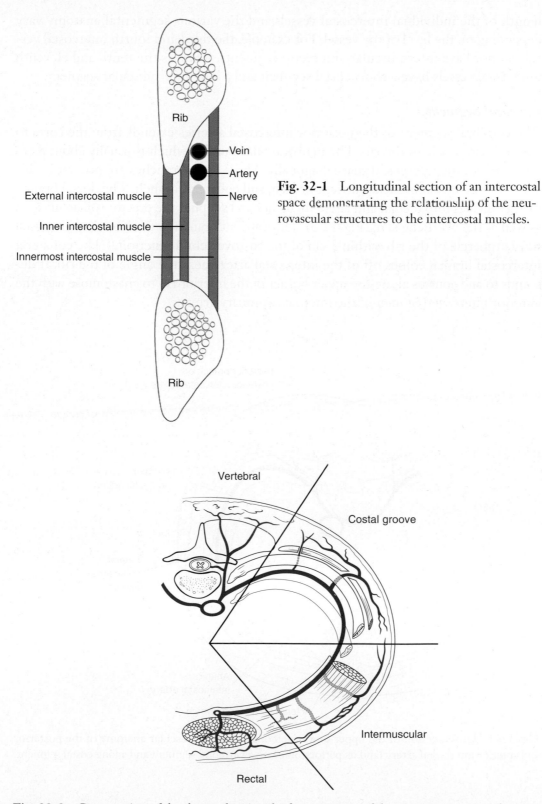

Fig. 32-1 Longitudinal section of an intercostal space demonstrating the relationship of the neurovascular structures to the intercostal muscles.

Rib

Vein

Artery

External intercostal muscle — Nerve

Inner intercostal muscle

Innermost intercostal muscle

Rib

Vertebral

Costal groove

Intermuscular

Rectal

Fig. 32-2 Cross section of the thorax showing the four segments of the posterior intercostal artery: vertebral, intercostal, intermuscular, and rectus.

length of the individual intercostal vessels and the various segmental anatomy vary depending on the level of the vessel. For example, the third and fourth intercostal vessels do not have intermuscular and rectus segments, whereas the tenth and eleventh intercostal vessels have a short costal segment and a long intermuscular segment.

Vertebral Segment

The vertebral segment of the posterior intercostal arteries extends from the aorta to the posterior angle of the rib. The neurovascular bundle, which is usually about 8 cm long, crosses the intercostal space diagonally. Three main branches are present in this segment: the dorsal branch, nutrient branch, and collateral branch. The dorsal branch further divides into medial and lateral branches and supplies the erector spinae muscles as well as the overlying skin (Fig. 32-3). The nutrient branch to the rib arises just distal to the tubercle of the rib within 3 cm of the costovertebral junction.[15] The collateral intercostal branch comes off of the intercostal artery near the angle of the rib. It descends to and courses along the upper border of the inferior rib to anastomose with the anterior intercostal branch of the internal mammary artery.

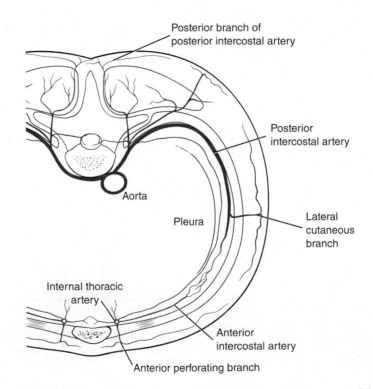

Fig. 32-3 Cross section of the upper thorax demonstrating the vascular anatomy of the posterior and anterior intercostal artery (and its perforators) with a vertebral segment and a long costal segment.

Costal Groove Segment

The costal groove segment of the posterior intercostal arteries extends from the posterior angle of the rib to the midaxillary line and is approximately 12 cm long. Two important branches, the dorsolateral musculocutaneous perforators and the lateral cutaneous branch arise from this segment of the posterior intercostal arteries.[3] Dorsolateral perforators are present on either side of the midscapular line. The lateral cutaneous branch is present in the midaxillary line. This branch divides into a small posterior and large anterior division accompanied by the sensory lateral cutaneous nerve. The anterior division may extend as far anteriorly as the lateral border of the rectus muscle.

Intermuscular Segment

The intermuscular segment of the posterior intercostal arteries extends from the origin of the abdominal musculature to the lateral border of rectus abdominis. It measures about 12 cm in length, depending on its level. The neurovascular bundle travels between transversus abdominis and internal oblique muscles. Small muscular and musculocutaneous branches are present in this segment.

Rectus Segment

The rectus segment of the posterior intercostal arteries is within the span of the rectus abdominis muscle. It measures about 8 cm in length. The neurovascular bundle enters the substance of the rectus abdominis muscle on the posterior surface and travels from lateral to medial within the muscle. The intercostal branches anastomose with superior and inferior epigastric arteries and give off several musculocutaneous perforators that pass through the rectus abdominis muscle and end in the overlying skin.

Anterior Intercostal Vessels

Anterior intercostal arteries from the first six intercostal spaces arise from the internal mammary artery. In the first two intercostal spaces, they are located between the pleura and inner intercostal muscle. In intercostal spaces three through six, they are between the inner intercostal muscle and the innermost intercostal muscle. The musculophrenic artery gives rise to anterior intercostal branches in intercostal spaces seven through nine. There are no anterior intercostal arteries in the inferior two intercostal spaces. The posterior intercostal arteries and their collateral branches supply the tenth and eleventh intercostal spaces. Anterior intercostal arteries anastomose with posterior intercostal arteries at the anteromedial third of the ribs. Perforators from the anterior intercostal arteries supply the intercostal muscles, pectoral muscles, breast, and skin (Fig. 32-4).

Oki et al[16] divided anterior intercostal arteries into three segments: upper, middle, and lower. The upper segment is located in the first through fourth intercostal spaces, the middle segment is from the fifth through eighth spaces, and the lower segment is from the ninth through twelfth spaces. In the upper segment, perforators were dominant in the parasternal regions, especially the second and third intercostal perforators which form a network around the nipple with the internal mammary artery perforators. The middle segment represents a "latticework" pattern of perforators between the intercostal spaces in horizontal and vertical directions that travel on average three to four intercostal spaces. In the lower segment, perforators anastomose with the superior and inferior epigastric vessels.

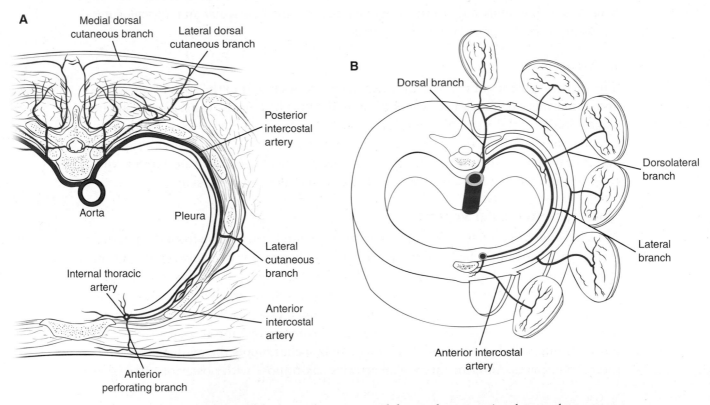

Fig. 32-4 A, Cross section of the lower thorax/upper abdomen demonstrating the vascular anatomy of the posterior and anterior intercostal arteries (and perforators) with a vertebral part, a short costal segment, a long intermuscular segment, and the terminal rectus segment. **B,** The course of the posterior intercostal artery and its communication with the anterior intercostal artery is shown, as well as various branches of the posterior intercostal artery and corresponding perforator flaps.

Subcostal Artery

The subcostal artery corresponds to the artery of the twelfth thoracic segment. In 1984, Badran et al[10] showed that the subcostal artery was absent in 5% of the intercostal spaces dissected and was replaced by the eleventh intercostal artery. However, in an anatomic study, Feinendegen et al[17] showed that the subcostal artery was present in all 28 dissected subcostal artery perforator flaps in 14 human cadavers. This was confirmed with Doppler ultrasonography in 15 healthy volunteers in the same study.

CLASSIFICATION OF FLAPS

Perforator flaps based on any of the cutaneous branches of the posterior or anterior intercostal arteries have in general been called and classified as *intercostal artery perforator* (ICAP) *flaps.*[1] Flaps based on dorsal rami are called *dorsal intercostal artery perforator* (DICAP) *flaps.* Flaps harvested on the dorsolateral branches of the costal segment of the posterior intercostal arteries are called *DLICAP flaps.*[3] LICAP flaps are based on the lateral branches of the costal segment of the posterior intercostal artery. The dorsal, dorsolateral, and lateral branches of posterior intercostal arteries are shown in an angiogram of the back (Fig. 32-5). Flaps based on anterior intercostal branches of the

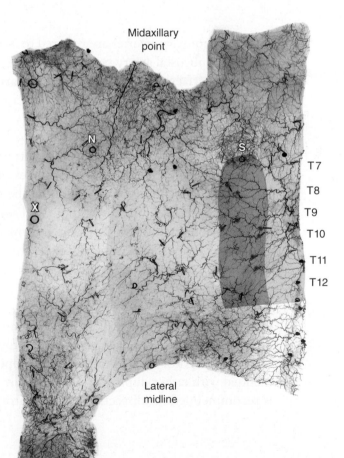

Fig. 32-5 Angiogram of the back demonstrating the different branches of the posterior intercostal artery. The perforators in the blue area are dorsal branches, those in the red area are dorsolateral branches, and those in the yellow area are lateral branches. Choke anastomoses are present between the different branches of the posterior intercostal arteries and also between the posterior intercostal arteries in the intercostal spaces above and below. (*N*, Nipple; *S*, inferior angle of scapula; *T7-T12*, thoracic vertebrae; *X*, xiphoid process.)

Table 32-1   Perforator Flaps Based on Cutaneous Branches of the Posterior or Anterior Intercostal Arteries

Intercostal Perforator Flap	Branches of Posterior Intercostal Artery	Branches of Anterior Intercostal Artery	Intercostal Spaces
Dorsal intercostal artery perforator (DICAP) flap	Dorsal (medial and lateral)		3-11
Dorsolateral intercostal artery perforator (DLICAP) flap	Dorsolateral		8-11
Lateral intercostal artery perforator (LICAP) flap	Lateral		3-11
Subcostal artery perforator (SCAP) flap	Subcostal		Subcostal space
Anterior intercostal artery perforator (AICAP) flap		Anterior	1-9

internal mammary arteries are referred to as *anterior intercostal artery perforator* (AICAP) *flaps.* The subcostal artery perforator (SCAP) flap is based on the subcostal artery. Table 32-1 summarizes this classification. The various perforator flaps based on branches of the posterior and anterior intercostal arteries are illustrated in Fig. 32-4, *B.*

SURGICAL TECHNIQUE

Perforator flaps based on the intercostal artery can be designed on any of the perforators in the four segments of the intercostal vessels (vertebral, costal groove, intermuscular, and rectus), depending on the wound to be reconstructed. The largest perforators are usually the lateral branches of the costal segment. These flaps can be used as pedicle flaps to reconstruct the defects on the trunk (anterior and posterior), axilla, and lumbar areas, or as a free flap. The reliability of the surgical procedure is directly related to the vascular anatomy and surface area of perfusion of the perforator of the flap. Badran et al[10] demonstrated with dye studies that the tenth and eleventh posterior intercostal arteries supplied an area of skin extending from the midline posteriorly to the lateral border of the rectus sheath anteriorly. The average width of the posterior intercostal artery territory is usually approximately four intercostal spaces. The ninth posterior intercostal territory is slightly smaller. Preoperative localization of perforators is recommended with either duplex ultrasonography or CT angiography. Loupe magnification is recommended for dissection of perforator flaps.

Dorsal Intercostal Artery Perforator Flap

- **Vessel** Dorsal branch of the posterior intercostal artery
- **Region** Either side of the midline of the back from the third through eleventh thoracic vertebrae
- **Applications** Reconstruction of defects of the midline of the back from the fourth through twelfth thoracic vertebrae.

Surface Landmarks

The DICAP flap is based on the dorsal branch of the posterior intercostal artery, which divides into medial and lateral branches. Medial branches are found 1 to 5 cm from the midline,[18,19] whereas lateral branches are found 5 to 8 cm from the midline posteriorly.[18]

Vascular Anatomy

In 2007, Minabe and Harii[2] described in detail the perforators of the dorsal rami of the posterior intercostal arteries. The dorsal branch usually measured 1.5 mm in diameter at the origin, and the perforators were 0.5 to 1.0 mm. Ogawa et al[18] concluded that the perforators of the sixth and seventh dorsal branches were dominant compared with their counterparts in adjacent intercostal spaces. This was later confirmed by Minabe and Harii.[2] Perforators of the dorsal branch of intercostal spaces four through six, ten, and eleven were dominant, whereas the perforators of intercostal spaces seven through nine were nondominant. Musculocutaneous perforators of the costal segment of intercostal spaces seven through nine were dominant. Perforators of the fourth, fifth, and sixth dorsal branches penetrated through the trapezius muscle at their origin and were cranial to the latissimus dorsi muscle. They also had extensive axial choke anastomoses with the circumflex scapular artery, thoracodorsal artery, and dorsolateral branches of the costal segment. Perforators in intercostal spaces seven through nine were less dominant compared with their counterparts in the spaces above and below. The tenth and eleventh dorsal intercostal artery perforators had choke connections with dorsolateral perforators of posterior intercostal artery and lumbar artery perforators; this facilitates the flap design extending to the iliac crest. The pedicle length increases from the fourth through eleventh dorsal branches.

Flap Design and Dissection

Perforator flaps based on the upper dorsal intercostal arteries can extend from the midline posteriorly to the midaxillary line. Flaps based on the lower dorsal intercostal arteries can extend to the iliac crest. The maximum dimensions of the flaps described by Minabe and Harii[2] were 31 by 13 cm and were based on two perforators. However, the maximum width of the flap was approximately 8 to 10 cm for primary donor site closure. The choke anastomoses between the dorsal branches of the posterior intercostal artery and circumflex scapular artery, thoracodorsal artery, and dorsolateral branches of the costal segment of the posterior intercostal artery can be used to harvest flaps extending up to the midaxillary line or the anterior border of latissimus dorsi muscle. After the perforator is located using either Doppler ultrasonography or CT angiography, an elliptical flap is designed (Fig. 32-6). Dissection proceeds from lateral to medial and caudal to cranial until the marked perforator is encountered. Pedicle length is increased by further dissection within the paraspinal muscles. The flap is then rotated into the defect, avoiding traction or kinking on the pedicle.

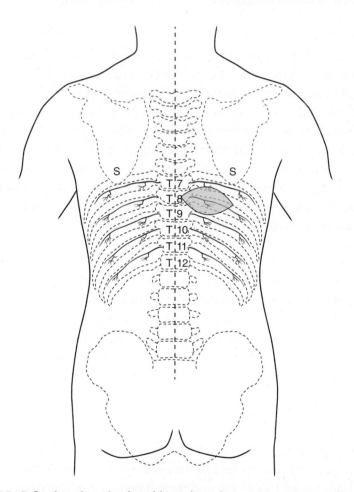

Fig. 32-6   A DICAP flap based on the dorsal branches of a posterior intercostal artery. (*S*, Inferior angle of scapula; *T7-T12*, thoracic vertebrae.)

Patient Example

This 72-year-old man presented with dermatofibrosarcoma protuberans of the central back (Fig. 32-7, *A*).[20] A wide local excision of the tumor was performed. After excision, the defect measured approximately 20 cm. A large perforator from the dorsal branch of a posterior intercostal artery was identified adjacent to the defect on the right side in the seventh intercostal space (Fig. 32-7, *B*). A DICAP flap measuring 40 by 15 cm was designed based on this perforator. The flap was dissected in a lateral to medial direction toward the perforator. It was rotated 180 degrees to reconstruct the defect (Fig. 32-7, *C* and *D*). The donor site was closed directly.

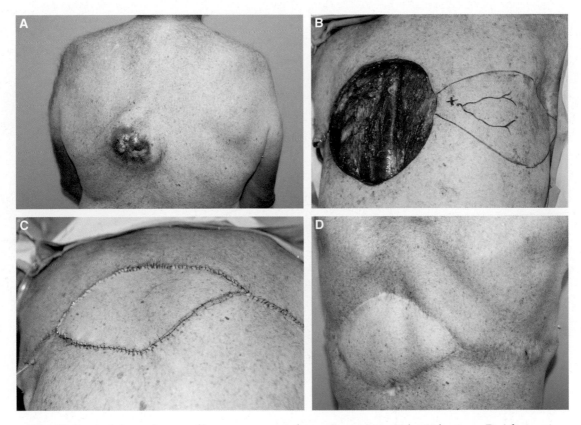

Fig. 32-7 A, A large dermatofibrosarcoma protuberans measuring 10 by 10 by 4 cm. **B,** After excision, the defect measured 20 cm in diameter. A propeller DICAP flap was designed. **C** and **D,** The immediate and 16-month postoperative results are shown. (From Prasad V, Morris S. Propeller DICAP flap for a large defect on the back: case report and review of the literature. Microsurgery, July 2012 [accepted for publication]).

Dorsolateral Intercostal Artery Perforator Flap

- **Vessel**   Dorsolateral branches of the posterior intercostal artery
- **Region**   Within 2 cm of the midscapular line in intercostal spaces eight through eleven
- **Applications**   Reconstruction of defects from the midscapular line to the midline of the back

Surface Landmarks

The landmarks of the DLICAP flap are the midline of the back, the inferior angle of the scapula, and the iliac crest (Fig. 32-8).

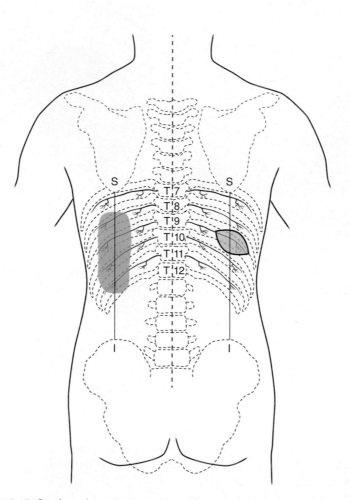

Fig. 32-8   A DLICAP flap based on the dorsolateral branches of the posterior intercostal artery on the right side. On the left, the *blue area* represents the dorsolateral branches of the costal segment of posterior intercostal arteries. The line from the tip of the inferior angle of the scapula *(S)* to the iliac crest *(I)* represents the midscapular line.

Vascular Anatomy

Musculocutaneous perforators of the costal segment of posterior intercostal arteries are named *dorsolateral perforators of the posterior intercostal arteries*.[3] These perforators are present segmentally and emerge through the latissimus dorsi muscle, and occasionally through the external oblique muscle, along the midscapular line in intercostal spaces eight through eleven. These perforators are located approximately 10 to 12 cm from the midline posteriorly. Offman et al[21] described the location of musculocutaneous perforators of the posterior intercostal arteries. They noted that these perforators were present segmentally through the latissimus dorsi along the midscapular line.

Beer et al[22] described the muscular branches from the costal groove segment of the posterior intercostal arteries to the latissimus dorsi. In another study, Beer and Manestar[23] followed the course of these musculocutaneous perforators of the costal segment from the surface of the latissimus dorsi muscle to the skin. Prasad et al[3] described these musculocutaneous perforators in intercostal spaces eight through eleven and proposed to call them *dorsolateral perforators*, because they are located between the dorsal and lateral branches of posterior intercostal arteries.

Dorsolateral perforators penetrate the latissimus dorsi muscle, giving off muscular and musculocutaneous branches in each of the intercostal spaces. There are no septo-cutaneous perforators in the costal groove segment of posterior intercostal arteries. At least one perforator was found in all intercostal spaces. Two or more perforators were found in 40% of the eighth and ninth intercostal spaces and in 60% of the tenth and eleventh intercostal spaces. Perforators are present perpendicular to the direction of the muscle fibers of the latissimus dorsi muscle. Cutaneous perforators are found one to two intercostal spaces below their origin from the posterior intercostal artery.

Flap Design and Dissection

The DLICAP flap can be applied as a pedicle or free perforator flap. Perforators are located with Doppler ultrasonography in a suitable intercostal space. An elliptical flap is designed based on the identified perforators (see Fig. 32-8). The latissimus dorsi muscle is split parallel to its fibers to follow the course of the perforator to the source vessel, the posterior intercostal artery. The average length of the pedicle from the integument to the intercostal space is approximately 4.6 ± 0.4 cm. The length of the pedicle can be increased by 6 to 12 cm by dissecting along the costal groove of the rib, between the internal intercostal muscle layer (middle muscle layer) and innermost intercostal muscle layer.

Patient Example

This 38-year-old man had positive frozen-section margins after removal and primary closure of a spinocellular carcinoma in the central back. After wide excision, a perforator was traced and located by Doppler ultrasound examination lateral to the defect on the left side (Fig. 32-9, *A*). A DLICAP flap was designed to cover the defect. The flap was elevated caudally and then laterally (Fig. 32-9, *B*). Dorsolateral intercostal artery perforators were differentiated from dorsal scapular artery perforators by their position relative to the trapezius muscle. Dorsal scapular artery perforators generally perforate the trapezius muscle, whereas DLICA perforators are mostly lateral to the trapezius muscle. Because of the short pedicle, the flap was rotated 180 degrees to cover the defect (Fig. 32-9, *C*). After a transient phase of hyperemia, which often occurs with intercostal flaps, healing was excellent in a tension-free environment (Fig. 32-9, *D*).

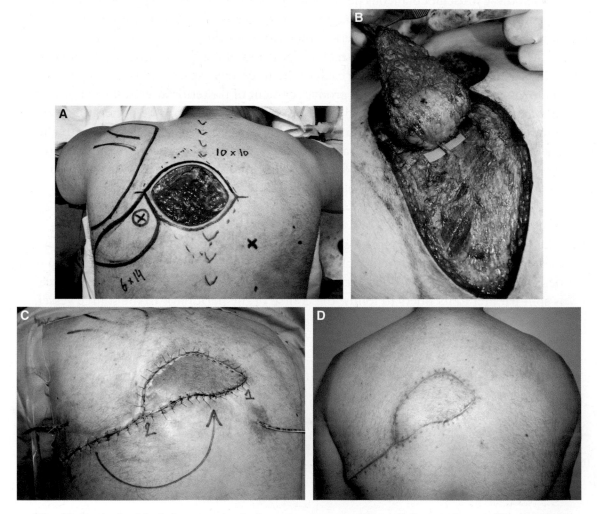

Fig. 32-9   A, A wide defect remained after resection of a spinocellular carcinoma. The DLICA perforator was indicated with an *X*, and the flap was outlined on the lateral left back. **B,** The flap was elevated and the perforator freed over a distance of a few centimeters to allow easy rotation. **C,** The flap was rotated 180 degrees, and the donor site was closed. Hyperemia is common and resolves after 24 to 48 hours. **D,** The long-term postoperative result is shown.

Lateral Intercostal Artery Perforator Flap

- **Vessel** Lateral (cutaneous) branches of the posterior intercostal artery
- **Region** Between the latissimus dorsi and pectoralis major muscles in intercostal spaces three through eleven (midaxillary line)
- **Applications** Partial mastectomy defects, especially of the lower outer quadrant; traumatic defects of the flank

In 1984, Badran et al[10] published an extensive anatomic and clinical study on the lateral intercostal free flap. Hamdi et al[1,4] described their clinical application of the lateral intercostal artery perforator flap for reconstructing defects in the lateral quadrants of the breast as an alternative to the pedicle latissimus dorsi flap or thoracodorsal artery perforator flap. Kwei et al[24] used a combination of a Wise-pattern mastopexy and a pedicle ICAP flap, although the perforators were not actually isolated, from the lateral side rolls for breast augmentation in massive-weight-loss patients. Hamdi et al[25] later described a true LICAP flap for autologous breast augmentation in massive-weight-loss patients. Recently, the LICAP flap was used to correct a deformity caused by overresection of breast tissue during surgery to correct gynecomastia.[26] Finally, LICAP flaps can be applied in a pedicle propeller fashion to cover defects of the flank and lateral iliac crest.

Surface Landmarks

The perforators of the lateral branches are found at the junction of the midaxillary line and the lower border of the corresponding rib (see Fig. 32-10, *A*). The mean distance from the anterior border of the latissimus dorsi muscle is 2.7 to 3.5 cm.[4] Perforators present between the fourth and sixth intercostal spaces are an ideal option for partial breast reconstruction, because they provide the maximum arc of flap rotation.

Vascular Anatomy

The main advantage of harvesting a flap on a lateral branch of the posterior intercostal artery is that it preserves the blood supply to the latissimus dorsi muscle for future use. A dominant perforator was present 94% of the time, with most of these located in the fifth to eighth intercostal spaces.[10] No dominant perforators were present in the third intercostal space.[4] The dominant perforator passes through a slip of the serratus anterior muscle and extends into the intercostal space to lie between the internal intercostal (middle layer of the intercostal space) and the innermost intercostal muscle (see Fig. 32-2). The dominant perforator has a smaller posterior branch that bifurcates above the serratus anterior muscle and anastomoses with thoracodorsal perforators. A pedicle length of 8 to 15 cm can be obtained with further dissection in the intercostal space. The diameter of the vessels is usually around 1.5 to 2 mm, adequate for microvascular anastomosis. Injection studies suggest that flaps as large as 25 by 20 cm can be raised safely, but safe, direct donor site closure is only possible with a maximum width of 12 cm.[10]

Flap Design and Dissection

LICAP flaps are based on the lateral branches of the posterior intercostal artery. Badran et al[10] showed that the flap based on the lateral branch of the posterior intercostal artery could extend from 5 cm posterior to the posterior axillary fold to the lateral border of the rectus abdominis muscle. LICAP flaps for breast reconstruction are located in the fourth, fifth, and sixth intercostal spaces, and the midaxillary line is the axis of rotation. The ninth, tenth, and eleventh intercostal vascular bundles are also used as pedicles for these flaps. An elliptical flap is designed over the midaxillary line extending 5 cm posterior to the posterior axillary line. Flap elevation begins with a horizontal incision between two perforators (Fig. 32-10, *A*). From this incision, midaxillary lateral intercostal artery perforators can be visualized cranially and caudally, and the plan can be adjusted. The latissimus dorsi muscle is exposed. The anterior border of the latissimus dorsi muscle is visualised, and the small posterior branch of the lateral branch of the posterior intercostal artery is identified (Fig. 32-10, *B*). Further dissection of this small posterior branch leads to the much larger anterior branch. The segments of the serratus anterior muscle are split to acquire satisfactory exposure of the lateral intercostal artery perforator bifurcation down to the underlying rib and intercostal muscles (Fig. 32-10, *C*). A pedicle length of 3 to 5 cm is adequate to reconstruct defects of the lateral breast, abdomen, or posterior trunk lateral to midline. The flap can be folded on itself to fill a quadrantectomy defect (only the lateral quadrants of the breast). Pedicle length can

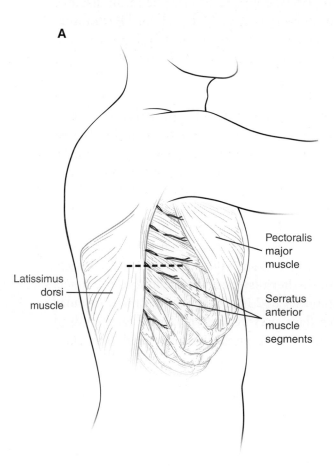

A

Latissimus dorsi muscle

Pectoralis major muscle

Serratus anterior muscle segments

Fig. 32-10   A, On the midaxillary line, between ribs two to eleven, the lateral intercostal artery perforators pierce the deep fascia. In the upper part they perforate between segments of the serratus anterior muscle. The first incision *(red line)* is made between two perforators down to the deep fascia.

be increased with further dissection of the posterior intercostal artery after identifying the junction of the lateral branch and main bundle (Fig. 32-10, *D*). The intercostal space is exposed with retraction of the latissimus dorsi muscle and splitting of the serratus anterior muscles in the direction of their muscle fibers, thereby reducing blood loss and donor site morbidity. Intercostal muscles are divided from the inferior end of the rib. Periosteum over the inferior end of the rib is incised and reflected downward to protect the neurovascular bundle. The neurovascular bundle lies between the internal intercostal muscle and the innermost intercostal muscles. Care must be taken to avoid entering the pleural cavity. Once the location and length of the perforator vessels are known, the remaining borders of the flap are incised, and the perforator flap is elevated above the muscle fascia (Fig. 32-10, *E*). The lateral intercostal cutaneous nerve can be harvested to provide a sensate flap.

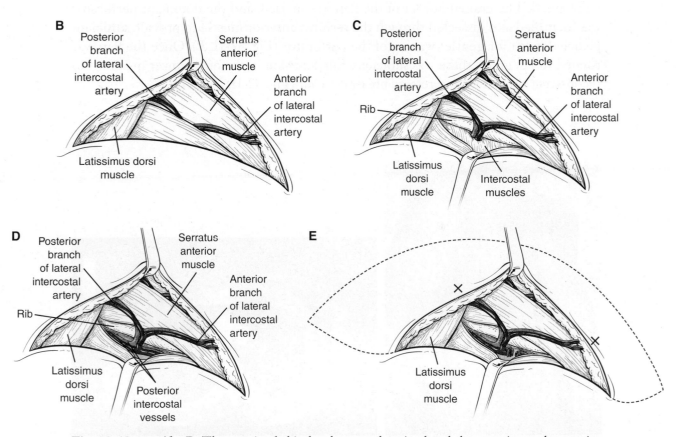

Fig. 32-10, cont'd   B, The proximal skin has been undermined and the anterior and posterior branches of the lateral intercostal artery perforator become visible anterior to the border of the latissimus dorsi muscle, and between two segments of the serratus anterior muscle. **C,** Once these segments are split along the muscle fibers, the common origin of the branches of the lateral intercostal artery perforator can be found. **D,** To expose the posterior intercostal vessels, the intercostal muscles need to be cut at the lower border of the rib. **E,** If more pedicle length is needed, the anterior intercostal vessels can be ligated and the pedicle followed in the subcostal space, after retracting the latissimus dorsi muscle. The entry points of the perforators in the flap are marked *(x)*. The skin pedicle is drawn and later incised as needed.

Patient Example

This 47-year-old woman presented with significant breast asymmetry after lower outer quadrantectomy of her left breast, which was followed by radiation therapy. In addition to volume, a large part of the skin envelope is lacking (Fig. 32-11, *A*). Therefore a pedicle LICAP flap was chosen over lipofilling. Preoperative MDCT angiography helped determine dominance of the intercostal or thoracodorsal system and the exact location of the dominant perforators (Fig. 32-11, *B*). An arbitrary grid was centered over the intersection between the midaxillary line and a horizontal line drawn through the inframammary fold (Fig. 32-11, *C*). The most important perforators were marked on the skin according to the coordinates on the grid, and their location was reconfirmed with a handheld Doppler device (Fig. 32-11, *D*). The flap was based on the dominant perforator located closest to the defect in the fifth intercostal space. By placing most of the skin island of the flap posterior to the perforator, a propeller-fashion rotation can be planned. The cranial border of the flap was incised, and the dominant perforator was identified and dissected through the serratus anterior muscle to provide sufficient pedicle length for gentle twisting of the perforator (Fig. 32-11, *E*). Once the flap was rotated 180 degrees, there was sufficient bulk and skin in the outer lower quadrant to reconstruct the defect and restore breast contour (Fig. 32-11, *F* and *G*).

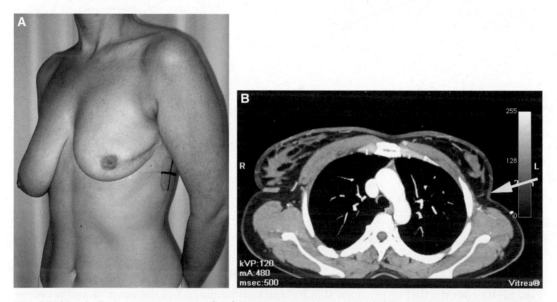

Fig. 32-11   A, Preoperative image after breast-conserving surgery of the left breast. **B,** An MDCT section demonstrated a lateral intercostal artery perforator at the fifth intercostal space *(arrow).*

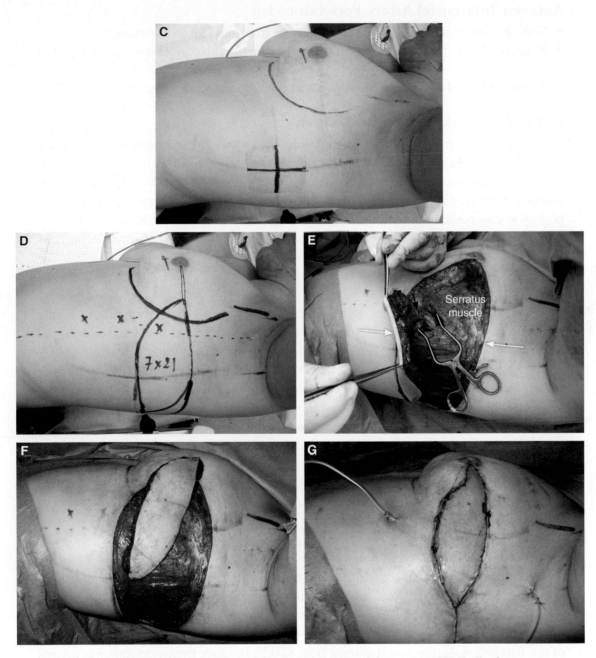

Fig. 32-11, cont'd   C, The axes of a cutaneous grid were used during MDCT. **D,** Perforators were marked and the flap designed. **E,** The LICAP flap was isolated on its perforator *(black arrow)*. The anterior border of the latissimus dorsi muscle is indicated between *white arrows.* **F,** The LICAP flap was rotated 180 degrees. **G,** Hyperemia is common during the first hours after skin closure because of pedicle twisting and changes in tension in the subcutaneous plexus.

Anterior Intercostal Artery Perforator Flap

- **Vessel**   Anterior intercostal branches of the internal mammary artery
- **Region**   1 to 3 cm from the lateral sternal border in intercostal spaces one through nine
- **Application**   Reconstruction of sternal, breast, thoracic, or epigastric areas

Surface Landmarks and Vascular Anatomy

The AICAP flap can be used for reconstructing the sternal, breast, thoracic, or epigastric region as a pedicle perforator flap.[5] Anterior intercostal perforators are usually located 1 to 3 cm from the lateral sternal border. Musculocutaneous anterior intercostal perforators pierce the upper 5 to 6 intercostal spaces between the internal mammary and posterior intercostal arteries. Perforators arising from the internal mammary artery are larger and closer to the sternum. The diameter of the anterior intercostal perforators is usually approximately 1 mm at the fascial level.

Flap Design and Dissection

The AICAP flap is designed around a selected perforator in a longitudinal or oblique direction toward the shoulder. The flap is dissected in a lateral to medial and caudal to cranial direction. After perforators are identified, the surrounding subcutaneous tissue is dissected to skeletonize the perforator. The perforator is dissected by splitting the muscle—either pectoralis major or rectus abdominis—depending on the location. Dissection proceeds in the direction of the anterior intercostal or internal mammary arteries. The pedicle length of the anterior intercostal bundle can be increased by further dissection in the intercostal space up to 1 to 2 cm lateral to the sternum. In this situation, intercostal muscles need to be divided and care must be taken to avoid entering the pleural cavity. Dissection through the costal cartilages may be necessary in lower intercostal spaces seven through nine. A sensate flap can be harvested with inclusion of the anterior cutaneous intercostal branch.

Patient Example

This 52-year-old man had recurrent colon cancer, with exposed mesh in the epigastric area after multiple midline laparotomies, and necrosis of the abdominal portion of the rectus abdominis muscles. A pedicle perforator flap was designed around the anterior intercostal artery perforator located at the left seventh intercostal space, with the axis of the flap following the costal margin (Fig. 32-12, *A*). Once the perforator was identified above the deep fascia, the borders of the flap were incised and the perforator followed down to the ribs (Fig. 32-12, *B*). A longer pedicle allows both transposition and rotation without pedicle kinking and is obtained by ligating the intercostal vessels in the subcostal space either medially or laterally and continuing the dissection in either direction (Fig. 32-12, *C*). The flap survived completely without problems, but later a skin graft was necessary for another wound. The donor site was closed primarily, leaving a subcostal scar (Fig. 32-12, *D*).

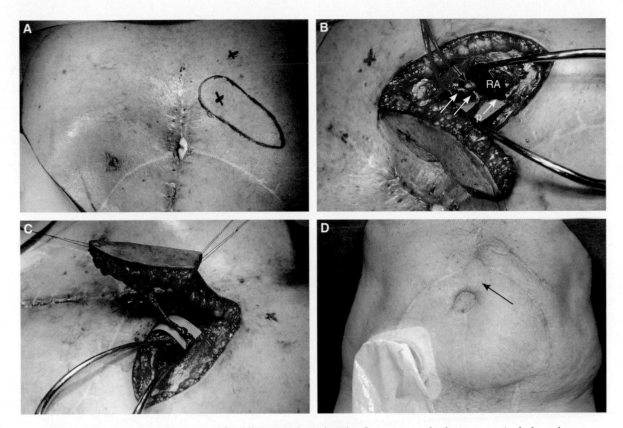

Fig. 32-12 A, A midline wound with exposed mesh. The flap was marked preoperatively based on an anterior intercostal artery perforator. **B,** The perforator *(p)* was dissected through rectus abdominis muscle *(RA)* (here held apart with a retractor), back to its origin from the anterior intercostal artery *(white arrows)* just inferior to the rib *(black arrow)*. **C,** The flap easily rotated into the defect after ligation of the anterior intercostal artery laterally. The pedicle was lengthened by dissection back toward the sternum. **D,** The flap *(arrow)* survived completely.

Subcostal Artery Perforator Flap

- **Vessel**   Subcostal artery
- **Region**   Subcostal space posteriorly
- **Application**   Reconstruction of lumbar defects

Feinendegen and Klos[27] first described the subcostal artery perforator flap for reconstruction of a lumbar defect.

Surface Landmarks

Feinendegen et al[17] showed that a constant perforator from the subcostal artery was present close to the junction of the anterior border of latissimus dorsi muscle and ex-

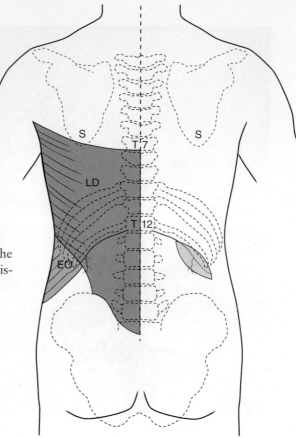

Fig. 32-13   The SCAP flap is based on the subcostal artery. The design of the flap is shown on the right. The perforator from the subcostal artery extends to the latissimus dorsi *(LD)* and external oblique *(EO)* muscles. *(S,* Inferior angle of the scapula.)

ternal oblique abdominis, 1 to 3 cm inferior to the end of the twelfth rib (Fig. 32-13). This perforator was found 10 to 18 cm (mean 14 cm) from the midline posteriorly.

Vascular Anatomy

The vascular basis of the subcostal artery perforator flap is the subcostal artery that corresponds to the twelfth thoracic segment (see Fig. 32-13). The vascular territory corresponds to the integument between the twelfth rib and anterior superior iliac spine. The average size of the source artery is approximately 2 mm. According to Badran et al,[10] the cutaneous territory of the subcostal artery does not reach the lateral border of the rectus (compared with the posterior intercostal artery). But the territory can extend to the anterior superior iliac spine, part of the upper thigh, and the lateral part of the inguinal region.

Flap Design and Dissection

The SCAP flap is indicated as a pedicle flap to cover dorsolumbar defects. Doppler ultrasound or CT angiography is recommended to identify the subcostal artery preoperatively. Subfascial dissection is performed from the edges of the defect, and the perforator is identified. A skin flap with a mean size of 10 by 14 cm (minimum 9 by 12 cm and maximum 11 by 16 cm) is designed, and retrograde dissection is performed to the source vessel.[17] In a clinical case, Feinendegen and Klos[27] reconstructed a lumbar defect (19 by

13 cm) resulting from excision of an angiosarcoma with a subcostal artery perforator flap. Additional pedicle length was obtained by freeing the subcostal artery deep to the latissimus dorsi muscle medially up to the lateral border of the erector spinae muscle.

Lumbar Artery Perforator Flap

Kroll and Rosenfeld[28] introduced flaps based on paraspinous and parasacral perforators in 1988. These perforator-based flaps were performed to reconstruct defects of the midline of the back and lumbosacral area. In 1980, Bostwick et al[29] described the "reverse" latissimus dorsi muscle musculocutaneous flap based on the lower intercostal and lumbar artery perforators. The transverse lumbosacral flap is based on lumbar artery perforators.[30] In 1999 Kato et al[31] described a pedicle lumbar artery perforator flap in an anatomic and clinical study. Lumbar artery perforators can be used as pedicle flaps to reconstruct defects of the lumbosacral area. The lumbar artery perforator flap can also be harvested as a free flap, but the pedicle is relatively short, though large, and almost always needs artery and vein grafts to overcome this shortage. Offman et al[21] analyzed the lumbar arteries in an anatomic study with angiograms and fresh cadaveric dissections (Fig. 32-14). Lui et al[32] described the three-dimensional anatomy of the lumbar artery perforator flap. Kiil et al[33] described lumbar artery perforators in a cadaveric and clinical anatomic study, performing CT angiography preoperatively as a virtual dissection tool.

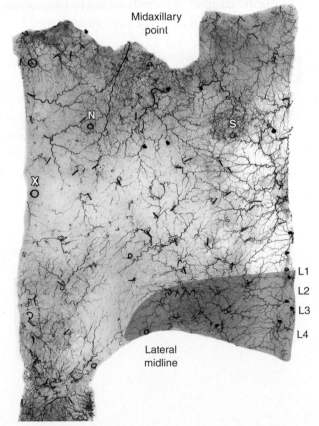

Fig. 32-14 Angiogram of the lumbar artery perforators. (*N*, Nipple; *L1-L4*, lumbar vertebrae; *X*, xiphoid process.)

ANATOMY

Lumbar arteries are somatic segmental branches of the abdominal aorta and correspond to the posterior intercostal arteries of the thoracic aorta. Lumbar artery perforators are located between the inferior margin of the twelfth rib and iliac crest. Lumbar arteries arise posterolaterally from the descending abdominal aorta at the level of the upper four lumbar vertebral bodies. The arteries on the right side pass posterior to the inferior vena cava. The upper two lumbar arteries run posterior to the corresponding crus of the diaphragm. Lumbar arteries on both sides travel inferior to the tendinous arches, from which the psoas major originates, and continue posterior to the psoas major and lumbar plexus. They cross the quadratus lumborum, with the upper three arteries running posteriorly and the fourth anterior to it (see Fig. 32-15, *A*). They cross the lateral border of the quadratus lumborum and pierce the posterior aponeurosis of the transversus abdominis muscle, and travel anteriorly between it and the internal oblique. Lumbar arteries anastomose with the lower posterior intercostal, subcostal, iliolumbar, deep circumflex iliac, and inferior epigastric arteries. In the study by Kato et al,[31] the first lumbar artery was absent in 9.5% of the specimens and was replaced with a branch from the subcostal artery. Perforators emerge lateral to the erector spinae muscle, giving a few cutaneous branches both medially and laterally.

SURGICAL TECHNIQUE

- **Vessel**   Lumbar artery perforators
- **Region**   First through fourth lumbar vertebrae area
- **Applications**   Reconstruction of lumbar and lumbosacral defects; option in breast reconstruction as a free perforator flap

Surface Landmarks and Vascular Anatomy

Lumbar artery perforators should be marked preoperatively with Doppler ultrasound or CT angiography (Fig. 32-15). Cutaneous perforators of the lumbar artery are located 5 to 9 cm from the midline.[31] Lumbar artery perforators are either musculocutaneous or septocutaneous. Although musculocutaneous perforators pass through the quadratus lumborum, septocutaneous perforators emerge between the erector spinae and quadratus lumborum muscles. Perforators of the fourth lumbar artery are more often septocutaneous, compared with those of the first through third lumbar arteries. Based on fluorescein injection results in a clinical case, Kato et al[31] showed that the skin territory of the second lumbar artery extends from the midline posteriorly to the lateral border of the rectus sheath and up to 10 cm above the anterior superior iliac spine. Perforators were not present in 14.3% of the first lumbar artery, 9.3% of the second lumbar artery, and 23.8% of the third lumbar artery. Perforators of the fourth lumbar artery were the largest and consistently present. Kiil et al[33] demonstrated variability of the lumbar artery and perforators with regard to diameter, course, and pedicle length. The diameter of perforators increases descending from the first to fourth lumbar artery. Lumbar arteries are accompanied by one or two veins throughout their course. Pedicle length decreases from the first (mean length 6.3 cm) to fourth (mean length 5.5 cm) lumbar artery. Because of the variability of the perforators, Kiil et al[33] recommended CT angiography of the lumbar region before surgery. According to Lui et al,[32] the average diameter and surface area supplied by lumbar artery perforators was 0.7 mm and 30 cm² (range from 14 to 64 cm²), respectively. Offman et al[21] found that lumbar arteries supplied a mean of 6 ± 2 perforators to a skin territory of 160 ± 50 cm². The mean diameter of the lumbar vessel at its origin was 2.1 ± 0.5 mm. A primary territory of 45 ± 23 cm² was found for a single lumbar artery.

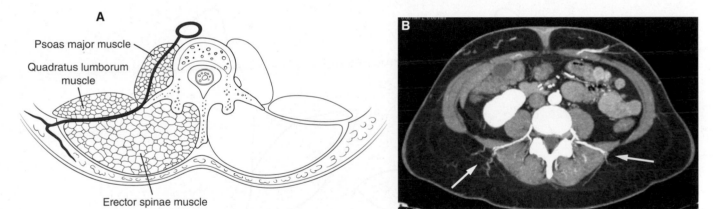

Fig. 32-15   A, Relationship of the lumbar artery to the quadratus lumborum and erector spinae muscles. **B,** MDCT angiography at the level of the umbilicus shows not only a large deep inferior epigastric artery perforator *(yellow arrow)*, but also a large lumbar artery perforator *(white arrow)* emerging just lateral to the quadratus lumborum and paravertebral muscles, and just above the iliac crest on both sides.

Flap Design and Dissection

Lumbar artery perforator flaps are designed with the axis in a transverse direction or obliquely from the midline posteriorly down to the anterior superior iliac spine (Fig. 32-16). The flap can extend from the posterior midline to beyond the midaxillary line. Patient positioning depends on the indication for the flap—prone for lumbosacral defects and lateral decubitus for breast reconstruction to facilitate a two-team approach.

Dissection begins from the anterior or superior margin of the flap. Lumbar fascia is included, and this results in inclusion of the cutaneous nerves. Dissection is continued until the perforator is identified. The arc of rotation cannot be extended with further dissection, because the lumbar artery passes obliquely and anteriorly from the lateral edge of the erector spinae muscles, and then beneath the transverse process of the vertebra. If wider arc of rotation is needed, the pivot point can be placed close to the transverse process after the erector spinae muscles are incised. However, this applies only to the first three lumbar arteries. The fourth lumbar artery passes anterior to the quadratus lumborum muscle. The flap is passed to the defect either through a subcutaneous tunnel or through an incision made between the defect and the donor site.

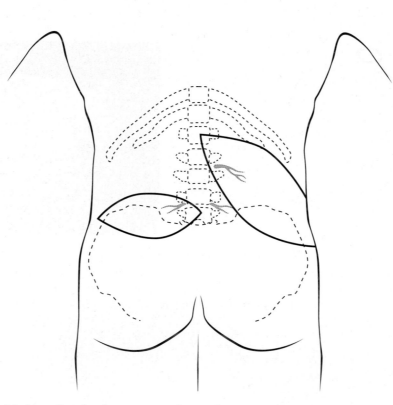

Fig. 32-16 Markings for a lumbar artery perforator flap oriented transversely *(left side)* and obliquely toward the iliac crest *(right side)*.

MODIFICATIONS

de Weerd and Weum[34] described a butterfly design of two pedicle lumbar artery perforator flaps to cover a large sacral defect. Each flap measured 12 by 27 cm. Cutaneous nerves were preserved in the flaps to provide protective sensation. de Weerd et al[35] used the lumbar artery perforator flap for breast reconstruction.

Patient Example

This 47-year-old paraplegic man had recurrent sacral and bilateral trochanteric pressure sores. A pedicle superior gluteal artery perforator (SGAP) flap from the right gluteus and a random-pattern rotation flap from the left gluteus had been used previously to cover sacral pressure sores (Fig. 32-17, *A*). A long pedicled lumbar artery perforator flap was designed on the right fourth lumbar artery perforator, extending to the midaxillary line (Fig. 32-17, *B*). The flap was isolated on its perforator and rotated 90 degrees to fill the entire defect (Fig. 32-17, *C*). The trochanteric pressure sores were treated with tensor fascia lata flaps. The sacral wound healed uneventfully.

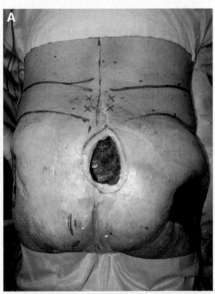

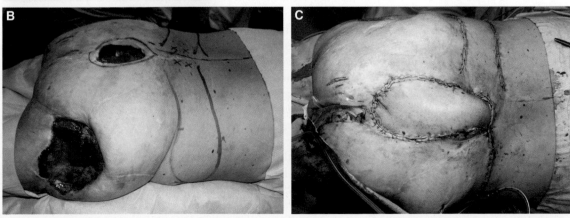

Fig. 32-17 **A,** Sacral and trochanteric pressure sores. **B,** A pedicle lumbar artery perforator flap was designed on the right fourth lumbar artery. **C,** The immediate postoperative result is shown. Wound healing was uneventful.

CONCLUSION

Perforator flaps of the intercostal and lumbar arteries are useful for reconstructing various defects of the torso, specifically in a pedicle fashion. Perforator flaps based on dorsal and dorsolateral branches of the posterior intercostal arteries can cover defects over the spine or posterior thoracic trunk. Flaps based on lateral branches are primarily useful for reconstructing partial mastectomy defects. Lumbar artery perforator flaps may be indicated for reconstructing pressure ulcer defects of the lumbar and lumbosacral areas and are an option for breast reconstruction.

References

1. Hamdi M, Van Landuyt K, de Frene B, et al. The versatility of the inter-costal artery perforator (ICAP) flaps. J Plast Reconstr Aesthet Surg 59:644-652, 2006.

   The authors harvested 20 pedicle ICAP flaps in 16 patients for immediate partial breast reconstruction following quadrantectomy for breast cancer (8); midline back and sternal defects following radical excision for a dermatofibrosarcoma or malignant melanoma (3); and autologous breast augmentation (four bilateral and one unilateral flap) after bariatric surgery. The average flap dimension was 18 by 8 cm². Two DICAP, two AICAP, and 16 LICAP flaps were performed. All but two flaps were based on one perforator. All flaps survived completely, and all donor sites were closed primarily. Underlying muscle was not sacrificed.

2. Minabe T, Harii K. Dorsal intercostal artery perforator flap: anatomical study and clinical applications. Plast Reconstr Surg 120:681-689, 2007.

   The authors developed a new flap, the DICAP flap. Five fresh human cadavers were injected with a lead oxide–gelatin mixture as a radiopaque agent. They were dissected, and angiographic studies were performed to map the dorsal intercostal artery perforators. Details of these studies were presented. They also performed 11 DICAP flaps in 10 cases, 9 of which had previously sacrificed the muscles of the latissimus dorsi, trapezius, or scapular circumflex artery. All flaps survived completely except for the largest flap, which had marginal necrosis.

3. Prasad V, Almutairi K, Kimble FW, et al. Dorsolateral musculocutaneous perforators of posterior intercostal artery: an anatomical study. J Plast Reconstr Aesthet Surg. 2012 Jun 8. [Epub ahead of print]

   The authors dissected 12 cadavers that were injected with a lead oxide–gelatine mixture to better understand the musculocutaneous perforators of the costal segment of the posterior intercostal arteries. Intercostal spaces eight through eleven were dissected. Angiograms were assembled with Adobe Photoshop. CT angiography was performed on two fresh cadavers, with three-dimensional reconstructions of the intercostal perforators. Details of their findings were provided. The authors proposed to call these unnamed musculocutaneous perforators "dorsolateral" branches of the posterior intercostal arteries.

4. Hamdi M, Spano A, Van Landuyt K, et al. The lateral intercostal artery perforators: anatomical study and clinical application in breast surgery. Plast Reconstr Surg 121:389-396, 2008.

   Twenty-four fresh cadavers were dissected to study lateral intercostal perforator anatomy. The field extended from the third to the eighth intercostal space and from the latissimus dorsi to the pectoralis major muscle. Their relationship with the anterior border of the latissimus dorsi muscle and serratus anterior vessels was examined. Details of the study were presented. The authors concluded that the LICAP flap is effective for treating challenging breast defects without sacrificing the pedicle of the latissimus dorsi muscle.

5. Hallock GG. The island anterior intercostal artery perforator flap as another option for the difficult epigastric abdominal wound. Ann Plast Surg 63:414-417, 2009.

   The AICAP flap was successfully used in two clinical cases as a pedicle island flap to close difficult subxiphoid wounds. Perforators of the anterior intercostal artery are diminutive, and dissection can be tedious; however, this flap is an option if a vascularized flap is needed.

6. Esser J. Biological or artery flaps of the face. Monaco: Institute Esser de Chirurgie Structive, 1931.

7. Dibbell DG. Use of a long island flap to bring sensation to the sacral area in young paraplegics. Plast Reconstr Surg 54:220-223, 1974.

8. Daniel RK, Kerrigan CL, Gard DA. The great potential of the intercostal flap for torso reconstruction. Plast Reconstr Surg 61:653-665, 1978.

9. Kerrigan CL, Daniel RK. The intercostal flap: an anatomical and hemodynamic approach. Ann Plast Surg 2:411-421, 1979.

    A good understanding of the anatomy of the intercostal arteries is essential for successful reconstructive surgery using intercostal island flaps. The authors studied human cadaver dissections, specifically the seventh through eleventh intercostal neurovascular bundles. They described four intercostal anatomic segments—vertebral, costal groove, intermuscular, and rectus—and their versatility for use in reconstructive surgery. Details of three clinical applications of the intercostal island flap were presented.

10. Badran HA, El-Helaly MS, Safe I. The lateral intercostal neurovascular free flap. Plast Reconstr Surg 73:17-26, 1984.

    The lateral intercostal flap is based on the lateral cutaneous branch of a single posterior intercostal neurovascular bundle. The donor area of the flap is the anterolateral skin of the abdomen. The authors shared their findings from dissections of 40 fresh cadavers and 11 clinical cases in which the noninnervated flap was used to treat defects in the neck, face, hands, and feet. Ten flaps were successful; one flap was partially lost, and one was completely lost.

11. Henderson J, Clibbon JJ, Haywood RM, et al. Inadvertent free intercostal artery perforator flaps. J Plast Reconstr Aesthet Surg 62:e140-e141, 2009.

12. Manchot C. Die Hautarterien des Menschlichen Korpers. Leipzig: FCW Vogel, 1889.

13. Salmon M. Artères des muscles de la tête et du cou. Paris: Masson, 1936.

14. Cormack GC, Lamberty BG. The Arterial Anatomy of Skin Flaps. London: Churchill Livingstone, 1986.

15. Daniel RK. Free rib transfer by microvascular anastomoses. Plast Reconstr Surg 59:737-738, 1977.

16. Oki K, Murakami M, Tanuma K, et al. Anatomical study of pectoral intercostal perforators and clinical study of the pectoral intercostal perforator flap for hand reconstruction. Plast Reconstr Surg 123:1789-1800, 2009.

    The authors performed an anatomic study of the anterior chest and abdominal regions in 13 cadavers to better understand the arterial networks used in pectoral intercostal perforator flaps. In the fifth to eighth intercostal spaces, perforators communicated to form a "latticework" pattern. Detailed results were presented. They also retrospectively analyzed 21 cases over 13 years. Aesthetic and functional results were satisfactory. Vascular territories of the intercostal perforators, the superior epigastric artery system, and the deep inferior epigastric artery system link with each other through choke vessels. The flap provides thinness and texture needed for hand reconstruction.

17. Feinendegen DL, Niederhauser T, Herrmann G, et al. The subcostal artery perforator flap; an anatomical study. J Plast Reconstr Aesthet Surg 61:1496-1502, 2008.

18. Ogawa R, Hyakusoku H, Murakami M, et al. An anatomical and clinical study of the dorsal intercostal cutaneous perforators, and application to free microvascular augmented subdermal vascular network (ma-SVN) flaps. Br J Plast Surg 55:396-401, 2002.

19. de Weerd L, Weum S. The sensate medial dorsal intercostal artery perforator flap for closure of cervicothoracic midline defects after spinal surgery: an anatomic study and case reports. Ann Plast Surg 63:418-421, 2009.

20. Prasad V, Morris S. Propeller DICAP flap for a large defect on the back: case report and review of the literature. Microsurgery, July 2012 (accepted for publication).

21. Offman SL, Geddes CR, Tang M, et al. The vascular basis of perforator flaps based on the source arteries of the lateral lumbar region. Plast Reconstr Surg 115:1651-1659, 2005.

    The focus of this study was to describe the vascular anatomy of the perforators of numerous source arteries in the lateral lumbar region to better explain the anatomy of donor sites in this area. Five fresh human cadavers were studied using a lead oxide–gelatin injection technique. The integument of the trunk was dissected, and origin, diameter, and pedicle length of perforating vessels were identified. Radiographs of tissue specimens were digitally analyzed to determine vascular territories. Detailed results were provided.

22. Beer GM, Lang A, Manestar M, et al. The bipedicled and bipartite latissimus dorsi free and perforator flap: an anatomic study. Plast Reconstr Surg 118:1162-1170, 2006.

23. Beer GM, Manestar M. The number of intercostal artery perforators over the distal latissimus dorsi muscle. Clin Anat 23:216-221, 2010.

24. Kwei S, Borud LJ, Lee BT, et al. Mastopexy with autologous augmentation after massive weight loss: the intercostal artery perforator (ICAP) flap. Ann Plast Surg 57:361-365, 2006.

25. Hamdi M, Van Landuyt K, Blondeel P, et al. Autologous breast augmentation with the lateral intercostal artery perforator flap in massive weight loss patients. J Plast Reconstr Aesthet Surg 62:65-70, 2009.

26. Salim F, Chana J, Salim F, et al. Intercostal adipofascial perforator flap for reconstruction of overcorrected gynaecomastia deformity. J Plast Reconstr Aesthet Surg 63:1385-1387, 2010.

27. Feinendegen DL, Klos D. A subcostal artery perforator flap for a lumbar defect. Plast Reconstr Surg 109:2446-2449, 2002.

28. Kroll SS, Rosenfield L. Perforator-based flaps for low posterior midline defects. Plast Reconstr Surg 81:561-566, 1988.

29. Bostwick J III, Scheflan M, Nahai F, et al. The "reverse" latissimus dorsi muscle and musculocutaneous flap: anatomical and clinical considerations. Plast Reconstr Surg 65:395-399, 1980.

30. Hill HL, Brown RG, Jurkiewicz MJ. The transverse lumbosacral back flap. Plast Reconstr Surg 62:177-184, 1978.

31. Kato H, Hasegawa M, Takada T, et al. The lumbar artery perforator based island flap: anatomical study and case reports. Br J Plast Surg 52:541-546, 1999.

     The authors studied 21 specimens of lumbar arteries in 11 cadavers and investigated the skin territory of the artery using fluorescein injection to detail the vascular anatomy of this region. They also performed four lumbar artery perforator–based island flaps to treat ulcers on the lower back. All flaps survived and donor site defects were closed primarily. Results of the cadaver dissection, injection study, and clinical cases were presented.

32. Lui KW, Hu S, Ahmad N, et al. Three-dimensional angiography of the superior gluteal artery and lumbar artery perforator flap. Plast Reconstr Surg 123:79-86, 2009.

33. Kiil BJ, Rozen WM, Pan WR, et al. The lumbar artery perforators: a cadaveric and clinical anatomical study. Plast Reconstr Surg 123:1229-1238, 2009.

34. de Weerd L, Weum S. The butterfly design: coverage of a large sacral defect with two pedicled lumbar artery perforator flaps. Br J Plast Surg 55:251-253, 2002.

35. de Weerd L, Elvenes OP, Strandenes E, et al. Autologous breast reconstruction with a free lumbar artery perforator flap. Br J Plast Surg 56:180-183, 2003.

33

Superior Gluteal Artery Perforator Flap

Robert J. Allen, Sr.
James L. Mayo
Robert Johnson Allen, Jr.
Maria M. LoTempio

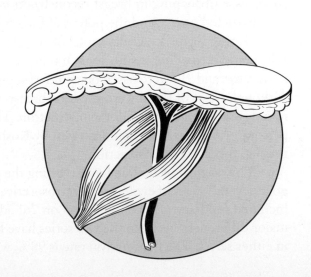

The microvascular transfer of gluteal tissue was introduced by Fujino et al[1] in 1975 and later championed by both Shaw[2] and Boustred and Nahai[3] in the form of gluteal musculocutaneous flaps. After three decades of experience with these techniques, certain advantages and disadvantages have become apparent. The main advantages include avoiding the morbidity associated with harvesting abdominal musculature and offering an option for free flap reconstruction in those in whom abdominal harvest is contraindicated. The main disadvantages of gluteal musculocutaneous flaps result from the bulky gluteal muscle mass. Including a gluteal muscle creates a shorter vascular pedicle, frequently necessitating vein grafts, with an increased risk of vascular complications. Consequently, the popularity of these flaps over time remained relatively low.

In 1993 Allen and Tucker[4] performed an alternative technique for harvesting gluteal tissue. Their findings were published in 1995. In this method, the skin and fat nourished by a perforating branch of the superior gluteal artery is harvested without sacrificing underlying structures. Gluteus maximus muscle function and bulk are preserved with this muscle-splitting approach. Additionally, dissection of the vascular structures through the muscle significantly increases the length of the pedicle, facilitating vascular anastomosis. Other advantages of the superior gluteal artery perforator (SGAP) flap include reliable anatomy, a ubiquitous donor site with good volume, firm fat consistency, low donor site morbidity, appropriate arc of rotation (with pedicle flaps) to cover sacral pressure sores, ease of shaping in breast reconstruction to help improve the projection of the reconstructed breast, and the potential for a neurosensory flap.[5-7]

During the past decade, a total of 503 gluteal artery perforator flaps were successfully completed at our institution. Of these, 293 were based on a superior gluteal artery perforator, and 210 were based on an inferior gluteal artery perforator (see Chapter 34). Although most of these were used for breast reconstruction (Fig. 33-1), we have also relied on this flap for trunk reconstruction. The true versatility of the gluteal artery perforator flap has been demonstrated by Koshima et al,[8] who successfully transferred the flap for facial reconstruction.

The original technique for harvesting the gluteal artery perforator flap has undergone several stages of evolution. A retrospective review of our first 9 years of experience included 142 flaps.[9] Since then, data on 261 additional flaps have been compiled. No major differences between the two series have been detected. No vein grafts were used in either series. The flap survival rate is 98%, with an overall complication rate of 19%.

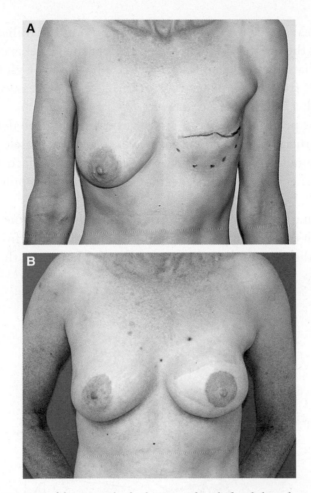

Fig. 33-1 A, This 49-year-old woman had a history of multifocal ductal carcinoma in situ in her left breast and had undergone a left mastectomy 3 months earlier. She had an inadequate volume of abdominal tissue; therefore an SGAP flap procedure was performed. **B,** Nipple-areola reconstruction and contralateral crescent mastopexy were performed 1 year after breast reconstruction. She is shown 3 years after breast reconstruction.

Most of the complications were minor; however, the microvascular complication rate was 6%. Advancements in imaging techniques have influenced surgical decision making, decreasing operative time and improving patient outcomes. Specifically, all flap candidates in our practice undergo preoperative imaging so that flaps are harvested on the ideal perforator or perforators, including septocutaneous perforators when available. In this chapter, we share important surgical refinements, advantages, disadvantages, and lessons learned in using the SGAP flap over the past decade.

ANATOMY

The superior gluteal artery is a terminal branch of the internal iliac artery and exits the pelvis through the greater sciatic foramen.[10] Here the vessel is encased by several distinct fat pads that dwell in a subfascial recess. The superior gluteal vein receives multiple tributaries from other pelvic veins at this level. The vessels continue toward the surface through a rent in the sacral fascia.

On exiting the pelvis, the superior gluteal artery divides into deep and superficial branches. The superficial branch continues above the piriformis muscle into the substance of the gluteus maximus muscle. As it travels toward the skin surface, the artery divides into multiple branches that perforate the muscle and go on to supply the overlying fat and skin (Fig. 33-2).

The perforating vessels travel in superior and lateral directions. The perforating vessels that nourish the medial portions of the skin paddle travel in a strictly superior direction toward the skin surface. The intramuscular length of these vessels is 4 to

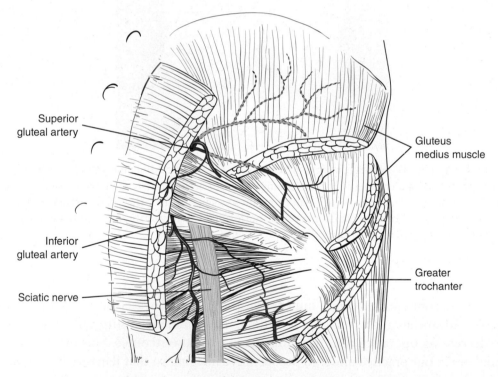

Fig. 33-2   Major branches of the superior and inferior gluteal arteries.

5 cm, depending on the thickness of the gluteus muscle mass. Perforators that nourish the lateral portions of the overlying skin paddle travel through the muscle substance in a more horizontal manner for 4 to 6 cm before turning upward toward the skin surface. Because they travel in a level plane through the muscle for relatively long distances, the vessels that feed the lateral portions of the overlying skin paddle are much longer than their medially based counterparts. The perforating vessels can be separated from the surrounding gluteus maximus muscle and fascia and traced down to the parent vessel, forming the basis for the superior gluteal artery perforator flap (see Fig. 33-2).

One to three perforators originating from the superficial branch of the superior gluteal artery are located in the upper half of each gluteal muscle (Fig. 33-3). Sensory innervation for the upper buttock originates from the dorsal branches of the lumbar segmental nerves.[7] Multiple nerve branches perforate the deep fascia just lateral to the posterior superior iliac crest and ascend toward the skin.

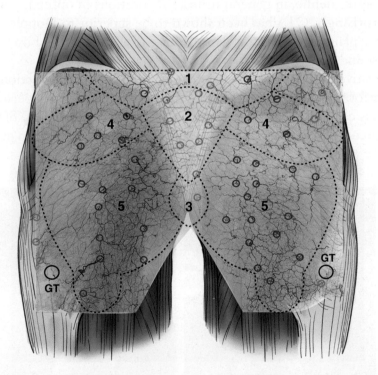

Fig. 33-3 The superior *(4)* and inferior *(5)* gluteal artery perforators and the skin territories they vascularize. (*1,* Dorsal cutaneous branches of lumbar arteries; *2,* lateral sacral artery; *3,* internal pudendal artery.)

SURGICAL TECHNIQUE
Surface Landmarks and Flap Design

The operative markings are typically placed the day before surgery, while the patient assumes standing and operative positions. The posterior superior iliac spine and the greater trochanter are palpated and marked. A line is drawn connecting these two points. The superficial branch of the superior gluteal artery emerges from the edge of the sacrum, near the junction of the first and second third of this line (closest to the posterior superior iliac spine). The perforating vessels can be identified near this line by a Doppler probe and followed laterally.

Preoperative imaging with either CTA or MRA helps guide this step by identifying for harvest those perforators with the most attractive features, including optimal diameter, length, and course. Preoperative imaging with these two modalities has become routine for every breast reconstruction case in our group. In the past, imaging was used only for more complex cases such as women with previous abdominal surgeries or liposuction; however, the logical progression has been to use imaging for each patient to create an individualized map for identifying and harvesting the best perforator or perforators. Numerous studies have evaluated the anatomy of gluteal perforators with imaging to better define, in general terms, the locations of optimal perforators.[11-16] And, not surprisingly, CTA has been shown to be superior to Doppler imaging for preoperatively planning perforator flaps because of a "miss rate" of up to 33.7% with duplex ultrasound.[17]

Preoperative imaging decreases operative time, facilitates selection of the most favorable perforator or perforators, and identifies septocutaneous perforators when available. Flaps can now be harvested in previous surgical sites because of the planning afforded by preoperative imaging (Fig. 33-4). Within our group, surgeon preference dic-

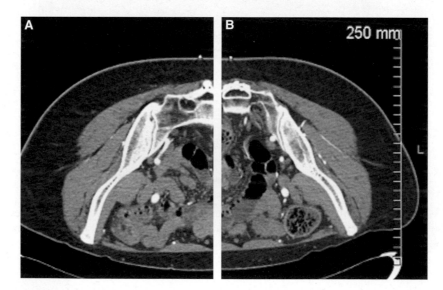

Fig. 33-4   A and **B,** CTA images showing bilateral septocutaneous perforator branches from the superficial branch of the superior gluteal artery. Preoperative imaging allows identification of septocutaneous perforators for planning SGAP procedures.

tates the use of CTA or MRA, though both modalities have been shown to be beneficial. Whereas CTA lacks the finer detail of MRA, it is less costly and more readily available.

With the adoption of preoperative imaging for all patients, there has been a focus on identifying septocutaneous perforators (Fig. 33-5). Septal perforators, when present, tend to be more laterally oriented, which adds length to the pedicle and preserves the shape of the buttock. Additionally, the presence of a septal perforator negates the need for any muscular dissection, eliminating the associated morbidity seen with muscular perforators. To date, our group has performed over 20 septocutaneous SGAP flaps, with an average decrease in associated operative time of 80 minutes.

The design of the SGAP flap varies from being angled upward or downward along the previously marked line, to a more horizontal design. The outline of the flap may be customized to almost any orientation, as long as it contains the perforating vessels. However, the obliquely oriented design with the lateral apex oriented slightly superiorly has proven advantages. This flap minimizes contour deformities and is more easily

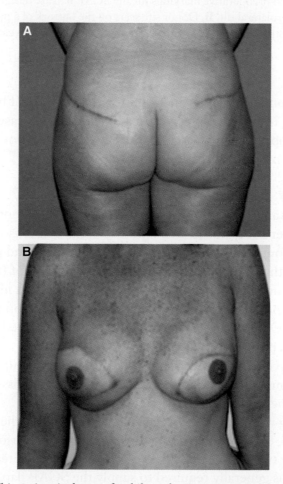

Fig. 33-5 A and **B,** This patient is shown after bilateral septocutaneous SGAP flaps. Perforators were identified preoperatively by CTA. Harvesting flaps based off known septal perforators has decreased operative time and allowed a more lateral flap, preserving buttock shape.

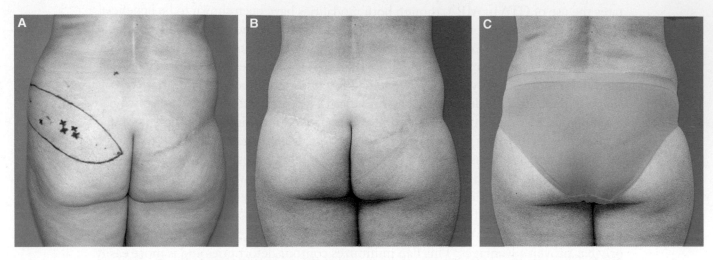

Fig. 33-6 A, This patient had a right SGAP flap for breast reconstruction and is marked for a left SGAP flap. Our preferred preoperative markings for the SGAP flap are designed as a horizontal skin paddle with a slight superolateral tilt. **B,** Donor site scars on the buttock of a patient who had bilateral SGAP flap breast reconstruction. **C,** The same patient is shown in underwear, with scars concealed.

hidden under most undergarments and swimwear (Fig. 33-6). The width of the skin paddle incorporated into the design averages 10 cm. In some cases, up to 12 cm may be included in the flap, still allowing closure of the donor area without undue tension. The length of the flap is usually 20 to 26 cm.

Vascular Anatomy

An incision is made and carried down to the fascia circumferentially. Laterally, the flap is positioned over the iliotibial tract, gluteal fascia, and tensor fascia lata muscle, and away from the nourishing vessels. Dissection begins here and proceeds swiftly but carefully to identify the proper plane of dissection. The fascia of the gluteus maximus muscle is identified and elevated along with the flap. This is an important step in the procedure that must not be omitted, because it allows the surgeon to enter the optimal plane for dissection. Once this relatively bloodless plane is entered, visualization of the perforating vessels is optimized (Fig. 33-7).

The gluteus maximus muscle inserts at the iliotibial tract and gluteal tuberosity of the femur; thus the muscular bundles lie parallel to the path of dissection. As dissection proceeds medially, the muscle bundles are encountered.

The perforating vessels travel between muscle bundles into the flap in the direction of the fibers (Fig. 33-8). Several perforators with an artery measuring 1 mm or more and accompanied by two venae comitantes can be found per gluteal muscle. Although only one perforator is generally required to supply the SGAP flap, a second large perforator is occasionally found as the dissection proceeds. This second vessel is included in the flap if it joins the first perforator; otherwise, the largest single perforating vessel ultimately carries the flap.

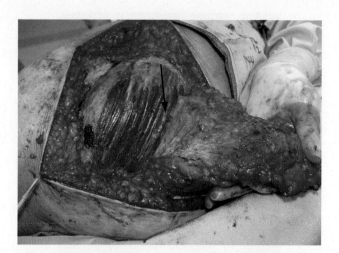

Fig. 33-7 The SGAP flap is dissected off the muscle from lateral to medial. The first large perforator is viewed between the muscle fibers *(arrow)*.

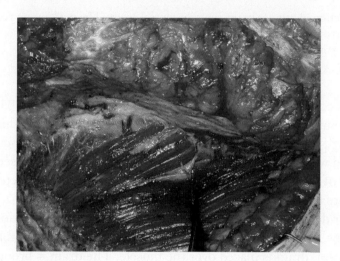

Fig. 33-8 The perforating vessel is traveling into the flap.

The chosen perforator is protected as the flap is islanded. If an innervated flap is desired, the superomedial skin bridge is maintained until the dorsal branches of the lumbar segmental nerves are identified and traced back to their origin. One large branch can be dissected and later anastomosed to the fourth intercostal nerve, providing sensation to the flap.[5] The space between the muscular bundles is broadened, and the vessel is followed. Before the sacral fascia is encountered, the deep branch is seen coursing on the surface of the iliac bone and should be ligated. The sacral fascia is opened to reveal a fatty recess. Multiple tributary veins are noted coming into the pedicle. Here dissection is delicate in an effort to carefully ligate the multiple branches.

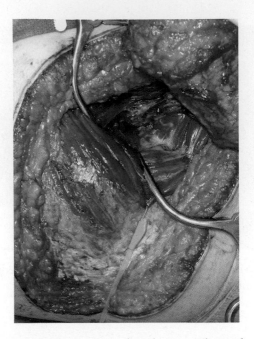

Fig. 33-9 Dissection continues to the superior gluteal artery. The perforating vessel has been separated from the surrounding muscle fibers. This vessel travels horizontally for some distance within the muscle. Harvesting this flap yields a pedicle length of 7 to 9 cm.

Dissection continues to the superior gluteal artery and vein (Fig. 33-9). The pedicle length at this point is usually 7 to 12 cm. The superior gluteal vein at this level is universally large enough in diameter (range 2.5 to 4.5 mm) to allow microvascular anastomosis to be performed without difficulty. The critical factor for ending dissection, therefore, is the diameter of the gluteal artery. Once the gluteal artery is dissected to a diameter of 2 mm or more (range 2.0 to 4.5 mm), the flap is harvested.

The donor defect should be closed with care to avoid complications. After undermining skin flaps, the gluteal muscle is reapproximated with absorbable sutures, and a single large suction drain is placed over the muscle. The drain is brought out through the lateral aspect of the incision to avoid uncomfortable positioning postoperatively. The superficial fascial system is identified and closed with sutures before final skin closure. At the end of the procedure, patients should be placed in a supportive girdle, which we recommend be worn for 2 weeks.

Neighboring Anatomic Structures

The most important regional structures encountered during the SGAP flap procedure are the greater sciatic nerve, inferior gluteal artery, internal pudendal artery, and posterior femoral cutaneous nerve. These structures exit caudal to the piriformis muscle and could be damaged with careless technique. The sciatic nerve is most commonly injured when traction is placed on the piriformis muscle to expose the superior gluteal vessels as they descend below the sacral fascia. If overzealous traction is transmitted to the sciatic nerve, patients experience irritation-type symptoms for some time. Good exposure is required to complete the procedure, but surgeons should be aware that this is a potential pitfall.

MODIFICATIONS
Preoperative Planning

Patient positioning is inherently important when using the SGAP flap. Consideration should be given to having both the donor and recipient sites exposed simultaneously to allow a two-team approach. This tactic is ideally suited for restorative breast surgery in which the patient is placed in the lateral decubitus position. The internal mammary vessels are the recipients of choice and can be harvested with the patient in this position with relative ease. Immediate mastectomy can be carried out in tandem with flap harvest. This approach saves operative time and potentially reduces morbidity. Normally, the arm ipsilateral to the breast being reconstructed is prepared and draped into the field so that it can be maneuvered to provide adequate exposure during mastectomy, internal mammary vessel dissection, and flap anastomosis. The patient is returned to a supine position after the flap is harvested, the donor site closed, and the dressing applied—and before flap anastomosis.

Technical Tips

When incising the SGAP flap, one should bevel out 1 to 2 cm in the fat to obtain more tissue bulk, depending on the volume requirements at the recipient site. Older patients tend to have increased skin laxity, which allows the donor site to be closed without tension even though greater volumes have been harvested. During breast reconstruction, the mastectomy specimen is weighed to gauge the volume needed. Flap dimensions are measured and flap weight (g) is estimated as follows:

$$\text{Width (cm)} \times \text{Length (cm)}/2 \times \text{Height or thickness (cm)}.$$

For example, an SGAP flap that is 20 cm long, 10 cm wide, and 4 cm thick would have an approximate weight of 400 g. When the flap is harvested, its weight is compared with this estimate. These weights and estimates are important to avoid overresection of volume from the donor site, which could increase the possibility of postoperative contour deformity.

During the dissection, the flap is islanded out completely, committing to the planned design. Care must be taken to protect the perforating vessels to avoid undue traction or avulsion during the dissection until the flap is ready for harvest. Insertion of the pedicle into the flap requires delicate handling, and special care is necessary.

Excellent exposure is required throughout the procedure but becomes critically important when ligating tributaries to the superior gluteal vein. Without adequate exposure, the risk of injury to the vein is magnified. To avoid this damage, we recommend placing the retractor so that it holds the piriformis and gluteus minimus muscles widely apart. The sacral fascia is opened around the vessels in a lateral direction with bipolar cautery to minimize bleeding. Fat pads in the immediate vicinity are resected, allowing unimpeded visualization of the vascular structures. Venous tributaries are ligated only when the gluteal vein is clearly visualized as it exits the pelvis.

In some cases, two gluteal artery perforator flaps are needed for bilateral breast reconstruction. Although bilateral flaps can be performed simultaneously, the procedure can be prolonged and burdensome. We prefer to perform two unilateral reconstructive procedures 1 week apart. We have found this schedule to be acceptable to patients and more comfortable for the operative team. Neither the incidence of anesthesia-related complications nor the need for blood transfusions has increased as a result of this staging.

PITFALLS
Time Management

Patient positioning is important for time management purposes and to aid with exposure of the recipient and donor sites. Appropriate padding is essential to prevent compression neuropathies. Sequential compression devices reduce the risk of deep venous thrombosis. These precautions can always be taken without compromising the time or energy required for the procedure.

Contour Deformity

A major contour deformity is very distressing for patients, requires corrective surgery, and should be avoided at all costs. The upper buttock scar may be objectionable to some patients, but with today's fashion styles it becomes a minor annoyance for very few patients. The horizontal or, preferably, the upwardly slanted oblique designs are superior to other designs in the gluteal area, because they result in minimal donor site concavity.[8] Closure of the superficial fascial system is also important for avoiding this complication. If a contour deformity does occur, lipoaspiration and infiltration can be performed at a second stage, when the patient returns for nipple reconstruction. During this procedure, attempts are made to transfer the fat cells into the gluteus maximus muscle to achieve the highest rate of viability.

Dissection Plane

The optimal plane of dissection is found below the gluteal fascia. To enter this relatively bloodless plane safely, we recommend beginning dissection laterally. In this way, visualization is optimized and dissection is carried out parallel to the muscle bundles. Consequently, the risk of injuring perforating vessels is reduced, because they run in the direction of the muscle fibers.

Short Pedicle and Anastomosis

Additional dissection through the muscle inevitably results in longer pedicles than those obtained with gluteal musculocutaneous flaps.[4] Adequate pedicle length can be achieved with either lateral or medial perforators, the largest one being chosen for flap perfusion. The advantages of using the perforator and eliminating muscle harvest are avoidance of vein grafts and facilitation of microvascular anastomosis.

Vessel Diameter Discrepancy

In some cases, a discrepancy in vessel diameter is unavoidable and most commonly occurs with the superior gluteal vein. Universally, the vein has a greater diameter than the artery, especially below the sacral fascia. The surgeon can be fooled into harvesting the flap at this time, only to find a miniscule artery accompanying the hefty vein. To bypass this potential hazard, we routinely employ a venous coupler device, which accommodates vessel caliber discrepancies and makes microvascular anastomosis easier and safer.

Recipient Vessels

The internal mammary vessels are the recipient vessels of choice at our institution. However, to reduce morbidity of the recipient site dissection, vessels are exposed between the ribs, with every effort made to avoid rib harvest. If perforators of the internal mammary vessels are identified with adequate caliber, they are used for anastomosis. Using internal mammary perforators allows less dissection at the donor site and can be advantageous, because the diameter of the artery is usually not as large (average 1.5 to 2.3 mm) and the pedicle length required to perform anastomosis comfortably is shorter.

References

1. Fujino T, Harasina T, Aoyagi F. Reconstruction for aplasia of the breast and pectoral region by microvascular transfer of a free flap from the buttock. Plast Reconstr Surg 56:178-181, 1975.
2. Shaw WW. Breast reconstruction by superior gluteal microvascular free flaps without silicone implants. Plast Reconstr Surg 72:490-501, 1983.

    The author reviewed his experience with 10 gluteus maximus myodermal free flap breast reconstructions in comparison with the current methods of reconstruction using silicone implants, latissimus dorsi flaps, regional skin flaps, and rectus abdominis myodermal flaps. The superior gluteal free flap can achieve a reliable, permanent, and aesthetic reconstruction of the breast without silicone implants. The softness, projection, natural appearance, and patient satisfaction are excellent compared with other methods. It is particularly useful in patients who object to the use of artificial implants, are not suitable candidates for regional flaps, or have disappointing results from previous reconstructions. Technical modifications of the flap design and selection of the recipient vessels are important.
3. Boustred AM, Nahai F. Inferior gluteal free flap breast reconstruction. Clin Plast Surg 25:275-282, 1998.

    The authors discussed the indications for and the anatomy, technique, and results of breast reconstruction with the inferior gluteal free flap. They also presented the results of their 25 inferior gluteal flap operations performed over a decade.
4. Allen RJ, Tucker C Jr. Superior gluteal artery perforator free flap for breast reconstruction. Plast Reconstr Surg 95:1207-1212, 1995.

    This article presented a new method of breast reconstruction using skin and fat from the buttock without sacrificing the muscle. Cadaver dissections were done to study the musculocutaneous perforators of the superior gluteal artery and vein. Eleven breasts were reconstructed successfully with skin-fat flaps based on the superior gluteal artery with its proximal perforators. Long flap vascular pedicles allow the internal mammary or thoracodorsal vessels to be used as recipient vessels. This new technique has several advantages over the previously described gluteus maximus musculocutaneous flaps, including a long vascular pedicle and no muscle sacrifice.
5. Koshima I, Moriguchi T, Soeda S, et al. The gluteal perforator-based flap for repair of sacral pressure sores. Plast Reconstr Surg 91:678-683, 1993.

    A gluteal perforator–based flap employing the gluteus maximus muscle perforators located around the sacrum was described. A cadaveric study disclosed the existence of several significant perforators all around the gluteal region. Among these, the parasacral perforators originating from the internal pudendal artery and lateral sacral artery have proved useful for the repair of sacral pressure sores. A total of eight decubitus ulcers in seven patients were treated with gluteal perforator–based flaps. There were no postoperative complications, such as flap necrosis and wound infection, with the exception of fistula formation in one case. This flap requires no transection or sacrifice of the gluteus maximus muscle, and elevation time for the flap is short. However, the perforators are located at various sites and thus require some careful dissection.

6. Blondeel PN. The sensate free superior gluteal artery perforator (S-GAP) flap: a valuable alternative in autologous breast reconstruction. Br J Plast Surg 52:185-193, 1999.

   The superior and inferior musculocutaneous gluteal free flaps have been considered as valuable alternatives to the latissimus dorsi or TRAM flap since 1975. The SGAP flap is the ultimate refinement of this musculocutaneous flap because no gluteus maximus muscle is harvested. The flap is vascularized by one single perforator originating from the superior gluteal artery. This study summarized the prospectively gathered data on 20 free SGAP flaps used for breast reconstruction in 16 patients. Immediate reconstruction was performed in six breasts and delayed reconstruction in 14 breasts. Mean follow-up time was 11.1 months. Two risk factors, Raynaud's disease and radiation therapy, were the cause of flap revision in two different patients. Total flap loss occurred in one case. Partial flap loss was not observed, and a small area of fat necrosis was diagnosed by mammography in one other patient. All flaps were anastomosed to the internal mammary vessels at the third costochondral junction. The anatomy of the sensate nerves of the SGAP flap is described. Two nervous repairs provided early sensory recovery. The free SGAP flap has become the author's second choice for autologous breast reconstruction after the deep inferior epigastric perforator artery (DIEAP) flap. The SGAP flap is indicated in patients with an asthenic body habitus or with excessive abdominal scarring. The advantages are the abundance of adipose tissue in this area, even in thin patients, a long vascular pedicle, a hidden scar, improved projection of the reconstructed breast compared with DIEAP and TRAM flaps, and preservation of the entire gluteus maximus muscle. Donor site morbidity is extremely low.

7. Verpaele AM, Blondeel PN, Van Landuyt K, et al. The superior gluteal artery perforator flap: an additional tool in the treatment of sacral pressure sores. Br J Plast Surg 52:385-391, 1999.

   The authors described the use of a large skin–subcutaneous tissue flap based on one perforator of the superior gluteal artery (SGA) to reconstruct large midline posterior defects in one stage. The integrity of the gluteus muscles is preserved, and these investigators stated that this is particularly important in nonparalyzed patients. Donor sites were always closed primarily. Use of the superior gluteal artery perforator (SGAP) flap preserves the entire contralateral side as a future donor site. On the ipsilateral side, the gluteal muscle itself is preserved, and all flaps based on the inferior gluteal artery are still possible. The authors recommended this flap in an area where reconstructive possibilities are limited, because it preserves other reconstructive flap options, both on the ipsilateral and contralateral sides.

8. Koshima I, Tsutsui T, Takahashi Y, et al. Free gluteal artery perforator flap with a short, small perforator. Ann Plast Surg 51:200-204, 2003.

   The introduction of supermicrosurgery has led to the development of a new gluteal perforator flap nourished only by a musculocutaneous perforator of the superficial gluteal artery system. This flap has a perforator that is short (3 to 4 cm in length) and small (less than 1 mm in diameter). The authors described successful transference of a free gluteal perforator flap for the coverage of soft tissue defects in the foot and face in two patients. With this flap, deeper and longer dissection for a pedicle vessel is unnecessary, flap elevation time is shorter, thinning of the flap with primary defatting and creation of an adiposal flap with customized thickness for tissue augmentation are possible, the donor site is in a concealed area with minimal donor site morbidity, and the flap can be used in reconstruction of scarring from previous operations in the gluteal region. The disadvantages of this flap include the necessity of dissection for a smaller perforator and anastomosis of small-caliber vessels less than 1 mm.

9. Guerra AB, Metzinger SE, Bidros RS, et al. Breast reconstruction with gluteal artery perforator (GAP) flaps: a critical analysis of 142 cases. Ann Plast Surg 52:118-125, 2004.

   Fujino was the first to introduce gluteal tissue as a free flap for breast reconstruction. The use of the musculocutaneous flap from the buttock in breast reconstruction was championed by Shaw. Despite the initial enthusiasm for this area as a donor site, few other large series exist on the subject. Two decades of experience with this region as a donor site led to recognition of advantages and drawbacks. Furthermore, the use of both the superior and inferior gluteal musculocutaneous flap was associated with certain important donor site complications and the use of vein grafts to allow for microvascular anastomosis. The evolution of free tissue transfer has progressed to the level of the perforator flap. This reconstructive technique allows elevation of tissue from any region consisting only of fat and skin. This minimizes donor site morbidity by allowing preservation of the underlying muscle and coverage of important structures, such as nerves, in the region. The authors have used superior and inferior gluteal perforator flaps for breast reconstruction since 1993. The superior gluteal artery perforator (SGAP) flap is the method of breast reconstruction they prefer when the abdomen is not available. They reported the results achieved with this flap over the past 9 years and discussed important surgical refinements, advantages, disadvantages, and lessons learned during this time.

10. Strauch B, Yu H. Gluteal region. In Strauch B, Yu H, eds. Atlas of Microvascular Surgery: Anatomy and Operative Approaches. New York: Thieme Medical Publishers, 1994.

11. Vasile JV, Newman T, Rusch DG, Greenspun DT, Allen RJ, Prince M, Levine JL. Anatomic imaging of gluteal perforator flaps without ionizing radiation: seeing is believing with magnetic resonance angiography. J Reconstr Microsurg 26:45-57, 2010.

    Preoperative imaging is essential for abdominal perforator flap breast reconstruction because it allows preoperative perforator selection, resulting in improved operative efficiency and flap design. The benefits of visualizing the vasculature preoperatively also extend to gluteal artery perforator flaps. Initially, our practice used computed tomography angiography (CTA) to image the gluteal vessels. However, with advances in magnetic resonance imaging angiography (MRA), perforating vessels of 1 mm diameter can reliably be visualized without exposing patients to ionizing radiation or iodinated intravenous contrast. In the authors' original MRA protocol to image abdominal flaps, they found the accuracy of MRA compared favorably with CTA. With increased experience with MRA, they decided to use MRA to image gluteal flaps. Technical changes were made to the MRA protocol to improve image quality and extend the field of view. Using the new MRA protocol, they have been able to image the vasculature of the buttock, abdomen, and upper thigh in one study. They have found that the spatial resolution of MRA is sufficient to accurately map gluteal perforating vessels, as well as provide information on vessel caliber and course. This article detailed their experience with preoperative imaging for gluteal perforator flap breast reconstruction.

12. Alonso-Burgos A, Garcia-Tutor E, Bastarrika G, et al. Preoperative planning of deep inferior epigastric artery perforator flap reconstruction with multislice-CT angiography: imaging findings and initial experience. J Plast Reconstr Aesthet Surg 59:585-593, 2006.

13. Lui KW, Hu S, Ahmad N, et al. Three-dimensional angiography of the superior gluteal artery and lumbar artery perforator flap. Plast Reconstr Surg 123:79-86, 2009.

    Three-dimensional angiography was first proposed by Cornelius and advanced by Voigt in 1975. Since then, a variety of improvements have been made. The three-dimensional evaluation of perforator flaps is no longer a clinical curiosity but an absolute necessity. By combining three-dimensional digital imaging and angiography, the authors have developed a new three-dimensional technique for visualizing blood vessels. This method produces a digitized model of the lumbar artery and superior gluteal artery musculocutaneous perforators that enables secure elevation of the lumbar and superior gluteal artery cross-boundary perforator flap. Two cadavers underwent whole-body lead oxide–gelatin injection. Spiral computed tomographic scanning was then performed on the cadavers and three-dimensional reconstructions were performed. Six fresh bodies were used, and underwent latex injection. Specimens were then dissected by layers to document the individual perforators. An average of five superior gluteal artery musculocutaneous perforators with a diameter of 0.6 mm were present in the specimens. The average diameter and area supplied by perforators from the lumbar arteries was 0.7 mm and 30 cm, respectively. The three-dimensional reconstructed model of the lumbar region can display the modality, spatial location, and adjacent relationship of the lumbar and superior gluteal arteries.

14. Saint-Cyr M, Schaverien M, Arbique G, et al. Three- and four-dimensional computed tomographic angiography and venography for the investigation of the vascular anatomy and perfusion of perforator flaps. Plast Reconstr Surg 121:772-780, 2008.

15. Chernyak V, Rozenblit AM, Greenspun DT, et al. Breast reconstruction with deep inferior epigastric artery perforator flap: 3.0-T gadolinium-enhanced MR imaging for preoperative localization of abdominal wall perforators. Radiology 250:417-424, 2009.

> *The authors reported on their study to prospectively evaluate 3.0-T gadolinium-enhanced magnetic resonance (MR) imaging for localization of inferior epigastric artery (IEA) perforators before reconstructive breast surgery involving a deep inferior epigastric perforator (DIEP) flap. This study was exempt from institutional review board approval, and the requirement for informed patient consent was waived. Data were collected and stored in compliance with HIPAA regulations. Nineteen patients (mean age 46.3 years) underwent three-dimensional gadolinium-enhanced 3.0-T MR imaging of the abdomen before undergoing DIEP flap breast reconstruction. Up to four of the largest perforators arising from the IEA on each side of the umbilicus were identified. The diameter, intramuscular course, and distance from the umbilicus of each perforator were recorded. One of the marked perforators on each side was labeled "the best" on the basis of an optimal combination of perforator features: diameter, intramuscular course, and location with respect to the flap edges. MR findings were compared with intraoperative findings. The two-tailed Student t-test was used to compare the mean diameters of all perforators with the mean diameters of the perforators labeled as the best. There were 30 surgical flaps, and 11 (58%) of the 19 patients underwent bilateral flap dissection. At surgery, 122 perforators were localized, and 118 (97%) of these perforators-with a mean diameter of 1.1 mm (range 0.8 to 1.6 mm) had been identified at preoperative MR imaging. Thirty perforators with a mean diameter of 1.4 mm (range 1.0 to 1.6 mm) were labeled as the best at MR imaging. Thirty-three perforators were harvested intraoperatively; all of these had been localized preoperatively. Twenty-eight (85%) of these 33 perforators were labeled as the best at MR imaging.*

16. Rozen WM, Ributto D, Atzeni M, et al. Current state of the art in perforator flap imaging with computed tomographic angiography. Surg Radiol Anat 31:631-639, 2009.

17. Scott JR, Liu D, Said H, Neligan PC, Mathes DW. Computed tomographic angiography in planning abdomen-based microsurgical breast reconstruction: a comparison with color duplex ultrasound. Ann Plast Surg 125:446-453, 2010.

34

Inferior Gluteal Artery Perforator Flap

Robert J. Allen, Sr.
James L. Mayo
Robert Johnson Allen, Jr.
Maria M. LoTempio

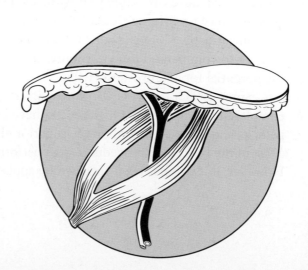

In 1975, Fujino et al[1] published their work on microvascular transfer of gluteal tissue as a free flap for reconstruction of aplasia of the heart and pectoral region. In 1978, Le-Quang[2] performed the inferior gluteal musculocutaneous flap. This work was published in 1992. Gluteal musculocutaneous flaps have been championed by Boustred and Nahai[3] and Shaw.[4] Boustred and Nahai preferred the inferior gluteal flap, because it provided a longer pedicle and more tissue bulk, and the incision was hidden in a more cosmetic location—the inferior gluteal crease. However, harvesting the gluteus muscle with this flap often left the sciatic nerve unprotected, and many patients suffered significant neurologic symptoms. Additionally, despite the proposed longer pedicle, many patients continued to require vein grafts with the increased risk of vascular complications.

To circumvent some of the drawbacks of musculocutaneous flaps, Allen and Tucker[5] performed an alternative method for harvesting gluteal tissue in 1993. Their work was published in 1995. With their technique, the skin–soft tissue envelope, nourished by perforators of the superior gluteal artery, was harvested without sacrificing the underlying structures. Gluteus maximus muscle function was preserved with a muscle-splitting approach. Dissecting the vascular structures through the muscle led to significantly longer pedicles. This method made vascular anastomosis a more common procedure without the need for additional vein grafts. The superior gluteal artery perforator (SGAP) flap was created (see Chapter 33). The technique was applied to the inferior gluteal vasculature that same year with equal success. Other advantages of the inferior gluteal artery perforator (IGAP) flap include a cosmetic location of the scar, reliable anatomy, usually a longer pedicle than that of the SGAP flap, a ubiquitous donor site with good volume and low morbidity, ease of shaping for breast reconstruction, and the potential for a neurosensory flap.

Since 1993 a total of 503 gluteal artery perforator flaps have been successfully completed by our group. Of these, 213 have been based on the inferior gluteal artery pedicle, and 290 were based on the superior gluteal artery perforator (see Chapter 33). Most of the IGAP flap procedures were performed for breast reconstruction (Fig. 34-1). However, this flap has been successfully applied for reconstruction of the trunk.

The IGAP flap was believed to be inferior to the SGAP flap for many years.[6] Early in our experience with the IGAP flap, we did not position the flap in the crease, and donor site aesthetics were not good. In 2004 we began designing the flap in the inferior gluteal crease, with excellent results.[7] After the initial excitement about the IGAP flap, our team has found some disadvantages. Our flap success rate is lower than that with the DIEP flap: 97% versus 99%. Complications include donor site pain and increased wound dehiscence from sitting on the wound. Others have reported similar "difficulties and limitations" with this flap.[7-8]

These factors should be considered when one is choosing the appropriate free flap for breast reconstruction. The DIEP flap remains the first option. However, for the ideal candidate—a pear-shaped woman with size B breasts and a large buttock—the IGAP remains an excellent option. In this chapter, we present important surgical refinements, advantages, disadvantages, and lessons learned in using the IGAP flap over the last two decades.

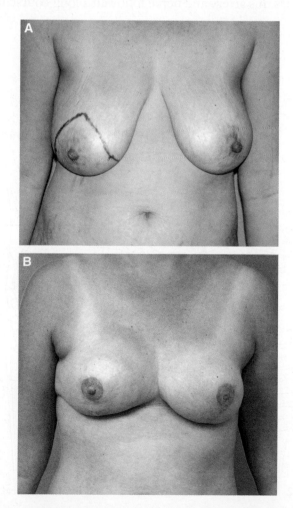

Fig. 34-1 A, This 38-year-old woman had a strong family history of breast cancer and tested positive for the *BRCA-2* gene mutation. **B,** She is shown 1 year after bilateral prophylactic mastectomy and bilateral IGAP breast reconstruction.

ANATOMY

The inferior gluteal artery is a terminal branch of the internal iliac artery and exits the pelvis through the greater sciatic foramen[9] (Fig. 34-2). The artery accompanies the greater sciatic nerve, internal pudendal vessels, and posterior femoral cutaneous nerve. Below the fascia of the sacrum, the inferior gluteal artery is also surrounded by several distinct fat pads. In this subfascial recess, the inferior gluteal vein receives tributaries from other pelvic veins. Of note, the coccygeal branch of the inferior gluteal artery develops here and pierces the sacrospinous ligament.[10] The inferior gluteal vasculature continues toward the surface by perforating the sacral fascia and exits the pelvis caudal to the piriformis muscle. Once under the inferior portion of the gluteus maximus muscle, perforating vessels of the inferior gluteal artery branch out through the substance of the muscle to supply the overlying skin and fat. A septocutaneous perforator may come around the medial or lateral border of the gluteal maximus muscle.

In 91% of the cases studied by Windhofer et al,[11] the inferior gluteal artery then descended into the thigh, accompanied by the posterior femoral cutaneous nerve (S1-2). They noted that this artery and nerve followed a long course together, eventually

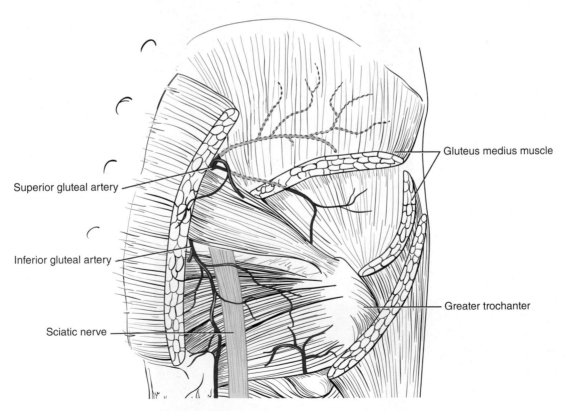

Fig. 34-2   Major branches of the superior and inferior gluteal arteries.

surfacing to supply the skin of the posterior thigh (Fig. 34-3). The posterior femoral cutaneous nerve (S1-2) also supplies the skin of the inferior buttock.[3] A neurosensory flap can be elevated if these nerves are preserved in the flap dissection.[3] The distance traveled by the inferior gluteal artery is longer than the distance traveled by its superior counterpart. The inferior gluteal artery also gives off more perforators than the superior gluteal artery.

The perforating vessels travel in superior, lateral, and inferior directions.[12] Perforating vessels that supply the medial and inferior portions of the buttock have a relatively short intramuscular course (5 to 7 cm), depending on the thickness of the muscle. Perforators that supply the lateral portions of the overlying skin paddle travel through the muscle substance in a horizontal manner for 4 to 6 cm before turning upward toward the skin surface. By traveling in a level plane through the muscle for relatively long distances, these vessels are much longer than their medially or inferiorly based counterparts. The perforating vessels can be separated from the underlying gluteus maximus muscle and fascia and traced down to the parent vessel, forming the basis for the IGAP flap. A total of two to four perforating vessels originating from the inferior gluteal artery are located in the lower half of each gluteal muscle. Pedicle length is usually 6 to 10 cm.

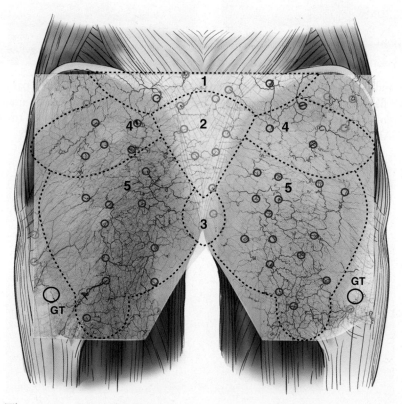

Fig. 34-3 The superior *(4)* and inferior *(5)* gluteal artery perforators and the skin territories they vascularize. (*1,* Dorsal cutaneous branches of lumbar artery; *2,* lateral sacral artery; *3,* internal pudendal artery.)

SURGICAL TECHNIQUE
Surface Landmarks and Flap Design

Markings are placed while the patient assumes standing and operative positions. The lateral edge of the sacrum, greater trochanter, and ischial tuberosity are palpated and marked. These marks identify the origin, insertion, and inferior extent of the gluteal muscle, respectively. A horizontal ellipse is diagrammed on the skin, with the lower incision in the inferior gluteal crease (Fig. 34-4). The width is usually 7 cm and the length 20 to 26 cm, beginning just lateral to the ischial tuberosity and extending toward the greater trochanter.

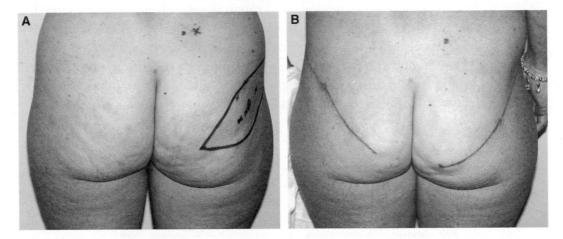

Fig. 34-4 A and **B,** Preoperative and postoperative images of the donor site of a patient who had bilateral IGAP flaps for breast reconstruction. The scars are well hidden beneath underwear or a bikini. This preoperative planning represents our markings before 2004, at which time we began performing IGAP flaps "in the crease."

For some patients with excess tissue in the saddlebag area, an IGAP flap may be chosen over an SGAP flap to make use of this extra tissue and provide desirable body contouring (Fig. 34-5).

The outline of the flap may be customized to almost any orientation, as long as it contains the perforating vessels. However, the upward obliquely oriented design has proved to be superior. Perforating vessels found in the lateral portion of the skin design can be chosen to carry the flap, because incorporating these distally based vessels results in longer pedicles. However, a medial perforator of adequate caliber can also be used. Preoperative imaging helps guide this process. The day before surgery either an MRA or CTA of the donor site area is performed. These studies allow the surgeon to choose the best perforator or perforators and course for the given flap. Doppler ultrasound is used to verify and mark the vessels in the office.

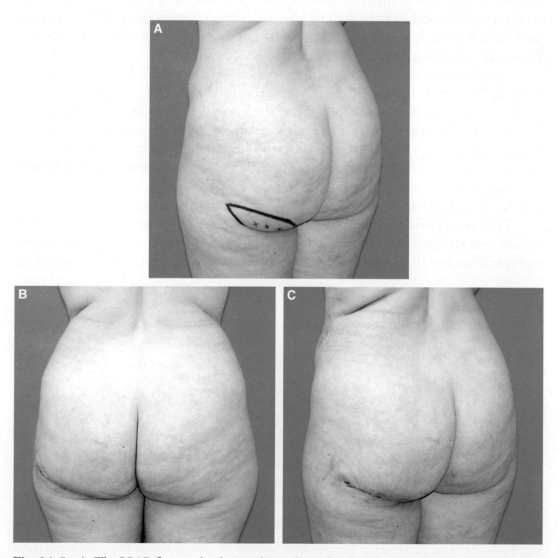

Fig. 34-5 **A,** The IGAP flap can be designed just above the gluteal crease if excess tissue exists in the saddlebag area. **B** and **C,** The resulting scar is well hidden within the gluteal crease.

Vascular Anatomy

Laterally the flap is positioned over the iliotibial tract and gluteal fascia, and away from the nourishing vessels. Dissection begins here and proceeds swiftly but carefully to identify the proper plane of dissection. The fascia of the gluteus maximus muscle is identified and elevated along with the flap. This is an important step in the procedure that must not be omitted, because it allows the surgeon to enter the optimal plane for dissection. Once this relatively bloodless plane is entered, visualization of the perforating vessels is optimized.

The gluteus maximus muscle inserts into the iliotibial tract and gluteal tuberosity of the femur; thus the muscular bundles lie parallel to the path of dissection. As dissection proceeds medially, the muscle bundles are encountered. The perforating vessels travel between muscle bundles into the flap. Several perforators with an artery measuring 1 mm or greater and accompanied by two venae comitantes can be found per gluteal muscle. Although only one perforator is generally required to supply the IGAP flap, occasionally a second large perforator is found as dissection proceeds. If it easily joins the first perforator, it is included; otherwise, the initial vessel ultimately carries the flap. Preoperative imaging has made perforator selection easier.

The chosen perforator is protected as the flap is islanded. The space between the muscular bundles is broadened, and the vessel is followed. The greater sciatic nerve courses below, into the thigh. Often the sciatic nerve is not exposed with the pedicle dissection. Great care is taken not to apply pressure on the nerve, and retractors placed into the wound must avoid direct contact with the nerve. To advance proximally, the femoral cutaneous nerve may need to be separated from the vascular structures; if sensory branches supplying the skin are found, these can be incorporated, creating a neurosensory flap. The femoral cutaneous nerve is usually not visualized with flap dissection.

The sacral fascia is opened to reveal a fatty recess. Tributary veins can be noted coming into the pedicle. Here dissection is delicate in an effort to carefully ligate the multiple branches (Fig. 34-6). The coccygeal branch of the gluteal artery should be

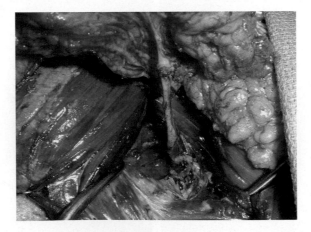

Fig. 34-6 After the perforator is dissected from between the gluteus muscle fibers, the sacral fascia is opened (held by left forceps). Numerous large tributary vessels need to be ligated with silk sutures before locating a vessel with an acceptable diameter.

ligated. The internal pudendal artery is seen medially and should not be injured. Dissection continues to the inferior gluteal artery and vein. The pedicle length at this point is usually 7 to 11 cm. The critical factor for ending dissection is the diameter of the gluteal artery. Once the gluteal artery is dissected to a diameter of at least 2 mm (range 2.0 to 4.5 mm), the flap is harvested.

The donor defect should be closed with care to avoid complications. The skin flaps are undermined, and the muscle is allowed to fall back together. A large suction drain is placed over the muscle and brought out through the lateral aspect of the incision. The superficial fascial system is identified and closed with sutures before final skin closure. At the end of the procedure, patients should be placed in a supportive garment.

Neighboring Anatomic Structures

The most important regional structures encountered are the greater sciatic nerve, inferior gluteal artery, and posterior femoral cutaneous nerve. These structures exit caudal to the piriformis muscle and could be damaged with careless technique. In this scenario, the nerve can be injured in two ways: directly or by traction injury. Retractors can injure the nerve when the ends penetrate the nerve substance and should be placed with extreme care in this situation. These potential hazards can be avoided by careful planning and meticulous operative technique. No sciatic nerve injuries have occurred in our series. In one case the posterior femoral cutaneous nerve was divided inadvertently and was repaired.

MODIFICATIONS
Preoperative Planning

Preoperative imaging with CTA or MRA has become routine for every breast reconstruction case in our group. CTA has been shown to be superior to Doppler imaging for preoperatively planning perforator flaps[13-19] and helps create an individualized map for identifying and harvesting the best perforator or perforators. Such imaging decreases operative time and facilitates selection of the most favorable perforator or perforators and identification of septocutaneous perforators when available. Within our group, the surgeon's preference determines whether CTA or MRA is performed. Both modalities have been shown to be beneficial for various perforator flaps. MRA avoids exposure to ionizing radiation or iodinated IV contrast. CTA may lack the finer detail of MRA but is less costly and more readily available.

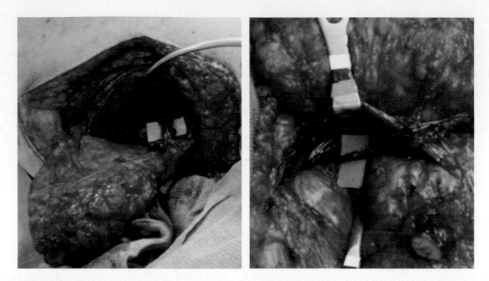

Fig. 34-7   The dissection of a septocutaneous IGAP flap allows a more lateral flap with more trochanteric fat. The operative time for dissection of septal perforators is significantly less than for musculocutaneous perforators.

With the adoption of preoperative imaging for all patients, there has been a focus on identifying septocutaneous perforators. We have performed six septocutaneous IGAP flaps, with operative time decreased by an average of 80 minutes (Fig. 34-7).

Patient positioning is inherently important with IGAP flaps. Both the donor and recipient sites should be exposed simultaneously, if possible, when a unilateral reconstruction is planned, allowing a two-team approach. This tactic is ideally suited for restorative breast surgery in which the patient is placed in the semilateral position. The internal mammary vessels are the recipients of choice and can be harvested with the patient in this position with relative ease. Immediate and delayed mastectomy can be carried out in tandem with flap harvest. This approach saves operative time and potentially reduces morbidity. For bilateral simultaneous IGAP procedures, the patient is positioned prone after mastectomy and recipient vessel preparation. With two microsurgeons present, both flaps are harvested simultaneously. The donor site is closed, and the patient is repositioned supine for anastomosis and insetting.

Technical Tips

When incising an IGAP flap, one should bevel out 1 to 2 cm in the fat to obtain more tissue bulk, depending on the recipient site requirements. When performing breast reconstruction, the mastectomy specimen is weighed to gauge the volume to be replaced. Flap dimensions are measured, and its weight (g) is estimated as follows: Width (cm) × Length (cm)/2 × Height or thickness (cm). When the flap is ultimately harvested, its weight is compared with this estimate. These weights and estimates are important to avoid overresecting volume from the donor site, which could increase the possibility of postoperative contour deformity.

During dissection, the skin is incised completely, islanding the flap around the chosen perforator. Care must be taken to avoid accidental avulsion or traction on the perforator, which can interrupt the intima and disrupt flow. Insertion of the perforator into the flap requires delicate handling and extreme care to avoid damaging this vessel.

Excellent exposure is required throughout the procedure. Without adequate exposure, dissecting the proximal pedicle is more difficult. The sacral fascia is opened around the vessels in a lateral direction for unimpeded visualization of the vascular structures. Once the perforator enters the descending inferior gluteal artery or an artery greater than 2 mm, it can be harvested. The vein at this level is usually 2.5 to 4 mm.

The greater sciatic nerve is rarely exposed during this procedure. Care is taken not to apply any sutures or clips near the location of the nerve. Additionally, the gluteus maximus muscle is normally allowed to fall back together into position, without the need for sutured closure. This protects the sciatic nerve.

PITFALLS
Time Management
Preoperative CTA or MRA reduces operating room time significantly. Patient positioning is important for time management during exposure of the recipient and donor sites. Bilateral procedures are longer than unilateral procedures, because the patient is repositioned twice intraoperatively. Appropriate padding must be placed to prevent compression neuropathies. Sequential compression devices reduce the risk of deep venous thrombosis. Heparin or Lovenox is routinely given for deep venous thrombosis prophylaxis. These precautions can always be taken without compromising time or energy during the procedure.

Contour Deformity
A major contour deformity at the donor site is very distressing for patients, requires corrective surgery, and should be avoided at all costs. This area can have contour depressions if the superficial fascial system is improperly closed. Upward oblique and horizontal designs produce fewer problems with contour deformities. Lipoinfiltration can be performed at a later stage to fill depressions or as a smoothing technique at the donor site.

Dissection Plane
The optimal plane of dissection is found deep to the gluteal fascia. To enter this relatively bloodless plane safely, we recommend beginning dissection laterally. Visualization is optimized and dissection is carried out parallel to the muscle bundles, reducing the risk of injury to the perforating vessels.

Short Pedicle
Additional dissection through the muscle inevitably results in longer pedicles than those obtained with gluteal musculocutaneous flaps.[6] Usually the IGAP flap provides a longer pedicle than the SGAP flap. To optimize pedicle length, effort should be focused on using the distal perforators. The rewards for using perforators and not harvesting muscle include avoidance of vein grafts and facilitation of microvascular anastomosis. With CTA and MRA, septocutaneous vessels are identified preoperatively, making dissection easier.

Vessel Diameter Discrepancy

In some cases, a discrepancy in vessel diameter is unavoidable. This most commonly occurs with the inferior gluteal vein. Great mismatches in vessel diameter were partially responsible for the 17% rate of vein graft use with gluteal musculocutaneous flaps reported by Boustred and Nahai.[3] The rate can be even greater with superior gluteal musculocutaneous flaps. To bypass this potential hazard, we routinely rely on a venous coupler device, which accommodates vessel size discrepancies and makes microvascular anastomosis easier and safer.

Gluteal Artery

The desired artery diameter is determined by the diameter of the recipient vessels. The internal mammary vessels are the recipient vessels of choice at our institution. To reduce morbidity at the recipient site, these vessels are exposed between the ribs, with every effort made to avoid rib harvest. If perforators of the internal mammary vessels are identified with adequate caliber, they are used as the recipient vessels. Using the internal mammary vessel perforators allows less dissection at the donor and recipient sites. In addition, the diameter of the inferior gluteal artery is usually not as large as that of the internal mammary artery (average 1.5 to 2.3 mm), and the pedicle length required to perform anastomosis comfortably is shorter. However, if the internal mammary vessels are used, large-caliber vessels are required. Universally, the gluteal vein has a greater diameter than the internal mammary vein, especially below the sacral fascia. Dissection should be continued more proximally to expose an artery with a diameter of at least 2 mm before harvesting the flap to ensure a favorable match with the recipient vessels. IGAP flap survival since 1993 has been 98%.

References

1. Fujino T, Harasina T, Aoyagi F. Reconstruction for aplasia of the breast and pectoral region by microvascular transfer of a free flap from the buttock. Plast Reconstr Surg 56:178-181, 1975.

2. Le-Quang C. Secondary microsurgical reconstruction of the breast and free inferior gluteal flap. Ann Chir Plast Esthet 37:723-741, 1992.

    A technique of secondary breast reconstruction by microsurgical transfer of an inferior gluteal flap was presented. Breast reconstruction with this flap was described in three operative steps. The advantages of this procedure include the natural curvature and softness of the reconstructed breast, moderate sequelae at the donor site, and a dissimulated scar in the gluteal fold.

3. Boustred AM, Nahai F. Inferior gluteal free flap breast reconstruction. Clin Plast Surg 25:275-282, 1998.

    The authors discussed the indications for and the anatomy, technique, and results of breast reconstruction with the inferior gluteal free flap. The results of their 25 inferior gluteal flap operations performed during one decade were presented.

4. Shaw WW. Breast reconstruction by superior gluteal microvascular free flaps without silicone implants. Plast Reconstr Surg 72:490-501, 1983.

    The author's experience with 10 gluteus maximus myodermal free flap breast reconstructions was compared with the current methods of reconstruction using silicone implants, latissimus dorsi flaps, regional skin flaps, and rectus abdominis myodermal flaps. The superior gluteal free flap can achieve a reliable, permanent, and aesthetic reconstruction of the breast without silicone implants.

5. Allen RJ, Tucker C Jr. Superior gluteal artery perforator free flap for breast reconstruction. Plast Reconstr Surg 95:1207-1212, 1995.

   A new method of breast reconstruction was presented using skin and fat from the buttock without muscle sacrifice. Cadaver dissections were done to study the musculocutaneous perforators of the superior gluteal artery and vein. Eleven breasts were reconstructed successfully with skin-fat flaps based on the superior gluteal artery with its proximal perforators. Long flap vascular pedicles allow the internal mammary or thoracodorsal vessels to be used as recipient vessels. The authors discussed the flap's advantages.

6. Guerra AB, Metzinger SE, Bidros RS, et al. Breast reconstruction with gluteal artery perforator (GAP) flaps: a critical analysis of 142 cases. Ann Plast Surg 52:118-125, 2004.

   Fujino was the first to introduce gluteal tissue as a free flap for breast reconstruction. The use of the musculocutaneous flap from the buttock in breast reconstruction was championed by Shaw. Despite the initial enthusiasm for this area as a donor site, few other large series existed on the subject. Two decades of experience with this region as a donor site led to recognition of advantages and drawbacks. Furthermore, use of both the superior and inferior gluteal musculocutaneous flap was associated with certain important donor site complications and the use of vein grafts to allow for microvascular anastomosis. The authors reported the results with this flap over 9 years and discussed important surgical refinements, advantages, disadvantages, and lessons learned during this time.

7. Mirzabeigi MN, Au A, Jandali S, et al. Trials and tribulations with the inferior gluteal artery perforator flap in autologous breast reconstruction. Plast Reconstr Surg 128:614e-624e, 2011.

8. Allen RJ. Discussion of Mirzabeigi MN, Au A, Jandali S, et al. Trials and tribulations with the inferior gulteal artery perforator flap in autologous breast reconstruction. Plast Reconstr Surg 128:625e, 2011.

9. Strauch B, Yu H. Gluteal region. In Strauch B, Yu H, eds. Atlas of Microvascular Surgery: Anatomy and Operative Approaches. New York: Thieme Medical Publishers 1994.

10. Thompson JR, Gibb JS, Genadry R, et al. Anatomy of pelvic arteries adjacent to the sacrospinous ligament: importance of the coccygeal branch of the inferior gluteal artery. Obstet Gynecol 94:973-977, 1999.

    The authors described the arterial vascular anatomy in the area of the sacrospinous ligament. Cadaver pelvises were dissected to reveal the anatomy of the sacrospinous ligament with emphasis on vascular and neuroanatomy. Flexible rulers were used to measure the coccygeal branch in five hemipelvises. The pudendal vessels and nerve pass immediately medial and inferior to the ischial spine (within 0.5 cm of the spine) and behind the sacrospinous ligament. The pudendal artery lies anterior to the sacrotuberous ligament, which passes behind the ischial spine to its attachment at the posterior ischial tuberosity. The inferior gluteal artery originates from the posterior or anterior branch of the internal iliac artery to pass behind the sciatic nerve and the sacrospinous ligament. There is a 3 to 5 mm window in which the inferior gluteal vessel is left uncovered above the top of the sacrospinous ligament and below the lower edge of the main body of the sciatic nerve plexus. The coccygeal branch of the inferior gluteal artery passes immediately behind the midportion of the sacrospinous ligament and pierces the sacrotuberous ligament in multiple sites. The main body of the inferior gluteal artery leaves the pelvis by passing posterior to the upper edge of the sacrospinous ligament and following the inferior portion of the sciatic nerve out of the greater sciatic foramen. Sutures placed through the sacrospinous ligament at least 2.5 cm from the ischial spine along the superior border of the sacrospinous ligament and without transgressing the entire thickness are in an area that is generally free of arterial vessels.

11. Windhofer C, Brenner E, Moriggl B, et al. Relationship between the descending branch of the inferior gluteal artery and the posterior femoral cutaneous nerve applicable to flap surgery. Surg Radiol Anat 24:253-257, 2002.

    The gluteal regions of 118 cadavers were studied to determine the relationship between the descending branch of the inferior gluteal artery and the posterior femoral cutaneous nerve. The results showed that a cutaneous or fasciocutaneous flap, either local or free, in this region can be reliably lifted on a cutaneous branch of the descending branch of the inferior gluteal artery without loss of sensitivity. However, the close relationship of the artery and nerve limits the arc of rotation in the case of a local flap.

12. Koshima I, Moriguchi T, Soeda S, et al. The gluteal perforator-based flap for repair of sacral pressure sores. Plast Reconstr Surg 91:678-683, 1993.

13. Scott JR, Liu D, Said H, Neligan PC, Mathes DW. Computed tomographic angiography in planning abdomen-based microsurgical breast reconstruction: a comparison with color duplex ultrasound. Ann Plast Surg 125:446-453, 2010.

14. Rozen WM, Phillips TJ, Ashton WM, Stella DL, Gibson RN, Taylor GI. Preoperative imaging for DIEA perforator flaps: a comparative study of computed tomographic angiography and Doppler ultrasound. Plast Reconstr Surg 121:9-16, 2008.

15. Alonso-Burgos A, Garcia-Tutor E, Bastarrika G, et al. Preoperative planning of deep inferior epigastric artery perforator flap reconstruction with multislice-CT angiography: imaging findings and initial experience. J Plast Reconstr Aesthet Surg 59:585-593, 2006.

16. Chernyak V, Rozenblit AM, Greenspun DT, et al. Breast reconstruction with deep inferior epigastric artery perforator flap: 3.0-T gadolinium-enhanced MR imaging for preoperative localization of abdominal wall perforators. Radiology 250:417-424, 2009.

17. Lui KW, Hu S, Ahmad N, et al. Three-dimensional angiography of the superior gluteal artery and lumbar artery perforator flap. Plast Reconstr Surg 123:79-86, 2009.

18. Saint-Cyr M, Schaverien M, Arbique G, et al. Three- and four-dimensional computed tomographic angiography and venography for the investigation of the vascular anatomy and perfusion of perforator flaps. Plast Reconstr Surg 121:772-780, 2008.

19. Vasile JV, Newman T, Rusch DG, et al. Anatomic imaging of gluteal perforator flaps without ionizing radiation: seeing is believing with magnetic resonance angiography. J Reconstr Microsurg 26:45-57, 2010.

INDEX